Third Edition

Laboratory and Diagnostic Tests with Nursing Implications

Third Edition

Laboratory and Diagnostic Tests with Nursing Implications

Joyce LeFever Kee, MSN, RN
Associate Professor
College of Nursing
University of Delaware
Newark, Delaware

APPLETON & LANGE
Norwalk, Connecticut/San Mateo, California

0-8385-5578-0

91 92 93 94 95 / 10 9 8 7 6 5 4 3 2 1

Prentice Hall International (UK) Limited, *London*
Prentice Hall of Australia Pty. Limited, *Sydney*
Prentice Hall Canada, Inc., *Toronto*
Prentice Hall Hispanoamericana, S.A., *Mexico*
Prentice Hall of India Private Limited, *New Delhi*
Prentice Hall of Japan, Inc., *Tokyo*
Simon & Schuster Asia Pte. Ltd., *Singapore*
Editora Prentice Hall do Brasil Ltda., *Rio de Janeiro*
Prentice Hall, *Englewood Cliffs, New Jersey*

Library of Congress Cataloging-in-Publication Data
Kee, Joyce LeFever.
    Laboratory and diagnostic tests with nursing implications / Joyce
LeFever Kee.—3rd ed.
        p. cm.
    Includes bibliographical references.
    Includes index.
    ISBN 0-8385-5578-0
    1. Nursing. 2. Diagnosis, Laboratory. I. Title.
    [DNLM: 1. Diagnosis, Laboratory—nurses' instruction. QY 4 K62L]
    RT48.5.K44 1990
    616.07′5—dc20
    DNLM/DLC
    for Library of Congress   90-749
                                                                  CIP

Acquisitions Editor: Marion K. Welch
Production Editors: Lauren Manjoney and Sandra K. Huggard
Designer: Michael J. Kelly

This book
I dedicate in
loving memory of
my mother
Esther Baker Lefever
for her years of
love, encouragement, and support

Contributors and Consultants

CONTRIBUTORS

Linda S. Farmer, MT, ASCP
Assistant Manager
Laboratory, St. Francis Hospital
Wilmington, Delaware

Evelyn R. Hayes, RN, PhD
Associate Professor
College of Nursing
University of Delaware
Newark, Delaware

Joyce LeFever Kee, MSN, RN
Associate Professor
College of Nursing
University of Delaware
Newark, Delaware

Ronald J. Lefever, BS
Coordinator of Emergency Room, Pharmacy Service
Medical College of Virginia
Richmond, Virginia

David C. Sestili, CRTT, RPFT
Manager
Pulmonary Laboratories
Medical Center of Delaware
Newark, Delaware

Jane P. Taylor, RN, MS
Associate Professor
Neumann College
Aston, Pennsylvania

CONSULTANTS

Catherine Balaguer, MT, ASCP
Supervisor, Chemistry Laboratories
Medical Center of Delaware
Newark, Delaware

Judith W. Fullhart, RN, BSN
Department of Gastroenterology
Veterans Administration Hospital
Elsmere, Delaware

Julie S. Lefever, MT, ASCP
Medical Technologist
Medical College of Virginia
Richmond, Virginia

John L. McCormack, MD
Neuroradiologist
MRI Department
Medical Center of Delaware
Newark, Delaware

Larry Purnell, RN, PhD
Assistant Professor
College of Nursing
University of Delaware
Newark, Delaware

Julie Waterhouse, RN, MS
Assistant Professor
College of Nursing
University of Delaware
Newark, Delaware

Contents

Preface

Nursing responsibilities are forever increasing. Nurses should understand laboratory and diagnostic tests and provide nursing implications through nursing assessment, judgement, implementation, teaching, and interaction.

Laboratory and Diagnostic Tests with Nursing Implications is designed to provide nurses and other health professionals with the pertinent information regarding laboratory and diagnostic tests and corresponding nursing implications.

ORGANIZATION

Each test is arranged in seven subsections: (1) **the name(s) of the test,** (2) **reference values/normal findings,** (3) **description,** (4) **clinical problems,** (5) **procedure,** (6) **factors affecting laboratory or diagnostic results,** and (7) **nursing implications with rationale.** Following the name(s) and initials for each test there may be names of other closely associated tests. Reference values/normal findings are given for children and adults. The **description,** brief and concise, focuses on background data, general purpose, and pertinent information related to the test. **Clinical problems** include disease entities, drugs, and foods that cause or are associated with abnormal test results. The procedure is explained with a rationale for the test and gives pertinent steps that the nurse and other health professionals can follow. **Factors affecting laboratory or diagnostic results** alert the nurse to the important factors that could cause an abnormal test result. The last subsection for each test and the most valuable part, concerns the **nursing implications with rationale.** For the laboratory test, nursing implications are listed for decreased and elevated abnormal results. For most of the **diagnostic tests,** nursing implications are given as "pre-test" and "post-test."

There are four parts in the text. Part I, Laboratory Tests; Part II, Diagnostic Tests; Part III, Laboratory/Diagnostic Assessments of Body Function; and Part IV, Therapeutic Drug Monitoring (TDM). Part III, entitled **Laboratory/ Diagnostic Assessments of Body Function,** should be most valuable to both the practicing nurse and the student. The section consists of 12 categories related to organ system and clinical conditions. These are: **Cardiac Function; Respiratory Function; Renal Function; Liver, Gallbladder, Pancreatic Functions; Gastrointestinal Function; Neurologic and Musculoskeletal Functions; Endocrine Function; Reproductive Function; Arthritic and Collagen Conditions; Shock; Neoplastic Conditions; and Hematologic Conditions.** Each category contains numerous laboratory and diagnostic tests ordered to assist in the diagnosis of disease entities and to determine organ function. These tests are briefly discussed with reference values as they relate to the organ or condition of that category. A few of the same tests (e.g., enzyme tests) can be found in more than one category (cardiac, muscle, liver). The nurse could determine if the test is more specific for one category or the other. **The nursing process with nursing diagnosis, nursing implications,** and **nursing evaluation** are to be found at the end of each category.

This third edition has more than 300 laboratory and diagnostic tests; some tests are combined with the test groups, such as differential white blood cells (neutrophils, eosinophils, basophils, lymphocytes, and monocytes). Additional drug toxicity tests have been added. All reference values and test procedures have been updated. A new subheading under nursing implications with rationale, patient teaching, provides the nurse with teaching instructions for patient understanding of the procedure, for test compliance, and for patient assessment following the test. The beginning section on **Importance of Specimen Collection,** has been condensed and only pertinent information is presented for understanding of specimen collection. The **Instructions for Laboratory and Diagnostic Tests** section provides an explanation of the six major subheadings and gives basic information that relates to most of the laboratory and diagnostic tests. A new section, Part IV entitled, **Therapeutic Drug Monitoring** (**TDM**), lists drugs that are monitored frequently by serum and urine for the purposes of achieving and maintaining therapeutic drug effects, and for preventing drug toxicity.

A list of references follows each part. The numbers that appear at the end of the **Description** section for each test are reference numbers. There are four appendices: **Abbreviations of Measurements Used for Normal Values, Abbreviations for Laboratory and Diagnostic Tests, Laboratory Test Groups** (laboratory profiles ordered for diagnosing clinical problems), and **Laboratory Test Values for Adults and Children.** The detailed index should be most helpful for locating the page of a test when the test name is different than the alphabetic listing used.

This text is appropriate for students in various types of nursing programs, that is, students in baccalaureate, associate degree, diploma and practical nursing. This book should be most valuable to the registered nurse and licensed practical nurse in hospital settings (ICU, Emergency Room, and general floors), clinics, and in independent nursing practice.

Acknowledgments

I wish to extend my sincere thanks and deep appreciation to the following people: Dr. Evelyn R. Hayes, Associate Professor, College of Nursing, University of Delaware, for reviewing and making the necessary corrections to the laboratory and diagnostic tests, the sections of specimen collection and instructions, and Part IV; Linda Farmer, Assistant Laboratory Manager at St. Francis Hospital, Wilmington, Delaware, for reviewing and correcting laboratory tests and the section on specimen collection; David Sestili, Manager, Pulmonary Laboratories, Medical Center of Delaware, for his contribution on pulmonary function tests, arterial blood gases, and bronchoscopy; Ronald J. Lefever, Coordinator of Emergency Room, Pharmacy Service, Medical College of Virginia, Richmond, Virginia, for correcting and giving suggestions to the drug toxicity tests in Part I, the laboratory section; and Jane Taylor, Associate Professor, Neumann College, Aston, Pennsylvania, for her contribution to the HIV test.

Other professionals who reviewed tests and gave suggestions include: Catherine Balaguer, Supervisor, Chemistry Laboratories, Medical Center of Delaware; Dr. John L. McCormack, Neuroradiologist, MRI Department, Medical Center of Delaware; Julie Lefever, Medical Technologist, Medical College of Virginia, Richmond, Virginia.

Many thanks to the following professionals for their input in this third edition: Julie Waterhouse, Assistant Professor, College of Nursing, University of Delaware; Dr. Larry Purnell, Assistant Professor, College of Nursing, University of Delaware; Patricia Pierce, Assistant Professor, College of Nursing, University of Delaware; Ann Lansu and Karen Andrea, educational instructors, VA Hospital, Elsmere, Delaware; the nursing staff in ICU at the VA Hospital, Elsmere, Delaware; and especially to Don Passidomo, Head Librarian and his assistant, June Akell, at the VA Hospital, Elsmere, Delaware, for their valuable assistance in making their services and talents available to me. Also, I wish to thank those acknowledged in my **Handbook of Laboratory and Diagnostic Tests with Nursing Implications,** 1990, for use of their corrected laboratory and diagnostic tests used for this edition.

My sincere appreciation also goes to Marion K. Welch, Executive Editor, Nursing, at Appleton and Lange, for her helpful suggestions and support, and to Dean Edith Anderson, College of Nursing, University of Delaware, for her support. To my dear husband, my love and appreciation for his support.

Introduction

THE IMPORTANCE OF SPECIMEN COLLECTION*

Nurses participate actively in laboratory testing protocols for patients. Historically and currently the nurses' role in laboratory testing has been considered by some persons to be that of ordering laboratory tests on requisition slips or computers. This is not the case. Nursing input is critical to obtaining valid and reliable laboratory test results. In the role of caregiver and teacher, nurses must communicate with the patient, physician, and laboratory personnel to obtain information that might affect test results. Nursing responsibilities include explaining the laboratory test, ensuring that both the patient and staff follow the procedure, assessing clinical findings with laboratory test results, noting pertinent information on the laboratory requisition slip (eg, drugs the patient is taking that might affect test results), and collecting the specimen.

Collection of specimens is the focus in this section. It is hoped that the nurse will gain an understanding of types of specimens, collection sites, position and patient activity affecting test results, time of collection, drug interference, labeling and handling of specimen, collection tubes, and types of reported laboratory measurement.

Types of Specimens

Blood is the most frequently analyzed specimen. When blood is withdrawn, it clots. The fluid contained in the clot mass is called *serum*. *Plasma* is the same as serum except that it also contains fibrinogen.

If the laboratory test requires plasma or whole blood for analysis, a tube containing an anticoagulant must be used so that the blood will not clot. However, most tests, such as electrolytes, use serum from clotted blood. Fre-

---

*Portions adapted from Tang, H.L. (1987). The importance of specimen collection and handling. In J.L. Kee(Ed.). *Laboratory and diagnostic tests with nursing implications* (2nd ed.). (pp. 1–30). East Norwalk, Conn: Appleton & Lange.

quently the terms serum and plasma are used interchangeably. However, the color of the tube top is different from serum (red) and plasma (lavender, green, gray, blue).

Collection of Specimen

Site of Collection: Venous blood is the commonest type of blood specimen taken and does not need to be noted on the laboratory slip; however, arterial blood and capillary blood should be recorded on the laboratory slip. Leg and feet sites for venipuncture are not used due to circulatory conditions.

When collecting the blood sample, the tourniquet should not be left on for longer than a minute. It can cause fluid shift from the vessel to the tissue spaces, leading to hemoconcentration and resulting in erroneous results. After collection, the blood specimen should be gently inverted several times to mix with anticoagulant if in the tube. Shaking the tube can cause hemolysis, thus damaging the red blood cells (RBCs) and possibly causing an inaccurate test result. Urine (random or 24 hour), cerebrospinal fluid (CSF), and synovial, pleural, peritoneal, fecal, sputum, and wound exudate are other types of specimens that are used for laboratory studies.

Position and Patient Activity: Standing or recent ambulation causes body fluid to shift from the vascular to the tissue spaces. Vascular hemoconcentration could result, affecting the concentration of proteins, enzymes, albumin, globulin, cholesterol, triglycerides, calcium, and iron. It takes 20 to 30 minutes for fluid levels to reestablish equilibrium after this shift in position. Exercise just prior to specimen collection can cause false results; this is especially true with enzyme testing.

Time: A time for routine blood collection needs to be established. Early morning before breakfast is the best time for blood collection so that food and fluid will not affect test results. Fasting, however, is required only for a few laboratory tests, such as glucose, triglycerides, cholesterol, potassium, vitamin B_{12}, folate, and thyroid studies. For fasting specimens, NPO for 8 to 12 hours is requested.

Drug Interference: Due to the increasing number of drugs taken by patients, there is an increased chance that the laboratory results can be affected. This is especially true if drugs are taken over a period of time and at high doses. Drugs affecting test results should be noted on the laboratory slip. Drugs with a short half-life are withheld until the blood is drawn and thereby do not affect adversely the laboratory test result.

Labeling and Handling: The laboratory requisition slip should include the patient's name, possible diagnosis, room location, identification number, age, sex, physician's name, test name (checked), time of collection, and special notation, such as drugs, food and fluids last taken.

Proper handling and prompt transport of the specimen to the laboratory is vitally important. Fresh specimens provide more accurate test results. With nonfresh blood specimen, hemolysis can occur, causing inadequate results; with nonfresh urine specimen that sits longer than 30 minutes, the pH of the urine becomes alkaline due to bacterial growth.

Collection Tubes: Tubes have color-coded stoppers that indicate the type of additives in the tube. The additives include anticoagulants such as oxalates, citrates, ethylenediaminetetraacetic acid (EDTA), and heparin. Blood-serum specimens are obtained in a red-top tube that does not contain an additive. Examples of the laboratory groups and color-top tubes follow.

RED: No additive, clotted blood. Serum is obtained from clotted blood mass. Laboratory groups that use red-top tubes are chemistry (electrolytes, proteins, enzymes, lipids, hormones), drug monitoring, radioimmunoassay (RIA) method, serology, and blood bank. Hemolysis should be avoided.

LAVENDER: Additive is EDTA. This color is used for plasma and blood specimens. Laboratory groups that use lavender-top tubes are hematology (Complete blood cell count [CBC], platelet count) and certain chemistry.

GREEN. Additive is heparin. This color is used for plasma-blood specimens. Laboratory groups that use green-top tubes are arterial blood gases, Lupus erythematosus (LE) test, and electrolytes and hormones (usually use red-top tubes).

BLUE: Additive is citrate. Blue is used for plasma-blood specimens. Laboratory groups that use blue-top tubes are coagulation studies (prothrombin time [PT], activated partial thromboplastin time APTT, partial thromboplastin time [PTT]) and hemoglobin.

GRAY. Additive is oxalate. Gray is used for plasma and blood specimens. Laboratory test for glucose uses gray-top tubes.

Types of Reported Laboratory Measurements

International System of Units: The World Health Organization (WHO) recommends that the medical and scientific community throughout the world adopt the International System of Units (SI units). The advantage is to establish a common international language for communicating laboratory measurements. Most clinical laboratories in Canada, Australia, western Europe, and some in the United States are now using SI units. Currently both metric and SI units are usually reported.

Reference Values: Reference values are determined based on "apparently healthy" individuals and the equipment and methods used in laboratories. Due to the methods and equipment used, reference values may vary among institutions.

Critical (Panic) Values: At times a patient's test results may fall outside the reference values, and a decision must be made as to whether the physician should be notified. Most laboratories have a list of critical-decision values. When a patient's results are in the range on this list, the physician or charge nurse must be notified immediately. A critical value policy and list are specific to each institution.

Joyce LeFever Kee

Consultants: Evelyn R. Hayes
Linda Farmer

INSTRUCTIONS FOR LABORATORY AND DIAGNOSTIC TESTS

This third edition of *Laboratory and Diagnostic Tests with Nursing Implications,* while a size comparable to the second edition, includes new and additional laboratory and diagnostic tests. Repetitive statements from the procedure and nursing implications, such as "instruct the patient that there are no food or fluid restrictions," will be omitted in the nursing implication section. With all laboratory and diagnostic tests, the nurse needs to explain the purpose and procedure of the test, both of which can be obtained from the description and the procedure. The following headings for laboratory and diagnostic tests help to clarify the changes.

Reference Values

Laboratory (norm) values can differ somewhat among institutions. The values given in this text are comparable to the reference values given in most institutions; however, nurses need to check the reference values at their institution.

Description

Information and purposes for the tests are included in the description of laboratory and diagnostic tests. Much of this information should be included when discussing the purpose of the test with the patient.

Clinical Problems

The disease entities that are associated with decreased and elevated test results are listed according to decreasing frequency of occurrence. Drugs that influence test results are given for both decreased and elevated levels. Drugs the patient is taking that can affect test results should be listed on the laboratory requisition slip.

Procedure

Procedure is an important part of the tests, and the nurse must discuss the procedure, step by step, with the patient. Most of the procedures for laboratory and diagnostic tests are similar among institutions. The following are helpful suggestions applicable to most tests.

Laboratory Tests
1. Follow institutional policy and procedure.
2. Collect recommended amount of specimen (blood, urine, etc).
3. Avoid using arm/hand with intravenous (IV) fluids for drawing venous blood specimen.
4. Label clearly specimen container with patient's identifying information.
5. Note significant drug data on label or laboratory requisition or both.
6. Avoid hemolysis; do not shake blood specimens.
7. Observe strict aseptic technique when collecting and handling each specimen.
8. Enforce food and fluid restriction only when indicated.

9. Collect 24-hour urine specimens:
   a. Have patient void prior to test, discard urine, and then save all urine for specified time, such as 24 hours.
   b. Refrigerate urine or keep on ice, unless preservatives are added or otherwise indicated.
   c. Instruct patient to avoid toilet paper and feces in urine specimens.
   d. Instruct patient *not* to urinate directly into the container.
   e. Label the urine collection bottle/container with the patient's name, date, and exact time of collection (eg, 6/21/93, 7 AM to 6/22/93, 7:01 AM).
10. List drugs and food the patient is taking that could affect test results.
11. When possible, hold medications and foods that could cause false test results until after the test. Before holding drugs, check with the physician. This may not be practical or possible; however, if the patient takes medication and the laboratory test is abnormal, this should be brought to the physician's attention.
12. Promptly send specimen to the laboratory.

Diagnostic Tests
1. A signed consent form is usually requested.
2. Food and fluid restriction is frequently ordered. Check with the procedure.
3. Institutional policies must be followed.

Factors Affecting Laboratory and Diagnostic Tests

Factors that affect test results should be identified and avoided when possible. When test results are abnormal, determine if factors stated could be contributing to the test results, and report to physician.

Nursing Implications

1. Be knowledgeable about laboratory and diagnostic tests.
2. Explain purpose and procedure of each test to the patient and family.
3. Provide time, and be available to answer questions. Be supportive to patient and family.
4. Follow procedure that is stated for each test. Label specimens with patient information.
5. Relate test findings to clinical problems and drugs. Test may be repeated to confirm a suspected problem.
6. Report abnormal results to physician.
7. Compare test results with other related laboratory and/or diagnostic tests.
8. Encourage patients to keep medical appointments for follow-up.
9. Provide health teaching related to clinical problem.
10. With diagnostic tests:
    a. Have patient void before premedication or before the test or both.
    b. Obtain history of allergies to iodine, seafood. Observe for severe allergic reaction to contrast dye.
    c. Obtain baseline vital signs. Monitor vital signs as indicated following the test.
    d. If sedative is used, instruct patient not to drive home.

Part I

Laboratory Tests

Acetaminophen (Serum)
Acetone, Ketone Bodies (Serum or
  Plasma)
Acid Phosphatase (ACP) (Serum)
Activated Partial Thromboplastin time
  (APTT)
ACTH
AIDS Virus
Alanine Aminotransferase (ALT)
  (Serum)
Albumin
Alcohol (Ethyl or Ethanol) (Serum or
  Plasma)
Aldolase (ALD) (Serum)
Aldosterone (Serum)
Aldosterone (Urine)
Alkaline Phosphatase (ALP), with
  Isoenzyme (Serum)
Alpha-1-Antitrypsin (α-1-AT) (Serum)
Alpha Fetoprotein (AFP) (Serum and
  Amniotic Fluid)
Ammonia (Plasma)
Amylase (Serum)
Amylase (Urine)
Anion Gap
Antibiotics/Aminoglycosides (Serum)
Antibiotic Susceptibility (Sensitivity)
  Test
Anticonvulsants (Blood, Serum,
  Plasma)
Antiglomerular Basement Membrane
  Antibody (AGBM) (Serum)

Antinuclear Antibodies (ANA) (Serum)
Antistreptolysin O (ASO) (Serum)
Arterial Blood Gases (ABGs)
Ascorbic Acid (Vitamin C) (Plasma
  and Blood)
Ascorbic Acid Tolerance (Blood and
  Urine)
Aspartate Aminotransferase (AST)
  (Serum)
Barbiturate (Blood)
Bilirubin (Indirect) (Serum)
Bilirubin (Total and Direct) (Serum)
Bilirubin and Bile (Urine)
Bleeding Time (Blood)
Blood Gases
Blood Urea Nitrogen (BUN) (Serum)
Blood Volume Determination/Studies
  (Blood Volume Measurement)
Bromide (Serum)
Calcitonin (hCT) (Serum)
Calcium (Ca) and Ionized Calcium
  (Serum)
Calcium (Ca) (Urine)
Calcium Channel Blockers (Serum)
Carbon Dioxide Combining Power
  (Serum or Plasma)
Carbon Monoxide,
  Carboxyhemoglobin (Blood)
Carcinoembryonic Antigen (CEA)
(Serum, Plasma)
Carotene (Serum)
Catecholamines (Urine)

Cerebrospinal Fluid (CSF)
Ceruloplasmin (Cp) (Serum)
Chlordiazepoxide (Librium) (Serum)
Chloride (Cl) (Serum)
Chloride (Sweat)
Cholesterol (Serum)
Cholinesterase (Red Blood Cells or
  Plasma)
Clot Retraction (Blood)
Coagulation Factors (Plasma)
Coagulation Time (CT) (Blood)
Cold Agglutinins (Serum)
Complement C3 Test (Serum)
Complement C4 Test (Serum)
Coombs Direct (Blood—RBC)
Coombs Indirect (Serum)
Copper (Cu) (Serum)
Cortisol (Plasma)
C-Reactive Protein (CRP) (Serum)
Creatine Phosphokinase (CPK)
  (Serum)
Creatinine (Serum)
Creatinine Clearance (Urine)
Cross Matching (Blood)
Cryoglobulins (Serum)
Cultures (Blood, Sputum, Stool,
  Throat, Wound, Urine)
Dexamethasone Suppression Test
Diazepam (Serum)
Differential White Blood Cell (WBC)
  Count
Digoxin (Serum)
Dilantin (Serum)
D-Xylose Absorption Test (Blood and
  Urine)
Erythrocyte Osmotic Fragility (Blood)
Erythrocyte Sedimentation Rate
  (ESR) (Blood)
Estradiol (E_2) (Serum)
Estriol (E_3) (Serum and Urine)
Estrogen (Serum)
Estrogens (Total) (Urine—24 Hours)
Factor Assay (Plasma)
FBS (Fasting Blood Sugar)
Febrile Agglutinins (Serum)
Ferritin (Serum)
Fibrin Degradation Products (FDP)
  (Serum)
Fibrinogen (Plasma)

Folic Acid (Folate) (Serum)
Follicle-Stimulating Hormone (FSH)
  (Serum and Urine)
FTA-ABS (Fluorescent Treponemal
  Antibody Absorption) (Serum)
Fungal Organisms: Fungal Disease,
  Mycotic Infections (Smear, Serum,
  Culture—Sputum, Bronchial, Lesion)
Gamma-Glutamyl Transferase (GGT)
  (Serum)
Gastrin (Serum or Plasma)
Glucagon (Plasma)
Glucose—Fasting Blood Sugar (FBS)
  (Blood)
Glucose—Postprandial (Feasting
  Blood Sugar) (Blood)
Glucose Tolerance Test—Oral (GTT)
  (Serum)
Glucose-6-Phosphate
  Dehydrogenase (G6PD or G-6-PD)
  (Blood)
Growth Hormone (GH, hGH) (Serum)
Haloperidol (Haldol) (Serum)
Haptoglobin (Hp) (Serum)
Hematocrit (Hct) (Blood)
Hemoglobin (Hb or Hgb) (Blood)
Hemoglobin Electrophoresis (Blood)
Hepatitis B Surface Antigen (HB_sAg)
  (Serum)
Heterophile Antibody (Serum, Mono-
  Spot)
Hexosaminidase (Serum, Amniotic
  Fluid)
Human Chorionic Gonadotropin
  (HCG) (Serum and Urine)
Human Immunosuppressive Virus
  (HIV) (Serum)
Human Leukocyte Antigen (HLA)
  (Serum)
Human Placental Lactogen (hPL)
  (Serum)
17-Hydroxycorticosteroids (17-
  OHCS) (Urine)
5-Hydroxyindolacetic Acid (5-HIAA)
  (Urine)
Immunoglobulins (Ig) (Serum)
Insulin (Serum), Insulin Antibody
  Test
Iron (Serum), Total Iron-Binding Ca-

pacity (TIBC), Transferrin, Percent Saturation (Serum)

Ketone Bodies, Acetone (Urine)

17-Ketosteroids (17-KS) (Urine)

Lactic Acid (Blood)

Lactic (Lactate) Dehydrogenase (LD or LDH), LDH Isoenzymes (Serum)

Lactose Tolerance Test

LDH Isoenzymes

Lead (Blood)

LE Cell Test, Lupus Erythematosus Test (Blood)

Lecithin/Sphingomyelin) (L/S) Ratio (Amniotic Fluid)

Legionnaire's Antibody Test (Serum)

Leucine Aminopeptidase (LAP) (Serum)

Lidocaine Hydrochloride (Blood, Serum, Plasma)

Lipase (Serum)

Lipoproteins, Lipoprotein Electrophoresis, Lipids (Serum)

Lithium (Serum)

Luteinizing Hormone (LH) (Serum and Urine)

Lyme Disease Test (Antibody)

Lymphocytes (T and B) Assay (Blood)

Magnesium (Mg) (Serum)

Malaria Smear (Blood)

5'Nucleotidase (5'N) (Serum)

Occult Blood (Feces)

Osmolality (Serum)

Osmalality (Urine)

Osmotic Fragility of Erythrocyte (Blood)

Ova and Parasites (O and P) (Feces)

Parathyroid Hormone (PTH) (Serum)

Partial Thromboplastin Time (PTT), Activated Partial Thromboplastin Time (APTT) (Plasma)

Phenothiazines (Serum)

Phenylketonuria (PKU) (Urine), Guthrie Test for PKU (Blood)

Phenytoin Sodium (Serum)

Phosphorus (P)—Inorganic (Serum)

Plasminogen (Plasma)

Platelet Aggregation and Adhesions (Blood)

Platelet Count (Blood—Thrombocytes)

Porphobilinogen (Urine)

Porphyrins—Coproporphyrins, Uroporphyrins (Urine)

Potassium (K) (Serum)

Potassium (K) (Urine)

Pregnanediol (Urine)

Pregnanetriol (Urine)

Procainamide Hydrochloride (Serum)

Progesterone (Serum)

Prolactin (PRL) (Serum)

Propranolol Hydrochloride (Blood, Serum, or Plasma)

Protein (Total) (Serum)

Protein (Urine)

Protein Electrophoresis (Serum)

Prothrombin Time (PT) (Plasma)

Quinidine (Serum)

Rapid Plasma Reagin (RPR) (Serum)

Red Blood Cell Indices (MCV, MCH, MCHC, RDW) (Blood)

Renin (Plasma)

Reticulocyte Count (Blood)

Rheumatoid Factor (RF), Rheumatoid Arthritis (RA) Factor, RA Latex Fixation (Serum)

Rh Typing (Blood)

Rubella Antibody Detection (Serum)

Salicylate (Serum)

Semen Examination

Serum Glutamic Oxaloacetic Transaminase (SGOT)

Serum Glutamic Pyruvic Transaminase (SGPT)

Sickle Cell (Screening) Test (Blood)

Sodium (Na) (Serum)

Sodium (Na) (Urine)

Testosterone (Serum or Plasma)

Theophylline (Serum)

Thyroglobulin Antibodies

Thyroid Antibodies (TA) (Serum)

Thyroid-Stimulating Hormone (TSH) (Serum)

Thyroxine (T_4) (Serum)

Torch Screen Test

Tricyclic Antidepressants (TCA, TAD) (Serum)

Triglycerides (Serum)

Triiodothyronine (T_3) (Serum)
Triiodothyronine Resin Uptake (T_3 RU) (Serum)
Uric Acid (Serum)
Uric Acid (Urine—24-Hour)
Urinalysis (Routine)
Urobilinogen (Urine)

Vanillylmandelic Acid (VMA) (Urine)
VDRL (Venereal Disease Research Laboratory) (Serum)
Vitamin B_{12} (Serum)
White Blood Cells (WBC) or Leukocytes (Total) (Blood)
White Blood Cell Differential (Blood)

ACETAMINOPHEN (SERUM)
(Tylenol, Tempra, Datril, Liquiprin, Paracetamol, Panadol, Aceta)

Reference Values

Adult: Therapeutic: 5–20 μg/mL, 31–124 μmol/L (SI units). *Toxic:* > 50 μg/mL, 305 μmol/L (SI units), > 200 μg/mL possible hepatotoxicity.

Child: Therapeutic: same as adult. *Toxic:* similar to adult

Description

Acetaminophen has a similar antipyretic and nonnarcotic analgesic effect to that of aspirin. Unlike salicylates (eg, aspirin), acetaminophen does not inhibit platelet aggregation, does not produce gastric distress and bleeding, and has only a weak anti-inflammatory response.

Overdose of acetaminophen can be dangerous, since it can lead to hepatotoxicity. It is metabolized in the liver to active metabolites and is absorbed rapidly from the gastrointestinal (GI) tract. Peak time occurs in ½ to 2 hours after oral ingestion. When there is an accumulation of acetaminophen in the body from massive dose(s) or chronic use, one of its metabolites tends to cause hepatotoxicity. Actually a single dose of 10 g or 30 tablets (325 mg each) could cause liver damage. Half-life of acetaminophen is about 3 hours. If the half-life is >4 hours, hepatic injury is likely to occur. After ingestion of a large amount of acetaminophen, either accidentally (children) or suicidal attempt, serum concentrations are plotted on a semilogarithmic scale. If the serum value is 200 μg/mL (1240 μmol/L) in 4 hours, or 50 μg/mL (310 μmol/L) in 12 hours after ingestion, hepatotoxicity could occur 3 to 6 days later. Antidote to acetaminophen toxicity is *N*-acetylcysteine. It must be administered soon after acetaminophen ingestion. Liver function tests (ie, AST [SGOT], ALT [SGPT]), bilirubin, prothrombin time (PT), electrolytes, should be closely monitored.[1–4]

Clinical Problems

Decreased Level: high carbohydrate meal

Elevated Level: acetaminophen overdose, liver disease. *Drug Influence:* phenobarbital

Procedure

- Collect 3 to 5 mL of venous blood in red-top tube.
- Record dose and time drug was taken on the laboratory requisition slip.
- There is no food or fluid restriction.

■ Factors Affecting Laboratory Results

None known

NURSING IMPLICATIONS WITH RATIONALE

- Explain to the patient that the purpose of the test is to monitor therapeutic level or toxic level of acetaminophen (give trade name).
- Suggest to the physician to order liver function tests periodically for patients on long-term acetaminophen therapy. Liver damage could result when taking the drug for weeks and/or months.
- Keep the acetaminophen bottle tightly closed and away from light.

Elevated Level

- Recognize that liver disease and acetaminophen overdose could result in hepatotoxicity.
- Observe for signs and symptoms of acetaminophen toxicity (ie, anorexia, nausea, vomiting, lethargy, generalized weakness, epigastric or abdominal pain).
- Observe for signs and symptoms of liver damage (ie, vomiting, jaundice, right upper quadrant tenderness, abnormal liver function tests).

Patient Teaching

- Inform the patient about the need for taking the prescribed dosage. An overdose or chronic use of acetaminophen could cause liver damage. Usually the drug should not be taken for more than 10 days at a time unless prescribed by the physician.
- Inform persons who consume large amounts of alcohol of the need to consult their physician before taking acetaminophen products. Usually these persons could be prone to liver damage, and ingestion of acetaminophen would compound the liver problem.
- Instruct the patient to keep acetaminophen products out of the reach of children. If a child ingests large amounts of the drug, call the poison center immediately, give syrup of ipecac if indicated by the center, and take the child to the emergency room. Acetylcysteine (Mucomyst) has been used as an antidote for adults within 16 hours after drug overdose.

ACETONE, KETONE BODIES (SERUM OR PLASMA)

Reference Values

Adult: Acetone: 0.3–2.0 mg/dL, 51.6–344.0 µmol/L (SI units). *Ketones:* 2–4 mg/dL

Child: Newborn to 1 Week: Slightly higher than adult. *Over 1 Week:* same as adult

Description

Ketone bodies are composed of three compounds—acetone, acetoacetic (diacetic) acid, and betahydroxybutyric acid—which are products of fat metabolism and fatty acids. Ketone bodies result from uncontrolled diabetes mellitus and starvation, causing increased fat catabolism instead of carbohydrate metabolism. In diabetic ketoacidosis, the serum acetone is > 50 mg/dL.

Ketones are small and excretable in the urine. However, the elevation is first apparent in the plasma or serum, then in the urine. Serum acetone (as ketones) is useful in monitoring acidosis caused by uncontrolled diabetes or starvation, since the serum level will decrease toward normal before the urine test (acetest) does.[5-8]

Clinical Problems

Elevated Level: diabetic ketoacidosis, starvation/malnutrition, vomiting and diarrhea, heat stroke, exercise

Procedure

- Collect 3 to 5 mL of venous blood in a red-top tube.
- There is no food or fluid restriction.

- Factors Affecting Laboratory Results

- Contamination can cause false-positive results.

NURSING IMPLICATIONS WITH RATIONALE

Elevated Level (> 2.0 mg/dL)

- Relate elevated serum acetone levels to diabetes acidosis and starvation. Many of the diet programs call for high-protein and low-carbohydrate diet. Daily carbohydrate intake of less than 100 g can result in ketosis (excess ketone bodies) caused by the substitution of fat metabolism for energy.
- Obtain a history from the patient concerning his or her diet. If the patient is on a reducing diet, the elevated serum level (ketosis) could be caused by a low carbohydrate diet.
- Assess for signs and symptoms of diabetic ketoacidosis, such as rapid, vigorous breathing; restlessness; confusion; sweet-smelling breath; and a serum acetone level greater than 50 mg/dL.
- Check the urine for ketone bodies. An acetest is usually performed and is positive.

ACID PHOSPHATASE (ACP) (SERUM)
Prostatic Acid Phosphatase (PAP)

Reference Values
Adult: 0.0–0.8 U/L at 37°C (SI units)

Child: 6.4–15.2 U/L

Description
The enzyme acid phosphatase (ACP) is found in the prostate gland and in semen in high concentration. It is found in lesser extent in bone marrow, red blood cells (RBCs), liver, and spleen. The highest rise in serum ACP occurs in prostatic cancer. In benign prostatic hypertrophy (BPH), the rise is also above normal level. A markedly elevated alkaline phosphatase level may cause a false-high serum ACP level.[1,6,8,9]

Clinical Problems
Decreased Level: Down's syndrome. *Drug Influence:* fluorides, oxalates, phosphates, alcohol

Elevated Level: carcinoma of the prostate, multiple myeloma, Paget's disease, cancer of the breast and bone, benign prostatic hypertrophy, sickle cell anemia, cirrhosis, chronic renal failure, hyperparathyroidism, osteogenesis imperfecta, myocardial infarction. *Drug Influence:* androgens in females, clofibrate (Atromid-S)

Procedure

- Collect 5 to 10 mL of venous blood in a red-top tube.
- Hemolysis should be prevented, and the specimen should be taken to the laboratory immediately. ACP is heat- and pH-sensitive. If the specimen is exposed to air and left at room temperature, there will be a decrease in activity after 1 hour.
- There is no food or fluid restriction.

■ Factors Affecting Laboratory Results

- Hemolysis of the blood sample can cause inaccurate test result.
- Certain drugs can decrease the serum ACP level (*See Drug Influence above.*)
- Blood specimen exposed to air and room temperature for longer than 1 hour can cause a decrease in ACP level.

NURSING IMPLICATIONS WITH RATIONALE

Decreased Level

■ Know which drugs can cause a decreased serum acid phosphatase.

Elevated Level

- Recognize clinical problems associated with an elevated serum ACP level. A high serum ACP level occurs with metastasized prostatic cancer.
- Indicate on the laboratory slip if the patient had a prostate examination 24 hours before the test. Prostatic massage or extensive palpation of the prostate can elevate the serum ACP.
- Check the serum ACP following treatment for carcinoma of the prostate gland. With surgical intervention, the serum level should drop in 3 to 4 days; following estrogen therapy (when the treatment is successful), it should drop in 3 to 4 weeks. If serum ACP has not been ordered, a reminder or suggestion to the physician may be necessary.
- Notify the laboratory before the serum ACP is drawn so that immediate attention will be given to the specimen.
- Encourage the patient to express concerns about the prostatic problem.

ACTIVATED PARTIAL THROMBOPLASTIN TIME (APTT)
See Partial Thromboplastin Time

ADRENOCORTICOTROPIC HORMONE (ACTH) PLASMA
Corticotropin, Corticotropin-Releasing Factor (CRF)

Reference Values

7 AM–10 AM, up to 80 pg/mL. ACTH is highest in early morning.

Description

Adrenocorticotropic hormone (ACTH) or corticotropin is stored and released from the anterior pituitary gland under the influence of corticotropin-releasing factor (CRF synthesized from the hypothalamus) and the plasma cortisol from the adrenal cortex. The negative feedback mechanism controls ACTH release: when plasma cortisol is low, ACTH is released; when plasma cortisol is high, ACTH release is inhibited. Stress caused by surgery, physical trauma, emotional trauma, or bacterial infections also increases the ACTH level. ACTH level follows a diurnal pattern, with its highest peak between 7 AM and 10 AM and its lowest level between 7 PM to 10 PM.

A plasma ACTH is performed to determine whether a decrease in plasma cortisol (corticosteroid) is due to adrenal cortex hypofunction or pituitary hypofunction. Two follow-up tests, ACTH suppression and ACTH stimulation, are ordered for identifying the origin of the clinical problem being from either the pituitary or the adrenal cortex.

ACTH Suppression Test: With the ACTH suppression test, a synthetic potent cortisol, dexamethasone (Decadron), is given to suppress the production of ACTH. If an extremely high dose is needed for ACTH suppression, the cause is of pituitary origin, such as pituitary tumor, producing an excess of ACTH secretion. However, if the plasma cortisol continues to be high with ACTH suppression, the cause could be adrenal cortex hyperfunction (Cushing's syndrome).

ACTH Stimulation Test: With the ACTH stimulation test, ACTH is administered, and the plasma cortisol level should double in 1 hour. If the plasma cortisol level remains the same or is lower, adrenal gland insufficiency (Addison's disease) is the cause. To check for pituitary hypofunction, the drug metyrapone is given to block the production of cortisol, thus causing an increase in ACTH secretion. If the ACTH level does not increase, the problem would be pituitary insufficiency.[1,6,10–12]

Clinical Problems

Decreased Level: adrenocortical hyperfunction (Cushing's syndrome), cancer of the adrenal gland. *Drug Influence:* steroids (cortisone, prednisone, dexamethasone), estrogen, amphetamines, alcohol

Elevated Level: stress (trauma, physical or emotional), pyrogens, adrenal cortical hypofunction, pituitary neoplasm, surgery, pregnancy

Procedure

- Collect 7 to 10 mL of venous blood in a green-top tube. Pack the tube in ice immediately and send to the laboratory. If ACTH level is not performed within 15 minutes, the plasma is frozen. Additional testing may be needed, since a single plasma value may be misleading.
- If adrenal hypofunction is suspected, blood sample is taken at the peak time, which is early morning. If adrenal hyperfunction is suspected, blood sample is usually taken at low level, which is early evening.
- Note on the laboratory label the time the blood sample was drawn.
- Food and fluid may be restricted. Low carbohydrate diet may be requested for 24 hours prior to the test.
- Restrict activity 8 to 12 hours before the test. When possible, restrict drugs such as cortisone until after the test.

■ Factors Affecting Laboratory Results

- Steroids, estrogen, oral contraceptives can decrease plasma ACTH.
- Physical activity prior to the blood test can affect results.
- Obesity can cause an elevated plasma level.
- Labeling the blood specimen with the wrong time can affect results.
- Failure to pack the blood sample in ice can affect results.
- Pregnancy and menstrual cycle can elevate plasma ACTH level.
- High carbohydrate diet can affect results.

NURSING IMPLICATIONS WITH RATIONALE

Decreased Level

■ Obtain a history of the patient's drug regimen. Recognize that steroid drugs (cortisone, prednisone) decreases ACTH secretion.

Elevated Level

■ Relate elevated plasma ACTH levels to clinical problems. Adrenal gland insufficiency or a pituitary tumor will increase ACTH secretion.

Patient Teaching

■ Instruct the patient to avoid physical activity and stress.
■ Explain to the patient having the ACTH suppression test with dexamethasone or ACTH stimulation with ACTH or metyrapone that drugs are used to confirm the cause of the hormonal imbalance.

AIDS VIRUS
(See Human Immunosuppressive Virus [HIV].)

ALANINE AMINOTRANSFERASE (ALT) (SERUM)
Serum Glutamic Pyruvic Transaminase (SGPT)

Reference Values

Adult: 5–35 U/mL (Frankel), 5–25 mU/mL (Wroblewski), 8–50 U/mL at 30°C (Karmen), 4–36 U/L at 37°C (SI units).

Child: Infant: could be twice as high as an adult. *Child:* similar to adult

Description

Alanine aminotransferase (ALT)/serum glutamic pyruvic transaminase (SGPT) is an enzyme found primarily in the liver cells and is effective in diagnosing hepatocellular destruction. It is also found in small amounts in the heart, kidney, and skeletal muscle.

Serum ALT levels can be higher than levels of its sister transferase (transaminase), aspartate aminotransferase (AST)/serum glutamic oxatoacetic transaminase (SGOT), in cases of acute hepatitis and liver damage from drugs and chemicals, with its serum levels reaching to 200 to 4,000 U/L. ALT is used for differentiating between jaundice caused by liver disease and hemolytic jaundice. With jaundice, the serum ALT levels of liver origin can be higher than 300 units; from causes outside the liver, the levels can be less than 300 units. Serum ALT levels usually elevate before jaundice appears.

ALT/SGPT levels are frequently compared with AST/SGOT levels for diagnostic purposes. ALT is increased more markedly than AST in liver necrosis and acute hepatitis, while AST is more markedly increased in myocardial necrosis (acute MI), cirrhosis, cancer of the liver, chronic hepatitis, and liver congestion. ALT levels are normal or slightly elevated in myocardial necrosis. The ALT levels return more slowly to normal range than AST levels in liver conditions.[1,5,6,9,10–12]

Clinical Problems

Decreased Level: exercise. *Drug Influence:* Salicylates

Elevated Level: Highest increase: acute (viral) hepatitis, necrosis of the liver (drug or chemical toxicity). *Slight or moderate increase:* cirrhosis, cancer of the liver, congestive heart failure, acute alcohol intoxication. *Drug Influence:* Antibiotics (carbenicillin, clindamycin, erythromycin, gentamicin, lincomycin, mithramycin, spectinomycin, tetracycline), narcotics (meperidine [Demerol], morphine, codeine), antihypertensives (methyldopa, guanethidine), digitalis preparations, indomethacin (Indocin), salicylates, rifampin, flurazepam (Dalmane), propranolol (Inderal), oral contraceptives (progestin-estrogen), lead, heparin.

Procedure

- Collect 5 to 7 mL of venous blood in a red-top tube. Avoid hemolysis, since RBCs have high concentration of ALT.
- There is no food or fluid restriction.
- Drugs administered to the patient that can cause false-positive levels should be listed on the laboratory slip along with the date last given.

■ Factors Affecting Laboratory Results

- Hemolysis of the blood specimen may cause false test results.
- Aspirin, can cause a decrease or increase of serum ALT.
- Certain drugs can increase the serum ALT level. (*See Drug Influence above.*)

NURSING IMPLICATIONS WITH RATIONALE

Elevated Levels (> 36 U/L [SI units])

- Relate the patient's serum ALT/SGPT to clinical problems. A high serum elevation (> 2000 U) can indicate liver necrosis from toxic agents or from acute viral hepatitis.
- Compare ALT and AST levels if both have been ordered. ALT is a better indicator of acute liver damage and will be at higher levels than AST in liver necrosis and acute hepatitis.
- Check for signs of jaundice. ALT levels rise several days before jaundice

---

begins if it is related to liver damage. However, if jaundice is present and serum ALT levels are normal or slightly elevated, the liver may not be the cause of the jaundice.

Patient Teaching

■ Instruct the patient to report signs of jaundice, such as yellow color in the sclera of the eyes.

ALBUMIN (SERUM)

Reference Values

Adult: 3.5–5.0 g/dL; 52% to 68% of total protein

Child: Newborn: 2.9–5.4 g/dL. *Infant:* 4.4–5.4 g/dL. Child: 4.0–5.8 g/dL

Description

Albumin, a component of proteins, makes up more than half of plasma proteins. Albumin is synthesized by the liver. It increases osmotic pressure (oncotic pressure), which is necessary for maintaining the vascular fluid. A decrease in serum albumin will cause fluid to shift from within the vessels to the tissues, resulting in edema.

A/G ratio is a calculation of the distribution of two major protein fractions, albumin and globulin. The reference value of A/G ratio is >1.0, which is the albumin value divided by globulin value (albumin ÷ globulin). A high ratio value is considered insignificant; low ratio value occurs in liver and renal diseases. Protein electrophoresis is more accurate and has replaced the A/G ratio calculation.[1,6,9,10,13]

Clinical Problems

Decreased Level (Hypoalbuminemia): Cirrhosis of the liver, acute liver failure, severe burns, severe malnutrition, preeclampsia, renal disorders, certain malignancies, ulcerative colitis, prolonged immobilization, protein-losing enteropathies, malabsorption. *Drug Influence:* penicillin, sulfonamides, aspirin, ascorbic acid

Elevated Level (Hyperalbuminemia): Dehydration, severe vomiting, severe diarrhea. *Drug Influence:* heparin

Procedure

■ Collect 5 to 10 mL of venous blood in a red-top tube.
■ There is no food or fluid restriction.

■ Factors Affecting Laboratory Results

■ Certain drugs could cause false negatives and false positives. (*See Drug Influence above.*)

NURSING IMPLICATIONS WITH RATIONALE

■ Check for peripheral edema and ascites when serum albumin is low. A low serum albumin decreases the oncotic pressure; thus fluid shifts from the vascular fluid to the tissue spaces, causing edema.
■ Assess for skin integrity if pitted edema or anasarca is present. Implement measures to avoid skin breakdown.
■ Offer foods high in protein (ie, meats, cheese, beans).

Patient Teaching

■ Teach the patient the importance of maintaining a good protein diet. In cases of protein deficit, the protein intake should be >50 g per day. Protein should increase the serum albumin level and decrease peripheral edema.

ALCOHOL (ETHYL OR ETHANOL) (SERUM OR PLASMA)

Reference Values

No Alcohol: 00.0% *No Significant Alcohol Influence:* <0.05% or 50 mg/dL. *Alcohol Influence Present:* 0.05%–0.10% or 50–100 mg/dL. *Reaction Time Affected:* 0.10%–0.15% or 100–150 mg/dL. *Indicative of Alcohol Intoxication:* >0.15% or >150 mg/dL. *Severe Alcohol Intoxication:* >0.25% or 250 mg/dL. *Comatose:* >0.30% or 300 mg/dL. *Fatal:* >0.40% or 400 mg/dL

Description

Ethyl alcohol (ethanol) in the blood is a frequently requested laboratory test for medical and legal reasons. In most states an alcohol level >0.10% or 100 mg/dL is considered by law to be proof of alcohol intoxication. On an empty stomach, plasma alcohol peaks in 40 to 70 minutes.

Serum/plasma alcohol may be used as a screening test on an unconscious patient. Nurses should check for any legal ramifications (state laws) in reference to drawing blood for plasma alcohol levels.[6,9,10,12]

Clinical Problems

Elevated Level: moderate to severe alcohol intoxication, chronic alcohol consumption, cirrhosis of the liver, malnutrition, folic acid deficiency, leukopenia, acute pancreatitis, gastritis, hypoglycemia, hyperuricemia. *Drug Influence:*

alcohol and drug interaction: (1) increases the effects of sedatives, hypnotics, narcotics, and tranquilizers (especially chlordiazepoxide [Librium] and diazepam [Valium]), depressing the CNS response; (2) antagonizes the action of warfarin (Coumadin) and phenytoin (Dilantin).

Procedure

- Obtain a consent form if required by law.
- Cleanse the venipuncture area with benzalkonium, and then wipe the solution off with a sterile swab or sponge. *Do not use* alcohol or tincture to cleanse the area.
- Collect 5 to 7 mL of venous blood in a red-top tube. A green or lavender or blue-top tube can be used. Avoid hemolysis.
- Write on the specimen and laboratory slip the date and time the blood specimen was drawn. The signatures of the collector and a witness must be included in the tube.

- **Factors Affecting Laboratory Results**

- Methyl alcohol (wood alcohol) and isopropyl alcohol (rubbing alcohol) can cause elevated serum alcohol levels and are very toxic.
- Cleansing the venipuncture site with alcohol or tincture can cause inaccurate results.
- Alcohol and drug interaction can affect results. (*See Drug Influence above*).

NURSING IMPLICATIONS WITH RATIONALE

Elevated Level (> 0.10% or 100 mg/dL)

- Provide safety measures to prevent physical harm to the patient when the serum alcohol level is greatly increased. Side rails may be needed while the patient is sleeping off the effects of alcohol.
- Follow legal ramifications in your state for drawing plasma alcohol level.

Patient Teaching

- Instruct the patient not to consume alcoholic beverages when taking sedatives, hypnotics, narcotics, tranquilizers (Valium, Librium), anticonvulsants (Dilantin), and anticoagulants (Coumadin). Alcohol and tranquilizers can depress respirations and might cause respiratory arrest.
- Encourage the patient to attend Alcoholics Anonymous (AA) meetings for chronic alcoholism. Listen to the patient's concerns.

ALDOLASE (ALD) (SERUM)

Reference Values

Adult: <6 U/L, 3–8 U/dL (Sibley-Lehninger), 22–59 mU/L at 37°C (SI units)
Child: Infant: 12–24 U/dL (four times). *Child:* 6–16 U/dL (two times)

Description

Aldolase is an enzyme present most abundantly in the skeletal and cardiac muscles. This enzyme monitors skeletal muscle diseases such as muscular dystrophy, dermatomyositis, and trichinosis. It is not elevated in muscle disease of neural origin, such as multiple sclerosis, poliomyelitis, and myasthenia gravis.

Serum aldolase is helpful in diagnosing early cases of Duchenne's muscular dystrophy before clinical symptoms appear. Progressive muscular dystrophy may cause elevated serum aldolase levels 10 to 15 times greater than normal. In late stages of muscular dystrophy, the enzyme level may return to normal or below normal. Serum aldolase is not the most effective diagnostic test for myocardial infarction (MI), since there is only a slight rise. Following an acute MI, it peaks (two times normal) in 24 hours and returns to normal in 4 to 7 days.[1,8,9]

Clinical Problems

Decreased Level: late muscular dystrophy

Elevated Level: early and progressive muscular dystrophy; trichinosis; dermatomyositis; acute MI; acute hepatitis; cancer of GI tract, prostate, and liver; lymphosarcoma; leukemia. *Drug Influence:* alcohol, cortisone, narcotics

Procedure

- Collect 3 to 5 mL of venous blood in a red-top tube. Unhemolyzed serum must be used when measuring for aldolase.
- There is no food or fluid restriction.

- Factors Affecting Laboratory Results

  - Hemolysis causes false-positive results.

NURSING IMPLICATIONS WITH RATIONALE

Elevated Level

- Recognize the purpose for monitoring aldolase levels. This is a useful test for diagnosing muscular disorders.
- List on the laboratory slip any drugs the patient is receiving that can elevate the serum aldolase level.
- Check serum aldolase results, and plan your nursing care according to symptoms present and psychologic needs.

ALDOSTERONE (SERUM)

Reference Values

Adult: 4–30 ng/dL (sitting position)

Description

Aldosterone is the most potent member of all mineralocorticoids produced by the adrenal cortex. Its major function is to regulate sodium, potassium, and water balance according to body needs. Aldosterone promotes sodium reabsorption from the distal tubules of the kidney and potassium and hydrogen excretion. With sodium reabsorption, water is retained. Eighty to 90% of aldosterone is inactivated in the liver.

This hormone responds to various changes in the body. When there is a sodium loss and a water loss, aldosterone is secreted for reestablishing sodium and water balance. Renin promotes aldosterone secretion, which causes more sodium and water to be retained and body fluid to be increased. Stress will increase aldosterone secretion. Hypernatremia (serum sodium excess) inhibits aldosterone secretion.

Serum aldosterone is not the most reliable test, since there can be fluctuations caused by various influences. If the patient is in a supine position, serum aldosterone will be lower than if he or she were in a sitting or standing position. A 24-hour urine test is considered more reliable than a random serum aldosterone collection. Several serum aldosterone levels may be requested.[7,11,13,14]

Clinical Problems

Decreased (< 1 ng/dL—supine position): overhydration with increased sodium, severe hypernatremia (sodium excess), high-sodium diet, adrenal cortical hypofunction, diabetes mellitus, licorice ingestion (excessive), glucose caused by excess infusion.

Elevated (> 9 ng/dL—supine position): dehydration, hyponatremia (sodium deficit), low-sodium diet, essential hypertension, adrenal cortical hyperfunction, cancer of the adrenal gland, cirrhosis of the liver, emphysema, severe congestive heart failure (CHF). *Drug Influence:* diuretics (furosemide [Lasix] and others), hydralazine (Apresoline), diazoxide (Hyperstat), nitroprusside.

Procedure

- Collect 5 mL of venous blood in a red-top tube. A green-top tube (heparinized) may also be used.
- The patient should be in a supine position for at least 1 hour before the blood is drawn.
- Write the date and time on the specimen. Aldosterone levels exhibit circadian rhythm, with peak levels occurring in the morning and lower levels in the afternoon.
- Food and fluids are not restricted, but excess salt and interfering substances (licorice) should not be consumed before the test. Normal salt intake is suggested.

■ Factors Affecting Laboratory Results

- A high- or low-salt diet can affect test results.
- Prolonged use of potent diuretics affect test results.
- Excessive licorice and glucose ingestion may decrease test results.
- Sitting or standing position when blood is drawn may cause false positive results.

NURSING IMPLICATIONS WITH RATIONALE

- Assess the patient for signs and symptoms of dehydration when the serum aldosterone is elevated, such as poor skin turgor, dry mucous membrane, shocklike symptoms, and for hyponatremia when the serum aldosterone is elevated.
- Compare the serum aldosterone and the 24-hour urine aldosterone results if both have been ordered.
- Record vital signs on the patient. A rapid pulse and later a drop in blood pressure (BP) could be indicative of hypovolemia (fluid volume deficit).

Patient Teaching

- Instruct the patient to remain in a supine position for at least 1 hour before blood is drawn to prevent false test results.

ALDOSTERONE (URINE)

Reference Values
Adult: 6–25 µg/24 hours

Description
(*See the Description for Aldosterone [Serum].*)
    Aldosterone causes sodium reabsorption and potassium excretion from the distal tubules of the kidney. Aldosterone secretion from the adrenal cortex influences sodium retention, fluid retention, fluid volume, and BP.

    A 24-hour urine aldosterone has an advantage over serum aldosterone, since fluctuation levels can be eliminated. Both urine and serum aldosterone will be increased by hyponatremia, a low-salt diet, and hyperkalemia. Likewise, hypernatremia, a high-salt diet, and hypokalemia will decrease urine and serum aldosterone. A urine sodium test may be ordered for comparison purposes.[7,11,13,14]

Clinical Problems
Decreased Level (<6 µg/24h): same as for serum aldosterone

Elevated Level (> 24 µg/24 h): tumors of the adrenal cortex or primary aldosteronism, same as for serum aldosterone

Procedure

- Collect a 24-hour urine specimen in a large container with a preservative (usually 1 g boric acid tablet).
- Have the patient void, and discard the urine before the test begins.
- Label the container with the exact date and time for the test (eg, 4/9/92, 7:35 AM to 4/10/92, 7:35 AM).

■ Factors Affecting Laboratory Results

- Failure to place all urine collected in a 24-hour period in the urine container can cause false results.
- Toilet paper and feces in the urine affect test results.

NURSING IMPLICATIONS WITH RATIONALE

- Check at specified times to determine whether the urine collection is being properly obtained.

Patient Teaching

- Instruct the patient on how to collect the 24-hour urine specimen. All urine should be saved after the initial urine is discarded. The urine may be kept on ice or refrigerated if indicated. Toilet paper or feces should not be in the urine.
- Answer the patient's questions concerning the test and the collection procedure.

ALKALINE PHOSPHATASE (ALP), WITH ISOENZYME (SERUM)

Reference Values

Adult: 30–120 IU/L 25–97 U/L at 37°C (SI units), 2–4 (U/dL Bodansky), 4–13 U/dL (King-Armstrong), 0.8–2.3 U/dL (Bessey-Lowry). ALP[1]: 20–120 U/L; ALP[2]: 20–110 U/L

Child: Infant and child (aged 0–12 years): 40–300 U/L. *Older child (13–18 years):* 30–165 U/L, 15–30 U/dL (King-Armstrong), 5–14 U/dL (Bodansky)

Elderly: slightly higher than adult

Description

ALP is an enzyme produced mainly in the liver and bone; it is also derived from the intestine, kidney, and placenta. The ALP test is useful for determining liver and bone diseases. In cases of mild liver-cell damage, the ALP level may be only slightly elevated, but it could be markedly elevated in acute liver disease. Once the acute phase is over, the serum level will promptly decrease, whereas the serum bilirubin would still remain increased. For determining liver dysfunction, several laboratory tests are performed (ie, bilirubin, leucine aminopeptidase [LAP], 5′-nucleotidase [5′-NT], and gamma-glutamyl transpeptidase [GGTP]).

With bone disorders, the ALP level is increased because of abnormal osteoblastic activity (bone cell production). In children it is not abnormal to find high levels of ALP during the prepuberty and puberty ages because of bone growth.

Isoenzymes of ALP are used to distinguish between liver and bone diseases, ALP[1] (liver origin), and ALP[2] (bone origin).[1,3,5,9,10]

Clinical Problems

Decreased Level: hypothyroidism, malnutrition, scurvy (vitamin C deficit), hypophosphatasia, pernicious anemia, placental insufficiency. *Drug Influence:* fluoride, oxalate, propranolol (Inderal)

Elevated Level: obstructive biliary disease (jaundice), cancer of the liver, hepatocellular cirrhosis, hepatitis, hyperparathyroidism, leukemia, cancer of the bone (breast and prostate), Paget's disease, osteitis deformans, healing fractures, multiple myeloma, osteomalacia, late pregnancy, rheumatoid arthritis (active), ulcerative disease. *Drug Influence:* IV albumin, antibiotics (erythromycin, lincomycin, oxacillin, penicillin), colchicine, methyldopa (Aldomet), allopurinol, phenothiazine tranquilizers, indomethacin (Indocin), procainamide, oral contraceptives (some), tolbutamide, isoniazid (INH), para-aminosalicylic acid (PAS).

Procedure

- Collect 5 to 10 mL of venous blood in a red-top tube. Avoid hemolysis.
- There is no food or fluid restriction. For ALP isoenzymes, fasting overnight might be indicated.
- Withhold for 8 to 24 hours drugs that can elevate ALP level, with physician's permission.
- List patient's age and drugs that may affect test results on laboratory slip.

■ Factors Affecting Laboratory Results

- Certain drugs that increase or decrease the serum ALP levels may cause false results. (*See Drug Influence above.*)
- Administered IV albumin can elevate the serum ALP to 5 to 10 times its normal value.
- Age of the patient (ie, youth and aged cause a serum increase).
- Late pregnancy to 3 weeks postpartum, which could cause a serum ALP elevation.

NURSING IMPLICATIONS WITH RATIONALE

- Know factors that can elevate serum ALP levels, such as drugs, IV albumin (can elevate serum ALP 5 to 10 times its normal value), age of patient (elevated in children and elderly), late pregnancy to 3 weeks postpartum, and blood drawn 2 to 4 hours after a fatty meal.
- Record pertinent information from procedure on laboratory slip.
- Assess for clinical signs and symptoms of liver disease or bone disease.
- Check the results of other ordered liver tests to determine the significance of the elevated serum ALP in liver disease.

Patient Teaching

- Inform the patient that other enzyme tests may be ordered to verify diagnosis.

ALPHA-1-ANTITRYPSIN (α-1-AT) (SERUM)
Alpha-1-Trypsin Inhibitor

Reference Values
Adult: 78–200 mg/dL, 0.78–2.0 g/L
Child: Newborn: 145–270 mg/dL *Infant:* similar to adult range

Description
Antitrypsin (α-1-AT) or trypsin inhibitor is a protein produced by the liver. It inhibits specific proteolytic enzymes that are released in the lung by bacteria or by phagocytic cells. A deficiency of homozygous antitrypsin (heredity linked) permits proteolytic enzymes to damage lung tissue, thus causing emphysema.

With inflammatory conditions, α-1-AT serum level can be increased. Following the inflammatory insult that could result from a surgical wound, the serum α-1-AT increases in 2 to 3 days and can remain elevated for 1 to 2 weeks. The serum level then returns to normal.[1,8–10,12]

Clinical Problems
Decreased Level: chronic obstructive lung disease (pulmonary emphysema), severe liver damage, malnutrition, severe protein-losing (nephrotic) syndrome

Elevated Level: acute and chronic inflammatory conditions, infections (selected), necrosis, late pregnancy, exercise (returns to normal in 1 day)/ *Drug Influence:* oral contraceptives

Procedure

- Collect 5 to 7 mL of venous blood in a red-top tube.
- Keep the patient NPO, except for water, for 8 hours before drawing blood.
- Hold oral contraceptives for 24 hours before the test, with the physician's permission. Any oral contraceptive taken should be listed on the laboratory slip.

■ Factors Affecting Laboratory Results

- Oral contraceptives can increase the α-1-AT level.
- Oral intake of food before the test can cause an inaccurate result, especially if the patient has an elevated serum cholesterol or serum triglycerides.

NURSING IMPLICATIONS WITH RATIONALE

Decreased Level

- Recognize clinical problems that are associated with α-1-AT deficiency (eg, emphysema).

Patient Teaching

- Explain to the patient that the test is ordered to determine whether there is an antitrypsin (protein) deficiency that can cause a lung disorder (disease). A nonsmoker with an α-1-AT deficiency can have emphysema. Antitrypsin inhibits proteolytic enzymes from destroying lung tissue; with a lack of this protein, the alveoli are damaged.
- Instruct the patient that he or she should have nothing by mouth except water for 8 hours before the blood test; this restriction before the blood test may vary among physicians.
- Instruct the patient with an α-1-AT deficit to use preventive methods in protecting his or her lungs (ie, avoid persons with upper respiratory infection [URI], seek medical care when having a respiratory infection).
- Encourage the patient to stop smoking and to avoid areas having high air pollution. Air pollution can cause respiratory inflammation and can promote chronic obstruction lung disease.

Elevated Level

- Check the serum α-1-AT level 2 to 3 days after extensive surgery. Inflammation can markedly increase the serum level. A base line serum level may be ordered before surgery for several reasons (eg, for determining lung disease and the effects of surgery).
- Report to the physician if the serum α-1-AT remains elevated 2 weeks after surgery.
- Note that serum α-1-AT can be markedly elevated during late pregnancy.

ALPHA FETOPROTEIN (AFP) SERUM AND AMNIOTIC FLUID

Reference Values

Nonpregnancy: <15 ng/mL

Pregnancy:

SERUM		AMNIOTIC FLUID	
Weeks of Gestation	ng/mL	Weeks of Gestation	ng/mL
8–12	0–39	14	11.0–32.0
13	6–31	15	5.5–31.0
14	7–50	16	5.7–31.5
15	7–60	17	3.8–32.5
16	10–72	18	3.6–28.0
17	11–90	19	3.7–24.5
18	14–94	20	2.2–15.0
19	24–112	21	3.8–18.0
20	31–122		
21	19–124		

Description

Serum alpha fetoprotein (AFP), a screening test, is usually done between 16 and 20 weeks' gestation to detect probability of twins, infant of low birth weight, or serious birth defects, such as open neural-tube defect. If a high serum AFP level occurs, the test should be repeated one week later. Ultrasound and amniocentesis may be performed to confirm elevated serum levels and to diagnose neural tube defect in the fetus.[1,3,6,9,10,15,16]

Clinical Problems

Decreased Level: Down's syndrome, absence of pregnancy

Elevated Level

Nonpregnant: Cirrhosis of the liver (not liver metastasis), germ cell tumor of gonads, such as testicular cancer

Pregnant: Neural tube defects (spina bifida, anencephaly, myelomeningocele), fetal death, fetal distress, Turner's syndrome, other anomalies (duodenal atresia, tetralogy of Fallot, hydrocephalus, trisomy 13), severe Rh immunization

Procedure

- Collect 7 mL of venous blood in a red-top tube. Avoid hemolysis.
- There is no food or fluid restriction.

- Factors Affecting Laboratory Results

  - Fetal blood contamination could cause an elevated amniotic AFP level.
  - Inaccurate recording of gestation week could affect results.
  - Multiple pregnancy or fetal death could cause a false-positive test.

- Hemolysis of blood sample could affect results.
- Body weight may be a factor (although not definitely confirmed). A heavier female tends to have a lower serum AFP level.

NURSING IMPLICATIONS WITH RATIONALE

- Explain that the test is for screening purposes. If the test is positive, genetic counseling might be necessary.
- Be supportive of individuals and family.

Patient Teaching

- Instruct the patient that it is essential to give the correct gestation date of the pregnancy, if known, to avoid a laboratory test error. Inform the patient that the test might be repeated in a week.
- If an ultrasound is performed, instruct the patient that it is usually done to confirm gestation age or to confirm the positive serum AFP and amniocentesis result(s).

AMMONIA (PLASMA)

Reference Values

Adult: 15–45 µg/dL, 11–35 µmol/L (SI units)
Child: Newborn: 64–107 µg/dL. *Child:* 21–50 µg/dL

Description

Ammonia, a by-product of protein metabolism, is formed from the bacterial action in the intestine and from metabolizing tissues. Most of the ammonia is absorbed into the portal circulation and is converted in the liver to urea. With severe liver decompensation or when blood flow is altered to the liver, the plasma ammonia level remains elevated.

Elevated plasma ammonia is best correlated with hepatic failure; however, other conditions that interfere with liver function (CHF, acidosis) may cause a temporary elevation of plasma ammonia.[7,10,11,13]

Clinical Problems

Decreased Level: renal failure, malignant hypertension, essential hypertension, *Drug Influence:* antibiotics (neomycin, tetracycline, kanamycin), monoamino oxidase inhibitors, diphenhydramine (Benadryl), potassium salts, sodium salts.

Elevated Level: hepatic failure, hepatic encephalopathy or coma, portacaval anastomosis, Reye's syndrome, erythroblastosis fetalis, cor pulmonale, CHF, pulmonary emphysema, high-protein diet with liver failure, acidosis, exercise. *Drug Influence:* ammonia chloride, diuretics (thiazides, furosemide [Lasix], ethacrynic acid [Edecrin]), ion exchange resin, isoniazid (INH).

Procedure

- Collect 5 mL of venous blood in a green-top tube. The blood sample should be delivered immediately in packed ice to the laboratory. Ammonia levels increase rapidly after blood is drawn.
- Minimize use of tourniquet for drawing blood.
- There is no food or fluid restriction unless indicated by the laboratory. Smoking should be avoided before the test.
- List drugs the patient is taking that could affect test results.

- ## Factors Affecting Laboratory Results

  - Failure to place the blood sample on ice and to analyze it immediately can result in false test.
  - High- or low-protein diet can cause false test result.
  - Exercise might increase the plasma ammonia level.
  - Certain antibiotics (neomycin and tetracycline) decrease the ammonia level.

NURSING IMPLICATIONS WITH RATIONALE

Elevated Level

- Identify clinical problems and drugs that can increase the plasma ammonia level.
- Notify the laboratory personnel when a plasma ammonia level is drawn so that it can be analyzed immediately to avoid false results.
- List antibiotics on the laboratory slip. Certain antibiotics (such as neomycin and tetracycline) can decrease the ammonia level, causing a false result.
- Observe for signs and symptoms of hepatic failure, especially when the plasma ammonia is elevated. There are many neurologic changes, such as behavioral and personality changes, lethargy, confusion, flapping tremors of the extremities, twitching, and, later, coma.
- Recognize that exercise may be a cause of an elevated plasma-ammonia level.
- Know various treatments used in decreasing the plasma ammonia level. A few of these are: low-protein diet, antibiotics (such as neomycin) to destroy intestinal bacteria, enemas, cathartics (such as magnesium sulfate) to prevent ammonia formation, and sodium glutamate and L-arginine in IV dextrose solution to stimulate urea formation.

Patient Teaching

- Explain to the patient why he or she may be NPO 8 hours before the test. Foods containing protein may cause a higher ammonia level.

AMYLASE (SERUM)

Reference Values

Adult: 60–160 Somogyi U/dL, 25–125 U/L (SI units)
Pregnancy: slightly increased
Child: not usually done
Elderly: slightly higher than adult

Description

Amylase is an enzyme that is derived from the pancreas, the salivary gland, and the liver. Its function is to change starch to sugar. In acute pancreatitis, serum amylase is increased to twice its normal level. Its level begins to increase 2 to 12 hours after onset, peaks in 20 to 30 hours, and returns to normal in 2 to 4 days. Acute pancreatitis is frequently associated with inflammation, severe pain, and necrosis caused by digestive enzymes (including amylase) escaping into the surrounding tissue.

Increased serum amylase can occur after abdominal surgery involving the gallbladder (stones or biliary duct) and stomach (partial gastrectomy). Following abdominal surgery, some surgeons order a routine serum amylase for 2 days to determine whether the pancreas has been injured.

The urine amylase level is helpful in determining the significance of a normal or slightly elevated serum amylase, especially when the patient has symptoms of pancreatitis. Amylase levels can also be obtained from abdominal fluid, ascitic fluid, pleural effusion, and saliva.[3,6,7,9]

Clinical Problems

Decreased Level: IV D5W, advanced chronic pancreatitis, acute and subacute necrosis of the liver, chronic alcoholism, toxic hepatitis, severe burns, severe thyrotoxicosis. *Drug Influence:* glucose (IV D5W), citrates, fluorides, oxalates

Increased Level: acute pancreatitis, chronic pancreatitis (acute onset), partial gastrectomy, peptic ulcer perforation, obstruction of pancreatic duct, acute cholecystitis, cancer of the pancreas, diabetic acidosis, diabetes mellitus, acute alcoholic intoxication, mumps, renal failure, benign prostatic hypertrophy, burns, pregnancy. *Drug Influence:* meperidine (Demerol), codeine, morphine, bethanechol chloride (Urecholine), pentazocine (Talwin), ethyl alcohol (large amounts), ACTH, guanethidine, thiazides, salicylates, tetracycline

Procedure

- Obtain 5 to 10 mL of venous blood in a red-top tube.
- Restrict food for 1 to 2 hours before the blood sample is drawn. If the patient has eaten or has received a narcotic 2 hours before the test, the serum results could be invalid.
- List on the laboratory slip drugs that could cause false amylase level.

■ **Factors Affecting Laboratory Results**

- Narcotic drugs can cause false-positive levels.
- IV fluids with glucose can result in false-negative levels.
- Contamination of the specimen with saliva can occur through coughing, sneezing, or talking when the tube is opened. This could cause false-positive results.

NURSING IMPLICATIONS WITH RATIONALE

Decreased Level

- Know that D5W administered intravenously can decrease the serum amylase level, causing a false-negative result.
- Identify drugs that give false-negative levels.
- Determine when the patient has ingested food or sweetened fluids. Blood should not be drawn until 2 hours after eating, since sugar can decrease the serum amylase level.

Elevated Level

- Know the disease entities related to increased levels, especially acute pancreatitis, abdominal surgery (partial gastrectomy, biliary resection), diabetes mellitus, cancer of the pancreas, acute alcoholic intoxication, and benign prostatic hypertrophy (BPH).
- Label the laboratory slip (for serum amylase) with the drugs the patient is receiving or has received in the last 24 hours. Morphine, meperidine, codeine, pentazocine, aspirin, and hydrochlorothiazide can cause a false-positive serum amylase level.
- Check serum amylase levels for several days after abdominal surgery. Surgery of the stomach or gallbladder might cause trauma to the pancreas and cause excess amylase to be released.
- Report symptoms of severe pain when pancreatitis is suspected. The physician may want to draw a serum amylase level before a narcotic is given. An elevated level may indicate an acute pancreatitis.
- Explain to the patient that blood is drawn for determining whether the severe pain is due to a pancreatic problem or to another cause.
- Ask the patient if he or she has had pancreatitis before and has taken narcotic analgesics. A report should be given to the physician.
- Report elevated serum amylase results occurring beyond 3 days. If the serum amylase levels remain elevated beyond 3 days (72 hours), pancreatic cell destruction could still be occurring.

Patient Teaching

- Instruct the patient to assume adequate health practices such as controlling alcohol intake and increasing protein and carbohydrates in the diet.

AMYLASE (URINE)

Reference Values

Adult: 4–37 U/L/2 h

Description

(See serum amylase.)

Amylase is an enzyme that is produced by the pancreas, salivary glands, and liver and is excreted by the kidneys. When there is an inflammation of the pancreas or salivary gland, more amylase goes into the blood and more amylase is excreted in the urine. The urine levels of amylase could remain elevated for a week, whereas the serum amylase level tends to remain elevated for a short time (peaks in 24 hours and returns to normal in 48 to 96 hours).

The urine amylase test is ordered at 1-hour, 2-hour, or 24-hour timed intervals, with the 2-hour urine specimen the most commonly ordered. A 24-hour specimen may be within normal range, whereas a 2-hour specimen shows an increase.

One drawback of urine amylase as well as of serum amylase values is their relation to renal function. A diminished renal function could lead to a decrease in urine amylase and increased serum amylase.[3,6,7,9]

Clinical Problems

Decreased Level: diminished renal function; *See Amylase—Serum.*

Increased Level: acute pancreatitis, choledocholithiasis; *See Amylase—Serum.*

Procedure

- A timed urine collection is required; thus the exact beginning and end of the urine collection should be recorded (date, hour, and minute—eg, 2/10/92, 9:02 AM to 2/10/92, 11:05 AM). First the patient voids and the urine is discarded.
- The urine specimen should be refrigerated or kept on ice. No preservative is needed.

- Factors Affecting Laboratory Results

  - Fecal material or toilet paper contamination can affect test results.
  - Diminished urine output affects test results.
  - Drugs that increase or decrease amylase levels are listed at drug influence.
  - Prolonged urine collection time affects test results.

NURSING IMPLICATIONS WITH RATIONALE

Decreased Level

- Check urinary output for 8 hours and 24 hours, BUN, and serum creatinine levels. A decrease in urine output and an increase in BUN and serum creatinine levels indicate poor kidney function. A decreased urine output could result in a decreased urine amylase.

Patient Teaching

- Explain to the patient the importance of collecting urine at a specified time. The patient should use a urinal or bedpan and should be instructed that all urine should be saved.
- Encourage the patient to drink water during the test unless water intake is restricted for medical reasons. A decreased urine output could result in no 2-hour specimen or a possible false result.

Increased Level

- Check urinary output and give fluids if the urine output is decreased. Encouraging fluids during the test should help in securing a urine specimen.
- Check the serum amylase level(s) and compare with the urine amylase level. A low serum amylase level and an increased urine amylase level could indicate that the acute problem is no longer present.
- List on the laboratory slip the drugs the patient is receiving that can increase amylase levels (eg, narcotics).
- Notify the physician when the patient is having severe abdominal pain. The physician may want to order a 2-hour or 24-hour urine specimen the next day.

ANION GAP

Reference Values

Adult: 11–17 mEq/L. *Average:* 14 mEq/L

Description

Anion gap is the interrelationship between electrolytes, the cations (sodium and potassium), and the anions (chloride and bicarbonate) in determining metabolic acid-base imbalances. Serum levels of these electrolytes are applied to the formula:

$$\text{Anion gap} = (\text{sodium} + \text{potassium}) - (\text{chloride} + CO_2 \text{ [bicarbonate]})$$

An elevated anion gap > 17 mEq/L is indicative of metabolic acidosis; a decreased anion gap < 11 mEq/L is indicative of metabolic alkalosis.[1,3,6,9,10]

Clinical Problems

Decreased Level (<11 mEq/L): High electrolyte values such as sodium, calcium, magnesium; multiple myeloma, nephrosis. *Drug Influence:* lithium, diuretics, chlorpropamide

Elevated Level (>17 mEq/L): Lactic acidosis, ketoacidosis (uncontrolled diabetes mellitus, starvation, anorexia nervosa), severe salicylate intoxication, renal failure, severe dehydration, antifreeze ingestion, paint thinner. *Drug*

Influence: penicillin and carbenicillin in high doses, salicylates, paraldehyde, diuretics (thiazides and loop diuretics), methanol ingestion

Normal Level Occurring in Metabolic Acidosis: Diarrhea, renal tubular acidosis, ureterosigmoidostomy, hyperalimentation, small bowel fistula, pancreatic drainage

Procedure

- Obtain serum electrolyte values of sodium (Na), potassium (K), chloride (Cl), and CO_2 (bicarbonate determinant) from the laboratory slip. If not available, collect 7 to 10 mL of venous blood in a red-top tube.
- There is no food or fluid restriction.

■ **Factors Affecting Laboratory Results**

- See "drug influence" under decreased and elevated levels.
- Hemolysis of blood sample increases potassium and bicarbonate levels.

NURSING IMPLICATIONS WITH RATIONALE

- Calculate anion gap from recently obtained electrolyte values of sodium, potassium, chloride, and serum CO_2. Use the formula given in "Description" above.
- Observe for signs and symptoms of metabolic acidosis (ie, rapid, vigorous breathing (Kussmaul's breathing), increased pulse rate, flushed skin).

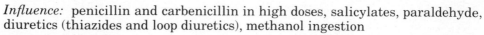

ANTIBIOTICS/AMINOGLYCOSIDES (SERUM)
Amikacin (Amikin), Gentamicin (Garamycin), Tobramycin (Nebcin)

Reference Values
Adult

Drug Name	THERAPEUTIC RANGE		Toxic Level
	Peak	**Trough**	
Amikacin	15–30 µg/mL	<10 µg/mL	>35 µg/mL
Gentamicin	5–10 µg/mL	<2 µg/mL	>12 µg/mL
Tobramycin	5–10 µg/mL	<2 µg/mL	>12 µg/mL

Child: same as adult

Description

Aminoglycosides are broad-spectrum antibiotics that are effective against gram-negative microorganisms. These agents are not well absorbed from the GI tract and so are given parenterally. Peak action after intramuscular (IM) injection is ½ to 1½ hours and after 30-minute IV infusion is ½ hour. Half-life is about 2 hours. Aminoglycosides cross the placental barrier but do not cross the blood-brain barrier. They are excreted mostly unchanged by the kidneys.

Ototoxicity and nephrotoxicity can result from overdose of aminoglycoside or from long-term administration. Renal function tests (ie, creatinine, creatinine clearance, and urinalysis) should be assessed periodically while the patient is receiving these agents. If patients with renal insufficiency receive any of these drugs, dosage should be adjusted (decreased). Drug half-life is usually 24 to 96 hours in patients having renal damage.[1,2,12,13]

Clinical Problems

Elevated Levels: overdose of aminoglycoside, renal insufficiency or failure.
Drug Influence: diuretics, cephalosporins (increase chance of nephrotoxicity)

Procedure

- Collect 3 to 5 mL of venous blood in red-top tube.
- Collect specimen during steady state, usually 24 to 36 hours after drug was started.
- Record on the laboratory requisition slip dose, route (IM or IV), and last time drug was administered.
- There is no food or fluid restriction.

■ Factors Affecting Laboratory Results

- Renal insufficiency or failure could cause an elevated serum aminoglycoside level.

NURSING IMPLICATIONS WITH RATIONALE

- Check serum aminoglycoside (amikacin, gentamicin, tobramycin) results, and report nontherapeutic levels to physician immediately.
- Assess intake and output. Notify the physician if urine output has greatly decreased. This could be a sign of aminoglycoside toxicity.
- Suggest renal function tests for patients receiving long-term aminoglycoside therapy and especially for those with renal insufficiency.
- Recognize that diuretics and cephalosporins coadministered with an aminoglycoside could enhance the risk of nephrotoxicity.
- Assess hearing status of the patient. Any hearing impairment, loss of high tone, while the patient is receiving aminoglycoside could indicate ototoxicity.

Elevated Level

- Recognize that overdose of aminoglycoside or renal insufficiency could cause an elevated serum aminoglycoside level.

- Observe for signs and symptoms of nephrotoxicity (ie, proteinuria, elevated creatinine, elevated BUN, decreased creatinine clearance test).
- Observe for signs and symptoms of ototoxicity (ie, nausea and vomiting with motion, dizziness, headache, tinnitus, decrease in ability to hear high-pitched tones).

ANTIBIOTIC SUSCEPTIBILITY (SENSITIVITY) TEST

Reference Values

Adult: Organism is sensitive or intermediate or resistant to antibiotics.

Child: same as adult

Description

(*See Cultures.*)

It is important to identify not only the organism responsible for the infection but also the antibiotic(s) that will inhibit the growth of the bacteria. The physician orders a culture and sensitivity test (C and S) when a wound infection, urinary tract infection, or other types of infected secretions are suspected. The choice of antibiotic depends on the pathogenic organism and its susceptibility to the antibiotics.

There are two methods employed to test antibiotic susceptibility: tube dilution and disk diffusion (also called agar diffusion), with the latter being the most commonly used method. A filter paper containing small antibiotic disks is placed in a Petri dish streaked with the single type of bacteria. If bacteria surround the disk, the organism is resistant to the antibiotic. If the bacteria growth around the disk is inhibited, the organism is susceptible to the antibiotic. Recently, the term *minimal inhibitory concentration* (MIC) has been used to express (in μg/mL) the lowest concentration of the antibiotics that will prevent visible growth of a cultured microorganism.

With the tube dilution method, bacteria are cultured in several tubes having various concentrations of antibiotic. The lowest concentration of antibiotic that inhibits the growth of the organism is the choice of antibiotic concentration for the patient.[1,5,7,10]

Clinical Problems

Resistant (R): The antibiotic is noneffective against the organism.

Intermediate (I): Bacterial growth retardation is inconclusive.

Sensitive (S): The antibiotic is effective against the organism.

Procedure

- It takes approximately 24 hours for bacterial growth and 48 hours for the test results.

- The specimen for C and S should be taken to the laboratory within 30 minutes of collection or else refrigerated.
- The specimen should be handled with care, preventing contamination and bacterial transmission (*See Culture Procedure*).

■ Factors Affecting Laboratory Results

- Antibiotics and sulfonamides could cause a false-negative reaction.

NURSING IMPLICATIONS WITH RATIONALE

- Collect specimen for C and S before preventive antibiotic therapy is started. Antibiotic therapy started before specimen collection could cause an inaccurate result.
- Record on the laboratory slip the antibiotic(s) the patient is receiving, the dosages, and how long the antibiotic(s) has (have) been taken.
- Check laboratory report for C and S result. If the patient is receiving an antibiotic and the report shows the organism is resistant to that antibiotic, the nurse should notify the physician.

Patient Teaching

- Inform the patient that the culture test results will be available in 48 hours.

ANTICONVULSANTS (BLOOD, SERUM, PLASMA)
Carbamazepine (Tegretol), Ethosuximide (Zarontin), Phenytoin (Dilantin) (See Phenytoin), Primidone (Mysoline), Valproic Acid (Depakene)

Reference Values
Adult

Drug Name	THERAPEUTIC RANGE		TOXIC LEVEL	
	µg/mL	µmoL/L	µg/mL	µmoL/L
Carbamazepine	4–12	16.9–50.8	>12–15	>50.8–69
(Child)	(Same as adult)		(Same as adult)	
Ethosuximide	40–100	283–708	>100	>708
(Child)	(2–4 per 1 mg/kg/day)		(Same as adult or higher)	
Phenytoin	10–20	39.6–79.3	>20	>79.3
Primidone	5–12	23–55	>12–15	>55–69
(Child <5 years)	(7–10)	(30–45)	(>12)	(>55)
Valproic acid	50–100	347–693	>100	>693
(Child)	(Same as adult)		(Same as adult)	

Description

The drugs listed as anticonvulsant agents are given to control or to alleviate grand mal, psychomotor, and/or petit mal seizures. Most of them have different therapeutic range, peak levels, and half-life.

Carbamazepine (Tegretol): This agent is used for grand mal seizures. Peak serum level occurs 4 to 8 hours after oral dose; half-life is about 10 to 26 hours in adults and 8 to 20 hours in children. Steady state is reached in 2 weeks. When carbamazepine is administered with phenytoin, phenobarbital, ethosuximide, primidone, or valproic acid, serum level of the drug might decrease. A serious side effect is bone marrow depression.

Ethosuximide (Zarontin). This agent is used for petit mal seizures. Peak serum level occurs 3 to 5 hours after oral dose; half-life is about 60 hours in adults and 30 hours in children. Steady state is reached in 7 to 10 days. When administered with carbamazepine or valproic acid, ethosuximide's serum level might decrease or increase. Side effects could include anorexia, nausea, vomiting, lupus erythematosuslike syndrome.

Phenytoin (Dilantin): (See separate listing.)

Primidone (Mysoline): This agent is used for grand mal and psychomotor seizures. Peak serum level occurs 7 to 8 hours after oral dose; half-life varies from 8 to 48 hours (shorter half-life with primidone and longer with the two active metabolites—phenobarbital and phenylethylmalonamide [PEMA].) Steady state is rapidly reached. When primidone is administered with carbamazepine, its serum level may increase. Side effects include sedation, nausea, dizziness, visual disturbance.

Valproic Acid: This agent is used alone or with other anticonvulsants for grand mal and petit mal seizures. Peak serum level occurs 1 to 4 hours after oral dose; half-life is 8 to 15 hours. Valproic acid inhibits phenobarbital metabolism. If primidone or phenobarbital are given with valproic acid, their dosage needs to be adjusted (lowered). Valproic acid can elevate ethosuximide and phenytoin levels when coadministered. It can cross the placenta. Valproic acid therapy may cause a false-positive urine ketone test. Side effects include anorexia, nausea, vomiting, fatigue, and altered liver function tests.[3,9,17]

Clinical Problems

Decreased Level

Carbamazepine: Drug Influence: barbiturates, benzodiazepines, ethosuximide, phenytoin, primidone, valproic acid

Ethosuximide: Drug Influence: carbamazepine, valproic acid

Valproic Acid Drug Influence: carbamazepine, phenytoin, phenobarbital, primidone

Elevated Level

Carbamazepine: overdose of carbamazepine. Liver disease, cardiovascular disease, bone marrow disease. *Drug Influence:* phenytoin, barbiturates, propoxyphene (Darvon), erythromycin

Ethosuximide: overdose of ethosuximide, liver disease. *Drug Influence:* carbamazepine, valproic acid

Primidone: overdose of primidone, liver disease. *Drug Influence:* pheno-barbital.

Procedure

- Collect 5 to 10 mL of venous blood in a red-top tube (valproic acid, carbamazepine), gray-top tube (primidone), green-top tube (ethosuximide). Check with laboratory for preferred collecting tube.
- Record name of drug, dose, route, and last time drug was administered on the laboratory requisition slip. Trough serum levels (drawn before next dose) are usually requested. List drugs the patient is taking that might interfere with test results on requisition slip.
- There is no food or fluid restriction.

■ Factors Affecting Laboratory Results

- Drugs (*see Drug Influence above*) that the patient is taking could increase or decrease test results.

NURSING IMPLICATIONS WITH RATIONALE

- Administer valproic acid with meals to reduce GI distress.
- Monitor serum drug levels, weekly, monthly, yearly during long-term drug therapy.
- Monitor CBC and platelet count prior to carbamazepine (Tegretol) therapy and at regular intervals—weekly, monthly. Bone marrow depression is rare; however, it could occur as a result of long-term carbamazepine therapy.
- Assess liver function tests (ie, aspartate aminotransferase AST, serum glutamic-oxaloacetic acid (SGOT), alanine aminotransferase ALT, serum glutamic-pyruvic transaminase (SGPT), bilirubin, alkaline phosphatase) while patient is receiving long-term anticonvulsant therapy. Compare test findings with base line levels. These drugs are metabolized in the liver, and hepatic damage could result.
- Assess serum amylase level while patient is receiving long-term valproic acid (Depakene) therapy. Pancreatitis could result.

Patient Teaching

- Inform the patient not to discontinue prescribed anticonvulsant agent abruptly without physicians's permission. Withdrawal of any anticonvulsant drugs could precipitate seizures.
- Inform patient that photosensitivity reaction could occur when taking anticonvulsants. While in the sun, use sunglasses and sunscreen lotion.

Elevated Level

- Relate clinical conditions and drugs (*see Clinical Problems above*) that could elevate serum and anticonvulsant levels.

- Observe for signs and symptoms of common side effects from anticonvulsant therapy (ie, anorexia, nausea, vomiting, fatigue, lethargy, dizziness, headache).
- Inform diabetic patient on valproic acid therapy that the drug could cause a false-positive urine ketone test.
- Report immediately symptoms of carbamazepine and primidone toxicity (ie, diplopia, blurred vision) to the physician.
- Report lupus erythematosuslike symptoms resulting from long-term ethosuximide therapy.
- Assess for bleeding or bruising (petechiae, ecchymosis, epistaxis, melena) while receiving valproic acid. Report findings to the physician. Check CBC for low platelet count and blood count.

ANTIGLOMERULAR BASEMENT MEMBRANE ANTIBODY (ANTI-GBM, AGBM) SERUM
Glomerular Basement Membrane Antibody

Reference Values

Negative or none detected

Description

This test is performed to detect circulating glomerular basement membrane (GBM) antibodies that can damage the glomerular basement membranes in the glomeruli. Beta hemolytic *Streptococcus* can cause an antibody response in the renal glomeruli.

Glomerulonephritis, caused by anti-GBM, is usually severe and rapidly progressive. Pulmonary hemorrhage often occurs due to cross-reactivity of anti-GBM with pulmonary vascular basement membrane.[3,10,18]

Clinical Problems

Positive Result: anti-GBM nephritis, tubulointerstitial nephritis, pulmonary capillary basement membranes

Procedure

- Collect 5 to 7 mL of venous blood in red-top tube. Test should be run immediately, and if not the blood should be frozen.
- There is no food or fluid restriction.
- Tissue from kidney biopsy might be the specimen. Tissue should be frozen after collection.

- Factors Affecting Laboratory Results

  - Improper care of specimen can result in inaccurate test results.

NURSING IMPLICATIONS WITH RATIONALE

- Obtain a history of a streptococcal throat infection.
- Monitor urine output. As the glomeruli are damaged, oliguria usually occurs.
- Assess for signs and symptoms of renal (glomerular) disease (ie, edema of the extremities, shortness of breath, proteinuria, hematuria, increased blood pressure, elevated serum BUN and creatinine, decreased urine output).

Patient Teaching

- Instruct patient to follow medical regimen of diet, drugs, and rest.

ANTINUCLEAR ANTIBODIES (ANA) (SERUM)
Anti-DNA Antibody, Anti-DNP Antibody

Reference Values

Adult: negative

Description

The ANA test is a screening test for diagnosing systemic lupus erythematosus (SLE) and other collagen diseases. ANAs are immunoglobulins (IgM, IgG, IgA) that react with the nuclear part of leukocytes. They form antibodies against deoxyribonucleic acid (DNA), ribonucleic acid (RNA), and others. Two antinuclear antibodies, anti-DNA and anti–D-nucleoprotein (Anti-DNP), are almost always present with SLE. Anti-DNA will fluctuate according to the disease process, with remission, and with exacerbation. It is normally present (95%) in lupus nephritis.

The total ANA can also be positive in scleroderma, rheumatoid arthritis, cirrhosis, leukemia, infectious mononucleosis, and malignancy. For diagnosing lupus, ANA test should be compared with other tests for lupus.[1,8–10,13]

Clinical Problems

Elevated—Positive (>1:20): SLE (most frequent cause), progressive systemic sclerosis, scleroderma, leukemia, rheumatoid arthritis, cirrhosis of the liver, infectious mononucleosis, myasthenia gravis malignancy. *Drug Influence:* antibiotics (penicillin, streptomycin, tetracycline), antihypertensives (hydralazine [Apresoline], methyldopa [Aldomet]), anti-TB (para-aminosalicylic acid [PAS], isoniazid [INH]), diuretics (acetazolamide [Diamox], thiazides [hydrochlorothiazide]), oral contraceptives, procainamide (Pronestyl), trimethadione (Tridione), phenytoin (Dilantin)

Procedure

■ Collect 5 to 7 mL of venous blood in a red-top tube. Take to the laboratory immediately.
■ There is no food or fluid restriction.
■ List drugs the patient is taking that could cause false-positive test results.

■ Factors Affecting Laboratory Results

■ Certain drugs cause false-positive results (*see Drug Influence above*).
■ The aging process can cause a slight positive ANA titer.

NURSING IMPLICATIONS WITH RATIONALE

Elevated—Positive Titer

■ Relate clinical problems and drugs to positive ANA results. With SLE, the ANA titer may fluctuate according to the severity of the disease.
■ Compare test result with other tests for lupus.
■ Assess for signs and symptoms of SLE (ie, skin rash over the cheeks and nose, joint pain).
■ Promote rest during an acute phase.

ANTISTREPTOLYSIN O (ASO) (SERUM)

Reference Values

Upper limit of normal varies with age, season, and geographic area.

Adult: <100 IU/mL

Child: Newborn: similar to mother's. *2 to 5 years:* <100 IU/mL. *12–19 years:* <200 IU/mL

Description

The beta-hemolytic *Streptococcus* secretes an enzyme known as streptolysin O, which is capable of lysing red blood cells (RBCs). Streptolysin O acts as an antigen and stimulates the immune system to develop antistreptolysin O (ASO) antibodies. A high titer of ASO indicates that streptococci are present and may cause rheumatic fever or acute glomerulonephritis. Increased serum ASO levels can also indicate a recent streptococcal infection.

The ASO antibodies appear approximately 1 to 2 weeks after an acute streptococcal infection, peak 3 to 4 weeks after onset, and could remain elevated for months. Many school-aged children have a higher ASO titer level than do preschool children or adults.

Other streptococcal antigens are antideoxyribonuclease (ADNase—titer > 10) and antistreptococcal hyaluronidase (ASH—titer > 128).[9,10,12,19]

Clinical Problems

Decreased Level: Drug Influence: antibiotics

Elevated Level: acute rheumatic fever, acute glomerulonephritis, streptococcal upper respiratory infections, rheumatoid arthritis (mildly elevated), hyperglobulinemia with liver disease, collagen disease (mildly elevated).

Procedure

- Collect 5 to 10 mL of venous blood in red-top tube. Avoid hemolysis.
- There is no food or fluid restriction.
- Repeated ASO testing (once or twice a week) is advisable to determine the highest level of increase.

■ Factors Affecting Laboratory Results

- Antibiotic therapy decreases the antibody response.
- Increased level may occur in healthy persons (carriers).

NURSING IMPLICATIONS WITH RATIONALE

- Note that antibiotic therapy could decrease antibody response.

Elevated Level

- Check serum ASO levels when the patient is complaining of joint pain in the extremities. A high elevated level could be indicative of acute rheumatic fever, and a slight elevation could be indicative of rheumatoid arthritis.
- Check the urinary output when the serum ASO is elevated. A urinary output of less than 600 mL/24 hours may be associated with acute glomerulonephritis.

Patient Teaching

- Instruct patient and family that when patient has a sore throat he or she should have a throat culture taken to check for beta-hemolytic streptococcus. A throat culture might need to be repeated if sore throat persists.

ARTERIAL BLOOD GASES (ABGs) ARTERIAL BLOOD
Blood Gases

Reference Values

Adult: pH: 7.35–7.45; Pco_2: 35–45 mm Hg; Po_2: 75–100 mm Hg; Sao_2: >95%; Svo_2: >70%; Hco_3: 24–28 mEq/L; base excess (BE): +2 to −2 mEq/L

Child: pH: 7.36–7.44. Other measurements are same as adult.

Description

Arterial blood gases (ABGs) are usually ordered to assess disturbances of acid-base (A-B) balance caused by a respiratory disorder and/or a metabolic disorder. The basic components of ABGs include pH, Pco_2, Po_2, o_2 saturation, bicarbonate (Hco_3), and BE.

pH: The pH, the negative logarithm of the hydrogen ion concentration, determines the acidity or alkalinity of body fluids. A pH less than 7.35 indicates acidosis, either respiratory acidosis or metabolic acidosis. A pH greater than 7.45 indicates alkalosis, either respiratory or metabolic alkalosis.

Pco_2: The partial pressure of carbon dioxide (Pco_2) reflects the adequacy of alveolar ventilation. When there is alveolar damage, Co_2 cannot escape. Carbon dioxide (Co_2) combines with water to form carbonic acid ($H_2o + Co_2 — H_2co_3$), causing an acidotic state. When the patient is hypoventilating, Pco_2 is elevated and respiratory acidosis results. Chronic obstructive lung disease is a major cause of respiratory acidosis. When the patient is hyperventilating (blowing off co_2 by rapid breathing), Pco_2 is decreased and respiratory alkalosis results.

Po_2: The partial pressure of oxygen (Po_2) determines the amount of oxygen that can bind with hemoglobin. The pH affects the combining power of oxygen and hemoglobin, and with a low pH, there will be less oxygen in the hemoglobin. Po_2 is decreased in respiratory diseases, such as emphysema, pneumonia, and pulmonary edema; in the presence of abnormal hemoglobin (Co Hb, Meth Hb, Sulfa Hb); and in polycythemia.

Oxygen Saturation (So_2): The oxygen saturation is the percentage of oxygen in the blood that combines with hemoglobin. It is measured indirectly by calculation of Po_2 and pH or measured directly by co-oximetry. The combination of oxygen saturation, partial pressure of oxygen, and hemoglobin indicates tissue oxygenation.

Hco_3 and BE: Bicarbonate (Hco_3) is an alkaline substance that comprises over half of the total buffer base in the blood. When there is a deficit of bicarbonate and other bases or an increase in nonvolatile acid such as lactic acid, metabolic acidosis occurs. If a bicarbonate excess is present, then metabolic alkalosis results. The bicarbonate plays a very important role in maintaining a pH of 7.35 to 7.45.

The base excess (BE) value is frequently checked with the Hco_3 value. A base excess of less than -2 is acidosis and greater than $+2$ is alkalosis.

Acid-base Imbalances: To determine the type of A-B imbalance, the pH, Pco_2, Hco_3, and BE are checked. The Pco_2 is a respiratory determinant, and Hco_3 and BE are metabolic determinants. Both Pco_2, Hco_3, and BE values are compared to the pH. A pH of less than 7.35 is acidosis and of greater than 7.45 is alkalosis.[3,9,10,18,20]

1) If the pH is <7.35, the Pco_2 is >45 mm Hg, and the Hco_3 and BE are normal, the A-B imbalance is respiratory acidosis.
2) If the pH is >7.45, the Pco_2 is <35 mm Hg, and the Hco_3 and BE are normal, the A-B imbalance is respiratory alkalosis.

3) If the pH is <7.35, the P_{CO_2} is normal, the H_{CO_3} and BE are < 24 mEq/L and <-2, the A-B imbalance is metabolic acidosis.

4) If the pH is >7.45, the P_{CO_2} is normal, the H_{CO_3} and BE are >28 mEq/L and >$+2$, the A-B imbalance is metabolic alkalosis.

ACID-BASE (A-B) IMBALANCE	pH	P_{CO_2}	H_{CO_3}	BE
Respiratory acidosis	↓	↑	N	N
Respiratory alkalosis	↑	↓	N	N
Metabolic acidosis	↓	N	↓	↓
Metabolic alkalosis	↑	N	↑	↑

Clinical Problems

Respiratory Acidosis: (pH <7.35; P_{CO_2} >45 mm Hg): Chronic obstructive lung disease (emphysema, chronic bronchitis, severe asthma), respiratory distress syndrome (ARDS), Guillain-Barré syndrome, anesthesia, pneumonia. *Drug Influence:* narcotics, sedatives

Respiratory Alkalosis: (pH >7.45; P_{CO_2} <35 mm Hg): Salicylate toxicity (early phase), anxiety, hysteria, tetany, strenuous exercise (swimming, running), fever, hyperthyroidism, delirium tremens, pulmonary embolism

Metabolic Acidosis: (pH <7.35; H_{CO_3} <24 mEq/L): Diabetic ketoacidosis, severe diarrhea, starvation/malnutrition, shock, burns, kidney failure, acute myocardial infarction

Metabolic Alkalosis: (pH >7.45; H_{CO_3} >28 mEq/L): Severe vomiting, gastric suction, peptic ulcer, potassium loss, excess administration of bicarbonate, hepatic failure, cystic fibrosis. *Drug Influence:* sodium bicarbonate, sodium oxalate, potassium oxalate

Procedure

- There is no food or fluid restriction.
- If the patient is receiving anticoagulant therapy or taking aspirin, the laboratory, nurse, or pulmonary technician drawing the blood should be notified.
- Collect 1 to 5 mL of arterial blood in a heparinized needle and syringe, remove the needle, make sure there is no air in the syringe, and apply an airtight cap over the tip of the syringe.
- Place the syringe with arterial blood in an ice-water bag (to minimize the metabolic activity of the sample), and deliver it immediately to the laboratory. Ice water is colder than ice.
- Indicate on the ABGs slip whether the patient is receiving oxygen and the flow rate, type of O_2 administration device (ie, cannula, mask), and the patient's current temperature.
- Apply pressure to the puncture site for 5 minutes; longer for persons on anticoagulants or streptokinase therapy.

◾ Factors Affecting Laboratory Results

- Improper handling of the blood sample, such as not using ice water, exposure of specimen to air, and not expelling all the heparin out of the collection syringe cause inaccurate results.
- Hemolysis of the blood sample cause false results.
- Narcotics and sedatives can contribute to the respiratory acidotic state and sodium bicarbonate, could cause metabolic alkalosis
- Inaccurate results can occur due to suctioning the patient, changes in O_2 therapy, and ventilators; patients exposed to carbon monoxide, nitrate, nitrate exposure; and patients receiving blood transfusion.

NURSING IMPLICATIONS WITH RATIONALE

Respiratory Acidosis

- Assess for signs and symptoms of respiratory acidosis, such as dyspnea, disorientation, and increased Pco_2 >45 mm Hg.
- Perform chest clapping to break up bronchial and alveolar secretions. CO_2 can be trapped in the lungs because of excess secretions and mucous plugs.
- Administer oxygen at a low concentration (2 to 3 L) when emphysema is present.
- Check for metabolic compensatory mechanism with respiratory acidosis—Hco_3 would be elevated, >28 mEq/L.

Patient Teaching

- Teach the patient breathing exercises to enhance Co_2 excretion from the lungs.
- Instruct the patient on how to properly use the intermittent positive-pressure breathing (IPPB) machine if ordered.
- Demonstrate the postural drainage procedure, if not contraindicated, by lowering the head of the bed or having the patient lie over the side of the bed. Secretions are mobilized and excreted by gravity.

Respiratory Alkalosis

- Relate a low Pco_2 value to clinical problems associated with tachypnea (overbreathing). Anxiety, hysteria, nervousness, and strenuous physical exertion can cause tachypnea. With rapid breathing, an excess of Co_2 is lost.
- Assess for signs and symptoms of respiratory alkalosis, such as tachypnea, dizziness, tetany spasms, and a Pco_2 less than 35 mm Hg.

Patient Teaching

- Instruct the patient to breathe slowly and deeply. Breathing into a paper bag will help to decrease hyperventilation.

Metabolic Acidosis

■ Relate decreased values of Hco_3 and BE to metabolic acidosis. When there is tissue breakdown from shock, malnutrition, and such, acid metabolites (eg, lactic acid) are released. Another cause of metabolic acidosis is ketone bodies (fatty acid) from diabetic ketoacidosis.

■ Assess for signs and symptoms of metabolic acidosis, such as rapid, vigorous breathing (Kussmaul's breathing), flushed skin, restlessness, decreased bicarbonate (Hco_3) value of less than 24 mEq/L, and decreased BE of less than −2.

■ Check for respiratory compensatory mechanism with metabolic acidosis— Pco_2 would be decreased, <35 mm Hg. The lung compensates by blowing off Co_2 to decrease carbonic acid in the blood and thereby decreasing the acidotic state.

Metabolic Alkalosis

■ Relate elevated Hco_3 and BE values to metabolic alkalosis. With severe vomiting and gastric suction, hydrogen and chloride-(hydrochloric acid) are lost, causing an alkalotic state. Drugs containing sodium bicarbonate taken in excess or over a long period of time could cause metabolic alkalosis.

■ Assess for signs and symptoms of metabolic alkalosis, such as shallow breathing, vomiting, elevated Hco_3 value of >28 mEq/L, and elevated BE value of >+2.

Patient Teaching

■ Instruct the patient not to ingest large quantities of antacids containing base substances like bicarbonate. An alkalotic state could result.

ASCORBIC ACID (VITAMIN C) (PLASMA AND SERUM)

Reference Values

Adult: 0.6–2.0 mg/dL (plasma), 34–114 μmol/L (SI units, plasma), 0.2–2.0 mg/dL serum, 12–114 μmol (SI units, serum)

Child: 0.6–1.6 mg/dL (plasma).

Description

(*See Ascorbic Acid Tolerance.*)

Ascorbic acid (vitamin C) is a water-soluble vitamin found in fresh fruits and vegetables. Deficiencies of vitamin C still occur, but the severe deficiency known as scurvy is rare.

Vitamin C is important for the formation of collagen substances and certain amino acids, in wound healing, and in withstanding the stresses of injury and infection. Since vitamin C is vitally important to the body's defense mechanisms in dealing with stress caused by injury and disease, the patient's ascorbic acid level should be known. This test can also be used to determine whether the ascorbic acid therapy is adequate. Excess ingestion of vitamin C is not considered toxic, as is excess ingestion of vitamins A and D, because excess vitamin C is water-soluble and is excreted in the urine.[9,11,13]

Clinical Problems

Decreased Level: scurvy, low vitamin C diet, malabsorption, pregnancy, infections, cancer, severe burns

Elevated Level: excess vitamin C ingestion. *Causes of False-Positive Readings:* clinitest, serum creatinine, serum uric acid, serum bilirubin, serum ALT and AST, blood glucose, serum cholesterol. *Causes of False-Negative Readings:* test for occult blood in stool, serum triglycerides

Procedure

- Collect 5 mL of venous blood in a gray-top tube (plasma) or a red-top tube (serum).
- There is no food or fluid restriction.

■ Factors Affecting Laboratory Results

- High doses of ascorbic acid can cause inaccurate results.

NURSING IMPLICATIONS WITH RATIONALE

- Recognize the functions of ascorbic acid in maintaining the state of wellness. Ascorbic acid has been taken by persons in large doses (> 1 g) to prevent colds. This has not been medically proven effective.
- Answer the patient's questions concerning the importance of vitamin C. It helps with the healing process.

Decreased Level

- Relate vitamin C deficit to certain clinical problems (eg, infections, burns). Vitamin C is lost during severe infections and burns.

Patient Teaching

- Teach the patient to eat foods rich in vitamin C (eg, oranges, grapefruits, strawberries, cantaloupe, pineapple, broccoli, cabbage, spinach, kale, turnips—all excellent to good sources). Approximately 25% of the population has an ascorbic acid deficit in the body.

Elevated Level

- Record on the patient's chart a habit of taking high doses of vitamin C continuously. High doses of ascorbic acid can cause false-positive laboratory results.

ASCORBIC ACID TOLERANCE (PLASMA AND URINE)
Vitamin C Tolerance

Reference Values

Adult: Plasma: >2.0 mg/dL. *Urine:* 4-, 5-, or 6-hour sample. *Oral:* 10% of administered amount. *IV:* 30%–40% of administered amount

Child: not usually done

Description

The ascorbic acid tolerance test is useful for determining the degree of ascorbic acid deficiency. Patients having severe burns, infections, or malignancy frequently have an ascorbic acid deficiency even when they are receiving vitamin C or having a diet adequate in vitamin C. With an ascorbic acid deficit, wound healing and recovery are prolonged.

The blood and urine tests are normally done together.[3,9]

Clinical Problems

Decreased Level (<2.0 mg/dL [plasma], <30% IV [urine]): infections, burns, cancer

Elevated Level (>2.0 mg/dL [plasma], >40% IV [urine]: excess vitamin C administration

Procedure

- Foods high in ascorbic acid should be omitted for 24 hours before the test (ie, fruits and vegetables). Water can be given.
- Have the patient void, and discard the urine before beginning the test.
- Administer ascorbic acid orally (11 mg/kg of body weight in a glass of water) or intravenously (10 mg/kg of body weight in saline solution).
- Collect 5 mL of venous blood in a gray-top tube 4 to 6 hours after the ascorbic acid is administered.
- Collect a 4-, 5-, or 6-hour urine specimen in a bottle containing acetic acid. The bottle should be kept on ice or refrigerated and taken to the laboratory immediately at the end of the specified time.

- Factors Affecting Laboratory Results

  - Oral high-potency vitamin supplements cause false test results
  - Ascorbic acid in IV fluids cause false test results
  - Inaccurate urine collection time and inaccurate labeling result in false test

---

NURSING IMPLICATIONS WITH RATIONALE

- Explain to the patient that the purpose of the test is to determine whether there is a vitamin C deficiency in the body.
- Explain to the patient that for 24 hours he or she should not eat foods high

---

in ascorbic acid (ie, oranges or orange juice, grapefruit, strawberries, or green vegetables). Drinking water is permissible.
■ Have the patient void, and discard the urine.
■ Administer ascorbic acid orally or intravenously according to body weight.
■ Instruct the patient that all urine should be saved for 4, 5, or 6 hours (according to the order or laboratory policy) in a bottle kept on ice or refrigerated. Following collection time, the urine specimen should be taken immediately to the laboratory.
■ Explain to the patient that blood will be drawn 4 to 6 hours after the ascorbic acid is administered.
■ Post the time for urine collection on the chart or Kardex or by the bedside. Visitors should not discard the patient's urine.

ASPARTATE AMINOTRANSFERASE (AST) (SERUM)
Serum Glutamic Oxaloacetic Transaminase (SGOT)

Reference Values

Adult: 5–40 U/mL (Frankel), 4–36 IU/L, 16–60 U/mL at 30°C (Karmen), 8–33 U/L at 37°C (SI units). Female values may be slightly lower than males. Exercise tends to increase values.

Child: Newborns: four times the normal level. *Child:* similar to adults.
Elderly: slightly higher than adults

Description

AST/SGOT is an enzyme found mainly in the heart muscle and liver, with moderate amounts in skeletal muscle, the kidneys, and the pancreas. Its concentration is low in the blood except when there is cellular injury, and then large amounts are released into the circulation.

High levels of serum AST are found following an acute myocardial infarction (MI) and liver damage. Six to ten hours after an acute MI, AST leaks out of the heart muscle and reaches its peak in 24 to 48 hours after the infarction. The serum AST level returns to normal 4 to 6 days later if there is no additional infarction. Serum AST is usually compared with other cardiac enzymes (CPK, LDH).

In liver disease, the serum level increases by ten times or more and remains elevated for a longer period of time.[6,9,10,21,44]

Clinical Problems

Decreased Level: pregnancy, diabetic ketoacidosis, *Drug Influence:* salicylates

Elevated Level: acute MI, hepatitis, liver necrosis, musculoskeletal diseases and trauma, acute pancreatitis, cancer of the liver, severe angina pectoris, strenuous exercise, IM injections. *Drug Influence:* antibiotics (ampicillin, carbenicillin, clindamycin, cloxacillin, erythromycin, gentamicin, lincomycin, nafcillin, oxacillin, polycillin, tetracycline), vitamins (folic acid, pyridoxine, vitamin A), narcotics (codeine, morphine, meperidine [Demerol]), antihypertensives (methyldopa [Aldomet], guanethidine), mithramycin, digitalis preparation, cortisone, flurazepam (Dalmane), indomethacin (Indocin), isoniazid (INH), rifampin, oral contraceptives, salicylates; theophylline

Procedure

- Collect 5 to 10 mL of venous blood in a red-top tube. Avoid hemolysis.
- Draw blood before drugs are given. The enzyme will remain stable for 4 days, refrigerated.
- List on the laboratory slip drugs the patient is taking that can cause false-positive levels with the date and time last given.
- There is no food or fluid restriction.

■ Factors Affecting Laboratory Results

- IM injections could increase serum AST levels.
- Hemolysis of the blood specimen could affect laboratory results.
- Drugs increasing the serum AST level (*See Drug Influence above*) could affect test results.
- Salicylates may cause false-positive or negative serum levels.

NURSING IMPLICATIONS WITH RATIONALE

Elevated Level

- Hold drugs causing an elevated serum AST for 24 hours prior to the blood test, with the physician's permission. Drugs that should not be withheld should be listed on the laboratory slip and charted.
- Compare serum AST levels with other cardiac enzyme results. Check serum ALT levels to determine if liver damage could be responsible for the abnormal value.
- Do not administer IM injections before the blood test. IM injections can increase the serum AST level. Few medications (eg, morphine) can be given intravenously without affecting the serum level.
- Assess the patient for signs and symptoms of MI (eg, chest and arm pain, dyspnea, or diaphoresis). Changes should be reported and charted.

Patient Teaching

- Instruct the patient to report symptoms of chest and arm pain, nausea, or diaphoresis immediately—day or night.

Aspirin
(See Salicylates)

BARBITURATE (BLOOD)

Reference Values

Adult

BARBITURATE	ACTION	THERAPEUTIC	TOXIC
Secobarbital (Seconal)	Short acting	1–5 μg/mL	>8 μg/mL
Pentobarbital (Nembutal)	Short acting	1–5 μg/mL	>8 μg/mL
Amobarbital (Amytal)	Intermediate acting	5–14 μg/mL	>20 μg/mL
Phenobarbital	Long acting	10–30 μg/mL 20–40 μg/mL (seizure control)	>60 μg/mL

Child: Phenobarbital: Therapeutic: 15–30 μg/mL; toxic: >35 μg/mL

Description

Barbiturate toxicity is a frequent cause of unconsciousness because of accidental or intentional barbiturate overdose. Barbiturates have different effects, and those that are short acting tend to be more potent and toxic than the long-acting types. Phenobarbital tends to be least toxic; however, this depends on the amount taken. This long-acting barbiturate peaks in 12 to 18 hours, and its serum half-life is 48 to 96 hours.

Alcohol and tranquilizers can intensify the effects of barbiturates. Blood barbiturate levels are usually measured on unconscious/comatose patients when the cause of unresponsiveness is unknown.[3,9,10,12]

Procedure

- Collect 5 to 10 mL of venous blood in a red- or lavender-top tube.
- There is no food or fluid restriction.
- Urine and gastric contents may be examined for barbiturates.

■ Factors Affecting Laboratory Results

- Alcohol and tranquilizers cause false results.
- Drugs: antipyrine and theophylline can elevate the barbiturate level.

NURSING IMPLICATIONS WITH RATIONALE

■ Observe for signs and symptoms of barbiturate toxicity (ie, depressed respirations, bradycardia, and loss of consciousness).

■ Obtain a history from the family or a friend to determine whether the patient has been taking a barbiturate and, if so, which type. Report the drug history to the physician.

■ Monitor the urinary output. Renal dysfunction caused by renal ischemia and tubular damage can prolong recovery. Diuretics, especially osmotic, have been used for correcting the effects of long-lasting barbiturates.

■ Report to the physician if the patient is taking tranquilizers and barbiturates. The combination of these two drugs could cause respiratory distress.

Patient Teaching

■ Inform the patient that it is important to keep medical appointments when taking barbiturates so that the physician can evaluate the effects of the drug and have the blood barbiturate levels checked.

■ Instruct the patient not to combine alcohol with barbiturates. Alcohol intensifies the effects of barbiturates, and respiratory distress could result.

BILIRUBIN (INDIRECT) (SERUM)
Van Den Bergh Test

Reference Values
Adult: 0.1–1.0 mg/dL, 1.7–17.1 μmol/L (SI units)

Child: same as adult

Description
(*See Bilirubin* [*Total and Direct*].)

Indirect-reacting or unconjugated bilirubin is protein bound and is associated with increased destruction of RBCs (hemolysis).

Elevated indirect bilirubin can occur in autoimmune or transfusion-induced hemolysis, in hemolytic processes caused by sickle cell anemia, in pernicious anemia, and with malaria and septicemia. Internal hemorrhage into soft tissues and the body cavity can cause the bilirubin to rise in 5 to 6 hours. With certain clinical problems, CHF, and severe liver damage, both indirect and direct bilirubin levels will increase. Indirect bilirubin frequently increases because the damaged liver cells cannot conjugate normal amounts, which leads to increased, unconjugated bilirubin.

Levels of indirect serum bilirubin may increase in hemolytic disease, such as erythroblastosis fetalis, in newborns. The newborn's liver is immature, and when extremely high levels of bilirubin occur, irreversible neurologic damage, referred to as kernicterus, could result.[1,8–10,12]

Clinical Problems

Decreased Level (<0.1 mg/dL): Drug Influence: See Bilirubin (Total and Direct).

Elevated-Level (>1.0 mg/dL): erythroblastosis fetalis, sickle cell anemia, transfusion reaction, pernicious anemia, malaria, septicemia, hemolytic anemias, CHF, decompensated cirrhosis, hepatitis. *Drug Influence:* aspidium, rifampin, phenothiazines. (*See Bilirubin [Total and Direct].*)

Procedure

■ There is no laboratory test for indirect bilirubin. Indirect bilirubin is calculated by subtracting direct bilirubin from the total bilirubin:

$$\text{Total bilirubin} - \text{direct bilirubin} = \text{Indirect bilirubin}$$

In newborn infants, only the total is determined, and this represents the indirect bilirubin only.

■ Factors Affecting Laboratory Results

■ (*See Bilirubin [Total and Direct].*)

NURSING IMPLICATIONS WITH RATIONALE

Elevated Levels (>1.0 mg/dL)

■ Check the patient's indirect serum bilirubin level, and compare it with the direct bilirubin result. If the indirect bilirubin is elevated and the direct is not, then the cause is a hemolytic problem.

Patient Teaching

■ Instruct the patient not to eat before blood is drawn. Carrots, yams, or foods high in fat should not be eaten the night before.

BILIRUBIN (TOTAL AND DIRECT) (SERUM)

Reference Values

Adult: Total: 0.1–1.2 mg/dL, 1.7–20.5 μmol/L (SI units). *Direct (conjugated):* 0.1–0.3 mg/dL, 1.7–5.1 μmol/L (SI units)

Child: Newborn: Total: 1–12 mg/dL, 17.1–205 μmol/L (SI units). *Child:* 0.2–0.8 mg/dL

Description

Bilirubin is formed from the breakdown of hemoglobin by the reticuloendothelial system and is carried in the plasma to the liver, where it is conjugated (directly) to form bilirubin diglucuronide and is excreted in the bile. There are two forms of bilirubin in the body: the conjugated, or direct-reacting (soluble), and the unconjugated, or indirect-reacting (protein bound). If the total bilirubin is within normal range, direct and indirect bilirubin levels do not need to be analyzed. If one value of bilirubin is reported, it represents the total bilirubin.

Direct or conjugated bilirubin is frequently the result of obstructive jaundice, either extrahepatic (from stones or tumor) or intrahepatic in origin. Conjugated bilirubin cannot escape in the bile into the intestine and thus backs up and is absorbed into the blood stream. Damaged liver cells cause a blockage of the bile sinusoid, increasing the serum level of direct bilirubin. With hepatitis and decompensated cirrhosis, both direct and indirect bilirubin may be elevated.

Serum bilirubin (total) in newborns can be as high as 12 mg/dL; panic range is >15 mg/dL. Jaundice is frequently present when serum bilirubin levels are greater than 3 mg/dL.[1,8–10,12]

Clinical Problems

Decreased Level (<0.1 mg/dL [adult total]): iron deficiency anemia. *Drug Influence:* barbiturates, salicylates (aspirin)—large amounts, penicillin, caffeine.

Elevated Level (>1.2 mg/dL [adult total]): obstructive jaundice caused by stones or neoplasms, hepatitis, cirrhosis of the liver, infectious mononucleosis, liver metastasis (cancer), Wilson's disease. *Drug Influence:* antibiotics (amphotericin B, clindamycin, erythromycin, gentamicin, lincomycin, oxacillin, tetracyclines), sulfonamides, anti-TB (para-aminosalicylic acid, isoniazid [INH]), allopurinol, diuretics (acetazolamide [Diamox], ethacrynic acid [Edecrin]), mithramycin, dextran, diazepam [Valium], barbiturates, narcotics (codeine, morphine, meperidine [Demerol]), flurazepam (Dalmane), indomethacin (Indocin), methotrexate, methyldopa (Aldomet), papaverine, procainamide (Pronestyl), steroids, oral contraceptives, tolbutamide (Orinase), vitamins A, C, and K.

Procedure

- Collect 5 to 10 mL of venous blood in a red-top tube. Avoid hemolysis.
- Keep the patient NPO except for water.
- Hold medications that would increase the serum bilirubin for 24 hours, with the physician's approval. If medications are given, list the drugs on the laboratory slip and the time they were last given.
- *Caution:* Whenever blood is drawn for liver function tests, avoid self-contamination to prevent possible infection (such as hepatitis). Use isolation technique. Protect the blood specimen from sunlight and artificial light, as light will reduce the bilirubin content. Blood should be sent to the laboratory immediately so that separation of serum from the cells can be performed as soon as possible to avoid hemolysis. Infants can have the blood taken from the heel of the foot. Two blood microtubes should be filled.

■ Factors Affecting Laboratory Results

■ A high-fat dinner prior to the test may affect bilirubin levels.
■ Carrots and yams may increase the serum bilirubin level.
■ Hemolysis of the blood specimen can give inaccurate results. The tube should not be shaken.
■ A blood specimen exposed to sunlight and artificial light will degrade the bile pigment. Certain drugs (*see Drug Influence*) can increase or decrease the serum bilirubin level.

NURSING IMPLICATIONS AND RATIONALE

Elevated Level

■ Check the serum bilirubin (total), and if it is elevated, check the direct and indirect bilirubin levels.
■ Check the sclera of the eyes and the inner aspects of the arm for jaundice.

Patient Teaching

■ Instruct the patient that he or she should have nothing by mouth except water before the test. If his or her medications are withheld, an appropriate explanation should be given. The nurse should emphasize that fats, carrots, and yams should not be eaten the night before the blood test.
■ Inform the mother whose baby is jaundiced that the bilirubin level will be closely monitored until the level is in normal range.

BILIRUBIN AND BILE (URINE)

Reference Values

Adult: Negative, 0.02 mg/dL

Description

Bilirubin is not normally present in urine; however, a very small quantity could be present without being detected by routine test methods. Bilirubin is formed from the breakdown of hemoglobin and is transported to the liver, where it is conjugated and is excreted as bile. Conjugated or direct bilirubin is water soluble and is excreted in the urine when there is an increased serum level. Unconjugated or indirect bilirubin is fat soluble and cannot be excreted in the urine.

Bilirubinuria (bilirubin in urine) indicates liver damage or biliary obstruction (eg, stones), and a large amount has a characteristic dark-amber color. When the amber-colored urine is shaken, it produces a yellow foam. It can frequently be tested by the floor nurse with a dipstick or tablet.[1,8–10]

Clinical Problems

Elevated Level (>0.02 mg/dL): obstructive biliary disease, liver disease (hepatitis, toxic agents), CHF with jaundice, cancer of the liver (secondary). *Drug Influence:* phenothiazines—chlorpromazine (Thorazine), acetophenazine (Tindal); chlorprothixene (Taractan); phenazopyridine (Pyridium); chlorzoxazone (Paraflex).

Procedure

- Use either bili-Labstix or Ictotest reagent tablets for the bilirubinuria test. The bili-Labstix is dipped in urine, and after 20 seconds is compared to a color chart on the bottle. For bili-Labstix and Ictotest tablets, follow the directions on the bottle.
- Test urine bilirubin within 1 hour. Keep urine away from ultraviolet light.
- There is no food or fluid restriction.

- Factors Affecting Laboratory Results

  - Certain drugs can give a false-positive result (*see Drug Influence above*).
  - Exposure of urine to light for 1 hour will cause deterioration of bile pigments.

NURSING IMPLICATIONS WITH RATIONALE

Elevated Level

- Check the serum bilirubin—total and direct—and report if it is elevated. Test the urine for bilirubinuria. Compare urine and serum findings.
- Assess the color of the urine. If it is dark amber in color, shake the urine specimen and note whether a yellow foam appears.
- Record the results of a bili-Labstix and the urine color on the patient's chart or Kardex.
- Notify the physician of amber urine with yellow foam and test results.

BLEEDING TIME (BLOOD)

Reference Values

Adult: Ivy Method: 3–7 minutes. *Duke Method:* 1–3 minutes. SI units for the Ivy and Duke methods are the same.

Description

Two methods, Ivy and Duke, are used to determine whether bleeding time is normal or prolonged. Bleeding time is lengthened in thrombocytopenia (decreased platelet count <50,000). The test is frequently performed when there is a history of bleeding (easy bruising), familial bleeding, or preoperative screening. The Ivy technique, in which the forearm is used for the incision, is the most popular method. Aspirins and anti-inflammatory medications can prolong the bleeding time.[1,7–10]

Clinical Problems

Decreased Rate: Hodgkin's disease

Prolonged Rate (7 minutes [Ivy]): thrombocytopenic purpura, platelet abnormality, vascular abnormalities, leukemia, severe liver disease, disseminated intravascular coagulation (DIC), aplastic anemia, factor deficiencies (V, VII, XI), Christmas disease, hemophilia. *Drug Influence:* salicylates (aspirins, others), dextran, mithramycin, warfarin (Coumadin), streptokinase (streptodornase; fibrinolytic agent)

Procedure

Ivy Method

- Cleanse the volar surface of the forearm (below the antecubital space) with alcohol and allow it to dry. Inflate the blood pressure cuff to 40 mm Hg, and leave it inflated during the test. Puncture the skin 2.5 mm deep on the forearm; start timing with a stopwatch. Blot blood drops carefully every 30 seconds until bleeding ceases. The time required for bleeding to stop is recorded in seconds.
- Test should *not* be performed while taking anticoagulant or aspirin; withhold medications for 3 to 7 days.

Duke Method

- The area used is the earlobe.
- There is no food or fluid restriction.

- Factors Affecting Laboratory Results

  - Method used; improper technique—the puncture wound might be deeper than required. Blotting the incision area and not the blood drops can break off fibrin particles, prolonging the bleeding time.
  - Aspirin and anticoagulants increase the bleeding time.

NURSING IMPLICATIONS WITH RATIONALE

Prolonged Rate

- Relate prolonged bleeding time to clinical problems and drugs. The nurse should be familiar with the methods used to obtain the bleeding time.
- Obtain a drug history of the last time (date) the patient took aspirin or anticoagulants. Aspirin prevents platelet aggregation, and bleeding can be prolonged by taking only one aspirin tablet (5 grains or 325 mg) 3 days prior to test. A history of taking "cold medications" should be recorded, since many cold remedies contain salicylates.
- Note whether the patient has been consuming alcohol. Alcohol increases bleeding time, and the bleeding may be difficult to stop.

■ Apply a dressing to the puncture wound site (Ivy method) to stop the bleeding.

Patient Teaching

■ Instruct the patient not to take aspirin and over-the-counter cold remedies for 3 days before the test. If the patient takes aspirins or anticoagulants, the laboratory should be notified and the drug names should be written on the laboratory slip.
■ Explain to the patient how the test is performed. In the Ivy method the forearm is used, and in the Duke method the earlobe is used. The step-by-step method of the procedure should be explained (*see Procedure above*). The nurse should check with the laboratory for changes in procedure.

BLOOD GASES
(See Arterial Blood Gases)

BLOOD UREA NITROGEN (BUN) (SERUM)

Reference Values
Adult: 5–25 mg/dL
Child: Infant: 5–15 mg/dL. *Child:* 5–20 mg/dL
Elderly: Could be slightly higher than adult

Description
Urea is formed as an end product of protein metabolism and is excreted by the kidneys. An elevated BUN level could be an indication of dehydration, prerenal failure, or renal failure. Dehydration from vomiting, diarrhea, and/or inadequate fluid intake can cause an increase in the BUN (up to 35 mg/dL). With dehydration, the serum creatinine level would most likely be normal or high normal. Once the patient is hydrated, the BUN should return to normal; if it does not, prerenal or renal failure would be suspected. Nephrons (kidney cells) tend to decrease during the aging process, and so older persons may have a higher BUN. Digested blood from GI bleeding is a source of protein and can cause the BUN to elevate. A low BUN value usually indicates overhydration (hypervolemia).

BUN/Creatinine Ratio is a calculation with reference value of 10:1 to 15:1. A decreased BUN/creatinine ratio occurs with malnutrition, liver disease, low-protein diet, excessive IV fluids, dialysis, or overhydration. An elevated BUN/creatinine ratio, >15:1, is found in renal disease, inadequate renal perfusion, shock, dehydration, GI bleeding, and drugs such as steroids and tetracyclines.[1,3,6,9,18,22]

Clinical Problems

Decreased Level (<5 mg/dL): severe liver damage, low-protein diet, overhydration, malnutrition (negative nitrogen balance), IV fluids (glucose). *Drug Influence:* phenothiazines.

Increased Level (>25 mg/dL): dehydration; high-protein intake; GI bleeding; prerenal failure (low renal blood supply caused by CHF, diabetes mellitus, acute myocardial infarction, renal insufficiency/failure from shock, sepsis, kidney diseases [glomerular nephritis, pyelonephritis]), licorice (excessive ingestion). *Drug Influence:* nephrotoxic drugs, diuretics (hydrochlorothiazide [Hydrodiuril], ethacrynic acid [Edecrin], furosemide [Lasix], triamterene [Dyrenium]), antibiotics, (bacitracin, cephaloridine [high doses], gentamicin, kanamycin, chloramphenicol [Chloromycetin], methicillin, neomycin, vancomycin), antihypertensive agents (methyldopa [Aldomet], guanethidine [Ismelin]), sulfonamides, propranolol, morphine, lithium carbonate, salicylates.

Procedure

- Collect 5–7 mL of venous blood in a red-top tube. Avoid hemolysis.
- It is preferable to have the patient remain NPO for 8 hours.

- **Factors Affecting Laboratory Results**

    - The hydration status of the patient should be known. Overhydration can give a false-low BUN level, and dehydration can give a false-high BUN level.
    - Drugs (ie, antibiotics, diuretics, and antihypertensive agents) raise the BUN level.

NURSING IMPLICATIONS WITH RATIONALE

- Compare serum BUN and serum creatinine results. If both BUN and creatinine are elevated, kidney should be highly suspected.

Decreased Level

- Assess the patient's dietary intake. A low-protein intake and a high-carbohydrate intake can decrease the BUN level.
- Report on patients receiving continuous dextrose intravenously without protein intake.
- Check the patient for signs and symptoms of overhydration (irritated cough, dyspnea, neck-vein engorgement, and chest rales) when the BUN is decreased. Overhydration (hypervolemia) causes hemodilution, diluting the urea in the blood.

Elevated Level

- Report urinary output less than 25 mL or 600 mL/day. Urea is excreted by the kidneys, and with a decreased urine output, urea accumulates in the blood.

- Check vital signs. A fast pulse, decreased BP, and increased respiration could indicate dehydration and, if severe enough, could lead to shock.
- Determine the hydration status of the patient. If dehydration is present, the elevated BUN may be attributed to hemoconcentration. Hydrating with IV fluids should correct the problem.
- Avoid overhydration with IV fluid. Rapid administration of IV fluids can overload the vascular system, especially in the aged, in children, and in heart patients, resulting in hypervolemia. This can lead to pulmonary edema.
- Assess the patient's dietary intake. A high-protein diet will increase the serum BUN. Individuals on a high-protein diet for dieting purposes will have an elevated BUN level unless adequate fluids are taken.
- Recognize drugs that increase the BUN (ie, antibiotics, diuretics, antihypertensive agents, and others; (see *Drug Influence*).

Patient Teaching

- Instruct patients with a slightly elevated BUN to increase fluid intake. Care should be taken in forcing fluids in patients with heart and kidney problems.

BLOOD VOLUME DETERMINATION/STUDIES
(Blood Volume Measurement)

Reference Values

Adult: Total Blood Volume: 55–80 mL/kg. Male: 7.5% body weight. Female: 6.5% body weight. *Red Cell Volume:* Male: 25–35 mL/kg. Female: 20–30 mL/kg. *Plasma Volume:* Male: 32–46 mL/kg. Female: 30–45 mL/kg.

Description

The blood volume determination is commonly used to determine the total blood, red cell, and plasma volumes. Two radioactive substances can be used for measurement: Cr-51–tagged red cells for RBC volume and I-131--or I-125–tagged human serum albumin for plasma volume. The patient's blood is mixed with the radioactive substance.

This test is useful for monitoring blood loss during surgery, evaluating GI or uterine bleeding, determining the cause of hypotension, determining the blood component lost (ie, RBCs, plasma) for replacement therapy, and diagnosing polycythemia vera.[8–10,14]

Clinical Problems

Decreased Volume: dehydration (total and plasma volume), hypovolemic shock, hemorrhaging

Elevated Volume: dehydration (RBC volume), polycythemia vera, overhydration (total volume)

Procedure

- Obtain the height and weight of the patient.
- Obtain a blood sample.
- Personnel from the nuclear medicine laboratory will obtain a blood sample and mix a radioisotope (radionuclide, ie, I-131, I-125, Cr-51) with the blood. After 15 to 30 minutes, the blood containing the radioactive substance will be reinjected into the patient.
- Collect another blood sample in 15 minutes.

■ Factors Affecting Diagnostic Results

- IV fluids can affect the test results.
- Prolonged time for blood sample collection can affect results. If I-131–tagged albumin is used, it will leave the plasma (intravascular fluid compartment) after 15 minutes and enter the extravascular fluid compartment.

NURSING IMPLICATIONS WITH RATIONALE

- Explain the procedure to the patient.
- Start IV therapy, if ordered, after the blood volume determination test has been completed.
- Explain to the patient that the radioactive substance he or she will receive is of low amount and should be harmless.
- Answer the patient's questions, or refer them to the appropriate health professionals.
- Observe for signs and symptoms of dehydration (ie, dry mucous membrane, poor skin turgor, and shocklike symptoms).
- Observe for signs and symptoms of shock (ie, tachycardia; tachypnea; pale, cold, clammy skin; and later a drop in BP).

BROMIDE (SERUM)

Reference Values

Adult: toxic levels—>100 mg/dL

Child: same as adult

Description

The use of bromides as a prescription drug for depression and sedation is seldom ordered; however, today many bromide-containing compounds in patent medicines are available to the public. Because of the cumulative effect of bromides, chronic bromide intoxication is becoming a common occurrence. Acute bromide intoxication is rare, since bromide can cause GI irritation.

The half-life of bromide is 12 days. Bromide is slowly excreted by the kidney, and the treatment for chronic bromide intoxication is to accelerate urinary excretion by chloride administration and mercurial diuretics.[8,11]

Procedure

- Collect 5 mL of venous blood in a green-top tube.
- There is no food or fluid restriction.
- A colorimetric test using gold chloride is an old but still useful test. The gold chloride reacts with the bromide in the plasma/serum, forming a yellow/red/orange color, depending on the bromide concentration.

- Factors Affecting Laboratory Results

  - An extremely high bromide level will cause a decreased chloride level, since both are anions.

NURSING IMPLICATIONS WITH RATIONALE

- Observe for signs and symptoms of chronic bromide intoxication (ie, anorexia, fever, skin rash, motor incoordination, tremors, delirium, impaired intellectual function, constipation, and weight loss).
- Obtain a history on over-the-counter drugs taken: when, for how long, and the daily quantity taken. If the bottle is available, read the label of the ingredients contained in the medicine.
- Check urine output. Bromides are excreted slowly by the kidneys, so "good" kidney function is extremely important.

Patient Teaching

- Teach patients to read labels on patent medicines. Explain the importance of contacting a physician before taking most patent medicines.

CALCITONIN (hCT) SERUM

Reference Values

Adult: Male: <40 pg/mL. *Female:* < 20 pg/mL

Child: Newborn: usually higher than in adults

Description

Calcitonin, a potent hormone secreted by the C cells of the thyroid gland, aids in maintaining normal serum calcium and phosphorus levels. This hormone is secreted in response to an elevated serum calcium level. It inhibits calcium reabsorption by the osteoclasts and osteocytes of the bones and increases calcium excretion by the kidneys. Calcitonin acts as an antagonist to the parathyroid hormone (PTH) and vitamin D, lowering serum calcium levels to maintain calcium balance in the body.

Excess calcitonin secretion occurs in the medullary carcinoma of the thyroid. A serum calcitonin level is frequently ordered to aid in the diagnosis of thyroid medullary carcinoma (> 500 to 2000 pg/mL [probable] and > 2000 pg/mL [definite]) and ectopic calcitonin-producing tumors of the lung and breast. Monitoring calcitonin levels after medullary carcinoma removal will help predict if the tumor reoccurs.

When the serum calcitonin level is slightly to moderately elevated (100 to 500 pg/mL), a *calcitonin stimulation test* might be performed in diagnosis of thyroid medullary carcinoma. This test consists of either a 4-hour calcium infusion or a 10-second pentagastrin infusion with measurement of serum calcitonin before and after the infusion.[1,3,9,10,12,13]

Clinical Problems

Elevated Level (> 500 pg/mL): medullary carcinoma of the thyroid, carcinoma of the lung or breast, chronic renal failure, parathyroid hyperplasia or adenoma, pernicious anemia, Zollinger-Ellison syndrome, acute or chronic thyroiditis, islet cell tumors, pheochromocytoma

Procedure

- NPO after midnight. A small amount of water could be given if needed.
- Collect 7 to 10 mL of venous blood in a green- or lavender-top tube or in a chilled red-top tube. Avoid hemolysis. Send blood specimen immediately to laboratory for analysis or freeze to avoid deterioration.

Calcitonin Stimulation Test
- Draw serum calcitonin level before administering IV calcium or IV pentagastrin.
- Administer IV calcium (15 mg/kg) over 4 hours to provoke calcitonin secretion.

OR
- Administer IV pentagastrin (0.5 μg/kg) over 5 to 10 seconds.
- After IV calcium infusion, draw serum calcitonin level 3 to 4 hours postinfusion. After pentagastrin infusion, draw serum calcium level at 2 minutes, 5 minutes, and 10 minutes.

- Factors Affecting Laboratory Results

  - Hemolysis could increase serum calcitonin level.
  - Levels may be increased during pregnancy and lactation.

NURSING IMPLICATIONS WITH RATIONALE

- Obtain a history of familial thyroid carcinoma. Record and report a positive history.
- Observe for signs and symptoms of hypercalcemia (ie, lethargy, headaches, weakness, muscle flaccidity, nausea and vomiting, and anorexia.

Patient Teaching

- Instruct the patient to remain NPO after midnight.
- Explain the calcitonin stimulating test (if ordered) to the patient. Refer to the procedure.
- Inform the patient that test results may take several days.

CALCIUM (Ca) (SERUM)

Reference Values

Adult Total Ca: 4.5–5.5 mEq/L, 9–11 mg/dL, 2.3–2.8 mmol/L (SI units). *Ionized Ca:* 4.4–5.0 mg/dL, 2.2–2.5 mEq/L, 1.1–1.24 mmol/L.

Child: *Newborn:* 3.7–7.0 mEq/L, 7.4–14.0 mg/dL. *Infant:* 5.0–6.0 mEq/L, 10–12 mg/dL. *Child:* 4.5–5.8 mEq/L, 9–11.5 mg/dL.

Description

Calcium is found most abundantly in the bones and teeth. Approximately 50% of the calcium is ionized, and only ionized calcium can be used by the body. Protein and albumin in the blood bind with calcium, thus decreasing the amount of free, ionized calcium. The ionized calcium level can be determined by using formulas that estimate the ionized calcium from total calcium. These formulas have been disputed. Only a few laboratories have the equipment to perform serum-ionized calcium levels. In acidosis, more calcium is ionized, regardless of the serum level, and in alkalosis, most of the calcium is protein bound and cannot be ionized.

Serum-ionized calcium (iCa) level is not affected by changes in serum protein/albumin concentration, and it reflects calcium metabolism better than total calcium values. A decrease in ionized calcium, <2.2 mEq/L or <4.5 mg/dL, might lead to neuromuscular irritability or tetany symptoms (tingling, twitching, spasmodic contractions).

Calcium is necessary for the transmission of nerve impulses and contraction of the myocardium and skeletal muscles. It causes blood clotting by converting prothrombin into thrombin. It strengthens capillary membranes. With a calcium deficit, there is an increased capillary permeability, which causes fluid to pass through the capillary.

A low serum-calcium levels is called hypocalcemia, and an increased level is called hypercalcemia. Calcium imbalances require immediate attention, for serum calcium deficit can cause tetany symptoms, unless acidosis is present, and serum calcium excess can cause cardiac arrhythmias.[1,3,9,13,23–25]

Clinical Problems

Decreased Level: diarrhea, malabsorption of calcium from the GI tract, extensive infections, burns, lack of calcium and vitamin D intake, hypoparathyroidism, chronic renal failure caused by phosphorous retention, alcoholism, pancreatitis. *Drug Influence:* cortisone preparations; antibiotics (gentamicin, methicillin), magnesium products (antacids), laxative (excessive use); heparin; insulin; mithramycin; acetazolamide (Diamox).

Elevated Level: hypervitaminosis D; hyperparathyroidism; malignant neoplasm of the bone, lung, breast, bladder, or kidney; multiple myeloma; prolonged immobilization; multiple fractures; renal calculi; exercise; alcoholism (alcoholic binge); milk-alkali syndrome. *Drug Influence:* alkaline antacids, estrogen preparations, calcium salts, vitamin D

Procedure

- Collect 5 to 10 mL of venous blood in a red-top tube.
- There is no food or fluid restriction, unless SMA12 or similar group test is ordered.

- Factors Affecting Laboratory Results

  - Drugs (*See Drug Influence*) can cause calcium excess or deficit.
  - A diet low in calcium or high in calcium and vitamin D can affect results.
  - IV saline (NaCl) solution can promote calcium loss.

NURSING IMPLICATIONS WITH RATIONALE

Decreased Level

- Observe for signs and symptoms of hypocalcemia (ie, tetany symptoms: muscular twitching and tremors, spasms of the larynx, parathesia [tingling in and numbness of fingers], facial spasms, and spasmodic contractions).
- Check serum calcium values, and report abnormal results to the physician, especially if tetany symptoms are present.
- Assess for positive Chvostek's and Trousseau's signs of hypocalcemia. To test for positive Chvostek's sign, tap the area in front of the ear and observe for spasms of the cheek and the corner of the lip. To test for positive Trousseau's sign, inflate the BP cuff for several minutes and observe for carpal spasms.
- Administer oral calcium supplements before or 1 to 1½ hours after meals.
- Observe for symptoms of hypocalcemia when the patient is receiving massive transfusions of citrated blood. Citrates prevent calcium ionization. The serum calcium level may be affected.
- Monitor the pulse regularly if the patient is receiving a digitalis preparation and calcium supplements. Calcium excess enhances the action of digitalis and can cause digitalis toxicity (nausea, vomiting, anorexia, bradycardia—arrhythmias).
- Administer IV fluids with 10% calcium gluconate slowly. Calcium should be administered in D5W and not in a saline solution, since sodium promotes calcium loss. Calcium should not be added to solutions containing bicarbonate, since rapid precipitation will occur.
- Monitor the electrocardiogram (ECG) during hypocalcemia for prolonged ST segments and lengthened QT intervals.

Patient Teaching

- Instruct the patient to avoid overuse of antacids and to prevent the chronic laxative habit. Excessive use of certain antacids could cause alkalosis, decreasing calcium ionization. In addition, many antacids contain magnesium, which could lower the serum calcium level. Many laxatives contain phosphates (phosphorous), which have an opposing effect on calcium, causing calcium loss. Chronic use of laxatives will decrease calcium absorption from the GI tract. Suggest fruits for improving bowel elimination.
- Encourage the patient to consume foods high in calcium, in milk and milk products, and/or in protein. Protein is needed to enhance calcium absorption.
- Teach the patient with hypocalcemia to avoid hyperventilation and crossing his or her legs, which could increase tetany symptoms.

Elevated Level

- Observe for signs and symptoms of hypercalcemia (ie, lethargy, headaches, weakness, muscle flaccidity, heart block, anorexia, nausea, and vomiting).
- Promote active and passive exercises for bedridden patients. This will prevent calcium loss from the bone.
- Identify symptoms of digitalis toxicity when the patient has an elevated serum calcium level and is receiving a digitalis preparation.
- Notify the physician if the patient is receiving a thiazide diuretic, since this will inhibit calcium excretion and promote hypercalcemia.
- Check the urine pH. Calcium salts are more soluble in acid urine (pH < 6.0) than in alkaline.
- Handle patients with long-standing hypercalcemia and bone demineralization gently to prevent pathologic fractures.

Patient Teaching

- Instruct patient to avoid foods high in calcium, to be ambulatory when possible, and to increase oral fluid intake. Increased fluid intake dilutes calcium in the serum and urine and prevents calculi formation.
- Encourage patient to eat acid-ash foods, as cranberry juice, meats, fish, poultry, eggs, cheese, and cereals to keep the urine acidic.

CALCIUM (Ca) (URINE)

Reference Values

Adult: 24-Hour: low-calcium diet: <150 mg/24 hours, <3.75 mmol/24 hours (SI units); average-calcium diet; 100–250 mg/24 hours, 2.50–6.25 mmol/24 hours; high-calcium diet; 250–300 mg/24 hours, 6.25–7.50 mmol/24 hours

Child: same as adult

Description

Urine calcium reflects the dietary intake of calcium, the serum calcium level, and the effects of disease entities (hypo- or hyperparathyroidism, multiple myeloma, bone tumors, etc). Hypercalciuria (increased calcium levels in the urine) usually accompanies an increased serum calcium level. Calcium excretion fluctuates and is lowest in the morning and highest after meals.

A 24-hour urine specimen for calciuria is useful for determining parathyroid gland disorders. In hyperparathyroidism, hyperthyroidism, and osteolytic disorders, the urinary calcium excretion is usually increased; it is decreased in hypoparathyroidism.[1,8–10,24]

Clinical Problems

Decreased Level: hypoparathyroidism, vitamin D deficiency, hypothyroidism, chronic renal failure, malabsorption syndrome. *Drug Influence:* thiazide diuretics

Elevated Level: hyperparathyroidism, osteoporosis, hyperthyroidism, malignancies (bone, breast, bladder), multiple myeloma, leukemias, hypervitaminosis D, amyotrophic lateral sclerosis (ALS), renal calculi acid-base imbalance. *Drug Influence:* cholestyramine resin, sodium- and magnesium-containing drugs, parathyroid injection, vitamin D

Procedure

- Label the bottle with the exact date and the times that the urine collection started and ended.
- Preservatives are required by some laboratories; however, in some institutions a preservative or refrigeration is not required.
- Indicate on the laboratory slip whether the patient's calcium intake has been limited in the last 3 days or whether the patient has had an average or high calcium intake.

- Factors Affecting Laboratory Results

- Discarded urine. All urine should be saved for the 24-hour urine collection.
- High or low in calcium content in diet may affect test results.
- Thiazide diuretics can decrease urine calcium level, and drugs containing sodium and magnesium can elevate urine calcium level.

NURSING IMPLICATIONS WITH RATIONALE

Decreased Level

- Observe for tetany symptoms if the patient's urine calcium is low. (*See Calcium [Serum] for tetany symptoms.*)
- Have available a 10% solution of calcium gluconate for emergencies. When administered, IV calcium should be diluted in D5W and not in saline solution.
- (*See Calcium [Serum] for other nursing implications.*)

Elevated Level

■ Observe patients for symptoms of renal calculi, especially if there is a history of renal calculi. Strain the urine, if indicated, and report severe low-back pain.
■ Prevent the possibility of a pathologic fracture by moving the patient gently. The patient should be encouraged to do active exercises.
■ (*See Calcium [Serum] for other nursing implications.*)

Patient Teaching

■ Instruct the patient & family members that urine is to be saved. Inform the patient not to put toilet paper or feces in the urine.

CALCIUM CHANNEL BLOCKERS (SERUM)
Verapamil (Calan, Isoptin), Nifedipine (Procardia), Diltiazem (Cardizem)

Reference Values

Adult

DRUG NAME	THERAPEUTIC RANGE	TOXIC LEVEL
Verapamil	100–300 ng/mL; 0.08–0.3 μg/mL	>300 ng/mL; >0.3 μg/mL
Nifedipine	50–100 ng/mL	>100 ng/mL
Diltiazem	50–200 ng/mL	>200 ng/mL

Note: Dosage is calculated according to mg/kg.

Description

Calcium channel blockers inhibit slow channel-calcium influx into the myocardial cells and vascular smooth muscle. As the result of these actions, a decrease in myocardial contraction and myocardial oxygen consumption and coronary and systemic vasodilation can occur. The calcium blockers were commercially available in the United States in the late 1970s for treating ischemic heart disease, or angina pectoris. Of the three calcium channel blockers, nifedipine (Procardia) is the most potent vasodilator, then verapamil (Calan, Isoptin), and, last, diltiazem (Cardizem). Calcium blockers are being prescribed more frequently for their antianginal actions.

Verapamil (Calan, Isopotin): This agent can be administered orally or intravenously. Verapamil has a negative inotropic effect and should be used with caution for patients with heart failure. Ninety percent is bound to plasma proteins; 70% of the metabolized drug is excreted in the urine, 15% is excreted in feces, and 4% to 5% is excreted unchanged in the urine. The peak

71

serum level is 5 hours for an oral dose and 10 to 15 minutes for an IV bolus. Half-life is 3 to 7 hours and after chronic therapy 8 to 10 hours.

Nifedipine (Procardia): This agent has potent coronary and peripheral vasodilator effects. Ninety percent of the drug is absorbed and bound to plasma proteins. About 75% of the metabolized drug is excreted in the urine and 15% through the GI tract. Peak serum level is 2 hours after the oral dose. Half-life is 4 to 5 hours.

Diltiazem (Cardizem): This agent is the newest calcium blocker and is not as potent as verapamil or nifedipine. It is absorbed rapidly in the GI tract, and 80% is bound to plasma protein. Metabolites of diltiazem are excreted in the urine and feces. Peak serum level is 2 hours.[2–4,9,26,27]

Clinical Problems

Elevated Level: overdose of verapamil, nifedipine, or diltiazem, liver or renal diseases. *Drug Influence:* beta blockers (ie, propranolol [Inderal]).

Procedure

■ Collect 5 to 10 mL of venous blood in a red-top tube. Check with your laboratory for the preferred collecting tube.

■ Record on the laboratory requisition slip name of drug, dose, route, and last time administered.

■ There is no food or fluid restriction.

■ Factors Affecting Laboratory Results

■ None known

NURSING IMPLICATIONS WITH RATIONALE

■ Check the patient's pulse rate and BP before each administered dose. The vasodilation effect of verapamil and diltiazem lowers pulse rate and BP. Nifedipine can decrease BP substantially without decreasing pulse rate.

■ Observe for signs and symptoms related to calcium blocking agents (ie, nausea, abdominal distress, headache, dizziness, lightheadedness, flushing, hypotension, bradycardia).

■ Monitor BP every 15 minutes for 1 hour after administering an IV bolus of verapamil. Transient asymptomatic hypotension could occur.

■ Monitor urine output. Decreased output could indicate renal insufficiency; toxicity could result.

■ Recognize that a calcium channel blocker administered with a beta blocker could cause severe hypotension.

Patient Teaching

■ Teach the patient how to take a radial pulse. Inform the patient that the pulse rate should be checked before each dose and changes reported to the physician.

- Instruct the patient not to abruptly discontinue a calcium blocking agent. Withdrawal symptoms (eg, severe hypotension) could result.
- Instruct a patient having constipation (verapamil induced) to eat foods high in fiber or take a mild laxative.
- Instruct a patient having palpitation and/or peripheral ankle or leg edema (nifedipine induced) to rest and to elevate leg(s). Report changes to the physician.

CARBON DIOXIDE COMBINING POWER (SERUM OR PLASMA)
CO_2 Combining Power

Reference Values
Adult: 22–30 mEq/L, 22–30 mmol/L (SI units)
Child: 20–28 mEq/L

Description
The serum CO_2 test, usually included with the electrolyte test, is performed to determine metabolic acid-base abnormalities. The serum CO_2 acts as a bicarbonate (Hco_3) determinant. When serum CO_2 is low, Hco_3 is lost, and acidosis results (metabolic acidosis). With an elevated serum CO_2, Hco_3 is conserved and alkalosis results (metabolic alkalosis).[7,9,23,24]

Clinical Problems
Decreased Level: metabolic acidosis, diabetic ketoacidosis, starvation, severe diarrhea, dehydration, shock, acute renal failure, salicylate toxicity, exercise. *Drug Influence:* diuretics (chlorothiazide [Diuril] hydrochlorothiazide [Hydrodiuril], triamterene [Dyrenium]), antibiotics (methicillin, tetracycline), nitrofurantoin (Furadantin), paraldehyde

Elevated Level: metabolic alkalosis, severe vomiting, gastric suction, peptic ulcer, hypothyroidism, potassium deficit, emphysema (hypoventilation). *Drug Influence:* barbiturates, steroids (hydrocortisone, cortisone), diuretics (mercurial agents, ethacrynic acid [Edecrin])

Procedure
- Collect 7 to 10 mL of venous blood in a green-top tube. A tourniquet should be used for a short time.
- There is no food or fluid restriction.

■ Factors Affecting Laboratory Results

- Drugs that can increase or decrease the serum CO_2 level (*see Drug Influence above.*)

NURSING IMPLICATIONS WITH RATIONALE

Decreased Level

- Know that a decreased serum CO_2 is related to an acidotic state. Whenever there is excess acid in the body and the kidneys cannot excrete it, metabolic acidosis results. There are many causes of acidosis (*see Clinical Problems above*).
- Assess for signs and symptoms of metabolic acidosis when the patient's serum CO_2 is decreased, especially when it is less, than 15 mEq/L. Symptoms include deep, vigorous breathing (Kussmaul's breathing) and flushed skin.
- Report clinical findings of metabolic acidosis to the physician.

Elevated Level

- Know that an increase serum CO_2 is related to an alkalotic state. Whenever there is an excess of HCO_3 in the body or a loss of acid, metabolic alkalosis occurs. There are many causes of alkalosis (*see Clinical Problems above*).
- Assess for signs and symptoms of metabolic alkalosis when the patient has been vomiting or has had gastric suction for several days. Signs and symptoms include shallow breathing, a serum CO_2 greater than 30 mEq/L, and a base excess greater than +2.

CARBON MONOXIDE, CARBOXYHEMOGLOBIN (BLOOD)

Reference Values

Adult: Nonsmoker: 2.5% of hemoglobin. *Smoker:* 2–5% saturation of hemoglobin. *Heavy Smoker:* 5%–9% saturation of hemoglobin. *Toxic:* >25% saturation of hemoglobin

Child: similar to adult nonsmoker

Description

Carbon monoxide (CO) combines with hemoglobin to produce carboxyhemoglobin, which can occur 200 times more readily than the combination of oxygen with hemoglobin (oxyhemoglobin). When CO replaces oxygen in the hemoglobin in excess of 25%, CO toxicity occurs.

CO is formed from incomplete combustion of carbon-combining compounds, as in automobile exhaust, fumes from improperly functioning furnaces, and cigarette smoke. Continuous exposure to CO, increasing carboxyhemoglobin by more than 60%, leads to coma and death. The treatment for CO toxicity is to administer a high concentration of oxygen.[7,8,10,14]

Clinical Problems

Elevated Level: smoking and exposure to smoking, automobile exhaust fumes, defective gas-burning appliances

Procedure

- Collect 5 to 10 mL of venous blood in a lavender-top tube.
- The commonest method of analysis is performed with an IL CO oximeter, a direct-reading instrument.
- There is no food or fluid restriction.

- Factors Affecting Laboratory Results

- Heavy smoking

NURSING IMPLICATIONS WITH RATIONALE

- Determine from the patient's history (obtained from the patient, family, or friends) whether CO inhalation could have occurred.
- Assess for mild to severe CO toxicity. Symptoms of mild CO toxicity are headache, weakness, malaise, dizziness, and dyspnea with exertion. Symptoms of moderate to severe toxicity are severe headache, bright-red mucous membranes, and cherry-red blood. When carboxyhemoglobin exceeds 40%, the blood's residue is brick red.
- Identify individuals who might be a candidate for CO poisoning. Persons complaining of continuous headaches or who are living (24 hours a day) in a house with an old heating system in the winter should have a blood CO test performed.

CARCINOEMBRYONIC ANTIGEN (CEA) (SERUM, PLASMA)

Reference Values

Adult: Nonsmokers: <2.5 ng/mL. *Smokers:* < 3.5 ng/mL. *Acute inflammatory disorders:* >10 ng/mL. *Neoplasms:* > 12 ng/mL

Child: not normally done; assumed to be low (level) after the child is several months old

Description

CEA has been found in the GI epithelium of embryos and has been extracted from tumors in the adult GI tract. Originally the CEA test was to detect colon cancer, especially adenocarcinoma. Elevated levels might occur when inflammation and tissue destruction are present. CEA should never be used as the sole criterion for diagnosis.

The CEA test is a nonspecific test; however, elevated levels have been found in approximately 70% of patients with known cancer of the large intestine and pancreas. The primary role of the CEA test is to monitor the treatment of colon and pancreatic carcinoma; it is also used for follow-up studies once cancer has been diagnosed. If the levels fall after treatment, the cancer is most likely under control. A CEA test may be ordered at 30- to 90-day intervals, and if a significant CEA level reoccurs, the physician may resume chemotherapy treatments or consider another form of therapy.[9,10,12,13]

Clinical Problems

Elevated Level: Cancer: GI tract (esophagus, stomach, small and large intestine, rectum), liver, pancreas, lung, breast, cervix, bladder, testes, kidney, leukemia; pulmonary emphysema; cirrhosis of the liver; bacterial pneumonia; chronic ischemic heart disease; acute pancreatitis; acute renal failure; ulcerative colitis; chronic cigarette smoking; neuroblastoma; inflammatory diseases; surgical trauma

Procedure

- Collect 10 mL of venous blood in a red-top or lavender-top tube. Avoid hemolysis.
- Heparin should not be administered for 2 days before the test, since it interferes with the results.
- There is no food or fluid restriction.

■ Factors Affecting Laboratory Results

- Heparin interferes with the result of the CEA test.
- Hemolysis can affect test results.

NURSING IMPLICATIONS WITH RATIONALE

Elevated Level

- Relate clinical problems to elevated CEA levels. CEA levels over 2.5 ng/mL do not always indicate cancer, nor do levels below 2.5 ng/mL indicate an absence of cancer. The CEA test is useful for management of cancer treatment.
- Be supportive of patient and family while awaiting test results.
- Hold heparin injections for 2 days before the test, with the physician's permission. If heparin is given, this fact should be noted on the laboratory slip.

CAROTENE (SERUM)

Reference Values

Adult: 60–200 µg/dL, 0.74–3.72 µmol/L (SI units)

Child: 40–130 µg/dL

Description

Carotene is a fat-soluble vitamin found in yellow and green vegetables and fruits. After absorption from the intestine, carotene is stored in the liver and can be converted to vitamin A, according to body needs. When fat absorption is decreased, the serum carotene level is decreased, which is indicative of fat malabsorption syndrome. Causes of serum carotene deficit include poor diet, malabsorption, high fever, and pancreatic insufficiency.[3,7,9,10]

Clinical Problems

Decreased Level: malabsorption syndrome, pancreatic insufficiency, protein malnutrition, febrile illness, severe liver disease, cystic fibrosis

Elevated Level: hyperlipidemia, diabetes mellitus, chronic nephritis, hypothyroidism, diet high in carrots, hypervitaminosis A (slight elevation), pregnancy, hypocholesterolemia

Procedure

- Collect 5 to 10 mL of venous blood in a red-top tube. Protect from light.
- Foods rich in carotene—yellow and green vegatables, vegetable juice, and fruits—should be omitted for 2 to 3 days before the test (check laboratory procedure). If the physician wishes to check the serum carotene level for determining the absorption ability, a diet high in carotene will be ordered for several days. Water is permitted.
- NPO, a diet low in carotene, or a diet high in carotene should be recorded on the laboratory slip.

- Factors Affecting Laboratory Results

  - Mineral oil will interfere with carotene absorption.
  - Foods rich in carotene can affect the serum results.

NURSING IMPLICATIONS WITH RATIONALE

Patient Teaching

- Explain to the patient that diet will be high or low in carotene, depending on the physician's clinical assumptions and orders. Drinking water is permitted.
- Explain to the patient that the test is to determine whether there is a vitamin (carotene) deficiency.
- Answer the patient's questions concerning what foods to avoid or to eat before the test. Vegetables and fruits are rich in carotene.

CATECHOLAMINES (URINE)

Reference Values

Adult: <100 μg/24 hours (higher with activity), <0.59 μmol/24 hours (SI units), 0–14 μg/dL (random), epinephrine <10 ng/24 hours, norepinephrine <100 ng/24 hours

Child: level less than adult because of weight differences

Description

Catecholamines are hormones (epinephrine and norepinephrine) secreted by the adrenal medulla. Catecholamine production increases after strenuous exercise; however, urinary levels are 3 to 100 times greater than normal in cases of pheochromocytoma (tumor of the adrenal medulla). In some psychiatric patients, the urine catecholamine level increases only slightly. In children, this test may be used to diagnose malignant neuroblastoma.

Certain drugs, coffee, and bananas cause elevated catecholamine levels. The urine catecholamine test is considered a more reliable test than a serum catecholamine test.[3,7,10,13]

Clinical Problems

Elevated Level (>100 μg/24 hours): pheochromocytoma, severe stress (septicemia, shock, burn, peritonitis), malignant neuroblastoma, acute myocardial infarction (first 48 hours), chronic ischemic heart disease, cor pulmonale, carcinoid syndrome, manic-depressive disorder, depressive neurosis, strenuous exercise. *Drug Influence:* antibiotics (ampicillin, demeclocycline, erythromycin, tetracyclines), antihypertensives (methyldopa [Aldomet], hydralazine [Apresoline]), vitamins (ascorbic acid [vitamin C], B complex), chlorpromazine (Thorazine), quinine, quinidine, isoproterenol (Isuprel) or epinephrine by inhalation

Procedure

- Collect urine for 24 hours in a large container with a preservative (10 mL of concentrated HCl), and keep the bottle refrigerated. The pH of the urine collection should be below 3.0.
- Drugs, chocolate, coffee, and bananas should not be taken for 3 to 7 days before the test. The number of days may vary among laboratories.
- Food and fluids other than those already mentioned are not restricted.
- Label the large container with the patient's name and the dates and exact times for the 24-hour urine collection (eg, 4/10/93 7:30 AM to 4/11/93, 7:30 AM).

■ Factors Affecting Laboratory Results

- Foods such as, bananas, coffee, chocolate, vanilla, could cause an inaccurate test result.
- Certain drugs can affect test results. (*See Drug Influence above.*)

NURSING IMPLICATIONS WITH RATIONALE

Patient Teaching

- Explain to the patient and family that all urine should be saved in the refrigerated container. Inform the patient that toilet paper and feces should not be put in the urine.
- Explain to the patient that there is a strong acid that acts as a preservative in the urine container and that he or she should not urinate directly in the container.
- Explain that fasting can increase catecholamine levels. Foods are not restricted except for those in the procedure.

Elevated Level

- Recognize causes of elevated urine catecholamines other than pheochromocytoma. These include severe stress, strenuous exercise, and acute anxiety and other psychiatric disorders. The highest levels occur in pheochromocytoma.
- Check vital signs and report rising BP readings.
- Report to the physician and record on the nurse's note or progress notes whether the patient has been involved in strenuous activity or has suffered from severe anxiety.

CEREBROSPINAL FLUID (CSF)
(Color, Pressure, Cell Count, Protein, Chloride, Glucose, Culture) Spinal Fluid

Reference Values

	COLOR	PRESSURE (mmH$_2$O)	CELL COUNT (LEUKOCYTES)— cu mm (mm^3, μL)	PROTEIN (mg/dL)	CHLORIDE (mEq/L)	GLUCOSE (mg/dL)
Adult	Clear, colorless	75–175	0–8	15–45	118–132	40–80
Child	Clear, colorless	50–100	0–8	14–45	120–128	35–75
Premature infant			0–20	<400		
Newborn	Clear		0–15	30–200	110–122	20–40
1–6 months				30–100		

Description

CSF, also known as spinal fluid, circulates in the ventricles of the brain and through the spinal cord. Of the 150 mL of CSF, approximately 100 mL are produced by the blood in the brain ventricles and reabsorbed back into circulation daily.

Spinal fluid is obtained by a lumbar puncture (spinal tap) performed in the lumbar sac at L3-4, or at L4-5. First CSF pressure is measured, then fluid is aspirated and placed in sterile test tubes. Data from the analysis of the spinal fluid is important for diagnosing spinal cord and brain diseases.

The analysis of spinal fluid usually includes color, pressure, cell count (leukocytes—WBC), protein, chloride, and glucose. In addition, the pH of the CSF is usually checked; it is usually slightly lower, about one tenth (0.1) of a point, than the pH of the serum. The CSF protein and glucose levels are lower than the blood levels; however, the CSF chloride level is higher than the serum chloride level. Normally a culture is done to detect any organism present in the spinal fluid.[1,8–10,13,18]

Clinical Problems

CSF	DECREASED LEVEL	ELEVATED LEVEL	COMMENTS
Color		Abnormal color: 1. Pink or red—subarachnoid or cerebral hemorrhage; traumatic spinal tap 2. Xanthochromia (yellow color)—previous subarachnoid hemorrhage	Yellow color indicates old blood (4 to 5 days after a cerebral hemorrhage), mixture of bilirubin and blood, or extremely elevated protein levels; fluid discoloration normally remains for 3 weeks.
Pressure	Dehydration, hypovolemia	Intracranial pressure due to meningitis, subarachnoid hemorrhage, brain tumor, brain abscess, encephalitis	Slight elevation can occur with holding breath or tensing of muscles.
Cell count (lymphocytes)		<500 mm³ (μL): viral infections—poliomyelitis, aseptic meningitis; syphilis of CNS; multiple sclerosis; brain tumor; abscess; subarachnoid hemorrhage (40% or more monocytes) >500 mm³ (μL): ↑ granulocytes, purulent infection	WBC differential count may be ordered to identify the types of leukocytes.
Protein		Meningitis: tuberculosis, purulent, aseptic	Protein and cell counts usually increase together.

CSF	DECREASED LEVEL	ELEVATED LEVEL	COMMENTS
		Guillain-Barré syndrome	
		Subarachnoid hemorrhage	
		Brain tumor	
		Abscess	
		Syphilis	
		Drug influence:	
		anesthetics	
		acetophenetidin	
		(phenacetin)	
		chlorpromazine	
		(Thorazine)	
		salicylates (aspirin)	
		streptomycin	
		sulfonamides	
Chloride	Tubercular meningitis Bacterial meningitis		IV saline or electrolyte infusion could cause an inaccurate result. Syphilis, brain tumors and abscess, and encephalitis do not affect the CSF chloride level.
Glucose	Purulent meningitis Presence of fungi, protozoa, or pyogenic bacteria Subarachnoid hemorrhage Lymphomas Leukemia	Cerebral trauma Hypothalamic lesions Diabetes (hyperglycemia)	Brain abscess or tumor and degenerative diseases have little effect on the CSF glucose. The CSF glucose is usually two thirds of the blood glucose. The blood glucose level is determined for comparative reasons.
Culture		Meningitis	Generally done when meningitis is suspected

Procedure

- Collect a sterile lumbar puncture tray, an antiseptic solution (ie, providone-iodine or iodine), a local anesthetic (ie, lidocaine), sterile gloves, and tape.
- Place the patient in a "fetal" position, with the back bowed, the head flexed on the chest, and the knees drawn up to the abdomen.
- Label the three test tubes 1, 2, and 3.
- The physician checks the spinal fluid pressure, using a manometer attached to the needle. The physician collects a total of 10 to 12 mL of spinal fluid—3 mL in a no. 1 tube, 3 mL in a no. 2 tube, and 3 mL in a no. 3 tube. The first tube could be contaminated (with blood from the spinal tap) and should *not* be used for cell count, culture, or protein determination.
- Label the tubes with the patient's name, date, and room number. Take the test tubes immediately to the laboratory.
- There is no food or fluid restriction.

Queckenstedt Procedure: The Queckenstedt procedure is performed during a lumbar puncture when spinal block is suspected. Temporary pressure is applied to the jugular veins while the CSF pressure is monitored. Normally the CSF pressure will rise when the jugular veins are compressed. In partial or total CSF block, the pressure fails to rise with jugular vein compression, or it takes 15 to 30 seconds for CSF pressure to drop after compression is released.[8,10]

■ Factors Affecting Laboratory Results

■ Refrigeration may affect the results of the culture.
■ A traumatic spinal tap could cause the presence of blood in the fluid specimen, which could be mistaken for a clinical problem.
■ Certain drugs could cause a false, increased, CSF protein level (*see Clinical Problems: Drug Influence above*).
■ IV fluid containing chloride could invalidate the CSF chloride level determination.
■ Hyperglycemia could increase the CSF glucose level.

NURSING IMPLICATIONS WITH RATIONALE

■ Explain the procedure for the lumbar puncture to the patient by giving a step-by-step detailed explanation.
■ Collect specimen in numerical order of tubes. Do not mix the numbers. The first tube may have some RBCs because of the needle insertion. For culture, the second or third test tube is used. For protein and cell count, the third specimen tube is used.
■ Check the vital signs before the procedure and afterwards at specified times (ie, ½, 1, 2, and 4 hours).
■ Assess for changes in the neurologic status after the procedure (ie, increased temperature, increased BP, irritability, numbness and tingling in the lower extremities, and nonreactive eye pupils).
■ Administer an analgesic as ordered to relieve a headache if it occurs.
■ Be supportive of the patient before, during, and after the lumbar puncture.

Patient Teaching

■ Instruct the patient to relax and to take deep and slow breaths with his or her mouth open. Hold the patient's hand to give reassurance, unless this is opposed by the patient.
■ Instruct the patient to remain flat in bed in the prone or supine position for 4 to 8 hours following the lumbar puncture. Headaches are common because of spinal fluid leaking from the site of the lumbar puncture, which can occur if the patient is in an upright position.

CERULOPLASMIN (Cp) (SERUM)

Reference Values

Adult: 18–45 mg/dL, 180–450 mg/L (SI units)

Child: Infant: <23 mg/dL, or may be normal. *Child:* similar to adult

Description

Ceruloplasmin (Cp) is a copper-containing glycoprotein known as one of the α_2-globulins in the plasma. Ceruloplasmin is produced in the liver and binds with copper. The principle role of ceruloplasmin is not clearly understood, except that when there is a serum deficit, there is an increased urinary excretion of copper and increased depositing of copper on the cornea, brain, liver, and kidney, causing damage and destruction of the organs. A deficit of ceruloplasmin or hypoceruloplasmin can result in Wilson's disease (hepatolenticular degeneration), commonly seen between the ages of 7 and 15 and in early middle age.[7,9,10,13]

Clinical Problems

Decreased Level: Wilson's disease (hepatolenticular degeneration), protein malnutrition, nephrotic syndrome, newborns and early infancy

Elevated Level: cirrhosis of the liver; hepatitis; pregnancy; Hodgkin's disease; cancer of the bone, stomach, lung; myocardial infarction; rheumatoid arthritis; infections and inflammatory process; exercise. *Drug Influence:* oral contraceptives, estrogen drugs

Procedure

- Collect 5 mL of venous blood in a red-top tube.
- There is no food or fluid restriction.
- Withhold drugs containing estrogen for 24 hours before the blood test, with the physician's permission.

■ Factors Affecting Laboratory Results

- Estrogen therapy, pregnancy, and exercise could cause an elevated serum ceruloplasmin level.
- In Wilson's disease with severe liver damage, a normal serum level could result.

NURSING IMPLICATIONS WITH RATIONALE

Decreased Level

- Relate hypoceruloplasmin (serum ceruloplasmin deficit) to Wilson's disease. The serum level is frequently below 15 mg/dL is commonly seen after the age of 7.

- Assess for signs and symptoms of Wilson's disease (ie, abnormal muscular rigidity [dystonia], tremors of the fingers, dysarthria, and mental disturbances).
- Check the cornea of the eye for a discolored ring (Kayser-Fleischer ring) from copper deposits.

Elevated Level

- Relate clinical problems of liver disorders, cancer, infections, inflammations, and drugs to hyperceruloplasmin (serum ceruloplasmin excess).
- Note whether the patient has been exercising in the last 24 hours, since a slight elevation could be due to strenuous exercise.

CHLORDIAZEPOXIDE (LIBRIUM, LIBRAX) SERUM

Reference Values

Adult: Therapeutic Range: 1.0–5.0 µg/mL. *Peak Time:* 1–3 hours. *Toxic Level:* > 5 µg/mL

Description

Chlordiazepoxide (Librium), a benzodiazepine and anxiolytic, is used mostly for the treatment of anxiety and alcohol withdrawal effects. It also suppresses seizure activity.[1,3,6,9,10]

Clinical Problems

Decreased Level: Drug Influence: Phenothiazine drug group

Elevated Level: overdose of chlordiazepoxide

Procedure

- Collect 7 mL of venous blood in a red-top tube.
- There is no food or fluid restriction.

■ Factors Affecting Laboratory Results

- Phenothiazines and taking other benzodiazepines with chlordiazepoxide could cause CNS depression.

NURSING IMPLICATIONS WITH RATIONALE

- Observe for side effects of chlordiazepoxide (ie, lethargy, drowsiness, slurred speech, tremors, transient hypotension, dizziness, bradycardia, dry mouth).

Patient Teaching

- Instruct the patient to report side effects. Many of the side effects will disappear after taking the drug for a few days.
- Advise the patient that if dizziness occurs he or she should rise slowly from a lying position.
- Inform the patient to avoid heavy smoking, since it could cause side effects. Heavy smoking can enhance the effect of chlordiazepoxide.
- Explain to the patient that antacids might delay absorption of Librium. Inform the physician if patient is taking antacids.

CHLORIDE (CI) (SERUM)

Reference Values

Adult: 95–105 mEq/L, 95–105 mmol/L (SI units)

Child: Newborn: 94–112 mEq/L. *Infant:* 95–110 mEq/L. *Child:* 98–105 mEq/L

Description

Chloride is an anion found mostly in the extracellular fluid. Chloride plays an important role in maintaining body water balance, osmolality of body fluids (with sodium), and acid-base balance. It combines with hydrogen ion to produce the acidity (hydrochloric acid [HCl]) in the stomach.

For maintaining acid-base balance, chloride competes with bicarbonate for sodium. When the body fluids are more acidic, the kidneys excrete chloride and sodium, and bicarbonate is reabsorbed. In addition, chloride shifts in and out of RBCs in exchange with bicarbonate.

Most of the chloride ingested is combined with sodium (sodium chloride [NaCl] or "salt"). The daily required chloride intake is 2 g. Hypochloremia means serum chloride deficit; hyperchloremia means serum chloride excess.[1,7,24]

Clinical Problems

Decreased Level: vomiting, gastric suction, diarrhea, hypokalemia ($\downarrow$ K), hyponatremia ($\downarrow$ Na), low-sodium diet, continuous IV D5W, gastroenteritis, colitis, adrenal gland insufficiency (Addison's disease), diabetic acidosis, heat exhaustion, hyperaldosteronism, acute infections, burns, excessive diaphoresis (sweating/perspiration), metabolic alkalosis. *Drug Influence:* diuretics (mercurials, thiazides, loop), bicarbonates

Elevated Level: dehydration, hypernatremia ($\uparrow$ Na), hyperparathyroidism, cancer of the stomach, multiple myeloma, adrenal gland hyperactivity, head injury, eclampsia, cardiac decompensation, excessive IV saline (0.9% NaCl), kidney dysfunction (glomerulonephritis, acute renal failure, pyelonephritis), hyperventilation, metabolic acidosis. *Drug Influence:* acetazolamide, ammonium chloride, boric acid, cortisone preparations, ion exchange resins, prolonged use of triamterene (Dyrenium).

Procedure

- Collect 5 to 10 mL of venous blood in a red- or green-top tube.
- There is no food or fluid restriction. This test may be combined with other tests (eg, for serum electrolytes), so the patient may be NPO. Check with the laboratory.

- Factors Affecting Laboratory Results

 - Drugs: *See Drug Influence above.*

NURSING IMPLICATIONS WITH RATIONALE

Decreased Level

- Assess for signs and symptoms of hypochloremia (hyperexcitability of the nervous system and muscles, tetany [twitching, tremors], slow and shallow breathing, and decreased BP resulting from fluid and chloride loss).
- Inform the physician when the patient is receiving IV D5W continuously. If no other solutes are given, the body fluids will be diluted, and the patient will not receive the daily required chloride intake.
- Check the serum potassium and sodium levels. Chloride is frequently lost with sodium and potassium (plentiful in the GI tract). With vomiting, potassium, hydrogen, and chlorides are lost, causing hypokalemic-hypochloremic alkalosis. Both potassium and chloride must be replaced, for if potassium is given and not chloride, hypokalemic alkalosis will persist.
- Observe for symptoms of overhydration when the patient is receiving several liters of normal saline (0.9% NaCl) for sodium and chloride replacement. Sodium holds water, and if there is history of heart or kidney disorder, water accumulation could occur. Symptoms of overhydration include a constant, irritated cough; dyspnea; neck and hand vein engorgement; and chest rales.

Patient Teaching

- Instruct the patient *not* to drink only plain water if there is a serum chloride deficit. Encourage the patient to drink fluids containing sodium and chloride (eg, broth, tomato juice, Pepsi Cola).
- Instruct the patient to drink and eat foods rich in chloride (ie, broth, seafoods, milk, meats, eggs, and table salt).

Elevated Level

- Assess for signs and symptoms of hyperchloremia (similar to acidosis)— weakness, lethargy, and deep, rapid, vigorous breathing.
- Notify the physician if the patient is receiving IV fluids containing normal saline. Check for symptoms of overhydration.
- Monitor daily weights and intake and output to determine whether fluid retention is present because of sodium and chloride excess.

Patient Teaching

■ Instruct the patient to avoid drinking or eating salty foods. Encourage the patient not to use the salt shaker and some salt substitutes.
■ Instruct the patient to read labels, since some salt substitutes contain calcium chloride or potassium chloride.

CHLORIDE (SWEAT)
Screening (Silver Nitrate); Iontophoresis (Pilocarpine)

Reference Values

Adult: <60 mEq/L

Child: <50 mEq/L; marginal: 50–60 mEq/L; abnormal: >60 mEq/L (possible cystic fibrosis)

Description

Sodium and chloride concentrations in sweat are higher in persons with cystic fibrosis, even though there usually is not an increased amount of sweat. Sweat chloride is considered more reliable than sweat sodium for diagnostic purposes. Some false negatives of sweat sodium have been reported in persons with cystic fibrosis.

There are two types of sweat chloride tests used: (1) screening tests, which use silver nitrate on agar or filter (special) paper and require contact with hand (palm or fingers), and (2) iontophoresis, in which pilocarpine is placed on the forearm to increase sweat gland secretion. A positive screening test is usually validated with iontophoresis, since the chloride level in the palm of the hand is usually higher than anywhere else. Some physicians feel that the screening should be routine in all children; however, others disagree.[10,13,14]

Clinical Problems

Elevated Level (>60 mEq/L): cystic fibrosis asthma

Procedure

Screening Test (Silver Nitrate)
■ Wash the child's hand and dry it. For 15 minutes, keep the hand from contacting any other part of the body.
■ Moisten the test paper containing silver nitrate compound with distilled water (*not saline*).
■ Press the child's hand on the paper for 4 seconds.
■ A positive result occurs when the excess chloride combines with the silver nitrate to form white silver chloride on the paper.
■ A heavy hand imprint is left by the child with cystic fibrosis.

Iontophoresis (Pilocarpine): usually performed by laboratory personnel.
■ Electrodes are placed on the skin of the forearm to create a small electric current for transporting pilocarpine (a stimulating drug) into the skin to induce sweating.
■ Sweat is collected and weighed. Chloride is measured.
■ There is no food or fluid restriction.

■ Factors Affecting Laboratory Results

■ Unwashed hands for the screening test affect test results.
■ Use of saline solution to moisten the test paper cause inaccurate test result.

NURSING IMPLICATIONS WITH RATIONALE

■ Explain the procedures (screening or iontophoresis or both) to the child and family. Answer questions if possible, or refer them to the physician or laboratory personnel.
■ Explain to the child and family that the tests are not painful.
■ Remain with the child during the procedure. Give comfort and reassurance as needed.

Elevated Level

■ Associate an elevated sweat chloride with cystic fibrosis. With cystic fibrosis, sweat chloride levels could be two to five times greater than normal.
■ Obtain a familial history of cystic fibrosis, when indicated.
■ Determine whether the child has washed and dried his or her hands before the screening test is performed. Dried sweat can leave a chloride residue, thus causing a false-positive result.

CHOLESTEROL (SERUM)

Reference Values

Adult: Desirable Level: <200 mg/dL *Moderate Risk:* 200–240 mg/dL. *High Risk:* >240 mg/dL. *Pregnancy:* high risk levels but returns to prepregnancy values 1 month after delivery

Child: Infant: 90–130 mg/dL. *Child: 2–19 years: Desirable Level:* 130–170 mg/dL; *Moderate Risk:* 171–184 mg/dL; *High risk:* >185 mg/dL

Description

Cholesterol is a blood lipid synthesized by the liver and is found in RBCs, cell membranes, and muscles. About 70% of cholesterol is esterified (combined with fatty acids), and 30% is in the free form. Cholesterol is used by the body to form bile salts fat digestion and for the formation of hormones by the adrenal glands, ovaries, and testes. Thyroid hormones and estrogen decrease the concentration of cholesterol, and an oophorectomy increases it.

Serum cholesterol is used as an indicator of atherosclerosis and coronary artery disease. Hypercholesterolemia causes plaque deposits in the coronary arteries, thus contributing to myocardial infarction. High serum cholesterol levels can be due to a familial (hereditary) tendency, biliary obstruction, and/or dietary intake. Approximately one third of Americans have a serum cholesterol level below 200 mg dL, which is desirable.[1,3,9,11,18,28,29]

Clinical Problems

Decreased Level: hyperthyroidism, Cushing's syndrome (adrenal hormone excess), starvation, malabsorption, anemias, acute infections. *Drug Influence:* antilipids (Lopid, Mevacor), thyroxine, antibiotics (kanamycin, neomycin, parmomycin, tetracycline), nicotinic acid, estrogens, glucagon, heparin, salicylates (aspirin), colchicine, oral hypoglycemic agents.

Elevated Level: acute myocardial infarction; atherosclerosis; hypothyroidism; biliary obstruction; biliary cirrhosis; cholangitis; familial hypercholesterolemia; uncontrolled diabetes mellitus; nephrotic syndrome; pancreatectomy; pregnancy (third trimester); types II, III, V hyperlipoproteinemia; heavy stress periods; high-cholesterol diet (animal fats). *Drug Influence:* aspirin, corticosteroids, steroids (anabolic agents and androgens), oral contraceptives, epinephrine and norepinephrine, bromides, phenothiazines (chlorpromazine [Thorazine], trifluoperazine [Stelazine], vitamins A and D, sulfonamides, phenytoin (Dilantin)

Procedure

- Keep the patient NPO (food, fluids, and medications) for 12 hours. The patient may have water.
- Collect 5 to 10 mL of venous blood in a red-top tube. Avoid hemolysis.
- List drugs the patient is taking that are not withheld on the laboratory slip.

- Factors Affecting Laboratory Results

- Aspirin and cortisone could cause decreased or elevated serum cholesterol levels.
- A high-cholesterol diet before the test could cause elevated serum cholesterol levels.
- Severe hypoxia could increase the serum cholesterol level.
- Hemolysis of the blood specimen may cause an elevation of the serum cholesterol level.

NURSING IMPLICATIONS WITH RATIONALE

Elevated Level:

- Relate clinical problems and drugs to hypercholesterolemia. An elevated cholesterol level can indicate liver disease as well as coronary artery disease.

■ Hold drugs that could increase the serum level for 12 hours before the blood is drawn, with the physician's permission.

Patient Teaching

■ Explain to the patient and family what is considered a normal serum cholesterol level and the effects of an elevated cholesterol level.
■ Encourage patient to lose weight if overweight and has hypercholesterolemia. Losing weight if obese can decrease serum cholesterol level.
■ Instruct the patient with hypercholesterolemia to decrease the intake of foods rich in cholesterol (ie, bacon, eggs, butter, fatty meat, certain seafood, coconut, and chocolate).
■ Teach the patient with severe hypercholesterolemia to keep medical appointments for follow-up care.

CHOLINESTERASE (RBCs OR PLASMA)
Acetylcholinesterase (True Cholinesterase of Blood Nerve Tissue—RBC); Pseudocholinesterase (Serum)

Reference Values

Adult: 0.5–1.0 U (RBC), 3–8 U/mL (plasma), 6–8 IU/L (RBC), 8–18 IU/L at 37°C (plasma)

Child: similar to adult

Description

There are two different cholinesterases (CHS): *acetylcholinesterase* (true cholinesterase), found in the RBCs (erthyrocytes) and nerve tissue, and *pseudocholinesterase,* or serum cholinesterase (PCHE). Cholinesterase is an enzyme that breaks down acetylcholine at the nerve synapse and neuromuscular junction.

Decreased cholinesterase levels may indicate insecticide poisoning caused by excess exposure to organic phosphate agents, liver disorders (hepatitis and cirrhosis), or an acute infection. This test is not used for assessment of liver function.[11–14]

Clinical Problems

Decreased Level: insecticide poisoning, liver disorders (hepatitis, cirrhosis, obstructive jaundice), malnutrition, acute infections, anemias, carcinomatosis

Elevated Level: nephrotic syndrome

Procedure

■ Collect 5 to 10 mL of venous blood in a green-top tube.
■ There is no food or fluid restriction.

■ Factors Affecting Laboratory Results

■ Nonheparinized tube for cholinesterase-RBC test affects test result.

NURSING IMPLICATIONS WITH RATIONALE

Decreased Level

■ Obtain a history of the patient's exposure to insecticides—kind, length of time, and amount. Excessive exposure to organic phosphate can cause acute or chronic toxicity, and the acetylcholinesterase level would be decreased.
■ Report to the physician and record on the chart if the patient has not been eating or has an acute infection.

CLOT RETRACTION (BLOOD)

Reference Values
Adult: 1–24 hours (retraction of clot)
Child: similar to adult

Description
The clot retraction (shrunken clot) test is useful in determining whether bleeding disorders are due to a decreased platelet count. This is a simple test (the rate and degree of contraction of a blood clot are measured) in which a clot of blood in a test tube will diminish in size because of fluid (serum) separating from the red cells. Platelets are responsible for the shrinkage of the blood clot. Frequently, when there is a platelet deficit, clot retraction will be slower and the clot formation will be softer.

In 1 hour the clot should be one half its original size (volume). The retraction should be near completion in 4 hours and definitely completed in 24 hours.[8,10,12,13]

Clinical Problems
Decreased Clot Formation: thrombocytopenia (decreased platelets), thrombasthenia (abnormal platelets), anemia (pernicious, folic acid, aplastic), Waldenström's macroglobulinemia

Procedure

■ Collect 5 mL of venous blood in a red-top tube.
■ There is no food or fluid restriction.

■ Factors Affecting Laboratory Results

- High hematocrit can cause poor clot retraction.
- Decreased fibrinogen can cause RBCs to spill out of the serum when retraction begins—poor cell retraction.
- Anticoagulants can inhibit clot formation.

NURSING IMPLICATIONS WITH RATIONALE

Decreased or Poor Clot Formation

- Report to the physician if bleeding time is prolonged.
- Note when the blood clot begins to separate from the tube wall. This usually begins to happen within 30 minutes to 1 hour. Note the length of time required for clot retraction (clot shrinking and fluid release).
- Check the consistency of the clot. Soft clots and shapeless clots may be due to abnormal or decreased platelets.
- Check the patient's hemoglobin, hematocrit, and platelet count. A high hematocrit resulting from hemoconcentration or polycythemia may cause decreased clot retraction. Clot retraction is influenced by the number of functional platelets and not necessarily by the total count.

COAGULATION FACTORS
(See Factor Assay)

COAGULATION TIME (CT) (BLOOD)
Lee-White Clotting Time, Venous Clotting Time (VCT)

Reference Values
Adult: *Three-Tube Method:* 5–15 minutes (average 8 minutes)
Child: similar to adults

Description
The coagulation time (CT), or the Lee-White test (clotting time), one of the oldest tests of coagulation, determines the time it takes for venous blood to clot in a glass test tube. CT, or the Lee-White test, should not be used as a screening test for diagnosing bleeding conditions, since it is not sensitive enough to detect mild to moderate coagulation problems, only severe ones. In addition, it is not specific for any one of the 13 coagulation factors. With a normal CT, there could still be a clotting problem.

CT is commonly used to monitor and to regulate patients receiving heparin therapy so as to keep the clotting time at approximately 20 minutes. Three glass test tubes are used and tilted at 30-second intervals to enhance clotting.[9,10,13,14]

Clinical Problems

Decreased Time: eclampsia. *Drug Influence:* Steroids (cortisone), epinephrine (adrenalin)

Prolonged Time: afibrinogenemia, hyperheparinemia, severe coagulation factor deficiencies, toxic effects of venom, heat stroke. *Drug Influence:* anticoagulants (heparin), antibiotics (carbenicillin, tetracycline), azathioprine (Imuran), mithramycin

Procedure

- A glass syringe and glass test tubes should be used. Plastic test tubes could lengthen the clotting time by 20 to 40 minutes.
- Test timing begins when blood enters the glass syringe. When using a plastic syringe, timing is started when the blood enters the glass test tube. Laboratory procedure differs from one institution to another and should be checked.
- For the Lee-White test, three glass test tubes at 37°C are used. Each tube should have 1 mL of venous blood, and the tubes should be tilted every 15 to 30 seconds to enhance clotting through the contact of the blood with the glass tube surface. When a firm clot has formed, the time should be recorded.

- Factors Affecting Laboratory Results

  - Use of plastic test tubes
  - Poor venipuncture procedure (ie, RBCs hemolyzed in the syringe as blood is drawn from the vein)
  - Improper tilting of test tubes and timing of blood samples
  - Drugs causing prolonged clotting time (*See Drug Influence above.*)
  - Due to difficulty in standardizing the technique, there are other tests of choice, such as the activated partial thromboplastin time (APTT) test.

NURSING IMPLICATIONS WITH RATIONALE

Prolonged (Increased) Time

- Relate prolonged or increased CT to clinical problems and drugs. Frequently, prolonged CT does not occur until there is a severe clotting problem. CT may be normal in mild hemophilia.
- Assess for signs and symptoms of bleeding due to a prolonged CT. Symptoms could include bleeding under the skin or from the nose, mouth, or rectum.

COLD AGGLUTININS (SERUM)
Cold Hemagglutinin

Reference Values

Adult: 1:8 antibody titer, >1:16 significantly increased, >1:32 definitely positive

Child: similar to adult

Elderly: Values are increased more than adults.

Description

Cold agglutinins (CAs) are antibodies that agglutinate RBCs at temperatures between 0°C and 10°C. Elevated titers (>1:32) are found frequently in patients with primary atypical pneumonia or with other clinical problems, such as influenza, pulmonary embolism, and cirrhosis. The cold agglutinins test is often done during the acute and convalescence phases of illness.[3,9,10,13]

Clinical Problems

Elevated Level: primary atypical pneumonia, influenza, cirrhosis of the liver, lymphatic leukemia, multiple myeloma, pulmonary embolism, acquired hemolytic anemias, malaria, infectious mononucleosis, frostbite, viral infections (cytomegalovirus), tuberculosis

Procedure

- Collect 7 mL of venous blood in a red-top tube. Keep specimen warm. Take immediately to the laboratory. The blood sample should not be refrigerated.
- The laboratory may rewarm the sample for 30 minutes before the serum is separated from the cells.
- There is no food or fluid restriction.

■ Factors Affecting Laboratory Results

- Antibiotic therapy may cause inaccurate results.
- Elevated cold agglutinins may interfere with typing and cross matching.
- Improper blood collection procedure may affect results.

NURSING IMPLICATIONS WITH RATIONALE

Elevated Level

- Relate elevated cold agglutinin levels to clinical problems, particularly primary atypical pneumonia.
- Answer the patient's questions concerning the significance of the test. Answers might include "most persons have an antibody titer level, but some have higher levels, such as older adults and those with viral infections; high titers may persist for years, and the test may be repeated at a later date."

COMPLEMENT C3 TEST (SERUM)
C3 Component of the Complement System

Reference Values

Adult: *Male:* 80–180 mg/dL. *Female:* 76–120 mg/dL

Child: Usually not performed

Description

C3 is the most abundant component of the complement system (a group of 11 proteins). The complement system has an important role in the immunologic system and the complements' components are activated when IgG and IgM antibodies are combined with their specific antigens.

The total complement system and C3 are decreased in lupus erythematosus, glomerulonephritis, and acute renal transplant rejection. Following onset of an acute or chronic inflammatory process or acute tissue destruction (necrosis), the total complement may be temporarily elevated. C3 and C4 of the complement system are best known, and the others (C1, C2, and C5 to C9) are still under study and intense research.[1,3,8–10,13]

Clinical Problems

Decreased Level: systemic lupus erythematosus (SLE), glomerulonephritis, acute poststreptococcal glomerulonephritis, acute renal transplant rejection, cirrhosis of the liver, multiple sclerosis (slightly lower), protein malnutrition, anemias (pernicious, folic acid), septicemia (gram-negative), bacterial endocarditis

Elevated Level: acute rheumatic fever; rheumatoid arthritis, early SLE, and malignant neoplasms of the esophagus, stomach, colon, rectum, pancreas, lungs, breast, cervix, ovary, prostate, and bladder

Procedure

- Collect 5 to 10 mL of venous blood in a red-top tube.
- Take the blood sample to the laboratory immediately.
- There is no food or fluid restriction.

- Factors Affecting Laboratory Results

  - Heat can destroy complement components.
  - C3 is unstable, and the serum value may decrease if the sample is left standing for 1 to 2 hours at room temperature.

NURSING IMPLICATIONS WITH RATIONALE

- Compare the serum C3 and C4 results.
- Be supportive of patient and family.

Decreased Level

- Relate a decreased C3 level to clinical problems such as lupus and kidney disorders.

- Check the serum C3 value with other laboratory studies that are ordered and related to disease process.

Elevated Level

- Relate an elevated C3 level to an acute or chronic inflammatory process and tissue necrosis, such as rheumatic fever, rheumatoid arthritis, and malignancies with metastasis.

COMPLEMENT C4 TEST (SERUM)
C4 Component of the Complement System

Reference Values

Adult: 15–45 mg/dL

Child: usually not performed

Description

(See Complement C3.)

    C4 is the second most abundant component of the complement system (a group of 11 serum proteins). A decrease in C4 as well as C3 is commonly found in diseases such as systemic lupus erythematosus (SLE), glomerulonephritis, and renal transplant rejection.

    An elevated serum C4 level is indicative of an acute inflammatory process; however, a well (healthy) person may have an elevated C4 level. With cancer, the C4 level is usually increased (with links to the stage of the disease), but the serum level drops significantly in the terminal phase of the malignancy.[3,9,12,14]

Clinical Problems

Decreased Level: lupus nephritis, systemic lupus erythematosus (C4 decreased time is longer than C3 decreased time), acute poststreptococcal glomerulonephritis (C4 usually lower than C3), cirrhosis of the liver, bacterial endocarditis

Elevated Level: rheumatoid spondylitis; juvenile rheumatoid arthritis; cancer of the esophagus, stomach, colon, rectum, pancreas, lung, breast, cervix, ovary, prostate, and bladder

Procedure

- Collect 5 to 10 mL of venous blood in a red-top tube.
- Take the blood sample to the laboratory immediately.
- There is no food and fluid restriction.

■ Factors Affecting Laboratory Results

- Heat will decrease complement C4.
- C4 is unstable and the serum level will decrease if it remains at room temperature for more than 1 to 2 hours.

NURSING IMPLICATIONS WITH RATIONALE

Decreased Level

■ Relate a decreased serum C4 level to clinical problems. With lupus nephritis and poststreptococcal glomerulonephritis, the serum C4 level is extremely low.

■ Compare the serum C3 and C4 results to determine which component of the complement system is involved.

COOMBS DIRECT (BLOOD—RBC)
Direct Antiglobulin Test

Reference Values
Adult: negative
Child: negative

Description
The direct Coombs test detects antibodies attached to RBCs that may cause cellular damage. This test can identify a weak antigen-antibody reaction even when there is no visible RBC agglutination. A positive Coombs test reveals antibodies present in RBC, but the test does not identify the antibody responsible.

This test is useful; for diagnosing early erythroblastosis fetalis of newborns, autoimmune hemolytic anemia, hemolytic transfusion reaction, and some drug sensitizations (ie, to levodopa and methyldopa).

The direct Coombs test is also known as the direct antiglobulin test, a method of detecting in vivo sensitization of RBCs.[3,10,12,13]

Clinical Problems
Positive (+1 to +4): erythroblastosis fetalis (hemolytic disease of newborns), acquired hemolytic anemia (autoimmune), transfusion reactions (blood incompatibility), leukemias (lymphocytic, myelocytic), systemic lupus erythematosus. *Drug Influence:* antibiotics (cephaloridine (Loridine), cephalothin (Keflin), penicillin, streptomycin, tetracycline), chlorpromazine (Thorazine), phenytoin (Dilantin), ethosuximide (Zarontin), hydralazine (Apresoline) isoniazid (INH), levodopa (Dopar), methyldopa (Aldomet), procainamide (Pronestyl), quinidine, rifampin (Rifadin), sulfonamides

Procedure
■ Collect 7 mL of venous blood in a lavender-top tube. Red-top tube could be used. Venous blood from the umbilical cord of a newborn may be used. Avoid hemolysis.
■ There is no food or fluid restriction.

97

■ Factors Affecting Laboratory Results

  ■ Certain drugs may cause a positive test result (*see Drug Influence above*).

NURSING IMPLICATIONS WITH RATIONALE

Positive Test

■ Report the drugs patient is receiving that could produce a positive direct Coombs test (ie, antibiotics, phenytoin, sulfonamides, chlorpromazine, methyldopa, and others (*see Drug Influence above*).

■ Observe for signs and symptoms of whole blood transfusion reactions (ie, chills, fever [slight temperature elevation], and rash).

■ Observe the newborn for symptoms of erythroblastosis fetalis, especially if the condition is suspected. The main symptom is jaundice of the skin, nails, and sclera.

COOMBS INDIRECT (SERUM)

Reference Values

Adult: negative

Child: negative

Description

The Coombs indirect test can detect free circulating antibodies in the patient's serum. This test is done in cross matching blood for transfusions to prevent transfusion reaction to incompatible blood caused by minor blood-type factors. As a result of previous transfusions, a recipient's blood may contain specific antibody (antibodies) that could cause a transfusion reaction.

The indirect Coombs test is also known as the indirect antiglobulin test, a method of detecting in vitro sensitization of RBCs.[3,7,10,13]

Clinical Problems

Positive (+1 to +4): incompatible cross-matched blood, specific antibody (previous transfusion), anti-Rh antibodies (detected during pregnancy), acquired hemolytic anemia. *Drug Influence:* same as for the direct Coombs test (*See Coombs Direct.*)

Procedure

■ Collect 5–7 mL of venous blood in a red-top tube. The blood bank will use the serum from the recipient's blood and select the compatible blood for proper transfusion.

■ There is no food or fluid restriction.

■ Factors Affecting Laboratory Results

  ■ Certain drugs can cause positive results. (*See Clinical Problems: Drug Influence under Coombs Direct.*)

NURSING IMPLICATIONS WITH RATIONALE

■ Obtain a history of previous transfusions and report any previous transfusion reactions.
■ Report any drugs the patient is receiving that could cause a positive result. Record drug information on the patient's chart in the nurse's notes or progress notes.

Patient Teaching

■ Explain to the patient that the donor and recipient's bloods are checked for antibodies prior to a blood transfusion to avoid a transfusion reaction.

COPPER (Cu) (SERUM)

Reference Values

Adult: *Male:* 70–140 μg/dL, 11–22 μmol/L (SI units). *Female:* 80–155 μg/dL, 12.6–24.3 μmol/L (SI units). *Pregnancy:* 140–300 μg/dL

Child: *Newborn:* 20–70 μg/dL. *Child:* 30–190 μg/dL. *Adolescent:* 90–240 μg/dL

Description

Copper is required for hemoglobin synthesis. Approximately 90% of the copper is bound to α_2-globulin, referred to as ceruloplasmin, which is the means of copper transportation in the body. In hepatolenticular disease (Wilson's disease), the serum copper level is less than 20 μg/dL, and the urinary copper level is greater than 100 μg/24 hours. There is a decrease in copper metabolism with Wilson's disease, and excess copper is deposited in the brain (basal ganglia) and liver, causing degenerative changes. A low-copper diet and D-penicillamine will promote copper excretion.

Hypercupremia (excess copper) can be observed during pregnancy, anemias, leukemia, collagen disease, and thyroid diseases. Serum copper and serum ceruloplasmin tests are frequently ordered together and compared. Both show decreased levels with Wilson's disease.[3,7,8,11]

Clinical Problems

Decreased Level (70 μg/dL [male]): hepatolenticular disease (Wilson's disease), protein malnutrition, chronic ischemic heart disease

Elevated Level (140 µg/dL [male]): cancer (bone, stomach, large intestine, liver, lung), Hodgkin's disease, leukemias, hypothyroidism, hyperthyroidism, anemias (pernicious and iron deficiency) rheumatoid arthritis, systemic lupus erythematosus, pregnancy, cirrhosis of the liver

Procedure

- Collect 5 mL of venous blood in a red-top or green-top tube.
- There is no food or fluid restriction.
- *Note:* A test for urinary copper may be requested simultaneously with the blood test.

■ Factors Affecting Laboratory Results

- A diet low or high in copper before the blood test may cause inaccurate result.
- Metallic contamination of collection tubes or equipment affects test result.

NURSING IMPLICATIONS WITH RATIONALE

Decreased Level

- Assess for signs and symptoms of hepatolenticular disease (Wilson's disease—ie, rigidity, dysarthria, dysphagia, incoordination, and tremors).
- Check for a Kayser-Fleischer ring (dark ring) around the cornea. This is a copper deposit that the body has not been able to metabolize.
- Compare the serum copper level with the serum ceruloplasmin level if both have been ordered. If hepatolenticular disease is present, the serum levels will be decreased.

Patient Teaching

- Explain to the patient with Wilson's disease that foods rich in copper (ie, organ meats, shellfish, mushrooms, whole-grain cereals, bran, nuts, and chocolate) should be avoided. Canned foods should be omitted. A low-copper diet and D-penicillamine promote copper excretion.

CORTISOL (PLASMA)
Hydrocortisone, Compound F

Reference Values

Adult: 8 AM–10 AM:5–23 µg/dL 138–635 nmol/L (SI units). 4 PM–6 PM 3–13 µg/dL, 83–359 nmol/L (SI units)

Child: 8 AM–10 AM: 15–25 µg/dL 4 PM–6 PM: 5–10 µg/dL

Description

Cortisol is a potent glucocorticoid release from the adrenal cortex in response to ACTH stimulation. Cortisol affects carbohydrate, protein, and lipid metabolism; acts as an anti-inflammatory agent; helps with maintenance of BP; inhibits insulin action; and stimulates glucogenesis in the liver.

Levels of plasma cortisol are higher in the morning and lower in the afternoon. When there is adrenal or pituitary dysfunction, the diurnal variation in cortisol function ceases.[3,9,10,13]

Clinical Problems

Decreased Level: anterior pituitary hypofunction, adrenal cortical hypofunction (Addison's disease), respiratory distress syndrome (low-birth-weight newborns), hypothyroidism, exercise (slight decrease) *Drug Influence:* androgens, phenytoin (Dilantin)

Elevated Level: cancer of the adrenal gland, benign tumor on the adrenal cortex, adrenal cortical hyperfunction (Cushing's syndrome), stress, pregnancy, obesity, acute myocardial infarction, acute alcoholic intoxication, diabetic acidosis, hyperthyroidism. *Drug Influence:* oral contraceptives, estrogens, spironolactone (Aldactone), triparanol

Procedure

- Collect 5 to 10 mL of venous blood in a green-top (heparinized) tube.
- Write the date and time the blood was drawn on the laboratory slip. If the patient has taken estrogen or oral contraceptives in the last 6 weeks, the drug(s) should be listed on the laboratory slip. Recommendation: Stop medication 2 months before test.
- Advise the patient to rest in bed for 2 hours before the blood is drawn.
- There is no food or fluid restriction.

- Factors Affecting Laboratory Results

  - Certain drugs can affect cortisol levels (see Drug influences).
  - Physical activity prior to the blood test might decrease cortisol level.
  - Obesity can cause an elevated serum level.
  - Inaccurate labeling of the blood specimen (ie, with the wrong time) can affect results.

NURSING IMPLICATIONS WITH RATIONALE

- Obtain a history on drugs taken prior to hospital admission or the test. Oral contraceptives and estrogen taken within 6 weeks of the test can cause false positive results.

Decreased Level

- Observe for signs and symptoms of Addison's disease (adrenal cortical insufficiency). Symptoms are anorexia, vomiting, abdominal pain, fatigue, dizziness, trembling, and diaphoresis.

Elevated Level

■ Observe for signs and symptoms of Cushing's syndrome (excess adrenal cortical hormone). Symptoms are fat deposits in the face (moonface), neck, and in the back of the chest; irritability; mood swings; bleeding under the skin; muscle wasting; and weakness.

Patient Teaching

■ Instruct the patient that he or she should be on bed rest for 2 hours prior to the test. Physical activity affects the cortisol level.

C-REACTIVE PROTEIN (CRP) (SERUM)

Reference Values

Adult: not usually present; > 1:2 titer, positive

Child: not usually present

Description

CRP appears in the blood 6 to 10 hours after an acute inflammatory process and tissue destruction, and it peaks within 48 to 72 hours. CRP is a nonspecific test ordered for diagnostic reasons similar to those for the erythrocyte sedimentation rate test (ESR), but CRP precedes ESR during inflammation and necrosis and returns to normal sooner. Serum CRP is also found in many of our body fluids (ie, pleural, peritoneal, and synovial).

The CRP test is used to monitor acute inflammatory phases of rheumatoid arthritis and rheumatic fever so that early treatment can be initiated before progressive tissue damage occurs. CPR elevates during bacterial infections but not viral infections.[1,3,7,9,10]

Clinical Problems

Normal Level: Drug Suppression: steroids (cortisone, prednisone), salicylates (asprin)

Elevated Level: rheumatoid arthritis, rheumatic fever, acute myocardial infarction, cancer (breast and with metastasis), inflammatory bowel disease, Hodgkin's disease, systemic lupus erythematosus, bacterial infections, late pregnancy, intrauterine contraceptive devices. *Drug Influence:* oral contraceptives

Procedure

■ Collect 5 to 7 mL of venous blood in a red-top tube. Avoid heat, since CRP is thermolabile.
■ Keep the patient NPO except for water for 8 to 12 hours before the test. Laboratory policies on NPO could vary and should be checked.

■ **Factors Affecting Laboratory Results**

- ■ Pregnancy (third trimester) could elevate CRP level.
- ■ Oral contraceptives and intrauterine contraceptive devices might elevate CRP level.

NURSING IMPLICATIONS WITH RATIONALE

Elevated Level

- ■ Recognize that an elevated serum CRP level is associated with an active inflammatory process and tissue destruction (necrosis). The CRP test is nonspecific; however, the CRP is elevated during acute rheumatic fever, rheumatoid arthritis, and acute myocardial infarction.
- ■ Assess for signs and symptoms of an acute inflammatory process, such as pain and swelling in joints, heat, redness, increased body temperature.
- ■ Notify the physician of a recurrence (exacerbation) of an acute inflammation. The physician may wish to order a serum CRP test.
- ■ Check the results of the serum CRP level. If the titer is decreasing, the patient is responding to treatment and/or the acute phase is declining. CRP may be compared to ESR. The serum CRP level will elevate and return to normal faster than the ESR level.

CREATINE PHOSPHOKINASE (CPK) (SERUM), CPK ISOENZYMES (SERUM)
Creatine Kinase (CK)

Reference Values

Adult: Male: 5–35 μg/mL, 30–180 IU/L, 55–170 U/L at 37°C (SI units). *Female:* 5–25 μg/mL, 25–150 IU/L, 30–135 U/L at 37°C (SI units)

Child: Newborn: 65–580 IU/L at 30°C. *Child:* Male: 0–70 IU/L at 30°C; Female: 0–50 IU/L at 30°C

CPK isoenzymes			
	CPK-MM:	94%–100%	(muscle)
	CPK-MB:	0%–6%	(heart)
	CPK-BB:	0%	(brain)

Description

Creatine phosphokinase (CPK), also known as creatine kinase (CK), is an enzyme found in high concentration in the heart and skeletal muscles and in low concentration in the brain tissue. Serum CPK/CK is frequently elevated by skeletal muscle disease, acute myocardial infarction, cerebral vascular disease, vigorous exercise, IM injections, and electrolyte imbalance-hypokalemia. CPK/CK has two types of isoenzymes: M, associated with muscle, and B, associated with the brain. Electrophoresis separates the isoenzymes into three subdivi-

103

sions: MM (in skeletal muscle and some in the heart), MB (in the heart), and BB (in brain tissue). When CPK/CK is elevated, a CPK electrophoresis is done to determine which group of isoenzymes is elevated. Increased isoenzyme CPK-MB could indicate damage to the myocardial cells.

Serum CPK/CK and CPK-MB rise within 4 to 6 hours after an acute myocardial infarction, reach a peak in 18 to 24 hours (> 6 times the normal value), and then return to normal within 3 to 4 days, unless new necrosis or tissue damage occurs. If medication for acute myocardial infarction has to be given parenterally, (for instance, morphine), it would be better to give it intravenously than intramuscularly so that mild muscle injury (from IM) would not elevate the CPK level; however, injections have little or no effect on CPK-MB. Draw blood for a serum CPK/CK level before giving an IM injection.[1,5,10–12,21]

Clinical Problems

Elevated Level: acute myocardial infarction (AMI), skeletal muscle disease, cerebrovascular accident (CVA), and with all, elevated CPK isoenzymes. *Drug Influences:* IM injections, dexamethasone (Decadron), furosemide (Lasix), aspirin (high doses), ampicillin, carbenicillin, clofibrate

CPK-MM isoenzyme: muscular dystrophy, delirium tremens, crush injury/ trauma, surgery and postoperative state, vigorous exercise, IM injections, hypokalemia, hemophilia, hypothyroidism

CPK-MB: AMI, severe angina pectoris, cardiac surgery, cardiac ischemia, myocarditis, hypokalemia, cardiac defibrillation

CPK-BB: CVA, subarachnoid hemorrhage, cancer of the brain, acute brain injury, Reye's syndrome, pulmonary embolism and infarction, seizures

Procedure

- Collect 5–7 mL of venous blood in a red-top tube. Avoid hemolysis.
- Note on the laboratory slip the number of times the patient has received IM injections in the last 24 to 48 hours.
- There is no food or fluid restriction.

■ Factors Affecting Laboratory Results

- IM injections can cause an elevated serum level of total CPK/CK.
- Vigorous exercise elevates the levels.
- Trauma and surgical intervention elevate serum levels.

NURSING IMPLICATIONS WITH RATIONALE

- Avoid giving IM injections until after blood is drawn for CPK.

Elevated Level

- Relate elevated serum CPK/CK and isoenzymes (CPK-MM, CPK-MB, and CPK-BB) to clinical problems. The CPK-MB is useful in making the differential diagnosis of myocardial infarction.

■ Indicate whether the patient has received an IM injection in the last 24 to 48 hours on the laboratory slip, and chart.

■ Assess the patient's signs and symptoms of an acute myocardial infarction. Symptoms include pain; dyspnea; diaphoresis (excess perspiration); cold, clammy skin; pallor, and arrhythmia.

■ Check the serum CPK/CK level at intervals, and notify the physician of serum level changes. The serum CPK/CK may be repeated every 6 to 8 hours during the acute phase. When the CPK/CK and CPK-MB are highly elevated, there may be extensive muscle damage to the myocardium. For acute myocardial infarction, also check results of the AST (SGOT) and LDH tests.

■ Compare serum AST/SGOT and LDH levels with CPK and CPK-MB.

■ Provide measures for alleviating pain.

CREATININE (SERUM)

Reference Values

Adult: 0.5–1.5 mg/dL; 45–132.3 μmol/L (SI units). Females may have slightly lower values due to less muscle mass.

Child: Newborn: 0.8–1.4 mg/dL. *Infant:* 0.7–1.7 mg/dL. *Child* (2–6 years): 0.3–0.6 mg/dL, 27–54 μmol/L (SI units). *Older Child:* 0.4–1.2 mg/dL, 36–106 μmol/L (SI units). Values increase slightly with age due to muscle mass.

Elderly: may have decreased values due to decreased muscle mass and decreased creatinine production.

Description

Creatinine, a by-product of muscle catabolism, is derived from the breakdown of muscle creatine phosphate. The amount of creatinine produced is proportional to the muscle mass. Creatinine is filtered by the glomeruli and it is excreted in the urine.

Serum creatinine is considered a more sensitive and specific indicator of renal disease than BUN. It rises later and is *not influenced by diet or fluid intake.* A slight BUN elevation could be indicative of hypovolemia (fluid volume deficit); however, a serum creatinine of 2.5 mg/dL could be indicative of renal impairment. BUN and creatinine are frequently compared. If BUN increases and serum creatinine remains normal, dehydration (hypovolemia) is present; and if both increase, then renal disorder is present. Serum creatinine is especially useful in evaluation of glomerular function.[3,6,10,13,22]

Clinical Problems

Decreased Level: pregnancy, eclampsia

Elevated Level: acute and chronic renal failure, shock (prolonged), systemic lupus erythematosus, cancer (intestine, bladder, testes, uterus, prostate), leukemias, Hodgkin's disease, essential hypertension, acute myocardial infarction, diabetic nephropathy, CHF (long standing), diet rich in creatinine (ie, beef [high], poultry and fish [minimal] effect). *Drug Influence:* amphotericin B, cephalosporins (cefazolin [Ancef], cephalothin [Keflin]), gentamicin, kanamycin, methicillin, ascorbic acid, barbiturates, lithium carbonate, mithramycin, methyldopa (Aldomet), glucose, protein, ketone bodies (increased), triamterene (Dyrenium)

Procedure

- Collect 5 to 10 mL of venous blood in a red-top tube.
- List any drugs the patient is taking that could elevate the serum level on the laboratory slip.
- There is no food or fluid restriction. Avoid red meats the night before the test.

■ Factors Afffecting Laboratory Results

- Certain drugs (*see Drug Influence*) may increase the serum creatinine level.
- Roast beef consumed in large quantities may affect results.

NURSING IMPLICATIONS WITH RATIONALE

- Relate the elevated creatinine levels to clinical problems. Serum creatinine may be low in patients with small muscle mass, in amputees, and in patients with muscle disease. Older patients may have decreased muscle mass.
- Hold medications (*see Drug Influence*) for 24 hours before the test, with the physician's permission. Certain medications that cannot be withheld should be listed on the laboratory slip and noted on the patient's chart.
- Check the amount of urine output in 24 hours. Less than 600 mL/24 hours can indicate renal insufficiency. Creatinine is excreted by the kidneys, and a continuous decrease in urine output could result in an increased serum creatinine level.
- Compare the BUN and creatinine levels. If both are increased, the problem is most likely kidney disease.

Patient Teaching

- Inform the patient to eat less beef, poultry, and fish if the serum creatinine level is extremely elevated. Normally food does not have an effect on the serum creatinine level.

CREATININE CLEARANCE (URINE)
Creatinine (Urine)

Reference Values

Adult: 85–135 mL/min. Females may have somewhat lower values

Child: similar to adult

Elderly: slightly decreased values than adult due to decreased glomerular filtration rate (GFR) caused by reduced renal plasma flow

Urine Creatinine: 1–2 g/24 hours

Description

Creatinine is a metabolic product of creatine phosphate in skeletal muscle, and it is excreted by the kidneys. Creatinine clearance is considered a reliable test for estimating glomerular filtration rate (GFR). With renal insufficiency, the GFR is decreased, and the serum creatinine is increased. GFR decreases with age, and with the older adult, the creatinine clearance may be diminished to as low as 60 mL/minute.

The creatinine clearance test consists of a 12- or 24-hour urine collection and a blood sample

The formula for calculating creatinine clearance test is:

$$\text{Creatinine clearance} = \frac{\text{Urine creatinine (mg/dL)} \times \text{Urine volume (dL)},}{\text{Serum creatinine (mg/dL)}}$$

A creatinine clearance less than 40 mL/minute is suggestive of moderate to severe renal impairment.[7,9,10,12,13]

Clinical Problems

Decreased Level: mild to severe renal (kidney) impairment, hyperthyroidism, progressive muscular dystrophy, amyotrophic lateral sclerosis (ALS). *Drug Influence:* Phenacetin, steroids (anabolic), thiazides

Elevated Level: hypothyroidism, hypertension (renovascular), exercise. *Drug Influence:* ascorbic acid, steroids, levodopa, methyldopa (Aldomet), phenolsulfonphthalein (PSP) test

Procedure

- Hydrate patient before test.
- Avoid meats, poultry, fish, tea and coffee for 6 hours before the test and during test with the physician's permission.
- List drugs patient is taking on the laboratory slip that could affect test results.
  Blood: collect 5 to 10 mL of venous blood in a red-top tube the morning of the test.
  Urine: Have the patient void and discard the urine before the test begins. Note the time. Save all urine during the specified time (12 hours or 24 hours) in a urine container, without any preservative, that is refrigerated or kept on ice.

■ Encourage water intake hourly during the test to have sufficient urine output.
■ Label the container with the exact time and date the urine collection started and ended.

■ Factors Affecting Laboratory Results

■ Phenacetin decreases the creatinine clearance.
■ Toilet paper and feces will contaminate the urine.

NURSING IMPLICATIONS WITH RATIONALE

■ Inform the physician of medications the patient is receiving that could cause false test results.

Patient Teaching

■ Explain to the patient the procedure for blood and urine collection. Blood is drawn in the morning. The patient voids and the urine is discarded. Then all urine is saved for 12 hours or 24 hours in a urine container. Toilet paper and feces should not be in the urine.
■ Instruct the patient not to eat meats, poultry, fish, tea, or coffee for 6 hours before the test or during the test, according to the physicians' orders.
■ Encourage water intake throughout the test—approximately 100 mL/hour.
■ Instruct patient not to do strenuous exercise during the test.

CROSS MATCHING (BLOOD)
Blood Typing Tests, Compatibility Test for RBC, Type and Cross Match

Reference Values
Adult: compatibility; absence of agglutination (clumping) of cells
Child: same as adult

Description
The four *major* blood types (A, B, AB, and O) belong to the ABO blood group system. RBCs have either antigen A, B, AB, or none on the surface of the cells. Type A has A antigen, B has B antigen, AB has A and B antigens, and O does not contain an antigen. These antigens are capable of producing antibodies. The AB blood person is the universal recipient (can accept all blood), since there are no antibodies; the O blood person is the universal donor (can give blood to all types).

ABO blood type and Rh factor are first determined. Then the compatibility of donor and recipient blood is determined by major crossmatch. The major crossmatch is between the donor's RBC and the recipient's serum and is checked to determine if the recipient has any antibodies to destroy the donor's RBC.[8,10,13]

Procedure

- Collect 7–10 mL of venous blood in a red-top tube.
- There is no food or fluid restriction.

■ Factors Affecting Laboratory Results

- Previously received incompatible blood can make blood cross matching difficult.

NURSING IMPLICATIONS WITH RATIONALE

- Observe the patient for signs and symptoms of fluid volume deficit (hypovolemia) such as tachycardia (pulse > 100), tachypnea (rapid breathing), pale color, clammy skin, and low BP (late symptoms). Crystalloid solutions (saline, lactated Ringer's) might be given rapidly to replace fluid volume until a transfusion can be administered. Usually 15 to 45 minutes are required to type and cross match blood.
- Check the date of the unit of blood. Usually blood should be used within 28 days. Blood that is older than 28 days should not be given to a patient having hyperkalemia.
- Monitor the recipient's vital signs before and during transfusions. Signs and symptoms of transfusion reaction include temperature > 1.1°C, chills and dyspnea.
- Start the blood transfusion at a slow rate for the first 15 minutes, stay with patient and observe for adverse reactions.
- Flush the transfusion set with normal saline if other intravenous solutions are ordered to follow the blood.

CRYOGLOBULINS (SERUM)

Reference Values
Adult: up to 6 mg/dL
Child: negative

Description
Cryoglobulins are serum globulins (protein) that precipitate from the plasma at 4°C and return to a dissolved status when warmed. They are present in IgG and IgM groups and are usually found in such pathologic conditions as leuke-

mia, multiple myeloma, systemic lupus erythematosus (SLE), rheumatoid arthritis, and hemolytic anemia.[8,9,13,14]

Clinical Problems

Elevated Level (> 2% precipitation): SLE, rheumatoid arthritis, polyarteritis nodosa, Hodgkin's disease, lymphocytic leukemia, multiple myeloma, acquired hemolytic anemias (autoimmune), cirrhosis (biliary), Waldenström's macroglobulinemia

Procedure

- Collect 5 to 10 mL of venous blood in a red-top tube.
- The blood sample should not be refrigerated before it is taken to the laboratory.
- There is no food or fluid restriction.

■ **Factors Affecting Laboratory Results**

- None reported

NURSING IMPLICATIONS WITH RATIONALE

Elevated Level

- Recognize that increased presence of cryoglobulins, might be caused by autoimmune diseases, collagen diseases, and leukemia.
- Observe for signs and symptoms of SLE (ie, "butterfly" rash [erythematosus rash on the cheeks and the bridge of the nose], arthritis, and urinary insufficiency).
- Observe for signs and symptoms of rheumatoid arthritis (ie, pain and stiffness in the joints [especially in the morning]; swollen, red, tender joints; joint deformities; and inability to make a fist and flexion contractures).
- Compare serum cryoglobulins with other laboratory tests.

CULTURES (BLOOD, SPUTUM, STOOL, THROAT, WOUND, URINE)

Reference Values

Adult: negative or no pathogen

Child: same as adult

Description

(*Also see Antibiotic Susceptibility Test.*)

Cultures are taken to isolate the microorganism that is causing the clinical infection. Most culture specimens are obtained using sterile swabs with medium (solid or broth), a sterile container (cup) with a lid, and a sterile syringe with a sterile bottle of liquid medium. The culture specimen should be taken immediately to the laboratory after collection (no longer than 30 minutes), since some organisms will die if not placed in the proper medium and incubated.

Most specimens for culture are either blood, sputum, stool, throat secretions, wound exudate, or urine. It usually takes 24 to 36 hours to grow the organisms and 48 hours for the growth and culture report.[5,7–10,12]

Clinical Problems

SPECIMEN	CLINICAL CONDITION OR ORGANISM
Blood	Bacteremia, Septicemia, Postoperative shock, Fever of unknown origin (FUO)
Sputum	Pulmonary tuberculosis, Bacterial pneumonia, Chronic bronchitis, Bronchiectasis
Stool	*Salmonella* species, *Shigella* species, Enteropathogenic *Escherichia coli, Staphylococcus* species
Throat	B-hemolytic streptococci (rheumatic fever), Thrush (*Candida* species), Tonsillar infection, *Staphylococcus aureus*
Wound	*Staphylococcus* species: *S aureus, Pseudomonas aeruginosa, Proteus* species, *Bacteroides* species, *Klebsiella* species, *Serratia* species
Urine	*Escherichia coli, Klebsiella* species, *Pseudomonas aeruginosa, Serratia* species, *Shigella* species, Yeasts: *Candida* species

Procedure

- Hand washing is essential before and after collection of the specimen.
- Send the specimen for culture to the laboratory *immediately* after collection.
- Obtain the specimen before antibiotic therapy is started. If the patient is receiving antibiotics, the drug(s) should be listed on the laboratory slip.
- Collection containers or tubes should be sterile. Aseptic technique should be used during collection. Contamination of the specimen could cause false-positive results and/or transmission of the organisms.
- Check with the laboratory for specific techniques used.

Blood: cleanse the patient's skin according to the institution's procedure. Usually the skin is scrubbed first with povidone-iodine (Betadine). Iodine can be irritating to the skin, so it is removed and an application of benzalkonium chloride or alcohol is applied. Cleanse the top(s) of the culture bottle(s) with iodine and leave it or them to dry. The bottle(s) should contain a culture medium. Collect 5 to 10 mL of venous blood and place in the sterile bottle. Special vacuum tubes containing a culture medium for blood may be used instead of a culture bottle.

Sputum: Sterile Container or Cup: Obtain sputum for culture early in the morning, before breakfast. Instruct the patient to give several deep coughs to raise sputum. Tell the patient to avoid spitting saliva secretion into the sterile container. Saliva and postnasal drip secretions can contaminate the sputum specimen. Keep a lid on the sterile container. The container *should not* be completely filled and should be taken immediately to the laboratory. The sputum sample should not remain for hours by the patient's bedside unless one needs a 24-hour sputum specimen (in this case, an extra sterile container should be left). *Acid-Fast Bacilli (TB Culture)*: Follow the instructions on the container. Collect 5 to 10 mL of sputum, and take the sample immediately to the laboratory or refrigerate the specimen. Three sputum specimens may be requested, one each day for 3 days. Check for proper labeling.

Stool: Collect an approximately 1-inch-diameter feces sample. Use a sterile tongue blade and place the stool specimen in a sterile container with a lid. The suspected disease or organism should be noted on the laboratory slip. The stool specimen should not contain urine. The patient should not be given barium or mineral oil, which can inhibit bacteria growth.

Throat: Use a sterile cotton swab or a polyester-tipped swab. The sterile culture kit could be used. Swab the inflamed or ulcerated tonsillar and/or postpharyngeal areas of the throat. Place the applicator in a culturette tube with its culture medium. Take the throat culture specimen immediately to the laboratory. Do *not* give antibiotics before taking the culture.

Wound: Use a culture kit containing a sterile cotton swab or a polyester-tipped swab and a tube with culture medium. Swab the exudate of the wound and place the swab in the tube containing a culture medium. Wear sterile gloves when there is an excess amount of purulent drainage.

Urine: Clean-Caught (Midstream) Urine Specimen: Clean-caught urine collection is the commonest method for collecting a urine specimen for culture. There are noncatheterization kits giving step-by-step instructions. Catheterizing for urine culture is seldom ordered. Usually the patient collects the urine specimen for culture, so a detailed explanation should be given, according to the instructions. The penis or vulva should be well cleansed. At times, two urine specimens (2 to 10 mL) are requested to verify the organism and in case of a possible contamination of the urine specimen. Collect a midstream urine specimen early in the morning, or as ordered, in a sterile container. The lid should fit tightly on the container and the urine specimen should be taken immediately to the bacteriology laboratory or refrigerated. Label the urine specimen with the patient's name, the date, and the exact time of collection (7/22/92 @ 8:00 A.M.). List any antibiotics or sulfonamides the patient is taking on the laboratory slip.

- **Factors Affecting Laboratory Results**

    - Contamination of the specimen cause inaccurate results.
    - Antibiotics and sulfonamides may cause false-negative results.
    - Urine in the stool collection may cause false test results.

NURSING IMPLICATIONS WITH RATIONALE

- Explain the procedure for obtaining the culture specimen. Answer questions. If the patient participates in the collection of the specimen (eg, urine), the procedure should be reviewed several times.

- Hold antibiotics or sulfonamides until after the specimen has been collected. These drugs could cause false negative results. If these drugs have been given, they should be listed on the laboratory slip and recorded on the patient's chart.
- Deliver all specimens immediately to the laboratory or refrigerate the specimen.
- Handle the specimen(s) with extreme care. Aseptic technique should be used. Prevent contamination of the specimen(s) or transmission of the organism to other patients or yourself. Observe strict aseptic techniques.
- Keep lids on sterile specimen containers. Sputum cups should not be uncovered by the bedside.
- Suggest a culture if a pathogenic organism is suspected. Check the patient's temperature.

DEXAMETHASONE SUPPRESSION TEST (DST)
ACTH Suppression Test

Reference Values

>50% reduction of plasma cortisol and urine 17-hydroxycorticosteroids (17-OHCS).

Rapid or Overnight Screening Test: plasma cortisol: 8 AM <10 μg/dL; 4 PM <5 μg/dL. Urine 17-OHCS (5-hour specimen): <4 mg/5 hours

Increased Dexamethasone Dose: Low Dose: plasma cortisol: one half of patient's base-line level. Urine 17-OHCS: <2.5 mg/24 hours/second day. *High Dose:* plasma cortisol: one half of patient's base-line level. Urine 17 OHCS: one half of patient's base-line level

Note: High dose is done if results do not change with low dose of dexamethasone.

Description

Dexamethasone (Decadron) is a potent glucocorticoid. The dexamethasone suppression test distinguishes between adrenal hyperplasia and adrenal tumor as the cause of adrenal hyperfunction, and is used to diagnose and to manage depression.

When given dexamethasone, there is a reduction (suppression) in ACTH secretion (negative feedback), thus causing a lower plasma and urine cortisol. Low-dose and high-dose dexamethasone are used to distinguish between adrenal hyperplasia and adrenal tumor (nonsuppress at low or high doses). Adrenal hyperplasia will suppress at high doses but not at low doses.

In psychiatry the DST is useful in diagnosing affective diseases, such as endogenous depression (melancholia). In approximately 50% of these patients, suppression of plasma cortisol does not occur.

The test could be a rapid or overnight screening test or a 2-day test (8 doses of dexamethasone) with low and/or high doses of the drug.[3,9,12]

Clinical Problems

No Plasma Cortisol or Urine 17-OHCS: adrenal adenoma (tumor), ectopic ACTH-producing tumor, bilateral adrenal hyperplasia (except with high steroid doses)

Procedure

- Obtain a baseline plasma cortisol and urine 17-OHCS 24 hours before the test.
- Avoid tea, caffeinated coffee, chocolates. No other food or fluid restriction is required.
- Refrigerate urine for 17-OHCS levels.

Rapid or Overnight Screening Test
- NPO after midnight. Check with laboratory policy.
- Give dexamethasone 1 mg or 5 μg/kg PO at 11 P.M.
- Obtain a base-line plasma cortisol and urine 17-OHCS. Draw blood at 8 AM for plasma cortisol. Obtain a urine OHCS at 12 noon.

Increased Dexamethasone Dose: Two days of low or high doses of dexamethasone (Decadron)

Low Dose
- Give dexamethasone 0.5 mg every 6 hours for 2 days (total of 4 mg).
- Obtain a plasma cortisol level at 8 AM, 4 PM, and 11 PM and 24-hour urine OHCS after 2-day low-dose test. If no suppression, the high-dose test may be recommended.

High Dose
- Give dexamethasone 2 mg every 6 hours for 2 days (total of 16 mg).
- Obtain a plasma cortisol level at 8 AM, 4 PM, and 11 PM and 24-hour urine OHCS after 2-day high-dose test.

■ Factors Affecting Laboratory Results

- Ingestion of excess coffee, tea, and chocolates could increase steroid release.
- Not refrigerating urine for 17-OHCS test could affect results.

NURSING IMPLICATIONS WITH RATIONALE

- Report anxiety, stress, fever, infection to the physician.
- Obtain a base line plasma cortisol and urine 17-OHCS 24 hours before the test. For the screening test, plasma cortisol should be obtained at 8 AM and urine 17-OHCS at 12 noon. For the 2-day dexamethasone test, plasma and urine test should be obtained after 2 days of low or high dexamethasone dosage.
- Administer dexamethasone at specified times *on time*. Milk or antacids may be required to decrease gastric irritation.
- Provide ample time for the patient to ask questions. Refer unknown answers to appropriate health professionals.

- Assess for side effects of dexamethasone resulting from high doses (ie, weight gain, gastric discomfort).
- Monitor electrolytes during test. Steroid causes serum potassium loss and serum sodium excess.
- Check blood glucose with Chemstrip bG for hyperglycemia while the patient is taking high doses of dexamethasone. This drug is a glucocorticosteroid and can elevate blood glucose levels.
- Be supportive to patient and family members during the test. This is a time-consuming test procedure. Cooperation from patient and family members is needed for accurate results.

Patient Teaching

- Instruct the patient to avoid caffeinated coffee, tea, and chocolate.

DIAZEPAM (SERUM)
(Valium)

Reference Values
Therapeutic: Adult: 0.5–2.0 mg/L, 400–600 ng/mL
Toxic: Adult: 3 mg/L, > 3000 ng/mL

Description
Diazepam (Valium), a benzodiazepine, has been one of the most commonly prescribed antianxiety agent in the United States. The clinical uses of diazepam include treatment of status epilepticus; alcohol withdrawal; induction of anesthesia for minor surgical procedures, endoscopic procedures; cardioversion; and muscle relaxation, especially for paraplegics, cerebral palsy, tetanus.

Diazepam is absorbed from the GI tract and is metabolized in the liver to a large number of metabolites. Peak blood level occurs 1 to 2 hours after the oral dose. After a single oral dose of 10 to 15 mg, peak value level usually is 200 to 300 ng/mL. Half-life is 10 to 40 hours (40 hours with continuous use). The major metabolite, *N*-desmethyldiazepam, has a half-life of 50 to 90 hours. Onset of action is 30 to 60 minutes after oral dose, 15 to 30 minutes after IM injection, and 1 to 5 minutes after IV dose. Diazepam is excreted in the urine as metabolites. This drug can cross the placenta and might cause teratogeny (birth defects).

Steady state for serum diazepam level may take 1 to 2 weeks. Monitoring the serum diazepam level should be continued after the steady state, and especially when daily dose is changed.[2,3,11,13]

Clinical Problems

Decreased Level: smoking

Elevated Level: diazepam overdose, liver disease, alcohol. *Drug Influence:* cimetidine (Tagamet), isoniazid (INH), valproic acid (Depakene)

Procedure

■ Collect 3 to 5 mL of venous blood in a red-top tube 2 hours after an oral dose or at trough level (before the next dose).

■ Record the dose, route, and last-administered dose on the laboratory requisition slip.

■ There is no food or fluid restriction.

■ Factors Affecting Laboratory Results

■ Drugs (*see Drug Influence above*) might cause an increased diazepam level.

■ Taking other benzodiazepines (ie, chlordiazepoxide [Librium], chlorazepate dipotassium [Tranxene], along with diazepam will interfere with correct test results, since these agents contain many of the same active metabolites.

NURSING IMPLICATIONS WITH RATIONALE

■ Record dose, route, and last time the drug was given on the requisition slip. Usually the blood specimen is drawn 2 hours after taking diazepam.

■ Elicit from a female patient if she is pregnant or intends to become pregnant before giving diazepam. This drug may have teratogenic effects.

■ Monitor frequently serum diazepam levels in children, in the elderly, and in debilitated adults. Small doses of diazepam should be given to these individuals to avoid diazepam toxicity.

■ Recognize that erratic absorption of diazepam could result from IM administration. Diazepam toxicity could occur after numerous injections.

Decreased Level

■ Recognize that smoking can decrease diazepam level.

■ Avoid administering diazepam in IV fluids. This drug could precipitate in the fluids or adhere to the IV bag or tubing, thus decreasing prescribed dosage.

Elevated Level

■ Recognize that diazepam overdose, liver disease, or alcohol could elevate serum diazepam level.

■ Check for signs and symptoms of diazepam toxicity (ie, drowsiness, ataxia, confusion, headache, slurred speech, tremors, hypotension, tachycardia, and circulatory collapse).

Patient Teaching

- Instruct the patient not to ingest alcohol or other CNS depressants while taking diazepam. The effects of taking these substances together could cause severe drowsiness, respiratory distress, or respiratory arrest.
- Explain to the patient that diazepam should never be abruptly discontinued. Diazepam is tapered to lower doses over 1 to 2 weeks to avoid withdrawal symptoms (ie, confusion, tremors, paranoia, ataxia, visual hallucinations, sweating, and abdominal and muscle cramps).

DIFFERENTIAL WHITE BLOOD CELL (WBC) COUNT
(See WBC Differential)

DIGOXIN (SERUM)
(Lanoxin)

Reference Values

Therapeutic: Adult: 0.5–2 ng/mL; 0.5–2 nmol/L (SI units). *Infants:* 1–3 ng/mL. *Child:* same as adult

Toxic: Adult: >2 ng/mL; >2.6 nmol/L (SI units). *Infants:* >3.5 ng/mL. *Child:* same as adult

Description

Digoxin, a form of digitalis, is a cardiac glycoside agent given to increase the force and velocity of myocardial contraction. More than 75% to 95% of the drug is absorbed through the GI tract, and a large amount of digoxin is excreted unchanged through the kidneys. The half-life of digoxin is 35 to 40 hours, with a shorter half-life in neonates and infants and a longer time in short-term infants/premature infants.

Serum plateau levels of digoxin occur 6 to 8 hours after an oral dose, 2 to 4 hours after IV administration, and 10 to 12 hours after IM administration. The most frequent routes used for administering digoxin are by mouth (oral) and IV.

Electrolyte imbalance (hypokalemia or hypomagnesemia), acid-base disturbances, and certain drugs predispose the person to digitalis toxicity. Common signs and symptoms of digitalis toxicity include pulse rate <60 per minute, anorexia, nausea, vomiting, headaches, and visual disturbance.[1–4,10]

117

Clinical Problems

Decreased Level: decreased GI absorption, decreased GI motility. *Drug Influence:* antacids, kaopectate, metoclopramide (Reglan), barbiturates, cholestyramine (Questran), spironolactone (Aldactone)

Elevated Level: digoxin overdose, renal disease, liver disease. *Drug Influence:* amphotericin B, diuretics (ethacrynic acid [Edecrin], furosemide [Lasix], thiazides), chlorthalidone (Hygroton), quinidine, reserpine (Serpasil), succinylcholine, sympathomimetics, corticosteroids

Procedure

- Collect 1 to 5 mL of venous blood in a red-top tube.
- Obtain a blood sample 6 to 10 hours after administration of oral digoxin, or, frequently preferred, take sample prior to next dose.
- There is no food or fluid restriction.

■ Factors Affecting Laboratory Results

- Administering digoxin intramuscularly might cause the absorption rate to be erratic, especially in a debilitated or elderly person with poor tissue perfusion.
- A low serum potassium (K) or magnesium (Mg) level could cause digitalis toxicity, and a high serum calcium (Ca) could cause digitalis toxicity.
- Hypothyroidism, severe heart disease, and renal function abnormalities may predispose a patient to digitalis toxicity.

NURSING IMPLICATIONS WITH RATIONALE

- Do not confuse digoxin with other digitalis glycosides (eg, digitoxin). Digitoxin has a longer half-life and cumulative effect.
- Check serum digoxin results and report nontherapeutic levels to the physician immediately.
- Keep digoxin bottle away from light.
- Obtain a blood sample for serum digoxin during predicted plateau levels for oral, IV, and IM administration.
- Take apical pulse for 1 minute prior to administering digoxin. If the pulse rate is below 60 per minute, do not give the digoxin, and notify the physician.

Decreased Level

- Associate GI disturbance and certain drugs (ie, antacids, kaopectate, barbiturates, Questran, Aldactone) with a decreased therapeutic serum-digoxin level. The digoxin dose might need to be increased if those drugs are being taken. If the digoxin dose has been increased while the person is on the drug(s) and later the drug has been discontinued, the digoxin dosage should be decreased.
- Inform the physician which drugs the person is taking that might decrease the effectiveness of the prescribed digoxin dose.

Elevated Level

- Check serum potassium, magnesium, and calcium levels. Hypokalemia, hypomagnesemia, and hypercalcemia enhance the action of digoxin and could cause digitalis toxicity.
- Observe for signs and symptoms of digitalis toxicity (ie, pulse rate <60 per minute, anorexia, nausea, vomiting, headache, visual disturbance).

Patient teaching

- Instruct the patient to take his or her pulse rate before taking digoxin and to call the physician if the rate is <60 per minute in adults or <70 per minute in children.

DILANTIN
(See Phenytoin.)

D-XYLOSE ABSORPTION TEST (BLOOD AND URINE)

Reference Values

Adult: Blood D-xylose: 25–40 mg/dL/2 hours. *Urine D-xylose:* Urine excretion: >3.5 g/5 hours; >5g/24 hours

Child: Blood D-xylose: 30 mg/dL/1 hour

Description

The D-xylose absorption test determines the absorptive capacity of the small intestine. After ingestion of D-xylose, a pentose sugar, serum and urine D-xylose levels are measured. Usually a low serum D-xylose level (<25 mg/dL) and a low urine D-xylose level (<3 gs) are indicative of malabsorption syndrome.

Abnormal test results occur in celiac disease, small-bowel ischemia, Whipple's disease, Zollinger-Ellison syndrome, enteritis, massive intestinal resection, and intestinal bacterial overgrowth.

Various clinical problems such as vomiting, hypomotility, dehydration, alcoholism, rheumatoid arthritis, severe congestive heart failure, ascites, and poor renal function could cause low urine D-xylose levels that are not secondary to intestinal malabsorption. Endoscopic examination and biopsy frequently are necessary to confirm the diagnosis of malabsorption.[3,9]

Clinical Problems

Decreased Level: celiac disease, small-bowel ischemia, Whipple's disease, Zollinger-Ellison syndrome, radiation enteritis, multiple jejunal diverticula, diabetic neuropathic, diarrhea, lymphoma, amyloidosis, scleroderma, massive intestinal resection, bacterial overgrowth.

Procedure

- Restrict foods for 8 hours for adults and for 4 hours for children prior to test. Foods that contain pentose, such as fruits, jams, jellies, and pastries, should be withheld for 24 hours prior to the test.
- The patient ingests 25 g of D-xylose dissolved in 8 oz (240 mL) of water. An additional 8 oz of water should follow the mixture of D-xylose and water. Some institutions use a 5-g dose instead of 25 g. Child dose is based on weight: 0.5 g/kg but not more than 25 g.
- Collect 10 mL of venous blood in a red-top tube. Blood specimens are drawn at 30, 60, and 120 minutes or at 2 hours only after D-xylose ingestion.
- Discard urine specimen before test. Keep all urine refrigerated; at the end of 5 hours, send the urine collection to the laboratory.
- Check order for the length of collection time (ie, 5 hours or 24 hours). Note on the laboratory slip the period of urine collection and the age of the patient. Older adults with mild renal impairment can have a decreased 5-hour test result and a normal 24-hour test.
- Indicate on the laboratory slip any drugs the patient is taking that could affect tests results. Nonsteroidal Anti-inflammatory drugs (NSAIDS) such as aspirin, indomethacin (Indocin); and atropine. These drugs should be withheld for 24 hours. Note the drug dose and the last time it was taken on the laboratory slip.

- Factors Affecting Laboratory Results

  - Drugs such as aspirin, indomethacin (Indocin), and atropine can decrease intestinal absorption.
  - Foods high in pentose (eg, fruits, jams, jellies and pastries) can affect serum and urine D-xylose results.
  - Hemolysis of the blood sample could cause inaccurate test results.
  - Renal impairment or insufficiency could decrease urine output, thus affecting urine test results.
  - Vomiting, dehydration, hypomotility, alcoholism, and other conditions (*see Description*) could cause a decreased urine D-xylose level that is not due to malabsorption.

NURSING IMPLICATIONS WITH RATIONALE

- Explain the blood and urine test procedures to the patient.
- Assess communications for verbal and nonverbal expressions of anxiety and fear concerning tests or the potential or actual problem.
- Report to the physician if the patient is having severe diarrhea, vomiting, and dehydration. These clinical problems could cause a decreased urine D-xylose level.
- Provide ongoing assessment before, during, and after procedure. Document and communicate alterations.

■ Be supportive to the patient and to family members. They might be most anxious about the test procedure and the unknown test results. Patient compliance during the procedure is essential for accurate test results.

Patient Teaching

■ Inform the patient that food is restricted, but fluids are not. Inform the patient not to eat foods high in pentose (jellies, jams, fruits) for 24 hours before the test.

■ Instruct the patient to save all urine during the 5- or 24-hour urine test. Refrigerate urine collection.

■ Instruct the patient to withhold aspirin, indomethacin (Indocin), and atropine or atropine products, with physician's approval, for 24 hours before the test. Aspirin could decrease D-xylose excretion and indomethacin and atropine could decrease intestinal absorption. Note on the laboratory slip the last drug dose and dosage that the patient received.

■ Be prepared to repeat information to the patient and family if anxiety or fear level is determined to be high. Provide written instructions to reinforce verbal instructions.

ERYTHROCYTE OSMOTIC FRAGILITY
(See Osmotic Fragility.)

ERYTHROCYTE SEDIMENTATION RATE (ESR) (BLOOD)
Sedimentation (SED) Rate

Reference Values

Adult: Westergren Method: Male <50 years: 0–10 mm/hour; *Female* <50 years: 0–20 mm/hour; *Male* >50 years: 0–20 mm/hour; *Female:* >50 years: 0–30 mm/hour. *Wintrobe Method: Male:* 0–7 mm/hour; *Female:* 0–15 mm/hour

Child: Newborn: 0–2 mm/hour; *4–14 years:* 0–20 mm/hour

Description

The ESR test (known also as the sedimentation rate or SED rate) measures the rate at which RBCs settle in unclotted blood in millimeters per hour (mm/hour). The ESR test is nonspecific. The rate can be increased in acute inflammatory process, acute and chronic infections, tissue damage (necrosis), rheumatoid collagen diseases, malignancies, and physiologic stress situations (eg, pregnancy). To some hematologists, the ESR test is unreliable, since it is nonspecific and is affected by physiologic factors that cause inaccurate results.

The C-reactive protein (CRP) test is considered more useful than the ESR test because CRP increases more rapidly during an acute inflammatory process and returns to normal faster than ESR. The ESR test is still an old standby used by many physicians as a rough estimate of the disease process and for following the course of illness. With an elevated ESR, other laboratory tests should be conducted to properly identify the clinical problem.[6,7,9,10,12]

Clinical Problems

Decreased Level: polycythemia vera, CHF, sickle cell anemias, infectious mononucleosis, factor V deficiency, degenerative arthritis, angina pectoris. *Drug Influence:* ethambutol (Myambutol), quinine, salicylates (aspirins), cortisone, prednisone

Elevated Level: rheumatoid arthritis, rheumatic fever, acute myocardial infarction, cancer (stomach, colon, breast, liver, kidney), Hodgkin's disease, multiple myeloma, lymphosarcoma, bacterial endocarditis, gout, hepatitis, cirrhosis of the liver, acute pelvic inflammatory disease, syphilis, tuberculosis, glomerulonephritis, systemic lupus erythematosus, hemolytic disease of newborns (erythroblastosis fetalis), pregnancy (second and third trimesters). *Drug Influence:* dextran, methyldopa (Aldomet), methysergide (Sansert), penicillamine (Cuprimine), procainamide (Pronestyl), theophylline, oral contraceptives, vitamin A

Procedure

- Collect 7 mL of venous blood in a lavender-top tube. Keep the specimen in a vertical position.
- Take the blood specimen to the laboratory immediately. Blood should not stand, since the SED rate could increase.
- If the blood specimen is refrigerated, it should be allowed to return to room temperature before it is tested.
- There is no food or fluid restriction.
- Hold medications that can cause false-positive results for 24 hours before the test with physician's permission.

- Factors Affecting Laboratory Results

  - Factors increasing the SED rate—pregnancy (second and third trimesters); menstruation; drugs (*see Drug Influence*); the presence of cholesterol, fibrinogen, and globulins
  - Factors decreasing the SED rate—newborns (decreased fibrinogen level); drugs (*see Drug Influence*); high blood sugar, serum albumin, and serum phospholipids

---

NURSING IMPLICATIONS WITH RATIONALE

Elevated Level

- Relate elevated ESR levels to clinical problems and drugs. The ESR test is a nonspecific test but it can indicate an inflammatory process occurring.
- Answer the patient's questions about the significance of an increased ESR

---

level. An answer could be that other laboratory tests are usually performed in conjunction with the ESR test for adequate diagnosis of a clinical problem.
■ Compare ESR with CRP test results.

ESTRADIOL (E$_2$) SERUM

Reference Values

Adult: Female: Follicular phase: 20–150 pg/mL; Midcycle: 100–500 pg/mL; *Luteal phase:* 60–260 pg/mL. Postmenopausal: <30 pg/mL. *Male:* 15–50 pg/mL

Child: 3–10 pg/mL

Description

Estradiol (E$_2$) evaluates gonadal dysfunction such as amenorrhea syndromes and testicular tumors. It is *not* used to evaluate fetal well-being in pregnant females.[1,3,6]

Clinical Problems

Decreased Level: primary amenorrhea, anorexia nervosa, ovarian failure, pituitary insufficiency (hypopituitarism), menopause

Elevated Level: ovarian tumors, testicular tumors, adrenal hyperplasia or tumors

Procedure

■ Collect 7 mL of venous blood in a red-top tube. In the female the blood sample may be drawn before ovulation occurs or at midcycle in the AM.
■ List on the laboratory slip the phase of the menstrual cycle.
■ There is no food or fluid restriction.

■ Factors Affecting Laboratory Results

■ Incorrect listing of the menstrual phase could affect the test result.

NURSING IMPLICATIONS WITH RATIONALE

■ Obtain the phase of the menstrual cycle from the patient. Record on the laboratory slip.
■ Ascertain patient's concern about the test result. Be supportive.

ESTRIOL (E₃) SERUM AND URINE

Reference Values
Pregnancy

SERUM		URINE	
Weeks of Gestation	**ng/dL**	**Weeks of Gestation**	**mg/24 hrs**
25–28	25–165	25–28	6–28
29–32	30–230	29–32	6–32
33–36	45–370	33–36	10–45
37–38	75–420	37–40	15–60
39–40	95–450		

Description

E_3 is a major estrogenic compound produced largely by the placenta. It increases in maternal serum and urine after 2 months of pregnancy and continues at high levels until term. If toxemia, hypertension, or diabetes is present after 30 weeks of gestation, E_3 levels are monitored. A decline in serum or urine E_3 levels suggests fetal distress caused by placental malfunction.

Serum estriol is replacing urine estriol due to the ease of specimen collection and since there is no 24-hour waiting period. The advantage of the 24-hour urine estriol is to avoid estriol value variations that usually occur within the day. A urine estriol averages out the "within-day" fluctuations of estriol. Repeated serum and/or urine estriol are frequently ordered.[1,3,6,9,10,13]

Clinical Problems

Decreased Level: fetal distress, placental dysfunction, diabetic pregnancy, pregnancy with hypertension, impending toxemia

Elevated Level: urinary tract infection, glycosuria. *Drug Influence:* antibiotics (ampicillin, neomycin), hydrochlorothiazide (Hydrodiuril), cortisone preparations

Procedure

■ There is no food or fluid restriction.

Serum

■ Collect 5 to 10 mL of venous blood in a red-top tube.

Urine

■ Collect urine for 24 hours in a large container with preservative.
■ Label the patients' name, and date, and the exact times of collection (eg, 3/28/93, 8 AM to 3/29/93, 8:03 AM).
■ Two 24-hour urine specimens (taken a day apart) are usually ordered for more valid results.

■ Factors Affecting Laboratory Results

■ Multiple pregnancy can increase levels.
■ Incorrect gestation week can cause false test result.
■ Glycosuria and urinary tract infection could give false urine-estriol results.

NURSING IMPLICATIONS WITH RATIONALE

■ Monitor the fetal heart rate, the patient's BP, and sugar in the urine. Hypertension and diabetes could cause placental dysfunction leading to fetal distress.
■ Report glycosuria and urinary tract infection during pregnancy; both could cause a false result.
■ Be supportive of patient and family.

Patient Teaching

■ Instruct the patient that several blood samples may be taken. If a urine collection is ordered, instruct the patient that all urine should be saved and that there may be more than one 24-hour urine specimen requested.

ESTROGEN (SERUM)

Reference Values

Adult: Female: Early menstrual cycle: 60–400 pg/mL; Midmenstrual cycle: 120–440 pg/mL; Late menstrual cycle: 150–350 pg/mL; Postmenopausal: <30 pg/mL. *Male:* 40–115 pg/mL. *Child:* 1–6 years: 3–10 pg/mL; 8–12 years: <30 pg/mL

Description

Estrogens are produced by the ovaries, adrenal cortex, and testes. There are over 30 estrogens identified in the body, but only three measurable types of estrogens: estrone (E_1), estradiol (E_2), and estroil (E_3). Total serum estrogen reflects E_1, mostly E_2, and some E_3. For fetal well-being during pregnancy, serum E_3 is used.[3,6,9]

Clinical Problems

Decreased Level: ovarian failure or dysfunction, primary hypogonadism, Turner's syndrome, intrauterine death in pregnancy, pituitary insufficiency, postmenopausal symptoms, anorexia nervosa, psychogenic stress

Elevated Level: ovarian tumors, precocious puberty, adrenal hyperplasia or tumors, testicular tumor, cirrhosis of the liver

Procedure

- Collect 5 to 10 mL of venous blood in a red-top tube. Avoid hemolipis.
- Indicate on the laboratory slip the phase of the patient's menstrual cycle.
- There is no food or fluid restriction.

■ Factors Affecting Laboratory Results

- Oral contraceptives can increase estrogen level; steroids can affect test results; and clomiphene, an estrogen antagonist, could decrease estrogen level.
- Shaking the blood sample could cause hemolysis.

NURSING IMPLICATIONS WITH RATIONALE

- Indicate on the laboratory slip if the patient is taking steroids, oral contraceptives, or estrogens.
- Note on the laboratory slip the phase of patient's menstrual cycle.
- Assess communications for verbal and nonverbal expressions of anxiety and fear concerning tests or the potential or actual problem.
- Encourage ventilation of feelings through provision of a private, calm environment. Use quiet, steady speech patterns when interacting with the patient. Employ touch if appropriate.

Decreased Level

- Note and record if the patient is postmenopausal.

Elevated Level

- Recognize clinical problems that increase estrogen level. Men can have increased estrogen level caused by adrenal or testicular tumors.
- Assess for signs and symptoms of estrogen excess in men, i.e., enlarged breast, voice change.
- Be supportive to patients, female and male, having excess estrogen levels. Encourage them to express their concerns.

ESTROGENS (TOTAL) (URINE—24 HOURS)

Reference Values

Adult: Female: Preovulation: 5–25 μg/24 hours; Follicular phase: 24–100 μg/24 hours; Luteal phase; 22–80 μg/24 hours; Postmenopause: 0–10 μg/24 hours.
Male: 4–25 μg/24 hours
Child: *<12 years:* 1 μg/24 hours; *Postpuberty:* same as adult

Description

Estrogens, hormones composed of estrone, estradiol, and estriol, are produced by the ovary, by the adrenal gland, and in pregnancy by the placenta. (*Also see Estriol.*) This 24-hour urine test is useful for diagnosing ovarian disorders and for the analysis of tumor tissue in breast cancer. To evaluate ovarian dysfunction, the age of the patient and the phase of the menstrual cycle should be known.[8,9,13]

Clinical Problems

Decreased Level: ovarian dysfunction, ovarian agenesis, infantilism, pregnancy (intrauterine death), menopausal and postmenopausal symptoms. *Drug Influence:* phenothiazines (in some cases), tetracyclines (in some cases), vitamins

Elevated Level: adrenocortical tumor, adrenocortical hyperplasia, ovarian tumor, some testicular tumors, pregnancy (gradual increase from the first trimester on). *Drug Influence:* phenothiazines, tetracyclines, vitamins (in some cases)

Procedure

- Collect a 24-hour urine sample in a refrigerated container. A preservative is usually added.
- There is no food or fluid restriction.
- Label the urine bottle with the patient's name, the date, and the exact time of collection (eg, 5/24/92 7:02 AM to 5/25/92, 7:01 AM.). Toilet paper or feces should not be in the urine.
- Record patient's age and phase of the menstrual cycle on the laboratory slip.

■ Factors Affecting Laboratory Results

- Certain drugs may cause a decrease or an increase in the estrogen level (*see Drug Influence above*).
- Saving only part of the 24-hour urine sample may cause an inaccurate result.

NURSING IMPLICATIONS WITH RATIONALE

- Check to see that a preservative is in the urine container. If not, notify the laboratory.
- Inform the patient and family that all urine should be saved and placed in the refrigerated container. Toilet paper and feces should not be in the urine.

Decreased Level

- Obtain a history of menstrual problems and the present menstrual cycle (eg, 14 days since the last menstrual period). The phase of the menstrual cycle has an influence on the result of the test.

Patient Teaching

■ Instruct the patient to keep accurate monthly records on the time of menstruation, how long each menstrual period lasts, and the amount of menstrual flow.

FACTOR ASSAY (PLASMA)
Factors I through XIII, Coagulation Factors, Blood Clotting Factors

Reference Values

Factor I (fibrinogen): 200–400 mg/dL, minimal for clotting 75–100 mg/dL

Factor II (prothrombin): minimal hemostatic level: 10%–15% concentration

Factor III (thromboplastin): variety of substances

Factor IV (calcium): 4.5–5.5 mEq/L or 9–11 mg/dL

Factor V (proaccelerin): 50%–150% activity; minimal hemostatic level: 5%–10% concentration

Factor VI: not used

Factor VII (proconvertin stable factor): 65%–135% activity; minimal hemostatic level concentration

Factor VIII (antihemophilic factor [AHF], VIII-A): 55%–145% activity; minimal hemostatic level: 30%–35% concentration

Factor IX (Christmas factor, IX-B): 60%–140% activity; minimal hemostatic level: 30% concentration

Factor X (Stuart factor): 45%–150% activity; minimal hemostatic level: 7%–10% concentration

Factor XI (plasma thromboplastin antecedent [PTA] XI-C): 65%–135% activity; 20%–30% minimal hemostatic level: 20%–30% concentration

Factor XII (Hageman factor): minimal hemostatic level: 0% concentration

Factor XIII (fibrin stabilizing factor [FSF]: minimal hemostatic level: 1% concentration

Description

Factor assays are ordered for identification of defects in the blood coagulation mechanism because of a lack of one or more of the 12 plasma factors (excluding factor VI). These 12 factors are important for clot formation, and these have been numbered according to the sequence of their discovery. To standardize clotting factors, the International Committee on Nomenclature of Blood Clotting Factors was established in 1954, and 12 clotting (coagulation) factors were given Roman numerals, named, and described.

FUNCTIONS OF COAGULATION FACTORS

Factor	Name	Source, Function
I	Fibrinogen	Manufactured by the liver; essential plasma protein; split by thrombin to produce fibrin strands necessary for clot formation
II	Prothrombin	Produced in the liver and requires vitamin K for its synthesis. Prothrombin is converted to thrombin by the action of extrinsic and intrinsic thromboplastin.
III	Thromboplastin	Thromboplastic activity is found in most tissues; this factor converts prothrombin to thrombin.
IV	Calcium	Absorbed in the GI tract from food. Inorganic ion is required in all stages of coagulation—thromboplastin generation, enzymatic conversion of prothrombin to thrombin, and stabilization of the fibrin clot.
V	Proaccelerin (labile factor)	Formed by the liver; for acceleration of thromboplastin generation; prompt conversion of prothrombin to thrombin; deteriorates rapidly in plasma at room temperature
VI		Not used
VII	Proconvertin (stable factor)	Manufactured in the liver and requires vitamin K for its synthesis; not destroyed or consumed in the clotting process; stable in heat; accelerates the conversion of prothrombin to thrombin. Use of antiocoagulants depresses factor VII in the plasma
VIII	Antihemophilic factor (A)	Produced by the reticuloendothelial cells; unstable at room temperatures; required for the generation of thromboplastin; essential for the conversion of the prothrombin to thrombin; sex linked
IX	Plasma thromboplastin component (PTC) (Christmas factor, antihemophilic factor B)	Manufactured in the liver and requires vitamin K for its synthesis; stable in plasma and serum; is not destroyed or consumed in the clotting process; essential for generating thromboplastin; sex linked
X	Stuart factor	Manufactured in the liver and requires vitamin K for its synthesis; stable in plasma and serum; not consumed in the clotting process; helps produce the thromboplastin-generating system
XI	Plasma thromboplastin antecedent (PTA) (antihemophilic C)	Synthesis unknown; present in serum and plasma; consumed during the clotting process; essential for plasma-thromboplastin formation
XII	Hageman factor	Synthesis unknown; activated in contact with glass and following injury; activated factor XII stimulates factor XI to continue the clotting process; converts plasminogen to plasmin in fibrinolysis
XIII	Fibrinase (fibrin stabilizing factor [FSF])	Synthesis unknown; enzyme (fibrinase) present in blood, tissue, and platelets and helps to stabilize fibrin strands to form a firm clot.[1,3,6,13]

Clinical Problems

A deficiency in one or more factors usually causes bleeding disorders. The associated clinical problems and the causes of these problems are outlined in the following table.

COAGULATION FACTOR DEFICIENCIES

Factor	Clinical Problems (Decreased Levels)	Rationale
I	Hypofibrinogenemia Leukemia Severe liver disease Disseminated intravascular coagulation (DIC)	Deficiency of fibrinogen and fibrinolysis
II	Hypoprothrombinemia Severe liver disease Vitamin K deficiency Drugs: salicylates (excessive), anti-coagulants, antibiotics (excessive), hepatotoxic drugs	Impaired liver function, vitamin K deficit
III	Thrombocytopenia	Low platelet count
IV	Hypocalcemia Malabsorption syndrome Malnutrition Hyperphosphatemia Multiple transfusions containing citrate	Low-calcium intake in diet
V	Parahemophilia (congenital) Severe liver disease DIC	Congenital problem, impaired liver function
VII	Hepatitis Hepatic carcinoma Hemorrhagic disease of newborn Vitamin K deficiency Drugs: antibiotics (excessive), anticoagulants	Impaired liver function, certain drugs affecting the clotting time, vitamin K deficit
VIII	Hemophilia A Von Willebrand's disease Disseminated intravascular coagulation (DIC) Multiple myeloma Lupus erythematosus	Congenital disorder (sex linked) occurring mostly in males; circulating factor VIII inhibitors
IX	Hemophilia B (Christmas disease) Hepatic disease Vitamin K deficiency	Congenital disorder (sex linked) occurring mostly in males; circulating factor IX inhibitors
X	Severe liver disease Hemorrhage disease of newborns DIC Vitamin K deficiency Drugs: anticoagulants	Impaired liver function; vitamin K deficit
XI	Hemophilia C Congenital heart disease Intestinal malabsorption of vitamin K Liver disease Drugs: anticoagulants	Congenital deficiency in both males and females; circulating factor XI inhibitors

Factor	Clinical Problems (Decreased Levels)	Rationale
XII	Liver disease	
XIII	Agammaglobulinemia Myeloma Lead poisoning Poor wound healing	Circulating factor XIII inhibitors; mild bleeding tendency.[1,8,13,14]

Procedure

- Collect 10 mL of venous blood in a blue-top tube (tube tops used may differ among laboratories).
- Mix the blood with an anticoagulant solution thoroughly, and avoid air bubbles.
- The tubes should be delivered to the laboratory immediately.
- There are no food or fluid restrictions.

- Factors Affecting Laboratory Results

  - Clotted blood can not be used for this laboratory test.
  - The factor assay results (factors I, V, and VIII) could be affected if the blood samples do not receive immediate attention in the laboratory.

NURSING IMPLICATIONS WITH RATIONALE

- Obtain a familial history of bleeding disorders and a history of the patient's bleeding tendency.
- Observe the venipuncture site for seeping of blood. Apply pressure to the site.
- Observe for signs of bleeding (ie, purpura, petechiae, or frank, continuous bleeding). Report your observations, and record them on the patient's chart.

FSB (FASTING BLOOD SUGAR)
(See Glucose—Fasting Blood Sugar.)

FEBRILE AGGLUTININS (SERUM)

Reference Values

Adult (febrile, titers): Brucella: <1:20, <1:20–1:80 (individuals working with animals), *Tularemia:* <1:40. *Widal (Salmonella):* <1:40 (nonvaccinated). *Weil-Felix (Proteus):* <1:40

Child: same as adult

Description

Febrile agglutination tests (febrile group) identify infectious diseases causing fever of unknown origin. Isolating the invading organism (pathogen) is not always possible, especially if the patient has been on antimicrobial therapy, so indirect methods are used to detect antibacterial antibodies in the serum. Detection of these antibodies is determined by the titer of the serum in highest dilution that will cause agglutination (clumping) in the presence of a specific antigen. The test should be done during the acute phase of the disease (maybe several times) and then done about 2 weeks later. A single agglutination titer is of minimal value. These tests can be used to confirm pathogens already isolated or to identify the pathogen present late in the disease (after several weeks).

Diseases commonly associated with febrile agglutination tests are brucellosis (undulant fever), salmonellosis, typhoid fever, paratyphoid fever, tularemia, and certain rickettsial infections (typhus fever).[1,7,13,14]

Clinical Problems

TEST	PATHOGEN(S) ANTIGEN(S)	ELEVATED LEVELS
Brucella	*Brucella abortus* (cattle) *B suis* (hogs) *B melitensis* (goats).	Brucellosis titer >1:160
Pasteurella (tularemia)	*Pasteurella tularensis*	Tularemia (rabbit fever) titer >1:80
Widal	*Salmonella* O (somatic)	Salmonellosis
	Salmonella H (flagellar)	Typhoid fever
	O and H portions of the organism act as antigens to stimulate antibody production.	Paratyphoid fever titer: O antigen— >1:80 suspicious, >1:160 definite; H antigen—>1:40 suspicious, >1:80 definite
	Salmonella vi (capular)	Nonvaccinated or vaccinated over 1 year before
Weil-Felix	*Proteus* X	Rickettsial diseases
	Proteus OX19	Epidemic typhus
		Tickborne typhus (Rocky Mountain spotted fever)
	Proteus OX2	Boutonneuse tick fever
		Queensland tick fever
		Siberian tick fever
	Proteus OXK	Scrub typhus titer—>1:80 significant, >1:60 definite

Procedure

- Collect 5 mL of venous blood in a red-top tube. Avoid hemolysis.
- Draw blood before starting antimicrobial therapy, if possible. If the patient is receiving drugs for an elevated temperature, write the names of the drugs on the laboratory slip.
- There is no food or fluid restriction.

■ The blood sample should be refrigerated if it is not tested immediately or frozen if it is to be kept 24 hours or longer.

■ Factors Affecting Laboratory Results

■ Vaccination could increase the titer level.
■ Antimicrobial therapy could decrease the titer level.
■ Leukemia, advanced carcinoma, some congenital deficiencies, and general debilitation could cause false-negative results.

NURSING IMPLICATIONS WITH RATIONALE

■ Obtain a history of the patient's occupation, geographic location prior to the fever, and recent vaccinations. Exposure to animals and ticks could be suggestive of the causative organism.
■ Record on the laboratory slip and in the patient's chart whether the patient has been vaccinated against the pathogen within the last year. Vaccinations can increase the antibody titer.
■ Monitor the temperature every 4 hours, when elevated.
■ Remind the physician of the need to repeat the tests when the fever persists and/or when the titer levels are suspicious. Titer levels could rise fourfold in 1 to 2 weeks.
■ Check to determine whether the blood sample has been taken before you give antibiotics or other drug agents to combat fever and the suspected organism. Antibiotic therapy could depress the titer level.

Patient Teaching

■ Instruct the patient to keep a record of temperatures and to notify the physician of changes in body temperature.

FERRITIN (SERUM)

Reference Values

Adult: Female: 10–125 ng/mL, 10–300 μg/L. *Male:* 35–300 ng/mL, 35–300 μg/L. *Postmenopausal:* 10–310 ng/mL

Child: 1–16 years: 8–140 ng/mL. *Infant:* 2–12 months; 30–200 ng/mL; 1 month: 200–550 ng/mL

Newborn: 20–200 ng/mL

Description

Ferritin, an iron-storage protein, is produced in the liver, spleen, and bone marrow. The ferritin levels are related to the amount of iron stored in the body tissues. It will release iron from tissue reserve as needed and will store excess iron to prevent damage effects from iron overload. One nanogram per milliliter of serum ferritin corresponds to 8 mg of stored iron.

Serum ferritin level is useful in evaluation the total body storage of iron. It can detect early iron deficiency anemia and anemias due to chronic disease that resemble iron deficiency. Serum ferritin is not affected by hemolysis and drugs.[1,3,6,9]

Clinical Problems

Decreased Level: iron deficiency, pregnancy, inflamed bowel disease, gastric surgery

Elevated Level: metastatic carcinomas, leukemias, lymphomas, hepatic diseases (cirrhosis, hepatitis, cancer of the liver), iron overload (hemochromatosis), hemosiderosis, anemias (hemolytic, pernicious, thalassemia), acute and chronic infection and inflammation (renal disease, neuroblastoma), tissue damage. *Drug Influence:* oral or injectable iron drugs

Procedure

- Collect 7 mL of venous blood in a red-top tube.
- There is no food or fluid restriction.
- List on the laboratory slip if patient is taking iron preparations.

- Factors Affecting Laboratory results

None known

NURSING IMPLICATIONS WITH RATIONALE

- Compare serum ferritin level with serum iron and transferrin percent saturation. Serum ferritin levels tend to be more reliable in determining iron deficiencies than serum iron levels. Serum ferritin levels decrease before iron stores are depleted.

FIBRIN DEGRADATION PRODUCTS (FDP) (SERUM)
Fibrin or Fibrinogen Split Products (FSP)

Reference Values

Adult: 2–10 µg/mL

Child: not usually done

Description

The FDP test is usually done in an emergency when the patient is hemorrhaging as the result of severe injury, trauma, and/or shock. Thrombin, which initially accelerates coagulation, promotes the conversion of plasminogen into plasmin, which, in turn, breaks fibrinogen and fibrin into FDP. The fibrin degradation (split) products act as anticoagulants, causing continuous bleeding from many sites. A clinical condition resulting from this fibrinolytic (clot-dissolving) activity is disseminated intravascular coagulation (DIC).[3,9,18]

Clinical Problems

Decreased Level: cerebral thrombosis

Elevated Level: DIC caused by severe injury, trauma, or shock; massive tissue damage; surgical complications; septicemia; obstetric complications (abruptio placentae, preeclampsia, intrauterine death, postcesarean birth), acute myocardial infarction, pulmonary embolism, acute necrosis of the liver, acute renal failure, burns, acute leukemia. *Drug Influence:* streptokinase, urokinase

Procedure

- Collect 10 mL of venous blood in a red-top tube. Avoid hemolysis
- Draw blood before administering heparin.
- There is no food or fluid restriction.

- Factors Affecting Laboratory Results

  - Hemolysis of the blood sample cause inaccurate test result.

NURSING IMPLICATIONS WITH RATIONALE

Elevated Level

- Monitor vital signs, and report shocklike symptoms, such as tachycardia, hypotension, pallor, and cold, clammy skin.
- Observe and report bleeding sites from the chest, the nasogastric tube, incisional or injured areas, and others.
- Report progressive discoloration of the skin (petechial, ecchymoses).
- Monitor infusion rates of IV fluids—crystalloids, colloids, and blood.
- Check urine output hourly. Report decreased urine output (<25 mL/h) and blood-colored urine.
- Provide comfort and support to the patient and family.

FIBRINOGEN (PLASMA)
Factor I

Reference Values

Adult: 200–400 mg/dL

Child: Newborn: 150–300 mg/dL. *Child:* same as adult

Description

Fibrinogen, a plasma protein synthesized by the liver, is split by thrombin to produce fibrin strands necessary for clot formation. A deficiency of fibrinogen results in bleeding. Low fibrinogen levels may be due to *disseminated intravascular coagulation* (DIC), which usually results from severe trauma or obstetric complications. Markedly prolonged prothrombin time (PT), an activated partial thromboplastin time (APTT), and a low platelet count suggest a fibrinogen deficiency and signs of DIC. Fibrin degradation products (FDP) are usually ordered to confirm DIC.[1,3,9,13]

Clinical Problems

Decreased Level: severe liver disease, hypofibrinogenemia, DIC, leukemia, obstetric complications

Elevated Level: acute infections, collagen diseases, inflammatory disease, hepatitis. *Drug Influence:* oral contraceptives, heparin

Procedure

- Collect 7 mL of venous blood in a blue-top tube. Mix blood well with the anticoagulant in the tube (invert tube several times). Avoid hemolysis by not shaking the tube.
- There is no food or fluid restriction.

- Factors Affecting Laboratory Results

- Postoperative surgery and third trimester of pregnancy could cause a false-positive fibrinogen elevation.
- Hemolysis of the blood sample cause inaccurate result.
- Oral contraceptives and heparin can elevate test result.

NURSING IMPLICATIONS WITH RATIONALE

- Report if patient had a blood transfusion within 4 weeks.
- Check laboratory results of PT, APTT, and platelet count. If FDP is ordered, check the laboratory result, since it confirms DIC.
- Monitor for signs and symptoms of of DIC (petechiae and ecchymoses, hemorrhage, tachycardia, hypotension).
- Notify the physician if active bleeding occurs.

Patient Teaching

- Instruct the patient to inform the physician of any current, acute infection or illness that might be contributing to the bleeding.

FOLIC ACID (FOLATE) (SERUM)

Reference Values

Adult: 3–16 ng/mL (bioassay), >2.5 ng/mL (radioimmunoassay [RIA]; serum), 200–700 ng/mL (RBC)

Child: same as adult

Description

Folic acid, one of the B vitamins, is needed for normal red and white blood-cell function. Folic acid is present in a variety of foods: milk, eggs, leafy vegetables, beans, liver, fruits (oranges, bananas), and whole wheat bread. Dietary deficiency is the commonest cause of a serum folic acid deficit, especially in children, older adults, and persons with chronic alcoholism. With a decreased folic acid intake, it takes approximately 3 to 4 weeks for folic acid deficiency to develop and 18 to 24 weeks before folic acid anemia will occur.

Usually the serum folic acid or folate test is performed to detect folic acid anemia, which is a megaloblastic anemia (abnormally large RBCs). Other causes of serum folic acid deficit are pregnancy (because of dietary deficiency and because the fetal requirement for folic acid is so great), alcoholism, and the aged.[3,10,12,13]

Clinical Problems

Decreased Level: folic acid anemia (megaloblastic anemia): *vitamin B₆* deficiency anemia; malnutrition; malabsorption syndrome (small intestine); pregnancy; malignancies; liver diseases; celiac sprue disease; *Drug Influence:* anticonvulsants—phenytoin (Dilantin), primidone (Mysoline); antineoplastic agents—methotrexate (folic acid antagonists); antimalaria agents; oral contraceptives

Elevated Level: pernicious anemia

Procedure

- Collect 7 to 10 mL of venous blood in a red-top tube. Avoid hemolysis. Send blood to the laboratory immediately.
- If an RBC folate determination is requested, collect 7 mL of venous blood in a lavender-top tube. Send this to the laboratory immediately. Ascorbic acid will be added in the laboratory.
- There is no food or fluid restriction. Avoid alcohol.

■ Factors Affecting Laboratory Results

- Drugs (*See Clinical Problems.*)
- Alcohol—persons who consume large quantities of alcohol usually have poor nutritional intake (folic acid deficiency).

NURSING IMPLICATIONS WITH RATIONALE

- Obtain a dietary history. Collaborate with the dietitian on formulating a diet high in folic acid, and have the dietitian plan the diet with the patient.
- Observe for signs and symptoms of folic acid deficiency, such as fatigue, pallor, nausea, anorexia, dyspnea, palpitations, and tachycardia.

Patient Teaching

- Encourage the patient to eat foods rich in folic acid, such as liver, lean meats, milk, eggs, leafy vegetables, bananas, oranges, beans, and whole wheat bread.

FOLLICLE-STIMULATING HORMONE (FSH) SERUM AND URINE

Reference Values

Serum

Adult: Female: Follicular phase: 4–30 mU/mL; Midcycle: 10–90 mU/mL; Luteal phase: 4–30 mU/mL; Menopause: 40–250 mU/mL. Male: 4–25 mU/mL
Child (Prepubertal): 5–12 mU/mL

Urine

Adult: Female: Follicular phase: 4–25 IU/24 h; Midcycle: 8–60 IU/24 h; Luteal phase: 4–20 IU/24 h. Menopause: 50–150 IU/24 h. Male: 4–18 IU/24 h
Child (Prepubertal): <10 IU/mL

Description

FSH, a gonadotropic hormone produced and controlled by the pituitary gland, stimulates the growth and maturation of the ovarian follicle to produce estrogen in females and to promote spermatogenesis in males. Infertility disorders can be determined by a serum and urine FSH test. Increased and decreased FSH levels can indicate gonad failure due to pituitary dysfunction.

Clinical Problems

Decreased Level: neoplasms of the ovaries, testes, adrenals; polycystic ovarian disease; hypopituitarism; anorexia nervosa. *Drug Influence:* estrogens, oral contraceptives, testosterone

Elevated Level: gonadal failure such as menopause, precocious puberty, FSH-producing pituitary tumor, Turner's syndrome, Klinefelter's syndrome, orchiectomy, hysterectomy, primary testicular failure

Procedure

- No food or fluid restriction is required.
- State phase of menstrual cycle or if menopausal on the laboratory slip.
- Note on the laboratory slip if the patient is taking oral contraceptives or any type of hormones.

Serum
- Collect 5 to 7 mL of venous blood in a red-top tube. Avoid hemolysis.
- Rest 30 minutes to 1 hour before blood is drawn.

Urine
- Collect a 24-hour urine specimen in a large container with a preservative. The pH of the 24-hour urine specimen should be maintained between 5 and 6.5 (glacial acetic acid or boric acid may be added).
- Avoid feces and toilet paper in the urine.

- Factors Affecting Laboratory Results

    - Alkaline urine can give an inaccurate test result.

NURSING IMPLICATIONS WITH RATIONALE

- Associate decreased or increased urine FSH with clinical problems. The excess production of estrogen with most ovarian tumors will decrease the production of FSH. After menopause, more FSH will be secreted to stimulate estrogen production.

Urine

- Label container with the patient's name, the dates, and the exact times of urine collection (eg, 5/10/93. 8AM to 5/11/93. 8:01 AM).

Patient Teaching

- Answer patient questions concerning the test. Be supportive of patient and family.
- Inform the patient to rest prior to a serum test, since exercise can increase FSH release.

FTA-ABS (FLUORESCENT TREPONEMAL ANTIBODY ABSORPTION) (SERUM)

Reference Values

Adult: nonreactive (negative)

Child: nonreactive (negative)

Description

The FTA-ABS test is the treponemal antibody test, which uses the treponemal organism to produce and detect these antibodies. This test is most sensitive, specific, and reliable for diagnosing all stages of syphilis. It is more sensitive than the venereal disease research laboratory (VDRL) and rapid plasma reagin (RPR) tests. The FTA-ABS test is useful for confirming or ruling out suspected false-positive serology tests for syphilis. The limitations of this test are that the stage and activity of the disease cannot be identified, the effectiveness of the therapy cannot be measured, and the test for syphilis remains positive even after treatment for a very long time or could remain positive forever.[1,9,10,12]

Clinical Problems

Reactive: Positive: primary and secondary syphilis. *False Positives (rare):* lupus erythematosus, pregnancy, acute genital herpes

Procedure

- Collect 5 mL of venous blood in a red-top tube. Avoid hemolysis.
- There is no food or fluid restriction.
- A borderline FTA-ABS should be repeated.

■ Factors Affecting Laboratory Results

- Medical treatment does not eliminate the treponemal antibodies. The test results may remain positive after treatment.

NURSING IMPLICATIONS WITH RATIONALE

- Be supportive of the patient and family. Keep conversation and information confidential except for what is required by law.
- Encourage the patient to have his or her sexual friend or spouse seek medical care if the test is positive.
- Check the results of other serology tests for syphilis. A positive VDRL could be false positive because of acute or chronic illness. The FTA-ABS test is reliable for syphilis, giving accurate results; however, many laboratories have to send the blood sample out for testing. Ask the patient if he or she has received treatment for syphilis. Positive FTA-ABS results can occur after treatment (penicillin, erythromycin) for months or several years or for the rest of the patient's life.
- Assess for signs and symptoms of syphilis. The primary stage begins with a small papule filled with liquid, which ruptures, enlarges, and becomes a chancre. With secondary syphilis, a generalized rash (macular and papular) develops and is found mainly on the arms, palms, soles of the feet, and face.

FUNGAL ORGANISMS: FUNGAL DISEASE, MYCOTIC INFECTIONS (SMEAR, SERUM, CULTURE—SPUTUM, BRONCHIAL, LESION)

Actinomyces, Histoplasma, Blastomyces, Coccidioides, Cryptococcus, Candida, Aspergillus

Reference Values

Adult: negative, serum: <1:8

Child: same as adult

Description

There are more than 45,000 species of fungi, but only 0.01%, or 45, are considered pathogenic to humans. Fungal infections are commoner today and can be classified as (1) superficial and cutaneous mycoses (tinea pedis [athlete's foot], tinea capitis [ringworm of the scalp], tinea barbae [ringworm of the beard], and tinea cruris [jock itch]), (2) subcutaneous mycoses, and (3) systemic mycoses (histoplasmosis, actinomycosis, and blastomycosis).

Most fungus organisms live in the soil and can be transmitted to man and animals by way of the lungs or a break in the skin. The persons most susceptible to fungal infections are those with debilitating or chronic diseases (eg, diabetes) or who are receiving drug therapy, such as steroids, prolonged antibiotics, antineoplastic agents, and oral contraceptives.[6,8,10,13]

Clinical Problems

ORGANISM	DISEASE ENTITY	COMMENTS
Actinomyces israelii	Actinomycosis	A gram-positive, non–acid-fast, anaerobic organism that can produce an abscess.
Histoplasma capsulatum	Histoplasmosis	The commonest systemic fungal infection. It is commonly found in the eastern part of the United States and in the Mississippi and Ohio valleys. Usually the organism is carried by birds (eg, starlings and chickens). In most patients histoplasmosis is a localized pulmonary disease and resembles pulmonary tuberculosis.
Blastomyces dermatitidis	Blastomycosis	It causes granulomatous lesions that involve the skin or visceral organs. Histologically it is similar to tuberculosis.
Coccidioides immitis	Coccidioidomycosis	It is commonly found in the Southwest and in the San Joaquin Valley of California. Usually the patient has respiratory symptoms and fever of unknown origin. If the infection is overwhelming, it resembles miliary tuberculosis.

(continued)

141

ORGANISM	DISEASE ENTITY	COMMENTS
Cryptococcus neoformans	Cryptococcosis Meningitis	Fungal disease usually begins as a pulmonary infection but disseminates to the central nervous system (CNS) (brain). The organism is usually carried by pigeons. Patients with decreased immunologic resistance (such as those with acute leukemia or Hodgkin's disease or who are receiving steroids or immunosuppressive agents) are susceptible to the disease.
Candida albicans, fungemia	Candidiasis (Moniliasis) Thrush	Patients with debilitating diseases or who are taking steroids, antineoplastic agents, or oral contraceptives are susceptible to this fungus.
Aspergillus fumigatus	Aspergillosis	Aspergillus organisms can cause severe respiratory infection. Fungus balls (aspergilloma) develop in the lung tissue. The sputum is golden brown and contains *Aspergillus hyphae*.[10,13]

Procedure

Serum

- Collect 7 to 10 mL of venous blood in a red-top tube.
- No food or fluid restriction is required. Suggest NPO for 12 hours. Check with your laboratory.
- Obtain serum antibody test 2 to 4 weeks after exposure to organism.

Culture

- Follow directions from the special laboratory on collection of the specimen.

ORGANISM	TESTS
Actinomyces israelii	Smear and culture of lesion Biopsy
Histoplasma capsulatum	Sputum culture Histoplasmin skin test Serum test: complement fixation or latex agglutination
Blastomyces dermatitidis	Culture Smear, wet-mount examination of the material from the lesion Biopsy—histologic examination Skin test Serum test: complement fixation
Coccidioides immitis	Culture Sputum smears Skin test Serum test: complement fixation (sensitive), latex agglutination (very sensitive)
Cryptococcus neoformans	Culture of CSF Serum test: latex agglutination (sensitive)
Candida albicans	Smear and culture of the skin, mucous membrane, and vagina
Aspergillus fumigatus	Sputum culture Skin test Serum IgE level and complement fixation

- Factors Affecting Laboratory Results
  - Contamination of the specimen affects results.

NURSING IMPLICATIONS WITH RATIONALE

- Associate mycotic infections with high-risk patients (ie, those patients having chronic illnesses [such as diabetes mellitus] or debilitating diseases [such as cancer] or who are receiving prolonged antibiotics, antineoplastic agents [anticancer chemotherapy], steroids, or oral contraceptives.
- Use aseptic technique when collecting a specimen for culture. Preventing the transmission of the organism is most important. Contamination of the specimen can give inaccurate results.
- Obtain a history from the patient—where he or she lives and occupation. Fungus organisms (eg, *Histoplasma, Coccidioides*) are more prevalent in selected parts of the country. Report if the patient works with chickens or pigeons.
- Teach the patient to wear a mask when exposed to chicken feces. Explain that the *H capsulatum* spores are in the feces and can be inhaled.
- Monitor the patient's temperature. With many of the fungal diseases, the temperature is elevated.
- Report clinical signs and symptoms of respiratory problems (ie, coughing up sputum, dyspnea, and chest pain).
- Check the color of the sputum. Certain fungi can be indentified by the color of their secretions. Golden brown sputum is characteristic of the *Aspergillus* organism.
- Assess the neurologic status when cryptococcosis is suspected. Report headaches and changes in sensorium, pupil size and reaction, and motor function.

GAMMA-GLUTAMYL TRANSFERASE (GGT) (SERUM)
Gamma-Glutamyl Transpeptidase (GGTP, or GTP; γ-Glutamyl Transpeptidase, γGT)

Reference Values 0–45 IU/L (overall average),
Adult: Male: 10–80 IU/L. *Female:* 5–25 IU/L, 5–40 U/L at 37°C (SI units)
Elderly: slightly higher than adult
Child: Newborn: 5 times higher than adult. *Premature:* 10 times higher than adult. *Child:* similar to adult

Description

The enzyme gamma-glutamyl transferase (GGT) is found primarily in the liver and kidney, with smaller amounts in the spleen, prostate gland, and heart

143

muscle. GGTP is sensitive for detecting a wide variety of hepatic (liver) parenchymal diseases. The serum level will rise early and will remain elevated as long as cellular damage persists.

High levels of GGT occur after 12 to 24 hours of heavy alcoholic drinking and may remain increased for 2 to 3 weeks after alcohol intake stops. Some alcoholic rehabilitation programs are using the GGTP level as a guide to planning care as they work with the alcoholic individuals.

The GGT test is considered more sensitive for liver dysfunction than the alkaline phosphatase (ALP) test.[1,3,7–10]

Clinical Problems

Elevated Level: cirrhosis of the liver, acute and subacute necrosis of the liver, alcoholism, acute and chronic hepatitis, cancer (liver, pancreas, prostate, breast, kidney, lung, brain), infectious mononucleosis, hemochromatosis (iron deposits in the liver), diabetes mellitus, hyperlipoproteinemia (type IV), acute myocardial infarction (fourth day), congestive heart failure, acute pancreatitis, acute cholecystitis, epilepsy, nephrotic syndrome. *Drug Influence:* phenytoin (Dilantin), phenobarbital, aminoglycosides, warfarin (Coumadin).

Procedure

- Collect 7–10 mL of venous blood in a red-top tube. Avoid hemolysis.
- There is no food or fluid restriction.

■ Factors Affecting Laboratory Results

- Phenytoin and barbiturates can cause a false-positive GGT test.
- Excessive and prolonged alcoholic intake will elevate the GGT level.

NURSING IMPLICATIONS WITH RATIONALE

Elevated Level

- Compare GGT with ALP, leucine aminopeptidase (LAP), and alanine aminotransferase (SGPT or ALT). The GGT test tends to be more sensitive for detecting liver dysfunction than the others.
- Report to the physician if the patient is receiving phenytoin or phenobarbital when the test is ordered. Usually these medications cannot be withheld. Note on the laboratory slip the names of the drugs (affecting GGT levels) and the dosages the patient is receiving.
- Assess the patient's diet.
- Observe for signs and symptoms of liver damage, such as restlessness, jaundice, twitching, flapping tremors, spider angiomas, bleeding tendencies (nose and rectal bleeding), purpura, ascites, and others.

Patient Teaching

- Instruct the patient to maintain a well-balanced diet (adequate protein and carbohydrate).

■ Encourage patients with an alcoholic problem to participate in Alcoholics Anonymous or a rehabilitation program.

GASTRIN (SERUM OR PLASMA)

Reference Values

Adult: *Fasting:* <100 pg/mL. *Nonfasting:* 50–200 pg/mL

Child: not usually done

Description

Gastrin is a hormone, secreted from the pyloric mucosa, that stimulates the secretion of gastric juices—mainly hydrochloric acid (HCl). Normally increased gastrin will cause hypersecretion of HCl, which in turn inhibits gastrin secretion.

This test is usually ordered to aid in the diagnosis of pernicious anemia, Zollinger-Ellison syndrome (a condition caused by a noninsulin-producing tumor of the pancreas that secretes excess amounts of gastrin), and stomach cancer.[7,9,10,12,13]

Clinical Problems

Elevated Level (>200 pg/mL): pernicious anemia, Zollinger-Ellison syndrome, malignant neoplasm of the stomach, peptic ulcer, chronic atrophic gastritis, cirrhosis of the liver, acute and chronic renal failure. *Drug Influence:* IV calcium gluconate

Procedure

■ Collect 10 mL of venous blood in a red-top or lavender-top tube.
■ Food and fluids (except water) are restricted for 12 hours before the test.

■ Factors Affecting Laboratory Results

■ IV infusion of calcium elevates the serum gastrin level.

NURSING IMPLICATIONS WITH RATIONALE

■ Inform the patient that food and beverages are restricted, with the exception of water, for 12 hours before the test. A fasting blood sample is required, but the length of the NPO time may differ among laboratories.

Elevated Level

■ Check the patient's serum gastrin value; in Zollinger-Ellison syndrome, the serum level can reach 2800 to 300,000 pg/mL. High levels are present in pernicious anemia and gastritis.
■ Observe for signs and symptoms of pernicious anemia (weakness, sore tongue, pallor of the gums and lips, anorexia, loss of weight, and numbness and tingling in the extremities).

GLUCAGON (PLASMA)

Reference Values

Adult: 50–200 pg/mL

Description

Glucagon is secreted by the alpha cells of the pancreas. It functions as a counter-regulatory hormone to insulin in regulating glucose metabolism. It increases blood glucose by converting glycogen to glucose in response to hypoglycemia.

Very high glucagon levels (500–1000 pg/mL) occur in glucagonoma, pancreatic alpha cell tumor.[3,9,10,18]

Clinical Problems

Decreased Level: glucose tolerance test during first hour, idiopathic glucagon deficiency, loss of pancreatic tissue

Elevated level (>200 pg/mL): glucagonoma, acute pancreatitis, severe diabetic ketoacidosis, infections, pheochromocytoma

Procedure

■ Collect 10 mL of venous blood in a lavender-top tube. Avoid hemolysis. Chill tube and take to laboratory immediately.
■ Food and fluids are restricted for 10 to 12 hours prior to the test.
■ Withhold drugs such as insulin, cortisone, growth hormones, and epinephrine with physician's permission until the test is completed.

■ Factors Affecting Laboratory Results

■ Vigorous exercise, undue stress, trauma, severe hyperglycemia affect test results.
■ Administer steroids and insulin after the test.

NURSING IMPLICATIONS WITH RATIONALE

■ Compare serum glucose and insulin levels. Glucose and insulin influence plasma glucagon levels.

- Record on the laboratory slip and report if patient has taken large doses of steroids in the last 24 hours.
- Observe for signs and symptoms of hyperglycemia.

Patient Teaching

- Instruct the patient to relax by lying down for 30 minutes to 1 hour prior to the test. Stress and activity could cause false-positive test results.

GLUCOSE—FASTING BLOOD SUGAR (FBS) (BLOOD)

Reference Values

Adult: *Serum and Plasma:* 70–110 mg/dL. *Whole Blood:* 60–100 mg/dL

Child: *Newborn:* 30–80 mg/dL. *Child:* 60–100 mg/dL

Elderly: 70–120 mg/dL

Description

Glucose is formed from dietary carbohydrates and is stored as glycogen in the liver and skeletal muscles. Insulin and glucagon, two hormones from the pancreas, affect the blood glucose level. Insulin is needed for cellular membrane permeability to glucose and for transportation of glucose into the cells. Without insulin, glucose cannot enter the cells. Glucagon stimulates glycogenolysis (conversion of stored glycogen to glucose) in the liver.

A decreased blood sugar (hypoglycemia) results from inadequate food intake or too much insulin. When elevated blood sugar (hyperglycemia) occurs, there is not enough insulin; this condition is known as diabetes mellitus. A fasting blood sugar greater than 125 mg/dL usually indicates diabetes, and to confirm the diagnosis when the blood sugar is borderline or slightly elevated, a feasting (postprandial) blood sugar and/or a glucose tolerance test may be ordered.

Dextrostix test is a rapid, simple, semiquantitative test for distinguishing hypoglycemia from hyperglycemia. The results are compared to a color chart with values between 40 and 240 mg/dL. This is a useful test in emergency situations. Chemstrip bG is the preferred method for checking blood sugar by finger stick.[6,9,10,12,13]

Clinical Problems

Decreased Level: hypoglycemic reaction (insulin excess); cancer (stomach, liver, lung), adrenal gland hypofunction, malnutrition, alcoholism, cirrhosis of the liver, strenuous exercise, erythroblastosis fetalis (hemolytic disease), hyperinsulinism, *Drug Influence:* insulin excess

Elevated Level: diabetes mellitus, diabetes acidosis, adrenal gland hyperfunction (Cushing's syndrome), acute myocardial infarction, stress, crushed injury, burns, infections, renal failure, hypothermia, exercise, acute pancreatitis, cancer of the pancreas, congestive heart failure, acromegaly, postgastrectomy (dumping) syndrome, extensive surgery. *Drug Influence:* ACTH; cortisone preparations; diuretics (hydrochlorothiazide [Hydrodiuril], furosemide [Lasix], ethacrynic acid [Edecrin]), anesthesia drugs, levodopa

Procedure

- Collect 5 to 10 mL of venous blood in a gray-top or red-top tube. Blood is drawn between 7 AM and 9 AM.
- NPO except water for 12 hours before the test.
- Give insulin as ordered and after the blood sample is taken.

■ Factors Affecting Laboratory Results

- Drugs—cortisone, thiazide, the "loop" diuretics can cause an increase in blood sugar.
- Trauma—stress can cause an increase in blood sugar.
- The Clinitest for determining urine glucose (glycosuria) may be falsely positive if the patient is taking excessive amounts of aspirin, vitamin C, and certain antibiotics (cephalosporin), since the test is not specific for glucose but for all reducing substances.
- High doses of vitamin C could cause false negative results when using Testape.

NURSING IMPLICATIONS WITH RATIONALE

- Hold morning insulin and drugs until blood specimen is taken.
- Record on the laboratory slip if the patient has been taking daily cortisone preparations, thiazides, or loop diuretics.

Decreased Level

- Recognize clinical problems associated with low blood sugar level. Excessive doses of insulin, skipped meals, and inadequate food intake are the common causes of hypoglycemia.
- Observe for signs and symptoms of hypoglycemia (nervousness, weakness, confusion, cold and clammy skin, diaphoresis, and increased pulse rate).

Patient Teaching

- Instruct the patient to carry lumps of sugar or candy at all times. Most diabetic persons have warnings when hypoglycemia occurs.
- Teach the patient to adhere to the American Dietetic Association (ADA) diet, as prescribed. Explain the Exchange Lists for meal planning.
- Encourage the patient to contact the American Diabetic Association for literature and information concerning their meeting dates.
- Explain to the patient that strenuous exercise can lower the blood sugar. Carbohydrate or protein intake should be increased before exercise or immediately after exercise; the physician should be contacted for food instruction.
- Encourage the patient to take insulin ½ to 1 hour before breakfast and to eat meals on time.

■ Teach patients with a hypoglycemic problem (blood sugar <50 mg/dL) to eat food high in protein and fat and low in carbohydrate. Too much sugar stimulates insulin secretion.

Elevated Level

■ Recognize clinical problems associated with high blood sugar levels. Diabetes mellitus, Cushing's syndrome, and stressful situations (trauma, burns, extensive surgery) are the common causes of hyperglycemia.

■ Consider drugs (such as cortisone, thiazides, and "loop" diuretics) as the cause of a slightly elevated blood sugar level. If blood sugar becomes too high, notify the physician—drug dosages may need to be decreased or insulin may need to be ordered or increased.

■ Observe for signs and symptoms of hyperglycemia (excessive thirst [polydipsia], excessive urination [polyuria], excessive hunger [polyphagia], and weight loss). If the blood sugar is greater than 500 mg/dL, Kussmaul's breathing caused by acidosis may be observed (rapid, deep, vigorous breathing).

Patient Teaching

■ Instruct the patient to test his or her blood before meals. Demonstrate how to use Chemstrip bG techniques or others.

■ Explain to the patient that infections can increase the blood sugar level and medical advice should be sought.

GLUCOSE—POSTPRANDIAL (FEASTING BLOOD SUGAR) (BLOOD)
Two-Hour Postprandial Blood Sugar (PPBS)

Reference Values

Adult: Serum or Plasma: <140 mg/dL/2 h. *Blood:* <120 mg/dL/2 h

Elderly: Serum: <160 mg/dL/2h. *Blood:* <140 mg/dL/2h

Child: <120 mg/dL/2 h

Description

A 2-hour PPBS or feasting sugar test in usually done to determine the patient's response to a high carbohydrate intake 2 hours after a meal (breakfast or lunch). This test is a screening test for diabetes, normally ordered if the fasting blood sugar was high normal or slightly elevated. A serum glucose greater than 140 mg/dL or a blood glucose greater than 120 mg/dL is abnormal, and further tests may be needed.[3,10,12]

Clinical Problems

Decreased Level: (See Glucose—Fasting Blood Sugar.)

Elevated Level: (See Glucose—Fasting Blood Sugar.)

Procedure

- A high-carbohydrate meal might be requested at breakfast or lunch.
- Collect 5–10mL of venous blood in a gray- or red-top tube 2 hours after the patient finishes eating breakfast or lunch. If the nurse does not draw the blood, the laboratory needs to be notified when the patient finished breakfast or lunch.
- Food is restricted for 2 hours after breakfast or lunch before the test, but water is not.

■ Factors Affecting Laboratory Results

- Smoking may increase the serum glucose level.
- *(See Glucose—Fasting Blood Sugar.)*

NURSING IMPLICATIONS WITH RATIONALE

- Determine the breakfast foods that the patient likes and dislikes and notify the dietary department.

Patient Teaching

- If the patient is not hospitalized, instruct the person to be at the laboratory 1½ to 2 hours after breakfast or lunch.

Elevated Level:

- (See Glucose—Fasting Blood Sugar.)

GLUCOSE TOLERANCE TEST—ORAL (GTT) (SERUM) AND IV GLUCOSE TOLERANCE TEST

Reference Values

Adult

ORAL GTT

Time	Serum (mg/dL)	Blood (mg/dL)
Fasting	70–110	60–100
½ hour	<160	<150
1 hour	<170	<160
2 hours	<125	<115
3 hours	Fasting level	Fasting level
Urine: negative		

IV GLUCOSE TOLERANCE TEST

Time	Serum (mg/dL)
Fasting	70–110
5 minutes	<250
½ hour	<155
1 hour	<125
2 hours	Fasting level

Urine: negative at fasting and at ½, 1, and 2 hours.

Child: Depends on the child's age. Infants normally have lower blood sugar levels (*See Glucose—Fasting Blood Sugar*). A child aged 6 or older has GTT results similar to those of the adult.

Description

A GTT is done to diagnose diabetes mellitus in persons having high-normal or slightly elevated blood sugar values. The test may be indicated when there is a familial history of diabetes, in women having babies weighing 10 lb or more, in persons having extensive surgery or injury, and in persons with obesity problems. The test should *not* be performed if the fasting blood sugar (FBS) is over 200 mg/dL. After the age of 60 years, the blood glucose level is usually 10 to 30 mg/dL higher than the "normal range."

The peak glucose level for the oral GTT is ½ to 1 hour after the ingestion of 100 g of glucose, and the blood sugar should return to normal range in 3 hours. Blood and urine samples will be collected at specified times.

The *intravenous glucose tolerance test (IV-GTT)* is considered by many to be more sensitive than the oral GTT, since absorption through the GI tract is not involved. The IV-GTT is usually done if the person cannot eat or tolerate the oral glucose. The blood glucose returns to the normal range in 2 hours. However, the values for oral GTT and IV-GTT slightly differ, since IV-glucose is absorbed faster.

Hyperinsulinism can be detected with the oral GTT. After 1 hour the blood glucose level is usually lower than in the FBS test. The person might develop severe hypoglycemic reactions—there is more insulin being secreted in response to the blood glucose.[6,9,10,13,18]

Clinical Problems

Decreased Level: hyperinsulinism, adrenal gland insufficiency, malabsorption, protein malnutrition

Elevated Level: diabetes mellitus, latent diabetes, adrenal gland hyperfunction (Cushing's syndrome), hyperlipoproteinemia, stress, infections, extensive surgery or injury, alcoholism, acute myocardial infarction, cancer of the pancreas, insulin resistance conditions (eclampsia, cancer metastases, acidotic conditions), duodenal ulcers. *Drug Influence:* corticosteroids (cortisone), oral contraceptives, estrogens, diuretics thiazides, salicylates, ascorbic acid

Procedure

OGTT

- A diet adequate in carbohydrate should be consumed 2 to 3 days prior to testing.
- The patient remains NPO for 12 hours before the test, except for water.
- No coffee, tea, or smoking are allowed during the test. No food should be eaten.
- Drugs that affect test results should not be taken for 3 days prior to the GTT, if possible.
- Collect 5 mL of venous blood in a red or gray top tube for FBS. Collect a fasting urine specimen.
- Give 100 g of glucose, either lemon-flavored solution or glucola. Some physicians will give glucose according to body weight (1.75 g/kg), as in pediatrics.
- Obtain blood and urine specimens ½, 1, 2, and 3 hours after glucose intake.

IVGTT

- NPO 12 hours before test.
- Administer infusion of 50% glucose over 3 to 4 minutes.
- Obtain blood and urine specimens at fasting, 5 minutes (blood only) ½, 1, and 2 hours.

■ Factors Affecting Laboratory Results

- Drugs (*See Drug Influence*).
- Age—older adults have higher blood sugars. Insulin secretion is decreased because of the aging process.
- Emotional stress, fever, infections, trauma, being bedridden, and obesity can increase the blood sugar level.
- Strenuous exercise and vomiting might decrease the blood sugar. Hypoglycemic agents will decrease the blood sugar.

NURSING IMPLICATIONS WITH RATIONALE

- Notify the laboratory of when (the exact time) the patient drank the glucose solution. Laboratory personnel will collect the blood samples at specified times.

Patient Teaching

- Explain to the patient the procedure for the test. Explain that food, alcohol, and medications are restricted for 12 hours prior to the test. Water is permitted.
- Explain to the patient that coffee, tea, and smoking are restricted during the test. Water is allowed and encouraged; however, in some institutions, only 240 mL is permitted.
- Explain to the patient that he or she may perspire or feel weak and giddy during the 2 to 3 hours of the test. This is frequently transitory; however, the nurse should be notified, and these symptoms should be recorded. They could be signs of hyperinsulinism.

■ Inform the patient to minimize his or her activities during the test. Increased activities could affect the glucose results.

Decreased Level

■ Observe for signs and symptoms of hypoglycemia, especially when hyperinsulinism is suspected. Symptoms include nervousness; irritability; confusion; weakness; pale, cold, clammy skin; diaphoresis (excessive perspiration); and tachycardia.
■ Obtain a history from the patient as to when hypoglycemic symptoms occur (eg, before meals). There may be periods of nervousness, "shakiness," and weakness.
■ Explain that eating candy to correct nervousness and weakness should be avoided with hyperinsulinism, since it will temporarily correct the problem (the need for glucose) but will stimulate insulin secretion. Sugar will temporarily correct an insulin reaction in a diabetic.

Elevated Level

■ Identify factors affecting glucose results (ie, emotional stress, infection, vomiting, fever, exercise, inactivity, age, drugs, and body weight). Most of these should be reported to the physician.
■ Check previous FBS results before the test. A known diabetic normally does not, and in some cases should not, have this test performed because diabetic coma may ensue.

GLUCOSE-6-PHOSPHATE DEHYDROGENASE
(G6PD or G-6-PD) (Blood)

Reference Values

Adult: Screen test: negative *Quantitative Test:* 8–18 IU/g Hb, 125–281 U/dL packed RBC, 251–511 U/10^6 cells, 1211–2111 mIU/mL packed RBC (varies with methods used)

Child: similar to adult

Description

G6PD is an enzyme in the RBCs or erythrocytes. It normally assists in glucose use in the RBCs, uses oxidative substances, and protects the integrity of the erythrocytes from injury.

A G6PD deficit is a sex-linked genetic defect carried by the female (X) chromosome, which will, in conjunction with infection, disease, and drugs, make a person susceptible to developing hemolytic anemia. With a moderate deficiency of G6PD enzyme, there is no apparent detectable RBC abnormality except for a decrease in the life-span of the RBCs. Metabolites from certain drugs possessing an oxidizing action in the RBCs will cause an increased need for G6PD for glucose metabolism. A lack of this enzyme results in hemolysis (destruction of the RBCs) and hemolytic anemia when augmented by an oxidative drug.[1,3,8–10]

Clinical Problems

Decreased Level: hemolytic anemia, diabetes acidosis, infections (bacterial and viral), septicemia. *Drug Influence:* acetanilid (acetylaniline), aspirin, ascorbic acid, nitrofurantoin (Furadantin), phenecetin, primaquine, thiazide diuretics, probenecid (Benemid), quinidine, quinine, chloramphenicol (Chloromycetin), sulfonamides, vitamin K, tolbutamide (Orinase). *Food:* fava beans

Procedure

- The laboratory methods used will vary. Screening tests for G6PD deficiency are methemoglobin reduction (Brewer's test), glutathione stability, dye reduction, and ascorbate and fluorescent spot tests. Check with the laboratory on whether capillary or venous blood is needed.
- Collect a small amount of capillary blood in a heparinized microhematocrit tube, or collect 5 mL of venous blood in a lavender- or a green-top tube.
- There is no food or fluid restriction.

- Factors Affecting Laboratory Results

  - Drugs can decrease level. (*See Drug Influence*)

NURSING IMPLICATIONS WITH RATIONALE

Decreased Level

- Obtain a familial history of RBC enzyme deficiency. Blacks are more prone to G6PD deficiency than whites; however, the degree of anemia is not as severe in blacks as it is in whites.
- Observe for symptoms of hemolysis, such as jaundice of the eyes and skin.
- Check for decreased urinary output. Urine should be voided at a rate of at least 25 mL/hour or 600 mL/day. Prolonged hemolysis (destruction of RBCs) can be toxic to the kidney cells, causing kidney impairment.
- Check the hemology results.
- Record oxidative drugs the patient is taking on laboratory slip. (*See Drug Influence*). Report your findings to the physician. Hemolysis usually occurs 3 days after the susceptible person has taken an oxidative drug. Hemolytic symptoms will disappear 2 to 3 days after the drug has been stopped.

Patient Teaching

- Instruct the susceptible person to read labels on patent medicines and not to take drugs that contain phenacetin and aspirin. Most of these drugs, if taken continuously, can cause hemolytic anemia.

GROWTH HORMONE (GH), HUMAN GROWTH HORMONE (hGH) SERUM
Somatotrophic Hormone (STH)

Reference Values

Adult: Male: <10 ng/mL. *Female:* <15 ng/mL. *Average:* <10 ng/mL (norms vary with method)

Child: <10 ng/mL

Description

Human growth hormone (hGH), hormone from the anterior pituitary gland, regulates growth of bone and tissue. Growth hormone levels are elevated by protein food, fasting, stress, exercise, and deep sleep.

A low serum hGH level might be the cause of dwarfism. Elevated hGH levels cause gigantism in children and acromegaly in adults. From a random growth hormone level, a positive diagnosis cannot be made; therefore *growth hormone stimulation or suppression challenge test* would be suggested. A glucose loading GH suppression test should suppress hGH secretion. Failure to suppress hGH levels confirms gigantism (children) or acromegaly (adult).[1,3,6,9,10]

Clinical Problems

Decreased Level: dwarfism in children, hypopituitarism. *Drug Influence:* cortisone preparations, phenothiazines, glucose

Elevated Level: gigantism (children), acromegaly (adult), major surgery, premature and newborn infants. *Drug Influence:* insulin, estrogens, amphetamines, beta-blockers, levodopa, methyldopa (Aldomet)

Procedure

- Collect 7 mL of venous blood in a 10-mL red-top tube, preferably in the early morning. Avoid hemolysis. Deliver the blood specimen immediately to the laboratory, since hGH has a short half-life.
- NPO for 8 to 10 hours except for water.
- Have the patient rest for 30 minutes to 1 hour before taking a blood sample.

- Factors Affecting Laboratory Results

- Stress, exercise, food (protein), and deep sleep could cause an elevated hGH level.
- Drugs listed in *Drug Influence* could decrease or elevate hGH levels.
- Hemolysis of the blood sample affect test result.

NURSING IMPLICATIONS WITH RATIONALE

- Maintain a quiet environment so that stress will not affect test results.
- Notify the physician or laboratory or both if patient is anxious, has eaten, or has exercised before the test.

155

Patient Teaching

■ Instruct the patient not to eat 8 to 10 hours before the test. Encourage the patient to rest and not to exercise prior to the test.
■ Inform the patient if the serum hGH is elevated, that follow-up testing may be necessary.

HALOPERIDOL (HALDOL) SERUM

Reference Values

Adult: Therapeutic Range: 3–20 ng/mL. *Peak Time:* PO: 2–6 hours. *Toxic Level:* >50 ng/mL

Description

Haloperidol is used in the treatment of acute and chronic psychosis, manic phase of manic-depressive psychosis, and in some cases of schizophrenia. It is a drug frequently used in psychiatry.[1–3,6]

Clinical Problems

Decreased Level: Drug Influence: anticholinergics (used for parkinsonism)
Elevated Level: overdose of haloperidol

Procedure

■ Collect 7 mL of venous blood in a red-top tube.
■ There is no food or fluid restriction.

■ Factors Affecting Laboratory Results

■ Anticholinergics used for the pseudoparkinsonism effect can decrease the effect of haloperidol.
■ Phenothiazines, benzodiazepines, or alcohol taken with haloperidol cause an additive CNS depressive effect.

NURSING IMPLICATIONS WITH RATIONALE

■ Observe for side effects of haloperidol (ie, dizziness, syncope, drowsiness, hypotension, pseudoparkinsonism, dry mouth, jaundice [due to large doses over a period of time]).
■ Check vital signs.

Patient Teaching

- Instruct the patient to avoid driving and activities that require alertness when taking haloperidol.
- Instruct the patient to avoid alcohol and other depressants that might cause side effects of haloperidol.
- Explain to the patient the importance of checking with the physician about taking over-the-counter (OTC) drugs. Some OTC drugs might cause side effects.

HAPTOGLOBIN (Hp) (SERUM)

Reference Values

Adult: 60–270 mg/dL; 0.6–2.7 g/L (SI units)

Child: Newborn: 0–10 mg/dL (absent in 90%). *Infant (1 to 6 months):* 0–30 mg/dL, then gradual increase

Description

Haptoglobins are α_2-globulins in the plasma. These globulin molecules combine with free (released) hemoglobin during RBC destruction (hemolysis). A decreased level of serum haptoglobin indicates hemolysis. Haptoglobins are decreased in severe liver disease, hemolytic anemia, and infectious mononucleosis and are elevated in inflammatory diseases, steroid therapy, acute infections, and malignancies. A hemolytic process may be masked in persons taking steroids.[3,9,10]

Clinical Problems

Decreased Level: hemolysis, anemias (pernicious, vitamin B_6 deficiency, hemolytic, sickle cell), severe liver disease (hepatic failure, chronic hepatitis), thrombotic thrombocytopenic purpura, disseminated intravascular coagulation (DIC), malaria

Elevated Level: inflammation, acute infections, cancer (lung, large intestine, stomach, breast, liver), Hodgkin's disease, ulcerative colitus, chronic pyelonephritis (active stage), rheumatic fever, acute myocardial infarction. *Drug Influence:* steroids (cortisone)

Procedure

- Collect 5 to 10 mL of venous blood in a red-top tube. Avoid hemolysis.
- There is no food or fluid restriction.
- Haptoglobin levels can be measured by electrophoresis, radioimmunodiffusion, or spectrophotometry.

■ Factors Affecting Laboratory Results

■ Steroids and inflammation may cause false results. Hemolysis could occur but the serum haptoglobin level may not indicate this.

NURSING IMPLICATIONS WITH RATIONALE

Decreased Level

■ Associate a decreased serum haptoglobin level with conditions causing hemolysis, such as hemolytic anemias, severe liver disease, and others.
■ Assess the patient's vital signs. Report abnormal vital signs, especially if the patient is having breathing problems. The oxygen capacity of hemoglobin may be reduced, causing a change in breathing pattern.
■ Assess the patient's urinary output. Excessive amounts of free hemoglobin may cause renal damage.

Elevated Level

■ Associate an elevated serum haptoglobin level with clinical problems, such as infections, inflammation, cancer, steroid therapy, and others.
■ Check the serum haptoglobin level. The haptoglobin level may be masked by steroid therapy and inflammation. If hemolysis is suspected, the serum level may be normal instead of low due to steroids or inflammation. Notify the physician of the findings.

HEMATOCRIT (Hct) (BLOOD)

Reference Values

Adult: Male: 40%–54%, 0.40–0.54 (SI units). *Female:* 36%–46%, 0.36–0.46 (SI units)

Child: Newborn: 44%–65%. *1 to 3 Years Old:* 29%–40%. *4 to 10 Years Old:* 31%–43%.

Description

The hematocrit (Hct) is the volume (in milliliters) of packed RBCs found in 100 mL (1 dL) of blood, expressed as a percentage. For example, a 36% hematocrit would indicate that 36 mL of RBCs were found in 100 mL of blood, or 36 vol/dL. The purpose of the test is to measure the concentration of RBCs (erythrocytes) in the blood.

Low hematocrit levels are found frequently in anemias and leukemias, and elevated levels are found in dehydration (a relative increase) and polycythemia vera. The hematocrit can be an indicator of the hydration status of the patient. As with hemoglobin, an elevated hematocrit level could indicate hemoconcentration because of a decrease in fluid volume and an increase in RBCs.[1,3,9,10,13]

Clinical Problems

Decreased Level: acute blood loss, anemias (aplastic, hemolytic, folic acid deficiency, pernicious, sideroblastic, sickle cell), leukemias (lymphocytic, myelocytic, monocytic), Hodgkin's disease, lymphosarcoma, malignancy of organs, multiple myeloma, cirrhosis of the liver, protein malnutrition, vitamin deficiencies (thiamine, vitamin C), fistula of the stomach or duodenum, peptic ulcer, chronic renal failure, pregnancy, systemic lupus erythematosus, rheumatoid arthritis (especially juvenile). *Drug Influence:* antineoplastic agents, antibiotics (chloramphenicol, penicillin), radioactive agents

Elevated Level: dehydration/hypovolemia, severe diarrhea, polycythemia vera, erythrocytosis, diabetic acidosis, pulmonary emphysema (later stage), transient cerebral ischemia (TIA), eclampsia, surgery, burns

Procedure

- No food or fluid is restricted.

Venous Blood

- Collect 7 mL of venous blood in a lavender-top tube. Mix well. Tourniquet should be on for less than 2 minutes.
- Do not take blood specimen from the same arm as IV.

Capillary Blood

- Collect capillary blood using the microhematocrit method. Blood is obtained from a finger prink, using a heparinized capillary tube.

- Factors Affecting Laboratory Results

  - If blood is collected from an extremity that has an IV line, the hematocrit will most likely be low. Avoid using such an extremity.
  - If blood is taken to check hematocrit levels immediately after moderate to severe blood loss and transfusions, the hematocrit could be normal.
  - Age of the patient—newborns normally have higher hematocrit levels because of hemoconcentration.

NURSING IMPLICATIONS WITH RATIONALE

- Explain the procedure of the test to the patient. If the microhematocrit method is used, explain that the finger will be cleansed with an alcohol sponge and pricked with a lancet or needle to obtain capillary blood.

Decreased Level

- Relate a decreased hematocrit level to clinical problems and drugs. Blood loss and anemias are the commonest causes of a low hematocrit. A hematocrit of 30% or less with no known bleeding frequently indicates a moderate to severe anemic condition.

- Assess for signs and symptoms of anemia (fatigue, paleness, and tachycardia).
- Assess changes in vital signs to determine whether shock is present because of blood loss. Symptoms could include rapid pulse, rapid respirations, and normal or decreased BP.
- Recommend a repeat hematocrit several days after moderate/severe bleeding or transfusions. A hematocrit taken immediately after blood loss and after transfusions may appear normal.

Elevated Level

- Relate an elevated hematocrit level to clinical problems. Dehydration and hypovolemia are common problems with hematocrit elevation because of hemoconcentration.
- Assess for signs and symptoms of dehydration/hypovolemia. A history of vomiting, diarrhea, marked thirst, lack of skin turgor, and shocklike symptoms (rapid pulse and respiration rates) could be indicative of a body fluid deficit.
- Administer IV or oral fluids according to the physician's order to reestablish body fluid volume.
- Avoid rapid administration of IV fluids to the older adult, child, or debilitated person so as to prevent overhydration and pulmonary edema. Signs and symptoms of overhydration are constant, irritated cough; dyspnea; hand and/or neck vein engorgement; and chest rales.
- Check the hematocrit daily, if ordered, when reestablishing body fluid volume. When an elevated hematocrit returns to normal, the elevation was due to hemoconcentration.
- Assess changes in urinary output. A urine output of less than 25 mL/hour or 600 mL daily could be due to dehydration/hypovolemia. Once body fluids are restored, urine output should be normal.

HEMOGLOBIN (Hb OR Hgb) (BLOOD)

Reference Values

Adult: *Male:* 13.5–18 g/dL. *Female:* 12–16 g/dL

Child: *Newborn:* 14–24 g/dL. *Infant:* 10–15 g/dL. *Child:* 11–16 g/dL

Description

Hemoglobin (Hb or Hgb), a protein substance found in RBCs, gives blood its red color. Hemoglobin is composed of iron, which is an oxygen carrier. Abnormally high hemoglobin levels may be due to hemoconcentration resulting from dehydration (fluid loss). Low hemoglobin values are related to various clinical problems.

The RBC count and hemoglobin do not always increase or decrease in value equally. For instance, a decreased RBC count and a normal or slightly decreased hemoglobin occur in pernicious anemia, and a normal or slightly decreased RBC and a decreased hemoglobin occur in iron deficiency (microcytic) anemia.[1,9,10,12,13]

Clinical Problems

Decreased Level: anemias (iron deficiency, aplastic, hemocytic), severe hemorrhage, cirrhosis of the liver, leukemias, Hodgkin's disease, sarcoidosis, excess IV fluids, cancer (large and small intestine, rectum, liver, bone), thalassemia major, pregnancy, kidney diseases. *Drug Influence:* antibiotics (chloramphenicol [Chloromycetin], penicillin, tetracycline), aspirin, antineoplastic drugs, doxapram (Dopram), hydantoin derivatives, hydralazine (Apresoline), indomethacin (Indocin), MAO inhibitors, primaquine, rifampin, sulfonamides, trimethadione (Tridione), vitamin A (large doses)

Elevated Level: dehydration/hemoconcentration, polycythemia, high altitudes, chronic obstructive lung disease, congestive heart failure, severe burns. *Drug Influence:* gentamicin, methyldopa (Aldomet)

Procedure

- There is no food or fluid restriction.
- Do not take the blood sample from a hand or arm receiving IV fluid. The tourniquet should be on less than a minute.

Venous Blood: Collect 7 mL of venous blood in a lavender-top tube. Avoid hemolysis.

Capillary Blood: Puncture the cleansed earlobe, finger, or heel with a sterile lancet. Do not squeeze the puncture site tightly, for serous fluid and blood would thus be obtained. Wipe away the first drop of blood. Collect drops of blood quickly in micropipettes with small rubber tops or microhematocrit tubes. Expel blood into the tubes with diluents.

■ Factors Affecting Laboratory Results

- Drugs could increase or decrease hemoglobin. (*See Drug Influence above.*)
- Taking blood from an arm or hand receiving IV fluids could dilute blood sample.
- Leaving the tourniquet on for more than a minute. Hemoglobin results could be falsely elevated due to hemostasis.
- Living in high altitudes will increase hemoglobin levels.
- Decreased fluid intake or fluid loss will increase hemoglobin levels due to hemoconcentration, and excessive fluid intake will decrease hemoglobin levels due to hemodilution.

NURSING IMPLICATIONS WITH RATIONALE

■ Explain to the patient the procedure of the test.

Decreased Level

■ Recognize clinical problems and drugs that could cause a decreased hemoglobin level (*see Clinical Problems*). Anemia is a common cause, but usually the patient is not considered anemic until the hemoglobin level is below 10.5 g/dL. Hemorrhage could cause a low hemoglobin level if the blood is not replaced; however, the hemoglobin level does not decrease immediately. It may remain normal for hours or even several days.
■ Observe the patient for signs and symptoms of anemia (ie, dizziness, tachycardia, weakness, dyspnea at rest). Symptoms depend on how low the hemoglobin level is (severe anemia).
■ Check the hematocrit level if the hemoglobin level is low.

Elevated Level

■ Recognize clinical problems and drugs that can cause an increased hemoglobin level (*see Clinical Problems*). Dehydration is a major transient cause of an elevated level. Once the patient is hydrated, the hemoglobin should return to the normal range.
■ Observe for signs and symptoms of dehydration (ie, marked thirst, poor skin turgor, dry mucous membranes, and shocklike symptoms [tachycardia, tachypnea, and, later, decreased BP]).

Patient Teaching

■ Instruct the patient to maintain an adequate fluid intake. Frequently older adults tend to drink less fluid.

HEMOGLOBIN ELECTROPHORESIS (BLOOD)
Hemoglobins A_1, A_2, F, C, S

Reference Values

Adult: Hemoglobin (Hb or Hgb) Electrophoresis: A_1, 95%–98% total Hb; A_2, 1.5%; F, <2%; C, 0%; D, 0%; S, 0%

Child: Newborn: Hb, F, 50%–80% total Hb. *Infant:* Hb F, 8% total Hb. *Child:* Hb F, 1%–2% total Hb after 6 months

Description

The normal types of hemoglobin are Hb A_1, comprising 95% to 98% of the total hemoglobin; Hb A_2, and Hb F (fetal). If Hb F comprises 5% or more of the total hemoglobin after the age of 6 months, thalassemia (Mediterranean anemia)

could be a factor. There are three clinical types of thalassemia; thalassemia major (Hb F is over 50%), thalassemia minor (increased Hb A_2 value), and thalassemia gene (combination of abnormal hemoglobins).

To identify normal hemoglobin types (A_1, A_2, and F) and abnormal hemoglobin types (Hb C, Hb M, Hb S, and others), a hemoglobin electrophoresis is usually ordered. It is not a routine test, but it is useful for identifying 150 or more types of hemoglobin. Many abnormal hemoglobin types do not produce harmful diseases; the common hemoglobinopathies are identified through electrophoresis.

Hemoglobin S: Hb S is the commonest hemoglobin variant. If both genes have Hb S, sickle cell anemia will occur; but if only one gene has Hb S, then the person simply carries the sickle trait. Approximately 1% of the black population in the United States has sickle cell anemia, and 8% to 10% carry the sickle cell trait.

Sickle cell anemia symptoms are usually not present until after the age of 6 months. In some cases Hb S is combined with another abnormal hemoglobin type, Hb C or Hb D. Hb S/C or Hb S/D produces RBCs (erythrocytes) that sickle as with Hb S/S. Those with sickle cell anemia have low oxygen tension (*also see Sickle Cell Test*).

Hemoglobin C: Hb C in the homozygous state (C/C) usually produces mild hemolytic anemia; in the heterozygous state (A/C), it produces the Hb C trait. This occurs more frequently in blacks.[1,10–13]

Clinical Problems

HEMOGLOBIN TYPE	ELEVATED LEVEL
Hemoglobin F	Thalassemia (after 6 months)
Hemoglobin C	Hemolytic anemia
Hemoglobin S	Sickle cell anemia

Procedure

- Collect 7 to 10 mL of venous blood in a lavender-top tube. Send immediately to the laboratory. Abnormal hemoglobin is unstable.
- There is no food or fluid restriction.

■ Factors Affecting Laboratory Results

- Blood transfusions given 4 months before hemoglobin electrophoresis may cause inaccurate results.
- Collection of the blood sample in the wrong color tube can affect results.

NURSING IMPLICATIONS WITH RATIONALE

- Observe for signs and symptoms of sickle cell anemia. Early symptoms are fatigue and weakness. Chronic symptoms are fatigue, dyspnea on exertion, swollen joints, bones that ache, and chest pains. Afflicted persons are susceptible to infection. Sickle cell crisis is usually due to small infarcts to

---

various organs. The crisis usually lasts 5 to 7 days, and immediate care is needed for the symptoms. Normally the hemoglobin level does not change.

Patient Teaching

- Encourage the patient to seek genetic counseling if he or she has sickle cell anemia or is a carrier of the sickle cell trait.
- Instruct the patient with sickle cell anemia to minimize strenuous activity and to avoid high altitudes and extreme cold. Encourage the patient to take rest periods.
- Encourage the patient to stay away from persons with infections.
- Suggest that the patient carry a medical alert bracelet and/or card.

HEPATITIS B SURFACE ANTIGEN (HB$_s$Ag) (SERUM)
Hepatitis-Associated Antigen (HAA)

Reference Values
Adult: negative
Child: negative

Description

The hepatitis B surface antigen (HB$_s$Ag) test was originally called the Australia antigen test and later the hepatitis-associated antigen (HAA) test. This test is done to determine the presence of hepatitis B virus in the blood in either an active or a carrier state (as in a hepatitis B carrier). Approximately 5% of persons with diseases other than hepatitis B (serum hepatitis) will have a positive HB$_s$Ag test.

The HB$_s$Ag test is routinely performed on the donor's blood to identify the hepatitis B antigen. Transmission of hepatitis B in blood transfusions has greatly diminished through HB$_s$Ag screening of the donor's blood and excluding donors with a history of hepatitis. Though transfusion-related hepatitis B has decreased, the occurrence of hepatitis B is still on the increase.

In hepatitis B, the antigen in the serum can be detected 2 to 24 weeks (average 4 to 8 weeks) after exposure to the virus. The positive HB$_s$Ag may be present 2 to 6 weeks after onset of the clinical disease. Approximately 10% of the patients with positive HB$_s$Ag are carriers, and their tests may remain positive for years.

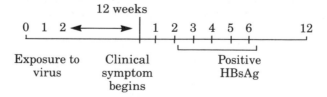

In 75% to 90% of the patients, antibody to hepatitis B surface antigen (called anti-HB$_s$Ag or HB$_s$Ab) is found 2 to 12 weeks after HB$_s$Ag occurs. Anti-HB$_s$Ag can be detected for years after the acute viral infection, but it does not guarantee immunity against future hepatitis infection.

HB$_s$Ag test does not diagnose hepatitis A virus. Two tests for hepatitis A are anti–HAV-IgM (indicates an acute infection) and anti–HAV-IgG (indicates a past exposure).[6,8–10,13]

Clinical Problems

Elevated Level (positive): hepatitis B, chronic hepatitis B. *Less Common:* hemophilia, Down's syndrome, Hodgkin's disease, leukemia. *Drug Influence:* drug addicts

Procedure

- Collect 5–7 mL of venous blood in a red-top tube. Careful handling of the blood sample and washing the hands are most important to keep from contacting the viral hepatitis B.
- There is no food or fluid restriction.

- Factors Affecting Laboratory Results

  - None known.

NURSING IMPLICATIONS WITH RATIONALE

- Explain to the patient the purpose of the test. If the person is a blood donor, the test is automatically done after the unit of blood is taken. Most of these persons do not know that the HB$_s$Ag test and other blood tests are done on donor's blood.
- Obtain a history of any previous hepatitis infection and report it to the physician.

Elevated Level (positive test)

- Handle blood obtained from the patient with care, avoiding blood contact with your skin (especially if skin and nail cuts are present). If you accidentally stick yourself with the used needle, you should, in most cases, receive gamma globulin as a preventive measure to avoid the disease.
- Discard all needles and syringes used on patients having hepatitis B. Follow the hospital's isolation procedure.
- Observe for signs and symptoms of hepatitis, such as lethargy, anorexia, nausea and vomiting, fever, dark-colored urine, and jaundice.

Patient Teaching

- Instruct the patient to get plenty of rest; a nutritional diet, if tolerated; and fluids (juice and carbonated drinks).

HETEROPHILE ANTIBODY (SERUM, MONO-SPOT)

Reference Values

Adult: normal, <1:28 titer; abnormal, >1:56 titer

Child: same as adult

Elderly: normal, slightly higher titer than adult

Description

This is a test primarily for infectious mononucleosis. Infectious mononucleosis is thought to be caused by Epstein-Barr virus (EBV).

Heterophiles are a group of antibodies that react to sheep and horse's RBCs, and if positive (titer), an agglutination occurs. Titers of 1:56 to 1:224 are highly suspicious of infectious mononucleosis; those of 1:224 or greater are positive for infectious mononucleosis. Elevated heterophile titers occur during the first 2 weeks, peak in 3 weeks, and remain elevated for 6 weeks. Sixty to 80% of persons with infectious mononucleosis have a positive heterophile antibody test.

Mono-Spot: There are several commercially prepared tests: Monospot by Ortho Diagnostics; Monoscreen by Smith, Kline and French; and Monotest by Wapole. Mono-Spot test is usually done first; if positive, then the titer test is performed.[1,9,10,12,13]

Clinical Problems

Elevated Level: Infectious mononucleosis, serum sickness, viral infections

Procedure

Heterophile Antibody

- ■ Collect 5 to 10 mL of venous blood in a red-top tube.
- ■ There is no food or drink restriction.

Mono-Spot Screening Test: Collect 2 mL of venous blood in a red-top tube. Use a monokit and follow directions. The patient's serum is mixed with the guinea pig tissue on one spot of a glass slide, and at another spot on the slide it is mixed with beef red-cell stromata. Unwashed horse red cells are added to both spots. Observe for 1 minute for agglutination. Results of the Mono-Spot test are as follows:

1. If agglutination is stronger at the guinea-pig–kidney-tissue spot, the test is positive for infectious mononucleosis.
2. If agglutination is stronger at the beef red cells, the test is negative for infectious mononucleosis.
3. If agglutination is present at both spots, the test is negative for infectious mononucleosis.
4. If no agglutination is present at either spot, the test is negative.

- ■ There is no food or drink restriction. Usually in infectious mononucleosis the WBC differential may have 10% to 25% atypical lymphocytes.

■ Factors Affecting Laboratory Results

■ Serum sickness and Forssman antibodies can cause positive titers.

NURSING IMPLICATIONS WITH RATIONALE

■ Explain to the patient the procedure for the heterophile antibody test and the Mono-Spot test.
■ Obtain a history of the patient's contact with any person or persons recently diagnosed as having infectious mononucleosis.
■ Observe for signs and symptoms of infectious mononucleosis, such as fever, sore throat, fatigue, swollen glands.
■ Determine when the symptoms (fever, fatigue, sore throat) first occurred. A repeat heterophile antibody or Mono-Spot test may be needed if the first was done too early. Elevated titers take 4 to 8 weeks to return to normal.

Patient Teaching

■ Encourage the patient to rest, drink fluids, and follow the physician's orders.

HEXOSAMINIDASE (TOTAL, A, AND A AND B) SERUM, AMNIOTIC FLUID

Reference Values

Adult: *Total:* 5–20 U/L. Hexosaminidase A: 55%–80%

Description

Hexosaminidase is a group of enzymes (isoenzymes A and B) responsible for the metabolism of gangliosides. It is found in brain tissue. Lack of the hexosaminidase A causes Tay-Sachs disease because of the accumulation of gangliosides in the brain. The total hexosaminidase may be normal or decreased. This test is used to confirm Tay-Sachs disease or to identify Tay-Sachs carriers.

Tay-Sachs disease is an autosomal-recessive disorder resulting in progressive destruction of the CNS cells. It is characterized by mental retardation, muscular weakness, and blindness. It affects primarily the Ashkenazic Jewish population. Death usually occurs before the age of 5 years.

Sandhoff's disease, a variant of Tay-Sachs, progresses more rapidly than Tay-Sachs disease. With this disorder there is a deficiency of hexosaminidase A and B. It is not prevalent in any ethnic group.[3,9,10]

Clinical Problems

Decreased Level: *Hexosaminidase A:* Tay-Sachs disease. *Hexosaminidase A and B:* Sandhoff's disease

167

Procedure

- Collect 7 mL of venous blood in a red-top tube for serum value. Avoid hemolysis.
- Collect cord blood from newborn.
- There is no food or fluid restriction.

■ Factors Affecting Laboratory Results

- Hemolysis of blood sample can cause inaccurate test result.
- Pregnancy could increase total hexosaminidase values. *Note:* Most laboratories will not perform the test on pregnant women.

NURSING IMPLICATIONS WITH RATIONALE

- Talk with physician and genetic counselor when both partners have a hexosaminidase A deficiency. It is important that correct information and answers are given to the couple.

Patient Teaching

- Inform the Ashkenazic Jewish couple that the hexosaminidase screening test is to determine if they are Tay-Sachs carriers. Explain to the couple that it is a recessive trait and that both must carry the gene for their offspring to get Tay-Sachs disease.

HUMAN CHORIONIC GONADOTROPIN (HCG) (Serum and Urine)
Pregnancy Test

Reference Values

Values may be expressed as IU/mL or ng/mL. Check with your laboratory.

Adult: SERUM: nonpregnant female: <0.01 IU/mL

PREGNANT (WEEKS)	VALUES	
1	0.01–0.04	IU/mL
2	0.03–0.10	IU/mL
4	0.10–1.0	IU/mL
5–12	10–100	IU/mL
13–25	10–30	IU/mL
26–40	5–15	IU/mL

- *URINE:* nonpregnant female: negative; pregnant: 1–12 weeks: 6000–500,000 IU/24 h. Many OTC pregnancy kits available. The woman is usually tested 3 days after missed menstrual period.[1]

Description

HCG is a hormone produced by the placenta. In pregnancy HCG appears in the blood and urine 14 to 26 days after the conception, and the HCG concentration peaks in approximately 8 weeks. After the first trimester of pregnancy, HCG production declines. HCG is not found in nonpregnant women, in death of the fetus, or after 3 to 4 days postpartum.

The immunologic test for pregnancy using anti-HCG serum is more sensitive, more accurate, less costly, and easier to perform than the older pregnancy test, which used live animals. The Aschheim-Zondek test and the Friedman test are no longer used.

Certain tumors (such as the hydatidiform mole, chorionepithelioma of the uterus, and choriocarcinoma of the testicle) can cause a positive HCG test. HCG may be requested on males for the determination of testicular tumor.[8–10,12,14]

Clinical Problems

Decreased Level (negative): nonpregnant, dead fetus, postpartum (3 to 4 days), incomplete abortion, threatened abortion (decreased serum value)

Elevated Level (positive): pregnancy, hydatidiform mole, chorionepithelioma, choriocarcinoma. *Drug Influence:* anticonvulsants, hypnotics, tranquilizers (phenothiazines), antiparkinsonism drugs

Procedure

- Perform the pregnancy test 2 weeks (no earlier than 5 days) after the first missed menstrual period. There are several commercially prepared kits for the immunologic pregnancy test.
- There is no food restriction.

Serum
- Perform the pregnancy test no earlier than 5 days after the first missed menstrual period.
- Collect 5 mL of venous blood in a red-top tube. Avoid hemolysis.

Urine
- NPO of fluid for 8 to 12 hours; no food is restricted.
- Take a morning urine specimen (60 mL) with specific gravity > 1.010 to the laboratory immediately. A 24-hour urine collection may be requested.
- Instruct patient to follow directions when using commercial kit.
- Avoid blood in the urine, as false positives could occur.

Note: There are many commercial kits; follow the directions on kit.

■ Factors Affecting Laboratory Results

- Diluted urine (specific gravity <1.010) could cause a false-negative test result.
- Certain drug groups can cause false-positive test results (*see Drug Influence*).
- Protein and blood in the urine could cause false-positive test results.
- During menopause, there may be an excess secretion of pituitary gonadotropin hormone, which could cause a false-positive result.

NURSING IMPLICATIONS WITH RATIONALE

■ Ask the patient when she had her last period. The test should be done 5 or more days after the missed period to avoid a false-negative result. Blood in the urine can cause a false-positive result.
■ Listen to patient's concerns.

Patient Teaching

■ Inform the patient who plans to use a commercially prepared pregnancy kit to follow the directions carefully.
■ Inform the patient that she will receive the results of the test within minutes. Some tests, such as a serum value, may take 1 to 2 hours.

HUMAN IMMUNOSUPPRESSIVE VIRUS (HIV) (SERUM)*
Human T-Cell Lymphotrophic Virus-III, Lymphadenopathy-Associated Virus (LAV)

Reference Values
Adult: seronegative (blood shows no evidence of HIV infection ie, no HIV antibodies found in serum)
Child: seronegative (same)

Description*
The retrovirus HIV has been identified as a cause of acquired immune deficiency syndrome (AIDS), which was first recognized in 1981. AIDS interferes with and destroys the immune system's T lymphocytes, creating increased susceptibility to opportunistic infections and rarer forms of cancer. It is believed that the infection starts once the virus invades the body, even though it may take approximately 6 weeks to more than a year for a positive antibody response to be found diagnostically. The virus is, however, transmittable during this period. Current studies have noted that HIV may remain latent in the body for up to 15 years (ie, without symptoms or clinical signs, although the infection does exist). Once an official diagnosis of AIDS has been made, although individual variations may occur in clinical course, over 80% die in 2 to 3 years.

HIV has been isolated in lymphocytes from blood, semen, saliva, tears, urine, brain, and breast milk. Transmission of the virus by tears is not known; exchange of saliva through "deep kissing" (which may also irritate mucous membrane is not currently viewed as a safe sex practice; "dry kissing" is considered safe. Infected lymphocytes carried by semen or vaginal fluid and/or blood can transmit the virus from an infected individual of either sex to a noninfected individual.

The incidence of positive HIV antibody in negative health care workers (nurses, physicians, and laboratory workers) directly exposed to blood from AIDS clients has been found to be statistically low. Investigation has revealed that exposure of most health care workers to the infection is preventable

It is estimated that by 1992, between 945,000 and 1.4 million Americans will have become infected with HIV; the Centers for Disease Control (CDC) also estimate that the annual number of *new* cases of AIDS in the United States is anticipated to rise from the 1989 figure of about 50,000 to approximately 70,000. By mid-1989, over 105,000 cases of AIDS had been reported *cumulatively,* with the number expected to increase to over 365,000 diagnosed cases by 1992. Estimates also include predictions that about 65,000 individuals who were earlier diagnosed with AIDS will die by the end of 1992.

In regard to pediatric clients, the CDC report a marked increase in new cases of AIDS in children under 13 years of age. Individual states also report increasingly large numbers of infants born infected with HIV. Some congenitally infected children have survived beyond the age of 10 years.

Individuals considered most at risk for contracting HIV infection include (1) *anyone* having unprotected sexual contact (vaginal, oral, or rectal) that involves exchange of vaginal fluid, semen, and/or blood with an infected person, particularly if unsafe practices such as sexual encounters with multiple partners or placing of a hand or "fist" into the rectum or mouth/anal contact ("rimming") involving subsequent body fluid exchange occurs; (2) IV drug abusers using infected needles; (3) the fetus exposed to the virus during gestation within an HIV infected mother; (4) persons who received blood transfusions prior to 1985. Since March 1985, all blood in banks is tested for HIV using the screening test enzyme-linked immunosorbent assay (ELISA); those donations that test positive are discarded. Transfusions with blood that has been screened is now considered a very minimal risk.[30–38]

Clinical Problems

Seropositive Test: Blood shows evidence of infection; HIV antibodies found in serum. (*Note:* For CDC to recognize and to diagnose AIDS, the client's history must fit with signs and symptoms agreed upon, *not* just the test result.)

Procedure

The diagnostic test developed for HIV identifies the presence of antibodies to HIV rather than the actual virus itself.

■ A signed consent form for HIV test is usually required from clients, except blood donors.
■ Collect 5 to 10 mL of venous blood in a red-top tube.
■ There are no food or fluid restrictions pre/post test.
■ ELISA, a nonspecific screening test to identify antibodies to the virus, is inexpensive and available in most laboratories. False-positive results can occur as a result of infections or reaction with another viral antigen. If positive, the ELISA is repeated, and if a second positive test occurs, the blood specimen is sent to a laboratory center for a more expensive confirmation test, usually the Western Blot procedure. It is only when the results of all three tests are positive that the client is considered to be HIV positive and is notified; if results are negative, usually the client is not notified of the

results of the tests. Blood donations with positive ELISA are discarded even if the Western Blot is negative.

■ Factors Affecting Laboratory Tests

   ■ None known

NURSING IMPLICATIONS WITH RATIONALE*

■ Obtain a client's signed, informed consent for HIV antibody testing in accordance with any existing state laws and/or hospital policy; consent, in writing, is preferable to verbal consent, should any dispute occur; document when information and/or counseling is provided.

■ Explain to the client that a positive HIV antibody test indicates possible exposure or possible presence of the virus. It does not always mean that the client has AIDS; repeat of test may be needed. A true-positive antibody test result (confirmation with Western Blot) means person is infected with HIV; in the future *may* become ill, exhibiting signs and symptoms; and that the client *can* cause others to become infected through sexual or blood contact.

■ Assess the client for signs or symptoms related to a depressed immune system related to infection with HIV, including tenderness and/or enlargement in lymph nodes in the cervical, axillary, and groin areas; fatigue; unexplained persistent fever; anorexia; weight loss (> 10 lb in 2 months); shortness of breath; cough; night sweats; persistent diarrhea; white spots or unusual mouth sores.

■ Refer the client to appropriate community resources that are known to assist in the areas of educational resources. Help client cope with stress, and promote activities of daily living.

■ Employ "universal precautions" (protective measures). Contact with blood, blood products, and/or body fluids is a possibility with *all* clients, irrespective of seropositive or seronegative status for HIV. A side benefit is that most clients will feel equally treated within a facility.

■ Protective measures include proper handwashing and use of intact latex or vinyl gloves prior to invasive procedures and if contact with blood or secretions (directly or indirectly) is possible; use of protective masks and goggles plus impervious gowns or aprons in conditions where blood may splatter; proper handling of laboratory specimens in accordance with infection control literature; proper disposal of soiled linens in leak-proof bags; proper handling of tubes, needles, and sharps (no recapping; no bending; no separating of needle from disposable syringes; disposal in puncture-free disposals); proper clean up of spills. Refrain from direct client care if caretaker's skin is nonintact.

■ Advise individuals not to use toothbrushes or razors of high-risk individuals known to be HIV positive because of the possibility of blood contamination due to bleeding gums.

---

*Contributed by Jane P. Taylor, R.N., M.S.

- Explain to members in the community that casual contact (talking to, shaking hands with, sharing glasses with, embracing, sharing spoons with, or being a household-sharing family member) with a HIV-positive person or one with AIDS, or with a person at high risk for AIDS does not put them at high risk for contacting AIDS. Intimate, unsafe sexual contact (oral, vaginal, rectal) with an infected person puts the individual at high risk to contact AIDS. The nurse needs to employ factual information to help address the high degree of anxiety and fear reactions within the public sector.
- Encourage clients with AIDS to voluntarily identify persons with whom they have had sexual contact. Clients may, at times, share names with the nurse before they tell the physician.
- Incorporate into teaching plans that the risks of infection rises with the number of male and/or female partners one has; thus it is important to stress the importance of one sexual partner.
- Incorporate into teaching plans that drug abuse with potentially infected needles and syringes used by someone else increases the risk of HIV infection. Attempt to counsel against drug abuse; however, be prepared to explain to addicts, if necessary, the proper procedure for cleaning needles and syringes.
- Inform seropositive women, if contemplating pregnancy, of the risk of infecting the fetus. Encourage them to talk with their health care professional about the risk of AIDS for their child.
- Encourage individuals to donate blood because sterile equipment is used and discarded with no risk of infection. Explain that donors have no contact with other blood.
- Assume a nonjudgmental position with AIDS clients and their families in regard to how the illness may have been acquired.

HUMAN LEUKOCYTE ANTIGEN (HLA) SERUM
HLA Typing, Organ-Donor Tissue Typing

Reference Values

Histocompatibility match or nonmatch; no norms

Description

Nucleated cells, including leukocytes, platelets, and many tissue cells, have antigens of the human leukocyte antigen (HLA) system on their surface membranes. These antigens are classified into five different series: A, B, C, D, and DR (D-related). There are many groups of these five series (20 A antigens, 40 B antigens, 8 C antigens, 12 D antigens, and 10 DR antigens) that can be HLA phenotyped to determine histocompatibility.[5]

Testing for HLA antigens is useful in determining tissue typing for recipients and donors for organ transplants, paternity testing, and genetic counseling associated with susceptibility to certain diseases. A putative father who does not have any antigen pair identical to one of the child's is excluded as the father.[1,3,9,10]

Clinical Problems

Positive Histocompatibility: tissue compatibility for grafts and organ transplants, father of child

Procedure

- Collect 10 mL of venous blood in a green-top tube. Avoid hemolysis. Blood samples should be tested immediately.
- There is no food or fluid restriction.

■ Factors Affecting Laboratory Results

- Hemolysis of the blood sample.
- Blood transfusion in the last 3 days could affect test results.

NURSING IMPLICATIONS WITN RATIONALE

- Encourage the patient to express concerns related to health problems.

HUMAN PLACENTAL LACTOGEN (hPL) SERUM
Chorionic Somatomammotropin

Reference Values

Adult: Nonpregnant Female: < 0.5 μg/mL

Pregnant Female

WEEKS OF GESTATION	REFERENCE VALUES
5–7	1.0 μg/mL
8–27	< 4.6 μg/mL
28–31	2.4–6.0 μg/mL
32–35	3.7–7.7 μg/mL
36–term	5.0–10.0 μg/mL

Male: < 0.5 μg/mL

Description

Human placental lactogen (hPL), a hormone produced by the placenta, can be detected in the maternal blood after 5 weeks of gestation. The hPL increases slowly throughout the pregnancy. This test is useful for evaluating placental function and fetal well-being in high-risk pregnancies, especially from the 28th week to term. A marked decrease in the serum hPL level during the third trimester of pregnancy is indicative of fetal distress; however, additional testing is recommended to determine fetal distress. A serum estriol and nonstress test are frequently ordered to verify the hPL test result.[1,3,9,10]

Clinical Problems

Decreased Level: fetal distress, toxemia of pregnancy, threatened-abortion, trophoblastic neoplastic disease (hydatidiform mole, choriocarcinoma)

Elevated Level: multiple pregnancy, diabetes mellitus, bronchogenic carcinoma, liver tumor, lymphoma

Procedure

- Collect 7 mL of venous blood in a red-top or green-top tube. Avoid hemolysis.
- hPL fluctuates; therefore the test might need to be repeated.
- There is no food or fluid restriction.

- Factors Affecting Laboratory Results

- Hemolysis of the blood sample.

NURSING IMPLICATIONS WITH RATIONALE

- Record the gestation week on the laboratory slip.
- Correlate the serum hPL result with the serum or urine estriol level. The human placental lactogen levels can fluctuate daily, so the hPL test is usually repeated, and other tests for detecting fetal distress are also ordered.

Patient Teaching

- Inform the patient that the test may be repeated due to frequently hPL fluctuations. Explain that other tests are usually ordered to monitor the fetal well-being.

17-HYDROXYCORTICOSTEROIDS (17-OHCS) (URINE)
Corticoids 17-OH, Porter-Silber Chromogens

Reference Values

Adult: Male: 5–15 mg/24 h. *Female:* 3–13 mg/24 h. Average 2–12 mg/24 h

Elderly: lower than adult

Child: Infant to 1 year: < 1 mg/24 h. *2 to 4 years:* 1–2 mg/24 h. *5 to 12 years:* 6–8 mg/24 h

Description

17-OHCS are metabolites of adrenocortical steroid hormones, mostly of cortisol, and are excreted in the urine. Since the excretion of the metabolites is diurnal, varying in rate of excretion, a 24-hour urine specimen is necessary for accuracy of test results. This test is useful for assessing adrenocortical hormone function. An increased urinary concentration of 17-OHCS may indicate hyperadrenalism, and a decreased urinary concentration may indicate hypoadrenalism.[3,9,10,13]

Clinical Problems

Decreased Level: Addison's disease, androgenital syndrome, hypopituitarism, myxedema (hypothroidism). *Drug Influence:* calcium gluconate, dexamethasone (Decadron), phenytoin (Dilantin), promethazine (Phenergan), reserpine (Serpasil)

Elevated Level: Cushing's syndrome, adrenal cancer, eclampsia, hyperpituitarism, hyperthyroidism, extreme stress, *Drug Influence:* antibiotics (cloxacillin, erythromycin), acetazolamide (Diamox), ascorbic acid, chloral hydrate, chlordiazepoxide (Librium), chlorothiazide (Diuril), chlorpromazine (Thorazine), colchicine, cortisone, digoxin, digitoxin, estrogen, hydroxyzine (Atarax), iodides, oral contraceptives, meprobamate (Equanil or Miltown), methenamine (Urex), paraldehyde, quinine, quinidine, spironolactone (Aldactone)

Procedure

- Collect urine in a large container/bottle, and add an acid preservative to prevent bacterial degradation of the steroids. The urine collection should be refrigerated if no preservative is added. No toilet paper or feces should be in the urine.
- Label container with patient's name, date, and exact time of collection (eg, 9/23/92, 7:20 AM to 9/24/92, 7:30 AM).
- Withhold drugs (with physician's approval) for 3 days before the test to prevent false results. Any drugs given should be listed on the laboratory slip.
- No food or fluid is restricted, except for coffee and tea. Fluid intake should be encouraged.

- Factors Affecting Laboratory Results

  - Drugs (*see Drug Influence*). Cortisone can elevate the urinary levels of 17-OHCS, and dexamethasone (Decadron), a potent cortisone derivative, can decrease the 17-OHCS level. The potent cortisone drug inhibits ACTH production, which causes a decrease in adrenocortical hormone secretion.
  - If the 24-hour urine sample is not refrigerated or does not contain a preservative, the results of the test could be inaccurate.

NURSING IMPLICATIONS WITH RATIONALE

- Encourage the patient to drink 6 to 8 glasses of water or other fluid (except coffee) during the 24-hour test.

■ Check the drugs the patient is receiving, and withhold drugs (with the physician's permission) that may interfere with test results. Many times, medication cannot be withheld; in such cases, the drugs given should be listed on the laboratory slip and reported.

■ Explain to the patient and family that all urine should be saved during a 24-hour period and that there should be no toilet paper or feces in the urine.

■ Label the urine bottle with the patient's name and the date and exact time for the urine collection (eg, 11/3/93, 7:20 AM to 11/4/93, 7:22 AM).

■ Post a notice of urine collection on the patient's door or bed and in the Kardex.

■ Check the results of the plasma cortisol and 17-ketosteroids tests.

Decreased Level

■ Observe for signs and symptoms of hypoadrenalism (Addison's disease). These symptoms include fatigue, weakness, weight loss, bronze coloration of the skin, postural hypotension, arrhythmia, craving of salty food, and fasting hypoglycemia. Report your findings to the physician.

Elevated Level

■ Observe for signs and symptoms of hyperadrenalism (Cushing's syndrome). These symptoms include fluid retention, "moon face," hirsutism, "buffalo hump," hypertension, hyperglycemia, petechiae, and ecchymosis. Report your findings to the physician.

5-HYDROXYINDOLEACETIC ACID (5-HIAA) (URINE)
5-OH-Indoleacetic Acid, Serotonin Metabolite

Reference Values

Adult: Qualitative Random Samples: negative. *Quantitative 24 Hours:* 2–10 mg/24 h

Child: not usually done—results would be similar to adult results

Description

5-HIAA, a metabolite of serotonin, is excreted in the urine as the result of carcinoid tumors found in the appendix or in the intestinal wall. Serotonin is a vasoconstricting hormone secreted by the argentaffin cells of the GI tract and is responsible for peristalsis. Carcinoid tumor cells, which secrete excess serotonin, are of low-grade malignancy. Early removal of this type of tumor ensures an 80% to 90% chance of cure. There have been reports of some noncarcinoid tumors producing high levels of 5-HIAA.

Certain foods may elevate the 5-HIAA urinary levels, and certain drugs may elevate or decrease the 5-HIAA urinary levels. More than one random sample of urine for the 5-HIAA test may be needed to avoid false-positive or false-negative results. The 24-hour urine test usually follows the random urine screening test.[6,8,10,13,14]

Clinical Problems

Decreased Level: Drug Influence (depresses 5-HIAA): ACTH, heparin, imipramine (Tofranil), isoniazid (INH), MAO inhibitors, methyldopa (Aldomet), phenothiazines (chlorpromazine [Thorazine]), promethazine (Phenergan)

Elevated Level: carcinoid tumors of the appendix and intestine, carcinoid tumor with metastasis (>100 mg/24 h), sciatica pain (severe), skeletal and smooth muscle spasm. *Drug Influence:* acetophenetidin (Phenacetin), glyceryl guaiacolate, methamphetamine (Methampex or Desoxyn), reserpine (Serpasil). *Foods:* banana, pineapple, avocados, plums, eggplant, walnuts

Procedure

■ Eliminate the food and drugs listed above for 3 days before the test, if possible.

Qualitative Random Urine Sample (for screening purposes): Collect a random urine sample and take it to the laboratory. If the urine sample is not tested immediately, it should be refrigerated. Collection of a random urine sample may need to be repeated to verify the results. The random urine screening test is usually done first, and if the test is positive, a 24-hour urine test for 5-HIAA is ordered.

Quantitative 24-Hour Urine Collection: Collect urine for 24 hours in a large container with a preservative. Some laboratories require no preservative, but the urine should be refrigerated during the 24-hour collection time. Label the bottle and laboratory slip with the patient's name and the date and exact times of the urine collection (eg, 6/24/93, 7:00 AM to 6/25/93, 7:00 AM).

■ Foods (except for those listed) and fluids are not restricted.

■ Factors Affecting Laboratory Results

   ■ Foods (*see Foods.*)
   ■ Drugs (*see Drug Influence.*)
   ■ A 24-hour urine sample that does not have a preservative and/or has not been refrigerated (Check with the laboratory about the urine preservative and refrigeration.)

NURSING IMPLICATIONS WITH RATIONALE

■ Instruct the patient not to eat bananas, pineapple, avocados, plums, eggplant, or walnuts for 3 days before the test. Foods and fluid other than those mentioned are permitted before and during the test.
■ Instruct the patient and family not to throw away any urine during the 24-hour collection time. Inform the patient not to discard toilet paper or feces in the urine.

- Inform the physician of any drugs the patient is taking that could cause a false-positive or false-negative result. These drugs should not be taken for 3 days before the test, if possible; if they are, the names of the drugs should be listed on the laboratory slip and recorded in the patient's chart.
- Check the 5-HIAA result of the random sample urine test and inform the physician if the result is unknown. A repeat test may be needed if the patient has taken drugs that can depress the 5-HIAA or if the test is negative. If the urine test is positive, the physician may order the 5-HIAA 24-hour urine test.

IMMUNOGLOBULINS (Ig) (SERUM)
IgG, IgA, IgM, IgD, IgE

Reference Values

	TOTAL Ig (99 %; mg/dL)	IgG 80 %; mg/dL	IgA (15%; mg/dL)	IgM (4 %; mg/dL)	IgD (0.2%; mg/dL)	IgE (0.0002% U/mL)
Adult	900–2200	650–1700	70–400	40–350	0–8	< 40 (IgE 0–120 mg/dL)
6–16 yr	800–1,700	700–1,650	80–230	45–260		<62
4–6 yr	700–1,700	550–1,500	50–175	22–100		<25
1–3 yr	400–1,500	300–1,400	20–150	40–230		<10
6 mo	225–1,200	200–1,100	10–90	10–80		
3 mo	325–750	275–750	5–55	15–70		
Newborn	650–1,450	700–1,480	0–12	5–30		

Description

Immunoglobulins (Ig) are classes (groups) of proteins referred to as antibodies; they can be divided into five groups found in gamma globulin. Immunoglobulin is produced by the action of B lymphocytes and plasma cells, and, as is characteristic of all antibody actions, immunoglobulin responds to invading foreign antigens. As individuals are exposed to antigens, immunoglobulin (antibody) production occurs. With further exposure to the same antigen, immunity results.

The five classes of immunoglobulins—IgG, IgA, IgM, IgD, and IgE—are separated by the process of immunoelectrophoresis. Of these five classes, IgG, IgA, and IgM are the important ones, since they make up most of the total gamma globulin.

The immunologic functions of the immunoglobulins are as follows:

IgG: IgG is the major immunoglobulin. IgG results from secondary exposure to the foreign antigen and is responsible for antiviral and antibacterial activity. This antibody passes through the placental barrier and provides early immunity for the newborn. The IgG response is longer and stronger than that of the other immunoglobulins.

IgA: This immunoglobulin is found in the secretions of the respiratory, GI, genitourinary tracts, tears, and saliva. Its purpose is to protect mucous membranes from invading organisms (viruses, certain bacteria—*Escherichia coli* and *Clostridium tetani*). IgA does not pass the placental barrier. Those having congenital IgA deficiency are prone to autoimmune disease.

IgM: IgM antibodies are produced 48 to 72 hours after an antigen enters the body and are responsible for primary immunity. This immunoglobulin produces antibody activity against rheumatoid factors, gram-negative organisms, and the ABO blood group. IgM activates the complement system by destroying antigenic substances. Since it does not pass the placental barrier, the serum value is low in newborns; however, it is produced early in life and the level increases after 9 months of age.

IgD: Unknown.

Ige: This immunoglobulin increases during allergic reactions and anaphylaxis.[1,9,10,14,36]

Clinical Problems

Ig	DECREASED LEVEL	ELEVATED LEVEL
IgG	Lymphocytic leukemia	Infections—all types
	Agammaglobulinemia	Severe malnutrition
	Preeclampsia	Chronic granulomatous infection
	Amyloidosis	Hyperimmunization
		Liver disease
		Rheumatic fever
		Sarcoidosis
IgA	Lymphocytic leukemia	Autoimmune disorders
	Agammaglobulinemia	Rheumatic fever
	Malignancies	Chronic infections
		Liver disease
IgM	Lymphocytic leukemia	Lymphosarcoma
	Agammaglobulinemia	Brucellosis
	Amyloidosis	Trypanosomiasis
		Relapsing fever
		Infectious mononucleosis
		Rubella virus in newborns
IgE		Allergic reactions (asthma)
		Skin sensitivity
		Drug influence
		Tetanus toxoid
		Tetanus antitoxin
		Gamma globulin

Procedure

- Collect 5 to 10 mL of venous blood in a red-top tube.
- Record on the laboratory slip the patient has received any vaccination or

immunization, including toxoid, within the last 6 months; or any blood transfusion, gamma globulin, or tetanus antitoxin injections in the last 6 weeks.
■ There is no food or fluid restriction. Some laboratories request NPO 12 hours before the test. Check with your laboratory.

■ Factors Affecting Laboratory Results

■ Immunization and toxoids received in the last 6 months and blood transfusions, tetanus antitoxin, and gamma globulin received in the last 6 weeks can affect immunoglobulin results.

NURSING IMPLICATIONS WITH RATIONALE

■ Obtain a history from the patient concerning previous vaccination or immunization, including toxoids (tetanus), received in the last 6 months and blood transfusions or injections of gamma globulin or tetanus antitoxin received in the last 6 weeks.
■ Report to the physician and record on the patient's chart and the laboratory slip if the patient has received recent blood transfusions, immunization or injections of toxoids, tetanus antitoxin, and gamma globulins.
■ Check the patient's temperature periodically.

Patient Teaching

■ Instruct the patient to avoid infections by using preventive measures (ie, to avoid being around persons with colds, to get adequate rest, to eat balanced meals, and to maintain an adequate fluid intake).

INSULIN (SERUM), INSULIN ANTIBODY TEST

Reference Values
Adult: Serum Insulin: 5–25 μU/mL, 10–250 μIU/mL
Insulin Antibody Test: < 4% serum binding of pork and beef insulin

Description
Insulin, hormone from the beta cells of the pancreas, is essential in transporting glucose to the cells for metabolism. Increased glucose levels stimulate insulin secretion.

Serum insulin and blood glucose levels are compared to determine the glucose disorder. Serum insulin is valuable in diagnosing insulinoma (islet cell tumor) and islet cell hyperplasia and in evaluating insulin production in diabetes mellitus. In insulinoma the serum insulin in high and blood glucose is <30 mg/dL. Hyperinsulinemia can occur in obesity as well as in insulinoma.

Insulin antibody test is ordered when a diabetic, taking pork or beef insulin, requires larger and larger insulin dosages. Insulin antibodies develop as the result of impurities in animal insulins. These antibodies are of immunoglobulin types (ie, IgG [most], IgM, IgE). The IgG antibodies neutralize the insulin, thus preventing glucose metabolism. IgM antibodies can cause insulin resistance, and IgE could be responsible for allergic effects.[3,9,10,18]

Clinical Problems

Decreased Level: diabetes mellitus. *Drug Influence:* Insulin

Elevated Level: insulinoma, insulin-resistant diabetic state, Cushing's syndrome, obesity. *Drug Influence:* cortisone preparations, oral contraceptives, thyroid hormones, epinephrine, levodopa

Procedure

- Collect 7 mL of venous blood in a red-top tube. Avoid hemolysis. Blood sample should be chilled. Serum must be separated within 30 minutes of collection. If blood glucose is needed, collect 7 mL in a gray-top or red-top tube.
- Food and fluids are restricted for 10 to 12 hours prior to the test. Insulin secretion reaches its peak in 30 minutes to 2 hours after meals.
- Withhold medications that could affect test results, such as insulin and cortisone, until after the test.

- Factors Affecting Laboratory Tests

   - Drugs such as insulin, cortisone, oral contraceptives, and hormones could increase serum insulin levels.
   - Hemolysis of the blood sample and not chilling the specimen could affect results.

NURSING IMPLICATIONS AND RATIONALE

- Obtain a history of glucose disorders from the patient or family. Report patient's complaints.
- Report if the patient's insulin dosage has increased over a period of time due to an increase in blood sugar.
- Be alert for signs and symptoms of hypoglycemia. If insulinoma is highly suspected, keep IV dextrose 50% available.

Patient Teaching

- Explain to the patient the importance of remaining NPO and resting (not exercising) before the test. Food and exercising increase blood glucose, thus increasing serum insulin level. Incorrect test results would occur.
- Teach patient to report signs and symptoms of insulin reaction (ie, nervousness, sweating, weakness, rapid pulse rate, confusion).

IRON (Fe), TOTAL IRON-BINDING CAPACITY (TIBC), TRANSFERRIN, PERCENT (TRANSFERRIN) SATURATION (SERUM)
Iron-Binding Capacity (IBC), Transferrin Saturation

Reference Values

	SERUM IRON	TIBC	SERUM TRANSFERRIN	SATURATION
Adult	50–150 μg/dL 10–27 μmol/L (SI units) Males slightly higher	250–450 μg/dL	250–430 mg/dL	30–50 (male) 20–35 (female)
Elderly	60–80 μg/dL			
Child				
Newborn	100–270 μg/dL	60–175 μg/dL		
Infant		100–400 μg/dL		
6 months–2 years:	40–100 μg/dL	100–135 μg/dL		
> 2 years:		40–100 μcg/dL		

Description

Iron is coupled with the iron-transporting protein transferrin. Transferrin is responsible for transporting iron to the bone marrow for the purpose of hemoglobin synthesis. The storage compound for iron is ferritin (*see ferritin*).

The total iron-binding capacity (TIBC) measures the amount of additional iron with which transferrin can bind. Normally TIBC is two to three times greater than serum iron level. When the serum iron is decreased, the TIBC is increased, and when serum iron is increased, the TIBC is decreased.

Transferrin can be measured as serum and as percent of saturation (transferrin saturation). The percent saturation is the ratio between serum iron and the transferrin that is available for binding with iron. The percent saturation and TIBC are helpful in determining the cause of abnormal serum-iron concentration. Serum iron, TIBC, transferrin, and percent (transferrin) saturation are needed to adequately diagnosis iron deficiency. The results of these tests indicating iron deficiency would be a low serum iron, high TIBC, high transferrin, and low percent saturation. Also serum ferritin would be low.[1,3,6,9,10]

Clinical Problems

Decreased Levels: Serum Iron: iron deficiency anemia; cancer of the stomach, intestine, rectum, breast; rheumatoid arthritis; bleeding peptic ulcer; protein malnutrition; low-birth-weight infants. *TIBC:* hemochromatosis; anemias: hemolytic, pernicious, sickle cell; hypoproteinemia; renal failure; cirrhosis of the liver; infections; cancer of the GI tract. *Transferrin:* anemia of chronic disease, hepatic damage, renal disease, cancer, acute or chronic infection. *Percent Saturation:* iron deficiency, anemia of chronic disease

Elevated Levels: *Serum Iron:* hemochromatosis (excessive iron deposits); anemias (hemolytic, pernicious, folic acid deficiency); liver damage; thalassemia; lead toxicity. *TIBC:* iron deficiency anemia, acute and chronic blood loss, polycythemia. *Transferrin:* iron deficiency. *Percent Saturation:* anemias (hemolytic, sideroblastic) hemochromatosis, iron overload. *Drug Influence:* oral contraceptives, iron preparations

Procedure

- Collect 7 to 10 mL of venous blood in a red-top tube. Avoid hemolysis, since it can cause false-positive readings.
- NPO for 8 hours before the test is preferred. Serum iron levels are usually higher in the morning and following food intake.

■ Factors Affecting Laboratory Results

- Hemolyis of the blood sample
- Oral iron medications and recent blood transfusion

NURSING IMPLICATIONS WITH RATIONALE

Decreased Level (Serum Iron)

- Observe for signs and symptoms of iron deficiency anemia (ie, pallor, fatigue, headache, tachycardia, dyspnea on exertion)
- Check with the laboratory or physician about NPO prior to test.

Patient Teaching

- Instruct the patient to eat foods rich in iron (ie, liver, shellfish, lean meat, egg yolk, dried fruits, whole grain, wines, and cereals). Milk has little or no iron. Nutritional instruction is particularly important for preschool and adolescent children and for pregnant women.
- Recommend rest and avoidance of strenuous activity before test.
- Instruct the patient on how to take iron supplements. Iron should be given following meals or snacks because it irritates the gastric mucosa. Orange juice and ascorbic acid promote iron absorption.
- Explain to the patient that iron supplements can cause constipation and that the stools will have a tarry appearance.

Elevated Level

- Observe for signs and symptoms of hemochromatosis (ie, bronze pigmentation of the skin, arrhythmias, and heart failure).

KETONE BODIES, ACETONE (URINE)

Reference Values

Adult: negative test

Child: negative test

Description

(*See Acetone, Ketone Bodies [Serum].*)

Ketone bodies are produced to provide energy when carbohydrates (CHO) cannot be used, as in diabetic acidosis and starvation/malnutrition. When these excess ketones are produced, ketosis (in the blood) results, thus exhausting the alkaline reserve (eg, bicarbonates) of the body, causing an acidotic state. Ketonuria (ketone bodies in the urine) occurs as a result of ketosis.

In testing for ketonuria, Acetest tablets are used to detect the two principle ketones (acetone and acetoacetic acid) in the urine. Ketostix can also be used, but this test method is more specific for acetoacetic acid.[9,10,13,14]

Clinical Problems

Positive Result: diabetic acidosis (ketoacidosis), starvation/malnutrition, reducing diet ($\downarrow$ CHO), fasting, severe vomiting, heat stroke, fetal death. *Drug Influence:* ascorbic acid, levodopa compounds, insulin, isopropyl alcohol, paraldehyde, pyridium, dyes used for the tests—bromsulfophthalein (BSP) and phenolsulfonphthalein (PSP)

Procedure

Collect a random urine specimen. Two tests are usually performed, as follows.

Acetest: Place an Acetest tablet on a clean surface (preferably a white paper towel), and put a drop of fresh urine on the tablet. Wait 30 seconds, and if the tablet changes color (lavender, medium purple, or dark purple), the result is positive for ketones.

The test is usually done on the same urine used for testing for glycosuria. The Clinitest is used for determining glycosuria and the Acetest for ketonuria.

Ketostix: Dip a reagent stick in fresh urine. Wait 15 seconds and compare it to the color chart. This test is more sensitive to acetoacetic acid than it is to acetone.

The urine should be fresh or refrigerated in a closed container. Waiting may cause false-negative results because of the instability of acetone.

There is no food or fluid restriction.

■ Factors Affecting Laboratory Results

- ■ A low-carbohydrate diet or a high-fat diet can cause false-positive results.
- ■ Certain drugs can cause false-positive results (*See Drug Influence*).
- ■ Urine kept at room temperature for 1 hour or more before testing may cause a false-negative result.

- Urinary tract infection—bacteria in the urine will cause a loss of acetoacetic acid.
- Juvenile diabetics are more prone to ketonuria (ketosis) than adults.

NURSING IMPLICATIONS WITH RATIONALE

Positive Result

- Relate ketonuria to diabetic acidosis (ketoacidosis), starvation, fasting, or a low-carbohydrate diet. In severe diabetic acidosis, both ketonuria and glycosuria may be present. This would not be true in severe vomiting, starvation, reducing diets, and heat stroke, since in such cases only ketonuria would be present.
- Explain to the patient that the urine should be freshly voided. Only 1 mL is needed. Acetone is lost in the urine if it stands at room temperature because it is volatile.
- Test and record the results of the Acetest and Clinitest on the patient's chart. Notify the physician if results are abnormal.
- Assess for signs and symptoms of diabetic acidosis, such as rapid, vigorous breathing; restlessness; confusion; sweet-smelling breath; and a positive Clinitest and Acetest.

Patient Teaching

- Instruct patient how to use the Acetest and Clinitest.
- Answer the patient's questions concerning urine testing and diabetes mellitus.

7-KETOSTEROIDS (17-KS) (URINE)

Reference Values

Adult: Male: 5–25 mg/24 h. *Female:* 5–15 mg/24 h.

Elderly: 4–8 mg/24 h

Child: Infant: <1 mg/24 h. *1–3 Years Old:* <2 mg/24 h. *3–6 Years Old:* <3 mg/24 h. *7–10 Years Old:* <4 mg/24 h. *10–12 Years Old:* Male: <6 mg/24 h; Female: <5 mg/24 h

Adolescent: Male: 3–15 mg/24 h. *Female:* 3–12 mg/24 h

Description

17-KS are metabolites of male hormones that are secreted from the testes and adrenal cortex. 17-KS are excreted in the urine. In men, approximately one third of the hormone metabolites come from the testes, and two thirds come from the adrenal cortex. In women, nearly all of the excreted hormones (androgens) are derived from the adrenal cortex.

Since most of the 17-KS is derived from the adrenal cortex and not from the testes, the 17-KS level is more useful for diagnosing adrenal cortex dysfunction. This test is also useful for determining pituitary and gonadal hormone function. Usually plasma cortisol and 17-OHCS determinations are requested at the same time to further confirm adrenal dysfunctions.[1,9–11,13,14]

Clinical Problems

Decreased Level: adrenal cortical hypofunction (Addison's disease), hypogonadism, hypopituitarism, nephrosis, myxedema, severe debilitating diseases. *Drug Influence:* thiazide diuretics, chlordiazepoxide (Librium), estrogen, oral contraceptives, paraldehyde, reserpine, probenecid (Benemid), promazine, meprobamate (Miltown),* quinidine, quinine

Elevated Level: ACTH therapy, adrenal cortical hyperfunction (adrenocortical hyperplasia, Cushing's syndrome, adrenocortical carcinoma), testicular neoplasm, ovarian neoplasm, hyperpituitarism, hirsutism, severe stress (burns, surgery, infectious diseases). *Drug Influence:* acetazolamide (Diamox); antibiotics (chloramphenicol [Chloromycetin], cloxacillin, erythromycin), chlorpromazine (Thorazine), hydralazine, meprobamate (Miltown),* phenothiazines, spironolactone (Aldactone), phenazopyridine, dexamethasone (Decadron)

Procedure

- There is no food or fluid restriction.
- Drugs that interfere with test results should not be given for 48 hours before the test. Check with physician first.
- Collect a 24-hour urine specimen in a large container and keep the container on ice or refrigerated. An acid preservative is usually added to keep the urine at a pH <4.5, thus preventing steroid decomposition by bacterial growth.
- List on the laboratory slip the patient's sex and age.
- Label container with the patient's name, date, and exact time of collection, such as 9/23/93, 7:30 AM to 9/24/93, 7:32 AM.
- Postpone test if female has her menstrual period. Blood in the urine can cause false-positive results.

■ Factors Affecting Laboratory Results

- Drugs (*See Drug Influence above*).

NURSING IMPLICATIONS WITH RATIONALE

- List on the laboratory slip the patient's sex and age. If the patient is a male, the laboratory results should be slightly higher than if the patient is a female. In addition, if the patient is over 65 years old, the test results should be low or low normal.
- Encourage the patient to increase fluid intake.

---

*Meprobamate may increase or decrease the 17-KS value.

Patient Teaching

■ Explain to the patient and family that all urine will be collected for 24 hours in the large urine container/bottle, which is on ice or refrigerated. Inform the patient that he or she should not put toilet paper or feces in the urine, and not to urinate directly into the collection container. The container could contain an acid preservative which could "splash" while urinating.

Decreased Level

■ Observe for the signs and symptoms of adrenal gland insufficiency (Addison's disease), such as weakness, weight loss, polyuria, hypotension, increased pulse rate, and shock (if severe).
■ Record fluid intake and output. Report if the patient's urine output is greater than normal (>2000 mL/24 h).
■ Monitor weight loss. In Addison's disease, sodium is not retained; therefore both sodium and water are lost. Weight loss and dehydration usually occur.

Patient Teaching

■ Encourage the patient to wear an identification bracelet containing emergency information.

Elevated Level

■ Observe for signs and symptoms of adrenal gland hyperfunction (Cushing's syndrome), such as moon face, hirsutism, weight gain, a cervicodorsal fat pad (buffalo hump), a bleeding tendency, hyperglycemia, and edema in the extremities.
■ Check serum potassium and blood glucose levels. Hypokalemia and hyperglycemia frequently occur; potassium supplements and insulin or a low-carbohydrate diet may be indicated.

LACTIC ACID (BLOOD)

Reference Values

Adult: Arterial Blood: 0.5–2.0 mEq/L, 11.3 mg/dL. *Venous Blood:* 0.5–1.5 mEq/L, 8.1–15.3 mg/dL. *Panic Range:* >5 mEq/L, >45 mg/dL

Description

Blood lactic acid or lactate is an indicator of the presence or absence of lactic acidosis. Lactic acidosis is suspected if the anion gap is >16 mEq/L and pH is decreased.

Shock and severe dehydration cause cell catabolism (cell breakdown) and an accumulation of acid metabolites, such as lactic acid. Excess lactic acid can decrease pH and cause lactic acidosis.[3,9,11]

Clinical Problems

Decreased Level: high lactic dehydrogenase (LDH) value

Elevated Level: shock, severe dehydration, severe trauma, ketoacidosis, severe infections, neoplastic conditions, hepatic failure, renal disease, alcoholism, salicylate toxicity (severe)

Procedure

- Collect 5 to 10 mL of blood in a green-top tube.
- Inform the patient to avoid hand clenching, which can lead to a buildup of lactic acid caused by a release of lactic acid from muscle of the clenched hand.
- Avoid using a tourniquet if possible. It could increase the blood lactic acid level.
- Deliver blood specimen on ice to the laboratory immediately.

- **Factors Affecting Laboratory Results**

  - Delivery to laboratory of arterial blood specimen not on ice could cause an inaccurate result.
  - Use of tourniquet could elevate lactic acid value.

NURSING IMPLICATIONS WITH RATIONALE

Elevated Level

- Associate an elevated lactic acid value with shock, severe dehydration, severe trauma, severe infection, and other conditions.
- Observe for signs and symptoms of acidosis, dyspnea or Kussmaus's breathing, increased pulse rate, decreased pH, decreased serum CO_2 value, and decreased arterial bicarbonate value.
- Be supportive of patient and family. If shock is present, anxiety and fear are common.

LACTIC (LACTATE) DEHYDROGENASE (LD OR LDH), LDH ISOENZYMES (SERUM)

Reference Values

Adult: Total LDH: 100–190 IU/L, 70–250 U/L

Isoenzymes: LDH_1, 14%–26%; LDH_2, 27%–37%; LDH_3, 20%–26%; LDH_4, 8%–16%; LDH_5, 6%–16%. Differences of 2% to 4% are considered normal.

Child: Newborn: 300–1500 IU/L. *Child:* 50–150 IU/L

Description

LDH is an intracellular enzyme present in nearly all metabolizing cells, with the highest concentrations in the heart, skeletal muscle, liver, kidney, brain, and erythrocytes. LDH has two distinct subunits—M (muscle) and H (heart). These subunits are combined in different formations to make five isoenzymes.

- LDH_1: cardiac fraction; H, H, H, H; in heart, RBCs, kidneys, brain (some)
- LDH_2: cardiac fraction; H, H, H, M; in heart, RBCs, kidneys, brain (some)
- LDH_3: pulmonary fraction; H, H, M, M; in lungs and other tissues: spleen, pancreas, adrenal, thyroid, lymphatics
- LDH_4: hepatic fraction; H, M, M, M; liver, skeletal muscle, kidneys and brain (some)
- LDH_5: hepatic fraction; M, M, M, M; liver, skeletal muscle, kidneys (some)

Serum LDH and LDH_1 are used for diagnosing acute myocardial infarction as well as other enzymatic tests, such as the creatine phosphokinase (CPK) and aspartate aminotransferase (AST) tests. A high serum LDH (total) level occurs 12 to 24 hours after the infarction, reaches its peak in 2 to 5 days, and remains elevated for 6 to 12 days, making it a useful test for delayed diagnosis of myocardial infarction. A flipped LDH_1/LDH_2 ratio with LDH_1 the highest indicates a myocardial infarction.

LDH_3 is linked to pulmonary diseases, and LDH_5 is linked to liver and skeletal muscle diseases. In acute hepatitis, total LDH rises, and the LDH_5 usually rises before jaundice develops and falls before the bilirubin level does.[10,11,13,18,21,23]

Clinical Problems

Elevated Level: acute myocardial infarction, CVA, cancer (lung, bone, intestines, liver, breast, cervix, testes, kidney, stomach, melanoma of the skin) acute leukemia, acute pulmonary infarction, infectious mononucleosis, anemias (pernicious, folic acid deficiency, sickle cell, acquired hemolytic), acute hepatitis, shock, skeletal muscular disease, heat stroke. *Drug Influence:* narcotics (codeine, morphine, meperidine [Demerol])

Procedure

- Collect 5–7 mL of venous blood in a red-top tube. Avoid hemolysis.
- List on the laboratory slip any narcotics or IM injections the patient received within 8 hours before the test.
- There is no food or fluid restriction.

■ Factors Affecting Laboratory Results

- Narcotic drugs and intramuscular (IM) injections can elevate serum LDH levels.
- Hemolysis of the blood sample can cause an elevated serum LDH level; the enzyme is plentiful in the RBCs (erythrocytes).

NURSING IMPLICATIONS WITH RATIONALE

Elevated Level

- Obtain a history of the patient's discomfort. A complaint of severe indigestion several days before could be indicative of a myocardial infarction. All information should be recorded and reported.
- Assess for signs and symptoms of an acute myocardial infarction (ie, pale or gray color, sharp stabbing pain or heavy pressure pain, shortness of breath, diaphoresis, nausea and vomiting, and indigestion).

Patient Teaching

- Instruct the patient to notify the nurse of any recurrence of chest discomfort or to seek medical care for indigestion of several days.

LACTOSE TOLERANCE TEST

Reference Values

Adult: Normal: 20–50 mg/dL rise from fasting blood glucose without abdominal symptoms of cramps and diarrhea. *Abnormal:* < 20 mg/dL of glucose rise from fasting blood glucose with abdominal cramps and diarrhea.

Description

Lactase, an enzyme from the small intestine, digests lactose, which is a sugar found in milk. The lactose tolerance test identifies patients with a deficiency of the enzyme lactase, which leads to an intolerance of lactose found in milk. With an absence of lactase, lactase cannot be absorbed from the small intestine and is excreted through the bowel undigested, causing the patient to have abdominal cramps and watery diarrhea.

This test is similar to a glucose tolerance test except that lactose is ingested instead of glucose. A flat curve of less than 20 mg/dL rise of the fasting glucose indicates lactose intolerance.[1,3,6,10,12]

Clinical Problems

Decreased Level of Glucose: lactose intolerance

Procedure

- NPO after midnight or at least 8 hours prior to the test.
- Collect 5 to 7 mL of a fasting venous blood specimen in a gray-top tube.
- The patient drinks 50 g to 100 g of lactose in 200 to 300 mL of water in 5 to 10 minutes. If severe lactase deficiency is suspected, lactose dosage may be decreased.

- Collect blood samples following lactose ingestion in 30 minutes and in 1, 2, and 3 hours.
- If the lactose tolerance test is abnormal, a glucose tolerance test may be ordered.

■ Factors Affecting Laboratory Results

- In the diabetic, an abnormal lactose tolerance can be due to abnormal carbohydrate metabolism.
- Twenty percent of individuals can have either a false-positive or false-negative test result.

NURSING IMPLICATIONS WITH RATIONALE

- Obtain a history from the patient of abdominal cramps and diarrhea that occur following ingestion of milk. Notify the physician of finding since this usually indicates lactose intolerance. The test may be cancelled.
- Explain the procedure to the patient.
- Assess the patient during and following the procedure for symptoms of abdominal cramps, pain, nausea, and watery diarrhea. Report findings.

Patient Teaching

- Instruct the patent with a lactose intolerance to buy lactose-free milk. It can be purchased in most grocery stores.

LDH ISOENZYMES
(See Lactic Dehydrogenase.)

LEAD (BLOOD)

Reference Values

Adult: Normal: 10–20 µg/dL. *Acceptable:* 20–40 µg/dL. *Excessive:* 40–80 µg/dL. *Toxic:* 80 µg/dL

Child: Normal: 10–20 µg/dL. *Acceptable:* 20–30 µg/dL. *Excessive:* 30–50 µg/dL. *Toxic:* 50 µg/dL

Description

Excessive lead exposure due to occupational contact is a hazard to adults; however, most industry will accept a 40 µg/dL blood lead level as a normal value. Lead toxicity can occur in children from eating chipped, lead-based paint found in old houses. Sources of lead include lead gasoline (fumes), lead-based paint, unglazed pottery, and "moonshine" whiskey prepared in lead containers.

Lead is usually excreted rapidly in the urine, but if excessive lead exposure persists, the lead will accumulate in the bone and soft tissues. Chronic lead poisoning is commoner than acute poisoning. Lead colic (crampy abdominal pain) occurs in both acute and chronic lead poisoning.[7,9,10,13,16]

Clinical Problems

Elevated Level: lead gasoline, including fumes; lead-based paint; unglazed pottery; batteries; lead containers used for storage; heat stroke (mobilizes lead stored in the body)

Procedure

- Collect 7 to 10 mL of venous blood in a lavender- or green-top tube.
- There is no food or fluid restriction.
- Urine may be requested for a 24-hour quantitative test; a lead-free container must be used.

- **Factors Affecting Laboratory Results**

  - None reported

NURSING IMPLICATIONS WITH RATIONALE

Elevated Level

- Obtain a history from the patient and/or parent concerning lead exposure. Record this history on the chart, and report the information to the physician.
- Observe for signs and symptoms of lead poisoning (lead colic [crampy abdominal pain], constipation, occasional bloody diarrhea, behavioral changes [from lethargy to hyperactivity, aggression, impulsiveness], tremors, and confusion).
- Monitor the urinary output, since lead toxicity can decrease kidney function. A urine output of less than 25 mL/h should be reported.
- Monitor the medical treatment for removing body lead such as chelation therapy. The principal chelating agent is calcium disodium edetate, which combines metal with calcium substance.
- Provide adequate fluid intake. Adequate hydration prevents hemoconcentration.

Patient Teaching

- Instruct patients/clients who are exposed to lead (in their occupations) that blood levels should be monitored. These persons should definitely keep medical appointments.

> ■ Suggest to parents ways of satisfying children's hunger through the attention method of providing psychologic satisfaction that will replace that gained by eating lead chips.

LE CELL TEST; LUPUS ERYTHEMATOSUS CELL TEST (BLOOD)
Lupus Test, LE Prep, LE Preparation, LE Slide Cell Test

Reference Values
Adult: negative, no LE cells
Child: negative

Description
LE cell test, a screening test for systemic lupus erythematosus (SLE), is a nonspecific test. Positive results have been reported in those having rheumatoid arthritis, scleroderma, and drug-induced lupus, such as penicillin, tetracycline, dilantin, oral contraceptives. The test is positive in 60% to 80% of those having SLE. Antinuclear antibodies (ANA) or antideoxyribonucleic acid (anti-DNA) are more sensitive tests for lupus and should be used to confirm SLE.[1,3,6,9]

Clinical Problems
Elevated Level: systemic lupus erythematosus (SLE), scleroderma, rheumatoid arthritis, chronic hepatitis. *Drug Influence:* hydralazine (Apresoline), procainamide (Pronestyl), quinidine, anticonvulsants (phenytoin [Dilantin], Mesantoin, Tridione), oral contraceptives, methysergide, antibiotics (penicillin, tetracycline, streptomycin), sulfonamides, methyldopa (Aldomet), isoniazid (INH), clofibrate, reserpine, phenylbutazone

Procedure
- ■ Collect 5 to 7 mL of venous blood in a red-top of green-top tube.
- ■ There is no food or fluid restriction.
- ■ List on the laboratory slip drugs taken that might affect test results.

■ Factors Affecting Laboratory Results

- ■ Certain drugs can cause false-positive test results (*See Drug Influence.*)
- ■ Hemolysis of the blood sample could affect test result.

NURSING IMPLICATIONS WITH RATIONALE

- ■ Compare LE test results with serum ANA or anti-DNA or both. LE test should not be the only test used to diagnose SLE.

■ Observe for signs and symptoms of SLE (ie, fatigue, fever, rash [butterfly over the nose], leukopenia, thrombocytopenia).
■ Be supportive of patient and family.

Patient Teaching

■ Instruct the patient to have daily rest periods, which help to decrease symptoms.

LECITHIN/SPHINGOMYELIN (L/S) RATIO (AMNIOTIC FLUID)

Reference Values

Before 35 Weeks of Gestation: 1:1. *Lecithin (L):* 6–9 mg/dL. *Sphingomyelin (S):* 4–6 mg/dL

After 35 Weeks of Gestation: 4:1. *Lecithin (L):* 15–21 mg/dL. *Sphingomyelin (S):* 4–6 mg/dL

Description

The L/S ratio can be used to predict neonatal respiratory distress syndrome (also called hyaline membrane disease) before delivery. Lecithin (L), a phospholipid, is responsible mostly for the formation of alveolar surfactant. Surfactant lubricates the alveolar lining and inhibits alveolar collapse, thus preventing atelectasis. Sphingomyelin (S) is another phospholipid, the value of which remains the same throughout pregnancy. A marked rise in amniotic lecithin after 35 weeks (to a level three or four times higher than that of sphinogomyelin) is considered normal, and so chances for having hyaline membrane disease are small. The L/S ratio is also used to determine fetal maturity in the event that the gestation period is uncertain. In this situation, the L/S ratio is determined at intervals of a period of several weeks.[9,12,13,15,16]

Clinical Problems

Decreased Ratio after 35 Weeks: respiratory distress syndrome, hyaline membrane disease

Procedure

■ The physician obtains amniotic fluid by the method of amniocentesis. The specimen should be cooled immediately to prevent the destruction of lecithin by certain enzymes in the amniotic fluid. The specimen should be frozen if testing cannot be done at a specified time (check with the laboratory).
■ Care should be taken to prevent puncture of the mother's bladder. If urine in the specimen is suspected, then the specimen should be tested for urea and potassium. If these two levels are higher than blood levels, the specimen

could be urine and not amniotic fluid. Ultrasound is frequently used when obtaining amniotic fluid.
■ There is no food, fluid, or drug restriction.

■ Factors Affecting Laboratory Results

■ Maternal vaginal secretions or a bloody tap into the amniotic fluid may cause a false, increased reading for lecithin.
■ The amniotic fluid specimen should be tested immediately to prevent inaccurate results.

NURSING IMPLICATIONS WITH RATIONALE

■ Check the procedures for amniocentesis. Explain the procedure to the patient. Assist the physician in obtaining amniotic fluid.
■ Obtain a fetal history of problems occurring during gestation. Also ask for and report information on any previous children born with respiratory distress syndrome.
■ Be supportive of the mother and her family before, during, and after the test. Remain with the patient and answer her questions, if possible, or refer her questions to appropriate professional personnel.
■ Assess the newborn at delivery for respiratory complications (substernal retractions, increased respiratory rate, labored breathing, and expiratory grunts).

LEGIONNAIRE'S ANTIBODY TEST (SERUM)

Reference Value

negative

Description

Legionnaire's disease, caused by a gram-negative bacillus, *Legionella pneumophila,* causes acute respiratory infection such as severe, consolidated pneumonia. This organism is in the soil and water (lakes, streams, reservoirs) and is passed by inhalation in aerosol form through plumbing fixtures (shower heads, whirlpool baths) and air conditioning systems (cooling towers and condensers). The bacteria can be isolated from blood, sputum, pleural fluid, and lung-tissue specimen.

A fourfold rise in antibody titer >1:128 during the acute and convalescent phase or a single titer >1:256 is evidence of the disease. Several blood samples and a tissue specimen are useful in confirming legionnaire's disease.[1,3,5,10,12]

Clinical Problems

Elevated Antibody Titer: Legionnaire's disease

Procedure

- Collect 7 mL of venous blood in a red-top tube. Tissue specimen from the lung or bronchiole site may be used.
- There is no food or fluid restriction.

■ Factors Affecting Laboratory Results

- None known

NURSING IMPLICATIONS WITH RATIONALE

- Obtain a history from the patient as to where he or she had been in the last week, such as hotel or other institutional site.
- Assess the patient's respiratory status by inspection, palpation, percussion, and auscultation.
- Observe for signs and symptoms of legionnaire's disease, such as malaise, high fever, chills, cough, chest pain, and tachypnea. Fever rises rapidly to 39°C to 41°C or to 102°F to 105°F.

Patient Teaching

- Inform the patient that legionnaire's disease is not transmitted from person to person but through aerosol means such as exhaust vents and fans.

LEUCINE AMINOPEPTIDASE (LAP) (SERUM)

Reference Values

Adult: 8–22 μU/mL, 12–33 IU/L (varies according to laboratory method).

Description

The LAP enzyme is produced by the liver and tends to parallel serum alkaline phosphatase (ALP), except that the LAP level is normal in bone disease or malabsorption syndrome. LAP is not an indicator of pancreatic carcinoma, as was once thought, but it is an indicator for biliary obstruction caused by liver metastases and choledocholithiasis.

This enzyme test is not frequently ordered but is useful as a supplement test in evaluating hepatobiliary disease.[7,8,11,13]

Clinical Problems

Elevated Level: cancer of the liver, extrahepatic biliary obstruction (stones), acute necrosis of the liver, viral hepatitis

Procedure

- Collect 5 to 10 mL of venous blood in a red-top tube.
- There is no food or fluid restriction.

■ Factors Affecting Laboratory Results

- None reported

NURSING IMPLICATIONS WITH RATIONALE

Elevated Level

- Compare LAP with other tests for liver dysfunction, such as alkaline phosphatase (ALP), alanine aminotransferase (ALT or SGPT), and gamma glutamyl transpeptidase (GGT) tests. The LAP test is frequently used to verify the results of other laboratory tests. It is not considered as sensitive as the other tests, and therefore it is not as commonly used.

LIDOCAINE HYDROCHLORIDE (BLOOD, SERUM, PLASMA)
(Xylocaine)

Reference Values

Therapeutic Range: *Adult:* 1.5–5.0 µg/mL; 6.0–22.5 µmol/L (SI units). *Child:* similar to adult

Toxic Level: *Adult:* >6 µg/mL. *Child:* similar to adult

Description

For treating acute ventricular arrhythmia, IV lidocaine is one of the drugs of choice. It obtains its antiarrhythmic effect by suppressing automaticity and increasing electrical stimulation threshold of the ventricle. Lidocaine is also used as a local anesthetic.

Lidocaine is metabolized in the liver to active metabolites; about 70% of the metabolites are bound to plasma protein. An initial bolus of parenteral lidocaine (50 to 100 mg) has a half-life of 10 minutes; however, the half-life is lengthened to 2 hours with continuous IV administration. Steady state occurs 6 to 12 hours after IV lidocaine infusion. Ninety percent of the drug is excreted in the urine as metabolites and 10% excreted unchanged.

Monitoring lidocaine levels is necessary to maintain therapeutic level and to avoid lidocaine toxicity. The maximum dose of lidocaine IV and bolus is 300 mg/h.[2-4,13]

Clinical Problems

Decreased Level: Drug Influence: barbiturates, phenytoin (Dilantin)
Elevated Level: Excess dosage of lidocaine: shock, liver and heart diseases.
Drug Influence: cimetidine (Tagamet), propranolol (Inderal)

Procedure

- Collect 5 to 10 mL in a red-top tube. Draw blood specimen 6 to 12 hours after starting lidocaine therapy for arrhythmia prophylaxis. Then check serum levels daily as ordered.
- Record dose, time, and route (bolus or infusion) of lidocaine administration on the laboratory requisition slip.
- There is no food or fluid restriction.

- Factors Affecting Laboratory Results
  - Incorrect blood-collecting tube. Check with the laboratory for the type of collecting tube.

NURSING IMPLICATIONS WITH RATIONALE

- Monitor therapeutic drug level every 12 hours, especially when cardiac or liver insufficiency exists. The maximum dose is 300 mg/h.
- Regulate IV rate using a microchamber tubing and infusion pump. Normally no more than 4 mg/min should be infused.

Elevated Level

- Observe for signs and symptoms of side effects of lidocaine and of lidocaine toxicity (drowsiness, dizziness, lightheadedness, confusion, disorientation, irritability, apprehension, double vision). High doses (>9 μg/mL, 38.4 μmol/L) may produce convulsions, hypotension, bradycardia, and shock.

LIPASE (SERUM)

Reference Values

Adult: 20–180 IU/L, 14–280 mU/mL, 14–280 U/L (SI units)
Child: Infant: 9–105 IU/L at 37°C. *Child:* 20–136 IU/L at 37°C

Description

Lipase, an enzyme secreted by the pancreas, aids in digesting fats. Lipase, like amylase, appears in the blood stream following damage to the pancreas. Acute pancreatitis is the commonest cause for an elevated serum lipase. Lipase and amylase levels increase early in the disease, but serum lipase can be elevated for up to 14 days after an acute episode, whereas the serum amylase returns to normal after approximately 3 days. Serum lipase is useful for a late diagnosis of acute pancreatitis.[3,9,12,13]

Clinical Problems

Decreased Level: late cancer of the pancreas, hepatitis

Elevated Level: acute and chronic pancreatitis, cancer of the pancreas (early stage), perforated ulcer, obstruction of the pancreatic duct, acute cholecystitis (some cases), acute renal failure (early stage) *Drug Influence:* codeine, morphine, meperidine (Demerol), bethanechol (Urecholine) steroids, guanethidine

Procedure

- Collect 5 to 10 mL of venous blood in a red-top tube. Avoid hemolysis.
- NPO except water for 8 to 12 hours.
- Narcotics should be withheld for 24 hours prior to the test. If narcotics are administered within the 24 hours, the drug and the time administered should be written on the laboratory slip.

■ Factors Affecting Laboratory Results

- Most narcotic drugs elevate the serum lipase level.
- Food eaten within 8 hours prior to the test may interfere with serum lipase levels.
- The presence of hemoglobin and calcium ions may cause a decreased serum lipase level.

NURSING IMPLICATIONS WITH RATIONALE

Elevated Level

- Relate elevated serum lipase and amylase levels to acute pancreatitis.
- Notify the physician when abdominal pain persists for several days. A serum lipase determination may be ordered, since it is an effective test for latent diagnosis of acute pancreatitis. Lipase levels may remain elevated in the blood for 2 weeks.

LIPOPROTEINS, LIPOPROTEIN ELECTROPHORESIS, LIPIDS (SERUM)

Reference Values

Adult: Total: 400–800 mg/dL, 4–8 g/L (SI units); *Cholesterol:* 150–240 mg/dL (see test on cholesterol). *Triglycerides:* 10–190 mg/dL (see test on triglycerides). *Phospholipids:* 150–380 mg/dL

LDL: 60–160 mg/dL. *Risk for CHD:* High: >160 mg/dL; Moderate: 130–159 mg/dL; Low: <130 mg/dL

HDL: 29–77 mg/dL. *Risk for CHD:* High: <35 mg/dL; Moderate: 35–45 mg/dL; Low: 46–59 mg/dL; Very low: >60 mg/dL

Child: *See tests on cholesterol and triglycerides.*

Description

Lipoproteins are lipids bound to protein, and the three main lipoproteins are cholesterol, triglycerides, and phospholipids. The two fractions of lipoproteins— alpha (α), high-density lipoproteins (HDL), and beta (β), low-density lipoproteins (chylomicrons, VLDL, LDL)—can be separated by electrophoresis. The β groups are the largest contributors of atherosclerosis and coronary artery disease. HDL, called "friendly lipids," are composed of 50% protein and do aid in decreasing plaque deposits in blood vessels.[3,6,7,11,28]

LIPOPROTEIN CLASSIFICATION

Subgroup Classes of Lipoproteins	Protein Composition (%)	Cholesterol (%)	Triglycerides (%)	Phospholipids (%)
Chylomicrons	2	3	90	5
Very low-density (VLDL, pre-β)	10	10	70	10
Low-density (LDL, β)	25	45	10	20
High-density HDL, α	50	20	Trace	30

Adapted from Henry, J. B. *Todd-Sanford-Davidsohn: Clinical diagnosis and management by laboratory methods* (17th ed., p. 183), Philadelphia: Saunders, 1984.

Increased lipoproteins (hyperlipidemia or hyperlipoproteinemia) can be phenotyped into five major types (I, IIA and IIB, III, IV, V). Cholesterol and triglycerides are the two lipids in each type found in varying amounts. With type II, the cholesterol is highly elevated, and the triglycerides are slightly increased. With type IV, the triglycerides are highly elevated, and the cholesterol is slightly increased. Types II and IV are the commonest phenotypes and are the most prevalent in atherosclerosis and coronary artery disease.

LIPOPROTEIN PHENOTYPE: HYPERLIPIDEMIA

Type	Lipid Composition*
I	Increased chylomicrons, increased triglycerides; rare pattern of hyperlipidemia
IIA	Increased beta (low-density) lipoproteins (LDL); increased cholesterol, slightly increased triglycerides or normal; common pattern of hyperlipidemia

(continued)

Type	Lipid Composition*
IIB	Increased beta and pre-beta lipoproteins; both cholesterol and triglycerides are elevated; common pattern of hyperlipidemia
III	Moderately increased cholesterol and triglycerides; uncommon pattern of hyperlipidemia
IV	Increase of pre-beta (very low-density) lipoproteins (VLDL); slightly increased cholesterol and markedly increased triglycerides; common pattern of hyperlipidemia
V	Increased chylomicrons, VLDL, and triglycerides, and slightly increased cholesterol; uncommon pattern of hyperlipidemia

Corbett (1987)
*Types II and IV are increased in atherosclerosis and coronary artery diseases.

Clinical Problems

Decreased Level: Tangier disease, chronic obstructive lung disease. *Drug Influence: See Cholesterol and Triglycerides.*

Elevated Level: hyperlipoproteinemia, acute myocardial infarction (AMI), hypothyroidism; diabetes mellitus, nephrotic syndrome, eclampsia, Laënnec's cirrhosis, multiple myeloma, diet (high in saturated fats). *Drug Influence: See Cholesterol and Triglycerides.*

Procedure

- NPO except for water for 12 to 14 hours prior to the test. The patient should be on a regular diet for 3 days before the test. No alcohol intake for 24 hours.
- Collect 7 to 10 mL of venous blood in a red-top tube.

■ Factors Affecting Laboratory Results

- A diet high in saturated fats and sugar could elevate   test results.
- Certain drugs can increase or decrease serum lipoproteins (*See Clinical Problems, Drug Influence for Cholesterol and Triglycerides.*)

NURSING IMPLICATIONS WITH RATIONALE

- Check the patient's serum cholesterol, serum triglyceride levels, LDL, and HDL. This information is helpful for teaching purposes and in answering the patient's questions.

Patient Teaching

- Instruct the patient with hyperlipoproteinemia to avoid foods high in saturated fats and sugar (ie, bacon, cream, butter, fatty meats, and candy).
- Answer patient's questions concerning risk of coronary heart disease related to LDL and HDL.

LITHIUM (SERUM)
(Eskalith, Lithobid, Esthalith CR, Lithotabs, Cibalith)

Reference Values

Adult: *Normal:* negative. *Therapeutic:* 0.5–1.5 mEq/L. *Toxic:* >2.0 mEq/L. *Lethal:* >4.0 mEq/L.

Child: not usually given to children.

Description

Lithium or lithium salt is used to treat manic-depressive psychosis. This agent is used to correct the mania in manic depression and to prevent depression. Since therapeutic and toxic lithium levels are narrow, serum lithium should be closely monitored.

Lithium salt was first used in the 1940s as a salt substitute; this practice was abandoned in the late 1940s because of its high toxicity. It was not used in the United States until after 1965 and then was used for treatment of manic depression.[1,2,4,7,9]

Clinical Problems

Elevated Level: *Toxicity:* lithium carbonate (Eskalith, Lithane, Lithonate), lithium bromide

Procedure

- Collect 5 to 7 mL of venous blood in a red-top tube 8 to 12 hours after the last lithium dose.
- There is no food or fluid restriction.
- The lithium tolerance test may be ordered instead of the conventional blood sample. A base blood specimen is obtained, and then the lithium dose is given. Blood specimens are collected 1, 3, and 6 hours after the lithium dose.

- Factors Affecting Laboratory Results

  - None reported

NURSING IMPLICATIONS WITH RATIONALE

- Observe for signs and symptoms of lithium overdose (slurred speech, muscle spasm, confusion, and nystagmus). Lithium dosage should be lower in the older adult (over 65 years) than in the middle-aged adult. Lithium test results should always be reported to the physician because of the narrow range of the "therapeutic" dosage.

Patient Teaching

■ Instruct the patient to take the prescribed lithium dosage daily and to keep his or her medical appointment. Periodic blood specimens will need to be drawn to determine lithium levels.

■ Suggest to the nursing mother taking lithium that the pediatrician should be notified before she breast-feeds the infant. Breast milk can contain high levels of lithium.

■ Encourage adequate fluid and sodium intake while the patient is maintained on lithium. Lithium inhibits ADH secretion, causing body water loss. Diuretics should be avoided.

LUPUS ERYTHEMATOSUS CELL TEST
(See LE test.)

LUTEINIZING HORMONE (LH) SERUM AND URINE
Interstitial Cell-Stimulating Hormone (ICSH)

Reference Values

Ranges vary among laboratories.

Serum
   Adult: Female: Follicular Phase: 3–30 mIU/mL; Midcycle: 30–100 mIU/mL; Luteal Phase: 2–25 mIU/mL. Postmenopausal: 40–100 mIU/mL. Male: 5–25 mIU/mL. *Child:* <10 mIU/mL

Urine
   Adult: Female: Follicular Phase: 5–25 IU/24 h; Midcycle: 30–90 IU/24 h; Luteal Phase: 2–24 IU/24 h. Postmenopausal: >40 IU/24 h. Male: 7–25 IU/mL.

Description

Luteinizing hormone (LH), gonadotropic hormone secreted by the anterior pituitary gland, is needed (with follicle-stimulating hormone [FSH]) for ovulation to occur. After ovulation, LH aids in stimulating the corpus luteum in secreting progesterone. FSH values are frequently evaluated with LH values. In men, LH stimulates testosterone production, and with FSH, they influence the development and maturation of spermatozoa.

LH is usually ordered to evaluate infertility in women and men. High-serum values are related to gonadal dysfunction, and low serum values are related to hypothalamus or pituitary failure. Women taking oral contraceptives have an absence of midcycle LH peak until the contraceptives are discontinued. This test might be used to evaluate hormonal therapy for inducing ovulation.[1,3,6,9,10]

Clinical Problems

Decreased Level: Hypogonadotropinism (defects in pituitary gland or hypothalamus), anovulation, amenorrhea (pituitary failure), hypophysectomy, testicular failure, hypothalamic dysfunction, adrenal hyperplasia or tumors. *Drug Influence:* oral contraceptives, estrogen compounds, testosterone administration

Elevated Level: amenorrhea (ovarian failure), tumors (pituitary, testicular), precocious puberty, testicular failure, Turner's syndrome, Klinefelter's syndrome, premature menopause, Stein-Leventhal syndrome, polycystic ovary syndrome, liver disease

Procedure

Serum

- Collect 7 mL of venous blood in a red-top or lavender-top tube. Avoid hemolysis. Daily blood samples must be taken at the same time each day to determine if ovulation occurs.
- There is no food or fluid restriction.
- Note on the laboratory slip the phase of the menstrual cycle, patient's age, and if patient is postmenopausal.
- Withhold 24 to 48 hours before the test medications that could interfere with test results (check with physician).

Urine

- Collect 24-hour urine specimen in a container with a preservative, or keep refrigerated if no preservative is added.
- Label the specimen with the patient's name, date, and time.

■ Factors Affecting Laboratory Results

- Hormones (estrogen, progesterone, and testosterone) and oral contraceptives could decrease plasma LH value.
- Hemolysis of the blood sample could affect test result.
- Collection of the daily specimen at different times of the day may cause inaccurate result.

NURSING IMPLICATIONS WITH RATIONALE

- Obtain a menstrual history from the patient. Record the menstrual phase on the laboratory slip.
- Check with the physician about withholding medications that could affect test results.
- Encourage the patient to express concerns about infertility or other health problems.
- Be supportive of patient and family.

Patient Teaching

- Instruct patient to express concerns to physician and to keep an accurate account of her menstrual cycle.

LYME DISEASE (Antibody) TEST

Reference Value
Titer: <1:256

Description
Borrelia burgdorferi is the spirochete that causes Lyme disease. Several tick vectors, primarily the deer tick, carry the spirochete. Lyme disease is most prevalent in the northeastern states, upper midwestern states, and western states.

A reddish, macular lesion usually occurs about 1 week after the tick bite. It can affect the CNS and the peripheral nervous system (PNS), causing a neuritis or aseptic meningitis. Also it can affect the heart and joints, causing transient ECG abnormalities, carditis, and problems in one or more joints, mostly the knees, leading to arthritis (may take from a few weeks to 2 years to become symptomatic.)[7,10]

Clinical Problems
Positive Titer: Lyme disease

Procedure

- Collect 5 mL of venous blood in a red-top tube.
- There is no food or fluid restriction.

■ Factors Affecting Laboratory Results

- Persons with a high rheumatoid factor could have a false-positive test result.

NURSING IMPLICATIONS WITH RATIONALE

- Report a history of a tick bite.
- Assess for a macular lesion at the site of the tick bite and elsewhere.
- Check titer level. A fourfold rise in titer is indicative of a recent infection.

Patient Teaching

- Instruct patient to wear clothing that covers entirely the extremities when in the woods and areas infested by ticks and deer.
- Instruct the patient to see physician immediately if bitten by a tick or if a macular lesion results from a tick bite. Antibiotic therapy is frequently started.
- Inform the patient that the commonest complication of Lyme disease is arthritis. Others are cardiac arrhythmias, carditis, and neuritis.

LYMPHOCYTES (T AND B) ASSAY (BLOOD)

T and B Lymphocytes; Lymphocyte Marker Studies; Lymphocyte Subset Typing

Reference Values

Adult: *T cells:* 60%–80%, 600–2400 cells/μL. *B cells:* 4%–16%, 50–250 cells/μL

Description

The two categories of lymphocytes are T lymphocytes and B lymphocytes. The T lymphocytes are associated with cell-mediated immune responses (cellular immunity) such as, rejection of transplant and graft, tumor immunity, microorganism (bacterial and viral) death. If the surface of the host's tissue cell is altered, the T cells might perceive that altered cell as foreign and attack it. This might be helpful if the altered surface is of tumor development; however, this T-cell attack might give rise to autoimmune disease.

The B lymphocytes, derived from bone marrow, are responsible for humoral immunity. The B cells synthesize immunoglobulins to react to specific antigens. An interaction between T and B lymphocytes is necessary for a satisfactory immune response.

Measurement of T and B lymphocytes is valuable for diagnosing autoimmune diseases (ie, immunosuppressive diseases such as AIDS, lymphoma, and lymphocytic leukemia). T and B cells can be used to monitor changes during the treatment of immunosuppressive diseases.[1,3,10]

Clinical Problems

Decreased Level

T lymphocytes: lymphoma, lupus disease (SLE), thymic hypoplasia (DiGeorge's syndrome), acute viral infections. *Drug Influence:* immunosuppressive agents. *B lymphocytes:* IgG, IgA, IgM deficiency, lymphomas, nephrotic syndrome, sex-linked agammaglobulinemia. *T and B lymphocytes:* immunodeficiency diseases

Elevated Level

T lymphocytes: autoimmune disorders such as Graves' disease. *B lymphocytes:* acute and chronic lymphocytic leukemias, multiple myeloma, Waldenström's macroglobulinemia

Procedure

■ Collect two 10-mL samples of venous blood in two lavender-top tubes. Refrigerate blood samples. *Check with laboratory procedure in your institution.*
■ There is no food or fluid restriction.

■ Factors Affecting Laboratory Result

■ Insufficient amount of blood for the test could affect test result.

NURSING IMPLICATIONS WITH RATIONALE

- Keep patient free from exposure to infection.
- Observe for signs and symptoms of lymphocytic leukemias (ie, fatigue, pallor, vesicular skin lesions, increased WBC).

Patient Teaching

- Teach the patient to stay away from persons with colds or communicable diseases.

MAGNESIUM (Mg) (SERUM)

Reference Values

Adult: 1.5–2.5 mEq/L, or 1.2–2.6 mEq

Child: Newborn: 1.4–2.9 mEq/L. *Child:* 1.6–2.6 mEq/L

Description

Magnesium is most plentiful in the cells (intracellular fluid). One third of the magnesium ingested is absorbed through the small intestine, and the remaining unabsorbed magnesium is excreted in the stools. The absorbed magnesium is eventually excreted through the kidneys.

As with potassium, sodium, and calcium, magnesium is needed for neuromuscular activity. Magnesium influences use of potassium, calcium, and protein, and when there is a magnesium deficit, there is frequently a potassium and calcium deficit. Magnesium is also responsible for the transport of sodium and potassium across the cell membranes. Another function of magnesium is its activation of enzymes for carbohydrate and protein metabolism.

Magnesium is found in most foods, so it would be difficult for a person who maintains a normal diet to have a magnesium deficiency. The daily required magnesium intake for an adult is 200 to 300 mg, or 0.2 to 0.3 g.

A serum magnesium deficit is known as hypomagnesemia, and a serum magnesium excess is called hypermagnesemia.[7,11,23,24,39]

Clinical Problems

Decreased Level: protein malnutrition, malabsorption, cirrhosis of the liver, alcoholism, hypoparathyroidism, hyperaldosteronism, hypokalemia ($\downarrow$ K), IV solutions without magnesium, chronic diarrhea, bowel resection complications, dehydration. *Drug Influence:* diuretics (mercurial, ethacrynic acid [Edecrin]), calcium gluconate, amphotericin B, neomycin, insulin.

Elevated Level: severe dehydration, renal failure, leukemia (lymphocytic and myelocytic), diabetes mellitus (early phase). *Drug Influence:* antacids (Maalox, Mylanta, Aludrox, DiGel), laxatives (epsom salts [$MgSO_4$], milk of magnesia, magnesium citrate)

Procedure

- Collect 5 to 10 mL of venous blood in a red-top tube. Avoid hemolysis.
- There is no food or fluid restriction.

■ Factors Affecting Laboratory Results

- Hypokalemia and hypocalcemia will decrease magnesium level.
- Drugs—Laxatives and antacids containing magnesium can cause hypermagnesemia, and diuretics, calcium gluconate, and insulin can cause hypomagnesemia. Insulin moves magnesium back into the cells, causing a serum-magnesium deficit.

NURSING IMPLICATIONS WITH RATIONALE

Decreased Level

- Observe for signs and symptoms of hypomagnesemia, such as tetany symptoms (twitching and tremors, carpopedal spasm, generalized spasticity), restlessness, confusion, and arrhythmia. Neuromuscular irritability can be mistakenly attributed to hypocalcemia.
- Check serum potassium, sodium, calcium, and magnesium levels. Electrolyte deficits may accompany a magnesium deficit. If hypokalemia and hypomagnesemia are present, potassium supplements will not completely correct the potassium deficit until the magnesium deficit is corrected.
- Check for a positive Chvostek's sign by tapping the facial nerve in front of the ear and observing for spasm of the cheek and twitching at the corner of the lip.
- Report to the physician if the patient has been NPO and receiving IV fluids without magnesium salts for weeks. Hyperalimentation solutions should contain magnesium.
- Check patients receiving digitalis preparations for digitalis intoxication (anorexia, nausea, vomiting, bradycardia). A magnesium deficit enhances the action of digitalis, causing digitalis toxicity.
- Assess renal function when the patient is receiving magnesium supplements. Excess magnesium is excreted by the kidneys.
- Assess ECG changes. A flat or inverted T-wave can be indicative of hypomagnesemia. It can also indicate hypokalemia.
- Administer IV magnesium sulfate in solution slowly to prevent a hot or flushed feeling.
- Have IV calcium gluconate available to reverse hypermagnesemia due to overcorrection. Calcium antagonizes the sedative effect of magnesium.

Patient Teaching

- Instruct the patient to eat foods rich in magnesium (fish, seafood, meats, green vegetables, whole grain, and nuts).

Elevated Level

■ Observe for signs and symptoms of hypermagnesemia, such as flushing, a feeling of warmth, increased perspiration (with the magnesium level at 3 to 4 mEq/L), muscular weakness, diminished reflex, respiratory distress, hypotension, a sedative effect (with the magnesium level at 9 to 10 mEq/L).

■ Monitor urinary output. Effective urinary output (>750 mL daily) will decrease the serum magnesium level.

■ Assess the patient's level of sensorium and muscle activity.

■ Assess ECG changes. A peaked T-wave and wide QRS complex can indicate hyperkalemia (↑ K) and hypermagnesemia, so the serum potassium and magnesium levels should be checked.

■ Provide adequate fluids to improve kidney function and to restore body fluids. Dehydration can cause hemoconcentration and, as a result, magnesium excess.

■ Check for digitalis intoxication if the patient is receiving calcium gluconate for hypermagnesemia. Calcium excess enhances the action of digitalis.

Patient Teaching

■ Instruct patients to avoid constant use of laxatives and antacids containing magnesium. Suggest to patients that they check drug labels.

MALARIA SMEAR (BLOOD)

Reference Values

Adult: negative

Child: negative

Description

Malaria is caused by malarial parasites transmitted by mosquitos. The parasites rupture the RBCs (hemolysis), causing the patient to have chills and fever.

Malarial parasites can be detected by blood smears (venous or capillary blood). Blood samples are usually taken in the presence of chills and fever daily for 3 days or at specified times—every 6 or 12 hours.[7,8,13]

Clinical Problems

Positive: malaria (*Plasmodium* species)

Procedure

■ Venous or capillary blood can be used for the malarial smear.

■ Collect 5 mL in a lavender-top tube.

■ There is no food or fluid restriction.

■ Factors Affecting Laboratory Results

   ■ None known

NURSING IMPLICATIONS WITH RATIONALE

■ Explain the procedure to the patient. The patient should inform the nurse when he or she is having chills and fever, since a blood sample is usually requested at that time. The blood sample may also be requested daily for 3 days or at specified times during the day.

■ Monitor the patient's temperature every 4 hours or as ordered. Record temperature changes.

■ Report chills and fever to the physician.

5′NUCLEOTIDASE (5′N or 5′NT) (SERUM)

Reference Values

Adult: < 14 U/L

Child: Values lower than adults

Description

This is a liver enzyme test that aids in the diagnosis of hepatobiliary disease. 5′Nucleotidase (5′N) is not elevated in bone disorders as is alkaline phosphatase (ALP); therefore it is useful in determining the origin of the problem. Elevated ALP and 5′N indicate liver disorder. Elevated ALP and normal 5′N indicate bone disorder. Usually several liver enzyme tests (ie, ALP, leucine aminopeptidase [LAP], gamma-glutamyl transferase [GGT]) are performed to evaluate liver function.[3,8,9]

Clinical Problems

Elevated Level: cirrhosis of the liver, biliary obstruction from calculi and tumor, and metastasis to the liver. *Drug Influence:* phenothiazines, narcotics (codeine, morphine, meperidine [Demerol])

Procedure

■ Collect 5 to 10 mL of venous blood in a red-top tube. Avoid hemolysis.

■ There is no food or fluid restriction.

■ Factors Affecting Laboratory Results

   ■ Hemolysis of the blood specimen

NURSING IMPLICATIONS WITH RATIONALE

■ Check the venipuncture site; patients with liver disorders tend to have prolonged clotting time.

Elevated Level

■ Compare 5′N levels with other liver enzyme levels. Elevated ALP, GGT, LAP, and 5′N values indicate that the problem is of liver origin.

Patient Teaching

■ Instruct the patient that there could be a tendency toward bleeding. If bleeding occurs from the mouth, rectum, or elsewhere, the physician should be notified.
■ Encourage the patient to eat well-balanced meals, especially if the condition is cirrhosis of the liver, cancer of the liver.

OCCULT BLOOD (FECES)

Reference Values

Adult: negative

Child: negative

Note: A diet rich in meats, poultry, fish, and drugs (cortisone, aspirin, potassium) could cause a false positive occult blood test.

Description

Occult (nonvisible or hidden) blood in the feces usually indicates GI bleeding. Bright red blood from the rectum can be indicative of bleeding from the lower large intestine (eg, hemorrhoids), and tarry black stools indicate blood loss of >50 mL from the upper GI tract.

Occult blood in the feces may be present days or several weeks after a single bleeding episode. False-positive occult blood test results may be due to ingestion of meats, poultry, fish, and certain drugs.[1,3,10,12]

Clinical Problems

Negative Results: Drug Influence: ascorbic acid (large amounts of vitamin C

Positive Results: bleeding, peptic ulcer, gastritis, gastric carcinoma, bleeding esophageal varices, colitis, intestinal carcinoma, diverticulitis. *Drug Influence:* aspirin, steroids (cortisone preparations), colchicine, iron preparations, iodine, indomethacin (Indocin), reserpine, potassium preparations, thiazide diuretics, bromides

Procedure

- There are a variety of blood-test reagents that may be used to test for occult blood. Some are more sensitive than others. Orthotolidine (Occultest) is considered the most sensitive test, more sensitive than the guaiac (least sensitive).
- Avoid meats, poultry, and fish for 3 days prior to stool specimen, especially if orthotolidine or benzidine tests are used.
- Obtain a single, random stool specimen and send it to the laboratory. Only a small amount of fecal material is needed. Stool may be obtained from a rectal examination. Many times the stool test is done on the nursing floor using a commercial kit.
- List on the laboratory slip drugs patient is taking that could affect test results.
- The stool specimen does not need to be kept warm or examined immediately.

- Factors Affecting Laboratory Results

    - Drugs (*See Drug Influence*).
    - Foods—Meats; poultry; fish; and green, leafy vegetables can cause a false-positive test result.
    - Urine and soap solution in the feces may affect the test result.

NURSING IMPLICATIONS WITH RATIONALE

Patient Teaching

- Instruct the patient not to eat meats, poultry, or fish for 3 days prior to the test. Green, leafy vegetables, if eaten in abundance, could cause a false-positive test.
- Instruct the patient not to take drugs that could cause false-positive results for 3 days before the test, if possible.

Positive Result for Occult Blood

- Obtain a history of recent or past bleeding episodes. Inform the physician of a history of GI bleeding.
- Inform the physician if the patient is receiving medication that could cause a false-positive test result (*see Drug Influence*).
- Determine whether the patient has had epigastric pain between meals. This type of pain could be indicative of a peptic ulcer.
- Be sure the stool is not contaminated with menstrual discharge.

Patient Teaching

- Encourage the patient to report abnormal-colored stools (eg, tarry stools). Oral iron preparations can cause the stools to be black.

OSMOLALITY (SERUM)

Reference Values

Adult: 280–300 mOsm/kg H_2O

Child: 270–290 mOsm/kg H_2O

Description

Serum osmolality is an indicator of serum concentration. It measures the number of dissolved particles (electrolytes, urea, sugar) in the serum and is helpful in the diagnosis of fluid and electrolyte imbalances. Sodium contributes 85% to 90% of the serum osmolality; changes in osmolality usually result from changes in the serum sodium concentration. Double the serum sodium can give a rough estimate of the serum osmolality.

The hydration status of the patient is usually determined by the serum osmolality. An increased value (>300 mOsm/kg) indicates hemoconcentration due to dehydration; a decreased value (<280 mOsm/kg) indicates hemodilution due to overhydration, or water excess. An osmometer is used in laboratories to determine serum osmolality; however, if the serum sodium, urea, and sugar are known, the serum osmolality can be calculated by the nurse as follows.[7–9,24,40,41]

$$\text{Serum osmolality} = 2 \times \text{Serum sodium} + \frac{\text{BUN}}{3} + \frac{\text{Sugar}}{18}$$

Clinical Problems

Decreased Level: excessive fluid intake, cancer of the bronchus and lung, adrenal cortical hypofunction, IV D_5W, syndrome of inappropriate diuretic hormone (SIADH)

Elevated Level: diabetes insipidus, dehydration, hypernatremia, hyperglycemia, uremia

Procedure

- Collect 5 to 10 mL of venous blood in a red-top tube. Avoid hemolysis.
- There is no food or fluid restriction.

■ Factors Affecting Laboratory Results

- Hyperglycemia increases the serum osmolality.

NURSING IMPLICATIONS WITH RATIONALE

Decreased Level

- Observe for signs and symptoms of overhydration, such as a constant, irritated cough; dyspnea; neck-and hand-vein engorgement; and chest rales.

■ Observe for signs and symptoms of water intoxication, such as headaches, confusion, irritability. Excessive amounts of hyposmolar solutions can "superdilute" the intravascular fluid.

Patient Teaching

■ Instruct the patient to decrease fluid intake.

Elevated Level

■ Assess for signs and symptoms of dehydration (thirst, dry mucous membranes, poor skin turgor, and shocklike symptoms).
■ Check for glycosuria. Increased sugar in the urine could indicate the presence of hyperglycemia.
■ Check the serum sodium, urea, and glucose for increased values. Calculate the serum osmolality by either doubling the serum sodium or using the formula given in the description.

Patient Teaching

■ Encourage the patient to increase fluid intake.

OSMOLALITY (URINE)

Reference Values

Adult: 50–1200 mOsm/kg/H_2O, average 200–800 mOsm/kg H_2O
Child: Newborn: 100–600 mOsm/kg/H_2O. *Child:* same as adult

Description

The urine osmolality test is more accurate than the specific gravity in determining the urine concentration, since its value reflects the number of particles, ions, and molecules and is not unduly influenced by large molecules. Specific gravity measures the quantity and nature of the particles, such as sugar, protein, and IV dyes (these elevate specific gravity but have little effect on osmolality).

The urine osmolality fluctuates in the same way that the urine-specific gravity does, and it can be low or high according to the patient's state of hydration. A dehydrated patient with normal kidney function could have a urine osmolality of 1000 mOsm/kg H_2O or more. When hemoconcentration occurs as a result of acidosis, shock, or hyperglycemia, the serum osmolality is elevated, and so should the urine osmolality be elevated.

If serum hyposmolality and hyponatremia occur with urine hyperosmolality, the problem is most likely SIADH. ADH causes water reabsorption from the kidney, thus diluting the serum.[12,18,23,41]

Clinical Problems

Decreased Level: excessive water intake, continuous IV D₅W, diabetes insipidus, glomerulonephritis, acute renal failure, sickle cell anemia, multiple myeloma. *Drug Influence:* diuretics

Elevated Level: high-protein diet, SIADH, Addison's disease (adrenal gland insufficiency), dehydration, hyperglycemia with glycosuria

Procedure

- Give a high-protein diet for 3 days prior to the urine osmolality test. Check with your laboratory.
- Restrict fluids for 8 to 12 hours before the test.
- Collect a random, morning, urine specimen. The first urine specimen in the morning is discarded, and the second specimen, taken 2 hours later, is sent to the laboratory. Urine osmolality should be high in the morning.
- Send the urine specimen to the laboratory.

■ **Factors Affecting Laboratory Results**

- Diuretics can cause urine hyperosmolality.
- A high-protein diet can cause urine hyperosmolality.

NURSING IMPLICATIONS WITH RATIONALE

- Explain to the patient that the purpose of the test is to determine the kidney's ability to concentrate urine.
- Explain the procedure of the test if it requires more than a random urine sample for urine osmolality. A high-protein diet is taken for 3 days before the test, and oral fluids are restricted the night before. The first urine specimen of the morning is discarded, and the second specimen, taken an hour or two later, is sent to the laboratory.

Decreased Level

- Determine whether the decreased urine osmolality could be caused by excessive intake of water (>2 quarts daily) or continuous IV administration of D₅W in water. A urine osmolality that remains less than 200 mOsm/kg after fluids are restricted could be indicative of early kidney impairment.
- Explain to the patient the need to decrease excessive water intake.
- Report to the physician when the patient is receiving D₅W continuously without any other solutes, such as saline (NaCl). The D₅W not only dilutes the urine, it can decrease the serum osmolality and cause water intoxication.
- Observe for signs and symptoms of water intoxication, such as headaches, confusion, irritability, weight gain, and, later, cerebral edema (if severe).

Elevated Level

- Determine the hydration status of the patient. Dehydration will cause an elevated urine osmolality as well as elevated serum osmolality. A urine

---

osmolality of 1000 mOsm/kg is not abnormal if the patient has a decreased fluid intake.

■ Check the serum osmolality. If the serum is hyposmolar and the urine is hyperosmolar, the problem could be due to SIADH. SIADH frequently occurs after surgery, trauma, or pain and will correct itself in a day or two. The function of ADH is to promote water reabsorption from the kidney tubules. The serum is diluted, and the decreased urine is concentrated.

■ Keep an accurate intake and output record. The fluid intake should be comparable to the urine output.

Patient Teaching

■ Instruct patients on high-protein diets to increase water intake.

OSMOTIC FRAGILITY OF ERYTHROCYTES (BLOOD)
Erythrocyte Osmotic Fragility, Red Cell Fragility

Reference Values

Adult

	% HEMOLYSIS	
% SALINE (NaCl)	**Fresh Blood (<3 hours)**	**Incubated at 37°C (24-hour blood)**
0.30	97–100	85–100
0.35	90–98	75–100
0.40	50–95	65–100
0.45	5–45	55–95
0.50	0–5	40–85
0.55	0	15–65
0.60	0	0–40

Child: similar to adult

Description

Water is normally exchanged between cells and extracellular fluid according to the osmolality (concentration) of fluid. RBC (erythrocyte) fluid and the plasma have similar ionic concentrations, iso-osmolar or isotonic. When there is an imbalance in one of the fluids, osmosis occurs. Fluid moves from the fluid with the lesser concentration to the fluid with the greater concentration. If erythrocytes are placed in a hypo-osmolar solution, fluid with less than the normal serum/plasma osmolality (<280 mOsm/L) will move into the erythrocytes, causing them to swell and eventually to rupture.

The erythrocyte osmotic fragility test determines the erythrocytes' ability to resist hemolysis (RBC destruction) in a hypo-osmolar solution. Erythrocytes are placed in various concentrations of saline. If hemolysis occurs at a slightly hypo-osmolar concentration of saline (0.36% to 0.73% solution), there is increased osmotic fragility, and if hemolysis occurs at a severely hypo-osmolar concentration of saline, there is decreased osmotic fragility. With increased fragility, the erythrocytes are usually spherical, and with decreased fragility, the erythrocytes are thin and flat.[1,3,10,12]

Clinical Problems

Decreased Level (<0.30%): anemias (iron deficiency, folic acid deficiency, vitamin B_6 deficiency, sickle cell), thalassemia major and minor (Mediterranean anemia or Cooley's anemia), hemoglobin C disease*, polycythemia vera, after splenectomy, acute and subacute necrosis of the liver, obstructive jaundice

Elevated Level (>0.46%): hereditary spherocytosis, transfusion (incompatibility—ABO and Rh), acquired hemolytic anemia (autoimmune), hemoglobin C disease*, chemical or drug poisonings, chronic lymphocytic leukemia, burns (thermal)

Procedure

- The test is usually performed on fresh blood less than 3 hours old and/or on 24-hour-old blood incubated at 37°C.
- Collect 7 to 10 mL of venous blood in a lavender-top or green-top tube. The tube should be filled to its capacity. A drop of blood is placed in tubes with decreasing saline concentration.
- Hemolysis is frequently determined by a colorimeter.
- There is no food or fluid restriction.

- Factors Affecting Laboratory Results

- Plasma pH, temperature, glucose concentration, and O_2 saturation of the blood affect the osmotic fragility.
- Older erythrocytes have increased osmotic fragility.
- A blood sample more than 3 hours old may show an increase in osmotic fragility.

NURSING IMPLICATIONS WITH RATIONALE

Decreased Level

- Identify clinical problems related to a decreased erythrocyte osmotic fragility. Normally complete hemolysis occurs with 0.30% saline. Thin, flat cells are usually resistant to hemolysis at 0.30%.
- Assess for signs and symptoms of anemias, such as fatigue, weakness, tachycardia, and dyspnea.

---

*Decreased or increased fragility may occur in hemoglobin C disease.

Elevated Level

- Identify clinical problems related to an increased erythrocyte osmotic fragility (ie, transfusion incompatibility, acquired hemolytic anemia, and chemical or drug poisoning [*see Clinical Problems*]).
- Monitor temperature when the patient receives a blood transfusion. A slightly elevated temperature is an early sign of transfusion reaction.
- Observe for signs and symptoms of transfusion reactions other than changes in temperature (ie, rash, difficulty in breathing, and an increased pulse rate).

OVA AND PARASITES (O AND P) (FECES)

Reference Values

Adult: negative

Child: negative

Description

Parasites may be present in various forms in the intestine, including the ova (eggs), larvae (immature form), cysts (inactive stage), and trophozoites (motile form) of protozoa. It is vitally important to detect parasites so that proper treatment can be ordered. Some of the organisms identified are amoeba, flagellates, tapeworms, hookworms, and roundworms. A history of recent travel outside the United States should be reported to the laboratory, since it may help in identifying the parasite.[1,10,12,13]

Clinical Problems

Positive Result: protozoa—*Balantidium coli, Chilomastix mesnili, Entamoeba histolytica, Giardia lamblia, Trichomonas hominis;* helminths (adults)—*Ascaris lumbricoides* (roundworm), *Diphyllobothrium latum* (fish tapeworm), *Enterobius vermicularis* (pinworm), *Necator americanus* (American hookworm), *Strongyloides stercoralis* (threadworm), *Taenia saginata* (beef tapeworm), *Taenia solium* (pork tapeworm)

Procedure

- Collect stool specimens for 3 days or every other day. Stool specimens should be taken immediately to the laboratory.
- Mark on the laboratory slip the countries the patient has visited outside the United States in the last 1 to 3 years.
- A loose or liquid stool is more likely to indicate that trophozoites are present. The stool must be kept warm and taken to the laboratory within 30 minutes. If the stool is semiformed or well formed, it does not need to be kept warm but should be taken to the laboratory at once.

■ If the stool is tested for tapeworm, the entire stool should be sent to the laboratory so that the head (scolex) of the tapeworm can be identified. The tapeworm will continue to grow as long as the head is lodged in the intestine.

■ Anal swabs are used to check for pinworm eggs, and the swabbing should be done in the morning before defecation or the morning bath.

■ No tissue paper or urine should be allowed in the fecal collection.

■ Avoid taking mineral oil, castor oil, Metamucil, barium, antacids, or tetracycline for 1 week before the test.

■ Laboratory results are available in 24 to 48 hours.

■ Factors Affecting Laboratory Results

■ Urine, toilet paper, soap, disinfectants, antibiotics, antacids, barium, harsh laxatives, and hypertonic saline enemas (Fleet) may affect the result of the test.

NURSING IMPLICATIONS WITH RATIONALE

■ Administer a mild laxative or normal saline enema, with the physician's approval, to obtain the stool specimen, if necessary.

■ Take the fresh stool specimen to the laboratory immediately.

■ Report to the physician if the patient is taking antacids and/or antibiotics or has received barium in the last 7 days. These agents can alter the stool examination for parasites and ova.

■ Obtain a history of the patient's recent travel. Certain parasites are common to certain countries, and the physician and laboratory should be notified of this information.

■ Handle the stool specimen with care to prevent parasitic contamination of yourself and other patients.

■ Check for occult blood in the stool. The worm attaches itself to the bowel's lining.

Patient Teaching

■ Explain to the patient the procedure for collecting the stool specimen. The stool should be collected in the morning, preferably before a bath. Explain to the patient that he or she should not use soap or a Fleet enema, for this may destroy the parasite. The stool specimen should be obtained before treatment is initiated.

■ Instruct the patient not to put urine or toilet paper in the sterile bedpan. Disinfectants should not be used, since they can cause the ova to deteriorate.

■ Instruct the patient to wash hands thoroughly after urinating and defecating.

PARATHYROID HORMONE (PTH) SERUM
Parathormone

Reference Values

Adult: *C-Terminal PTH:* 400–900 pg/mL. *N-Terminal PTH:* 200–600 pg/ml

Description

Parathyroid hormone (PTH), secreted by the parathyroid glands, regulates the concentration of calcium and phospohorus in the extracellular fluid. The main function of PTH is to promote calcium reabsorption and phosphorus excretion. Serum calcium levels affect the secretion of PTH: low serum-calcium levels stimulate the secretion of PTH; high serum-calcium levels inhibit PTH secretion.

Two forms of PTH, inactive C-terminal PTH and active N-terminal PTH, are used in diagnosing parathyroid disorders. C-terminal assays (PTH-C) are an effective indicator of chronic hyperparathyroidism. N-terminal assays (PTH-N) detect acute changes in the PTH secretion, can differentiate between hypercalcemia due to malignancy or parathyroid disorder, and are useful for monitoring patient's response to PTH therapy. Both assays and serum calcium values are used in diagnosing early and borderline parathyroid disorders.[1,3,6,9,10]

Clinical Problems

Decreased Level: PTH-C levels: hypoparathyroidism, nonparathyroid hypercalcemia. *PTH-N levels:* hypoparathyroidism, nonparathyroid hypercalcemia, certain tumors, pseudohyperparathyroidism. *PTH (serum):* hypoparathyroidism, nonparathyroid hypercalcemia, Graves disease, sarcoidosis

Elevated Level: PTH-C levels: secondary hyperparathyroidism, tumors, hypercalcemia, pseudohypoparathyroidism. *PTH-N levels:* primary and secondary hyperparathyroidism, pseudohypoparathyroidism. *PTH (serum):* primary and secondary hyperparathyroidism, hypercalcemia, chronic renal failure, pseudohyperparathyroidism (defect in renal tubular response)

Procedure

■ NPO for 8 hours prior to the test.
■ Collect 7 to 10 mL of venous blood in a red-top tube in the morning. Morning PTH is usually at its lowest point. Avoid hemolysis. Two tubes may be required (5 mL each). N-terminal PTH is unstable and needs to be chilled or frozen if test is not immediately run.
■ N-terminal PTH levels decrease during hemodialysis; therefore, collect blood specimens prior to dialysis.

■ Factors Affecting Laboratory Results

■ Nonchilled tube for N-terminal PTH affects test result.
■ Food, especially milk products, might lower PTH level.
■ Hemolysis of the blood sample could cause inaccurate result.

Nursing Implications and Rationale

■ Check with the laboratory to verify the procedure for collecting blood sample(s).
■ Assess for signs and symptoms of hypocalcemia (tetany; ie, muscular twitching and tremors, paresthesia [tingling and numbness of fingers], spasmodic contractions).
■ Assess for signs and symptoms of hypercalcemia (ie, lethargy, muscle flaccidity, weakness, headaches, nausea and vomiting).

Patient Teaching

■ Instruct the patient not to eat until after the blood sample is taken. Explain to patient that foods high in calcium can affect test results.

PARTIAL THROMBOPLASTIN TIME (PTT), ACTIVATED PARTIAL THROMBOPLASTIN TIME (APTT) (PLASMA)

Reference Values

Adult: Results vary in accordance with equipment and laboratory values. *PTT:* 60–70 seconds. *APTT:* 20–35 seconds.

Child: increased above adult level

Anticoagulant Therapy: 1.5–2.5 times the control in seconds.

Note: most laboratories do APTT only.

Description

The partial thromboplastin time (PTT) is a screening test used to detect deficiencies in all clotting factors except VII and XIII and to detect platelet variations. It is more sensitive than the prothrombin time (PT) in detecting minor deficiencies but is not as sensitive as the activated partial thromboplastin time (APTT).

The PTT is useful for monitoring heparin therapy. Heparin doses are adjusted according to the PTT test.

The APTT is more sensitive in detecting clotting factor defects than the

PTT, since the activator added in vitro shortens the clotting time. By shortening the clotting time, minor clotting defects can be detected.

The APTT is similar to the PTT, except that the thromboplastin reagent used in the APTT test contains an activator (kaolin, celite, or ellagic acid) for identification of deficient factors. This test is commonly used to monitor heparin therapy.[1,3,6,9,10,13,14]

Clinical Problems

Decreased Level: extensive cancer

Increased Level: factor deficiency (factors V, VIII [hemophilia], IX [Christmas disease], X, XI, XII), cirrhosis of the liver, vitamin K deficiency, hypofibrinogenemia, prothrombin deficiency, von Willebrand's disease (vascular hemophilia), disseminated intravascular coagulation (DIC) leukemias (myelocytic, monocytic), malaria. *Drug Influence:* heparin, salicylates

Procedure

- Collect 7 to 10 mL of venous blood in a blue-top tube. The tube should be filled to its capacity. The blood sample should be packed in ice and taken to the laboratory immediately.
- An activated thromboplastin mixture (thromboplastin reagent and an activator, such as kaolin) is added to the patient's plasma sample and the control sample. When a small amount of calcium solution is added, the stopwatch is started; it is stopped when fibrin strands are noted. The tests are usually duplicated and should agree to within 1 to 1.5 seconds. The test can also be done using a "fibronmeter."
- There is no food or fluid restriction.

■ Factors Affecting Laboratory Results

- A clotted blood sample
- A test (collection) tube without an anticoagulant

NURSING IMPLICATIONS WITH RATIONALE

- Check the APTT or PTT and report the results to the physician. The heparin dosage may need to be adjusted. The APTT range for heparin therapy is 1.5 to 2.5 times the normal value.
- Assess the patient for signs and symptoms of bleeding (purpura [skin], hematuria, and nosebleeds).
- Administer heparin subcutaneously or intravenously through a heparin lock. Do not aspirate when giving heparin subcutaneously, since a hematoma (blood tumor) could occur at the injection site.

PHENOTHIAZINES (SERUM)

Reference Values

Adult

DRUG	THERAPEUTIC RANGE	PEAK TIME	TOXIC LEVEL
Chlorpromazine (Thorazine)	50–300 ng/mL	2 to 4 hours	>750 ng/mL
Prochlorperazine (Compazine)	50–300 ng/mL	2 to 4 hours	>1000 ng/mL
Thioridazine (Mellaril)	100–600 ng/mL 0.2–2.6 mg/L	2 to 4 hours	>2000 ng/mL >10 mg/L
Trifluoperazine (Stelazine)	50–300 ng/mL	2 to 4 hours	>1000 ng/mL

Description

Phenothiazines are major tranquilizers (neurolytics) used for the treatment of psychosis and emesis. The phenothiazines have many active metabolites that are excreted in the urine. Thus phenothiazines can be measured in the urine and also in gastric fluids. Since phenothiazines are metabolized to many metabolites, the serum value is difficult to measure.

The phenothiazines have a wide therapeutic index. Consequently large dosage or large overdoses are relatively safe. However, extremely large overdoses can cause drug toxicity.[2–4,6,9,26]

Clinical Problems

Decreased Level: Drug Influence: antacids, anticholinergics (for pseudoparkinsonism)

Elevated Level: phenothiazide overdose.

Procedure

- Collect 7 mL of venous blood in a red-top tube.
- There is no food or fluid restriction.

■ Factors Affecting Laboratory Results

- Barbiturates and other antipsychotic agents enhance the phenothiazine effect.
- Antacids slow down the phenothiazine absorption, and anticholinergics taken for the pseudoparkinsonism effect can decrease the phenothiazine effect.

NURSING IMPLICATIONS WITH RATIONALE

■ Obtain a history from the patient concerning drug dosage and frequency.
■ Determine if the patient smokes. Smoking increases metabolism of the drug, and the drug dosage might need to be increased.
■ Check liver enzyme laboratory tests, especially if the patient is taking chlorpromazine (Thorazine). Taking chlorpromazine for a long period of time could have an effect on the liver.
■ Observe for side effects of phenothiazines, especially the common, pseudo-parkinsonism effect (muscle rigidity, tremors, bent-over position when walking).

Patient Teaching

■ Explain to the patient the importance of taking the prescribed drug dosage. Desired effect from the drug would not be obtained if the patient were underdosed.
■ Inform the patient to use protective suntan lotion, since photosensitivity is common with phenothiazines.
■ Advise the patient to check with the physician before taking OTC drugs to avoid side effects.
■ Inform the patient that the urine may be pink or red-brown when taking chlorpromazine (Thorazine).

PHENYLKETONURIA (PKU) (URINE), GUTHRIE TEST FOR PKU (BLOOD)

Reference Values

Adult: PKU and Guthrie test not usually done

Child: Phenylalanine: 0.5–2.0 mg/dL. *PKU:* negative, but positive when the serum phenylalanine is 12–15 mg/dL. *Guthrie:* negative, but positive when the serum phenylalanine is 4 mg/dL

Description

The urine PKU and Guthrie (blood) tests are two screening tests used for detecting a hepatic enzyme deficiency, phenylalanine hydroxylase, that prevents the conversion of phenylalanine (amino acid) to tyrosine in the infant. Phenylalanine from milk and other protein products accumulates in the blood and tissues and can lead to brain damage and mental retardation.

At birth the newborn's serum phenylalanine level is less than 2 mg/dL because of the mother's enzyme activity. After the third day of life or after 48 hours of milk ingestion, the serum level increases if phenylalanine is not metabolized.

The Guthrie procedure is the test of choice because a positive test result occurs when the serum phenylalanine reaches 4 mg/dL at 3 to 5 days of life after milk ingestion. A positive Guthrie test does not always indicate PKU, but if it is positive, a specific blood phenylalanine test should be performed. The PKU urine test is done after the infant is 3 to 4 weeks old and should be repeated a week or two later. Significant brain damage usually occurs when the serum level is 15 mg/dL. If either the Guthrie test or the urine PKU is positive, the infant should be maintained on a low phenylalanine diet for 6 to 8 years.[9,10,12,13]

Clinical Problems

Elevated Level: PKU, low-birth-weight infants, hepatic encephalopathy, septicemia, galactosemia. *Drug Influence:* aspirin and salicylate compounds, chlorpromazine (Thorazine), ketone bodies

Procedure

Guthrie Test **(Guthrie bacterial inhibition test):** Phenylalanine promotes bacterial growth (*Bacillus subtilis*) when the serum level is greater than 4 mg/dL.

■ Cleanse the infant's heel, and prick it with a sterile lancet. Obtain several drops of blood on the filter paper. The surface of the filter paper is streaked with *Bacillus subtilis,* and if the bacillus grows, the test is positive. Check the procedure outlined by your institution.
■ The test should not be done before 2 to 4 days of milk intake, either cow's milk or breast milk, and is preferably done on or after the fourth day.
■ Note on the laboratory slip the date of birth and the date the first milk was ingested.

Urine PKU: There are several urine tests for detecting phenylpyruvic acid. All use the reagent ferric chloride, which causes the urine specimen to turn green when positive. The Phenistix is a dipstick with ferric salt in the filter paper; it is dipped in fresh urine or pressed against a wet diaper. The dipstick will turn green if positive.

■ The urine PKU test should be done 3 to 6 weeks after birth, preferably at the fourth week. It is usually not positive for PKU until the serum phenylalanine levels are between 10 and 15 mg/dL.
■ The infant should be receiving milk for accurate Guthrie and urine PKU test results.

■ Factors Affecting Laboratory Results

■ Urine that is not fresh can cause inaccurate result.
■ Vomiting and/or decreased milk intake may cause a normal serum phenylalanine level in the infant with PKU.
■ Aspirins and salicylate compounds can cause a false-positive result.
■ Early PKU testing before the infant is 3 days old (Guthrie) or 2 weeks old (Phenistix) may cause false-negative test result.

NURSING IMPLICATIONS WITH RATIONALE

Elevated Level

- Relate positive Guthrie and urine PKU test results to the clinical problem, phenylketonuria.
- Explain to the mother the screening tests used to detect PKU. The Guthrie test is normally done while the mother and infant are in the hospital. Many pediatricians want the urine PKU done at home by the parent or in the doctor's office 3 to 4 weeks after birth as a follow-up test.
- Determine whether the infant has been taking adequate feedings (cow's milk or breast milk) before performing the Guthrie test. Vomiting and/or refusing to eat are common problems of PKU infants. This may cause a normal serum phenylalanine level.
- Obtain history if mother was a "PKU baby." If so, the mother should be on a low-phenylalanine diet before and during pregnancy.

Patient Teaching

- Instruct the mother how to perform a urine PKU test accurately. A fresh, wet diaper or a fresh urine specimen should be used.
- Instruct the mother that the baby should not receive aspirin or salicylate compounds for 24 hours before testing the urine. A false-positive test could result. Tylenol should be given instead of aspirin.
- Tell the mother which foods the baby should and should not have. The preferred milk substitute is Lofenalac (Mead Johnson and Co), an enzymic casein hydrolysate with vitamins and minerals. It provides a balanced nutritional formula. Other low-phenylalanine foods are fruits, fruit juices, vegetables, cereals, and breads. High-protein foods should be avoided (eg, as milk shakes, ice cream, and cheese). It is thought that after the age of 6 to 8 years, 90% of the brain growth has occurred, and the diet does not need to be as restrictive.

PHENYTOIN SODIUM (SERUM)
Diphenylhydantoin (Dilantin)

Reference Values

Therapeutic Range: Adult: as an anticonvulsant, 10–20 μg/mL, 39.6–79.3 μmol/L (SI units); As an antiarrhythmic, 10–18 μg/mL, 39.6–71.4 μmol/L (SI units). *In saliva:* 1–2 μg/mL, 4–9 μmol/L.

Toxic Level: Adult: >20 μg/mL, >79.3 μmol/L (SI units). *Child:* >15–20 μg/mL, 56–79 μmol/L (SI units)

Description

Phenytoin (Dilantin) reduces voltage, frequency, and spread of electrical discharges within the motor cortex. It is used to prevent and control grand-mal seizures. Phenytoin is also used as an antiarrhythmic drug for decreasing force of myocardial contraction, improving atrioventricular conduction depressed by a digitalis preparation, and prolonging the refractory period of the heart contraction.

Phenytoin sodium is absorbed from the GI tract within 3 to 12 hours. Foods and antacids can decrease its absorption rate. Neonates and infants during their first 2 to 3 months of age cannot absorb phenytoin, so other anticonvulsants should be used during that period of time.

Approximately 90% to 95% of phenytoin is bound to plasma proteins, and the remainder is free. About 5% to 10% of the drug is excreted unchanged in the urine. Half-life in adults is an average of 24 hours and in children is an average of 15 hours. Frequent monitoring of serum phenytoin levels is indicated for checking therapeutic level and for avoiding toxic level. It takes about 5 to 10 days to obtain steady state. With a change in phenytoin dosage, resampling is suggested in 48 hours.

General signs and symptoms of phenytoin toxicity include nystagmus (rapid movement of the eyeball), slurred speech, gingival hyperplasia, ataxia, drowsiness, lethargy, and confusion. IM injection might cause a slow and erratic absorption. Oral and IV routes (not to exceed 50 mg/min push) are preferred.[1,2–4,6,26]

Clinical Problems

Decreased Level: pregnancy, infectious mononucleosis. *Drug Influence:* alcohol, carbamazepine (Tegretol), folate

Elevated level: phenytoin overdose, uremia, liver disease. *Drug Influence:* aspirin, phenylbutazone (Butazolidin), dicumarol, chloramphenicol (Chloromycetin), sulfisoxazole (Gantrisin), chlorothiazide (Diuril), tranquilizers (chlordiazepoxide [Librium], chlorpromazine [Thorazine], prochlorperazine [Compazine], diazepam [Valium]), isoniazid (INH), phenobarbital, propoxyphene (Darvon)

Procedure

- Collect 5 to 7 mL of venous blood in a red-top tube. Avoid hemolysis.
- Record the dose, route, and last dose administered on the laboratory requisition slip. List drugs patient is taking that could affect test results.
- There is no food or fluid restriction.

■ Factors Affecting Laboratory Results

- Hemolysis of the blood specimen
- Drugs that increase serum phenytoin level (*See Drug Influence above.*)

NURSING IMPLICATIONS WITH RATIONALE

- Check serum phenytoin (Dilantin) result and immediately report nontherapeutic levels to the physician.
- Record dose, route, and last time the drug was given on the requisition slip.
- Note the method of drug administration. The oral and IV routes are commonly chosen methods for administration. The IM route might cause a slow and erratic absorption.

Elevated Level

- Observe for signs and symptoms of phenytoin toxicity, such as nystagmus, slurred speech, ataxia, drowsiness, lethargy, confusion, and rash.

PHOSPHORUS (P)—INORGANIC (SERUM)
Phosphate (PO$_4$)

Reference Values

Adult: 1.7–2.6 mEq/L or 2.5–4.5 mg/dL; 0.78–1.52 mmol/L (SI units)

Child: Newborn: 3.5–8.6 mg/dL. *Infant:* 4.5–6.7 mg/dL. *Child:* 4.5–5.5 mg/dL

Elderly: slightly lower than adult

Description

Phosphorus is the principal intracellular anion; however, most of phosphorus exists in the blood as phosphate. From 80% to 85% of the total phosphates in the body are combined with calcium in the teeth and bones.

Phosphorus is the laboratory term used, since phosphates are converted into inorganic phosphorus for the test. Functions of phosphorus include metabolism of carbohydrates and fats, maintenance of the acid-base balance, use of B vitamins, promotion of nerve and muscle activity, and transmission of hereditary traits.

Phosphorus (P) metabolism is associated with calcium (Ca) metabolism. Both ions need vitamin D for their absorption from the GI tract. Phosphorus and calcium concentrations are controlled by the parathyroid hormone. Usually there is a reciprocal relationship between calcium and phorphorus, since when serum phosphorus levels increase, serum calcium levels decrease, and when serum phosphorus levels decrease, serum calcium levels increase. In certain neoplastic bone diseases, this relationship is no longer true, since both calcium and phosphorus are increased.

A high serum phosphorus level is called hyperphosphatemia, which is usually associated with kidney dysfunction (poor urinary output). Hypophosphatemia means a low serum phosphorus level.[1,9,12,24]

Clinical Problems

Decreased Level: starvation, malabsorption syndrome, hyperparathyroidism, hypercalcemia, hypomagnesemia, chronic alcoholism, vitamin D deficiency, diabetic acidosis, myxedema, continuous IV fluids with glucose. *Drug Influence:* antacids such as aluminum hydroxide (Amphojel), epinephrine (adrenalin), insulin, mannitol

Elevated Level: renal insufficiency, renal failure, hypoparathyroidism, hypocalcemia, hypervitaminosis D, bone tumors, acromegaly, fractures (healing). *Drug Influence:* antibiotics (methicillin, tetracyclines), phenytoin (Dilantin), heparin, Lipomul, laxatives with phosphate

Procedure

- Collect 5 mL of venous blood in a red-top tube. Avoid hemolysis.
- The patient should be NPO except for water for 8 hours before the test. Some laboratories will require NPO for 4 hours. Carbohydrate lowers serum phosphorus levels because phosphate goes into the cells with glucose.
- The blood sample should be taken to the laboratory within 30 minutes. The serum should be separated from the RBCs quickly.

■ Factors Affecting Laboratory Results

- A high-carbohydrate diet and IV fluids with glucose can lower the serum phosphorus level; hence a fasting specimen is needed.
- Hemolysis of the blood sample can increase the serum phosphorus level. When RBCs rupture, they release intracellular phosphate into the serum.
- Late delivery of the blood sample (longer than 30 minutes) may cause the release of phosphorus from the blood cells into the serum. The serum should be separated from the blood clot within 30 minutes.
- Drugs (*see Drug Influence above*). Amphojel can lower the serum phosphorus level.

NURSING IMPLICATIONS WITH RATIONALE

- Hold medications in the morning until the blood sample is taken.
- Hold IV fluid with glucose for 4 to 8 hours before the blood test, if possible. Glucose can lower the serum phosphorus level by promoting the shift of phosphate back into the cells.

Decreased Level

- Check the serum phosphorus, calcium, and magnesium levels, and report changes to the physician if the serum levels are unknown. An elevated calcium level causes a decreased phosphorus level.
- Monitor oral and IV phosphorus replacements. Some of the oral phosphate salts (Neutrophos) come in capsules, which are indicated if nausea is present. Administer IV phosphate (KH_2PO_4) slowing to prevent hyperphosphatemia.

- Observe for signs and symptoms of hypophosphatemia, such as anorexia and pain in the muscles and bone.
- Observe for signs and symptoms of hypocalcemia (tetany) while the patient is receiving phosphate supplements.

Patient Teaching

- Instruct the patient to eat foods rich in phosphorus (ie, meats [beef, pork, turkey], milk, whole grain cereals, and almonds) if the decrease is caused by malnutrition. Most carbonated drinks are high in phosphates.
- Instruct the patient not to take antacids that contain aluminum hydroxide (Amphojel). Phosphorus binds with aluminum hydroxide; a low serum phosphorus level results.

Elevated Level

- Check the serum phosphorus, calcium, and magnesium levels. Observe for signs and symptoms of hypocalcemia (tetany); with an increased phosphorus level, calcium is usually low.
- Monitor urinary output. A decreased urine output (<25 mL/h or <600 mL/day) can increase the serum phosphorus level. Notify the physician of changes in urinary status.

Patient Teaching

- Instruct the patient to eat foods that are low in phosphorus (ie, vegetables). Instruct the patient to avoid drinking carbonated sodas that contain phosphates.

PLASMINOGEN (PLASMA)

Reference Values

Adult: 2.5–5.2 U/mL, 20 mg/dL[5]; 3.8–8.4 CTA (Council on Thrombolytic Agents)[24]

Description

Plasminogen, inactive precursor of plasmin, is converted to plasmin that activates the fibrinolytic process, a breakdown of fibrin clots in prevention of coagulation. Since plasmin cannot be measured in its active form in blood, plasminogen is measured to evaluate fibrinolysis. A decrease in plasminogen concentrate can indicate a tendency for thrombosis and also a serious secondary disease process (disseminated intravascular coagulation [DIC]).

Plasminogen is frequently monitored during administration of thrombolytic agents, such as streptokinase and urokinase, that are used to dissolve blood clots following an acute myocardial infarction. This test is also helpful in evaluating DIC.[1,3,6,9]

Clinical Problems

Decreased Level: DIC, liver disease (cirrhosis), thrombolytic therapy, tumors, preeclampsia. *Drug Influence:* streptokinasse

Elevated Level: acute infection, myocardial infarction, stress, surgery, trauma, malignant disease. *Drug Influence:* oral contraceptives

Procedure

- Collect 7 mL of venous blood in a blue-top tube. Avoid hemolysis. Avoid leaving the tourniquet on too long.
- There is no food or fluid restriction.

■ Factors Affecting Laboratory Results

- Hemolysis of the blood sample can affect results.
- Prolonged use of tourniquet could decrease plasma plasminogen level.
- Drugs (see *Drug Influence*).

NURSING IMPLICATIONS WITH RATIONALE

- Assess for bleeding tendencies, apprehension, petechiae, bleeding from orifices, tachycardia, and, later, hypotension.
- Check other laboratory findings (eg, fibrin degradation products [FDP]).
- Monitor vital signs.

PLATELET AGGREGATION AND ADHESIONS (BLOOD)

Reference Values

Adult: aggregation in 3 to 5 minutes

Description

Platelet aggregation test measures the ability of platelets adhering to each other when mixed with an aggregating agent such as collagen, ADP, or ristocetin. This test is performed to detect abnormality in platelet function and to aid in diagnosing hereditary and acquired platelet deficiencies such as von Willebrand's disease. Increase bleeding tendencies result from a decrease in platelet aggregation time.

Platelet adhesion test, like platelet aggregation, evaluates platelet function and helps to confirm hereditary diseases such as von Willebrand's disease. This test is also performed on patients taking large doses of aspirin for several weeks and on persons having a prolonged bleeding time. It is not performed in many laboratories because of the difficulty in standardizing the technique.[1,9,13,20]

Clinical Problems

Decrease Platelet Aggregation: von Willebrand's disease, Bernard-Soulier syndrome, Glanzmann's disease (thrombasthenia), leukemia, idiopathic thrombocytopenia purpura, platelet release defects, afibrinogenemia, cirrhosis of the liver, uremia. *Drug Influence:* aspirin and aspirin compounds, anti-inflammatory agents (ibuprofen [Motrin], indomethacin [Indocin], phenylbutazone [Butazolidin]), 5-Fluorouracil, phenothiazines, tricyclic antidepressants, diazepam (Valium), antihistamines, dipyridamole (Persantine), cortisone preparations, theophylline, cocaine, marijuana

Elevated Platelet Aggregation: diabetes mellitus, hyperlipemia, hypercoagulability

Procedure

- Collect 7 mL of venous blood in a blue-top tube. Avoid hemolysis.
- NPO, including no medications, after midnight, except for water.
- Allow no aspirin or aspirin compounds for 7 to 10 days prior to the test. List drugs patient is taking on the laboratory slip.

- Factors Affecting Laboratory Results

  - Foods high in fat content eaten before the test—Hyperlipemia increases platelet aggregation.
  - Drugs that inhibit platelet aggregation (*See Drug Influence.*)

NURSING IMPLICATIONS WITH RATIONALE

- Obtain a drug history from the patient. Record and underline names of drugs the patient is taking that could prolong platelet aggregation.
- List names of drugs the patient is taking that could affect test results on the laboratory slip.
- Check for bleeding tendencies, petechiae, purpura.

Patient Teaching

- Instruct the patient about the importance of not taking aspirin and aspirin compounds 7 to 10 days before the test (check with the physician about the time period to avoid aspirin intake). Aspirin inhibits clotting time or prolongs bleeding time, thus the test could be invalidated.
- Inform the patient that no medications, food, or fluids, except water, should be taken after midnight before the test (it may be necessary to take some medications before test; check with physician).

PLATELET COUNT (BLOOD—THROMBOCYTES)

Reference Values

Adult: 150,000–400,000 μL (mean, 250,000 μL), 0.15–0.4 $\times$ 10^{12}/L (SI units)

Child: Premature: 100,000–300,000 μL. *Newborn:* 150,000–300,000 μL. *Infant:* 200,000–475,000 μL

Description

Platelets (thrombocytes) are basic elements in the blood that promote coagulation. Platelets are much smaller than erythrocytes. They clump and stick to rough surfaces and injured sites when blood coagulation is needed. A decrease in circulating platelets of less than 50% of the normal value will cause bleeding; if the decrease is severe (<50,000 μL), hemorrhaging might occur.

Thrombocytopenia means platelet deficiency or a low platelet count. It is commonly associated with leukemias, aplastic anemia, and idiopathic thrombocytopenic purpura. Increased platelet counts (thrombocytosis) occur in polycythemia, in fractures, and after splenectomy.[1,3,8,10,12,13]

Clinical Problems

Decreased Level: idiopathic thrombocytopenic purpura, multiple myeloma, cancer (bone, GI tract, brain), leukemias (lymphocytic, myelocytic, monocytic), anemias (aplastic, iron deficiency, pernicious, folic acid deficiency, sickle cell), liver disease (cirrhosis, chronic active hepatitis), systemic lupus erythematosus, disseminated intravascular coagulopathy, kidney diseases, eclampsia, acute rheumatic fever. *Drug Influence:* antibiotics (chloromycetin, streptomycin), sulfonamides, aspirin (salicylates), quinidine, quinine, acetazolamide (Diamox), amidopyrine, thiazide diuretics, meprobamate (Equanil), phenylbutazone (Butazolidin), tolbutamide (Orinase), vaccine injections, chemotherapeutic agents

Elevated Level: polycythemia vera, trauma (surgery, fractures), postsplenectomy, acute blood loss (peaks in 7 to 10 days), metastatic carcinoma, pulmonary embolism, high altitudes, tuberculosis, reticulocytosis, severe exercise. *Drug Influence:* epinephrine (adrenalin)

Procedure

■ There is no food or fluid restriction.

Venous Blood: Collect 5 mL of venous blood in a lavender-top tube.

Capillary Blood: Discard the first few drops. Collect a drop of blood from a finger puncture, and dilute the blood immediately with the appropriate diluting solution.

■ Factors Affecting Laboratory Results

■ Chemotherapy and x-ray therapy can cause a decreased platelet count.
■ Drugs (*See Drug Influence.*)

NURSING IMPLICATIONS WITH RATIONALE

■ Explain to the patient that the purpose of the blood test is to determine the platelet count, or give a similar explanation.
■ Check the platelet count, especially with bleeding episodes, and report abnormal levels to the physician if results are not known by the physician.

Decreased Level

■ Observe for signs and symptoms of bleeding (skin [purpura, petechiae] or GI [hematemesis, rectal bleeding]). Record findings on the chart, and report them to the physician.
■ Monitor the platelet count, especially when the patient is receiving chemotherapy or radiation therapy for cancer.

Patient Teaching

■ Instruct the patient to avoid injury, if possible. Mild injury could cause bleeding.

PORPHOBILINOGEN (URINE)

Reference Values

Adult: *Random (qualitative):* negative. *24-Hour (quantitative):* 0–2 mg/24h
Child: same as adult

Description

Porphobilinogen is one of the precursors of porphyrins, and large amounts are excreted during an acute attack of porphyria. Between attacks there may not be an appreciable amount of porphobilinogen present. The test should be conducted during the acute phase.

The urine porphobilinogen test is ordered to detect the presence of porphyrias. Porphyrias are inherent metabolic disorders that affect the synthesis of heme of hemoglobin. Congenital porphyria (erythropoietic porphyria) is characterized by pinkish brown-stained teeth, pinkish yellow to reddish black urine, and skin photosensitivity. Uroporphyrin and coproporphyrin I are excreted.

Hereditary hepatic porphyria can be divided into three types: acute intermittent porphyria, variegate porphyria, and herditary coproporphyria. During an acute attack of porphyria, the urine becomes deep red and there are mental disturbances and severe abdominal pain. These attacks mimic various diseases such as appendicitis and pancreatitis; the leukocyte (WBC) count becomes elevated. Barbiturates, alcohol, and estrogen can precipitate an acute attack of porphyria.[3,7,10,13,14]

Clinical Problems

Elevated level: acute intermittent porphyria, variegate porphyria, secondary malignant neoplasm, Hodgkin's disease, cirrhosis of the liver (occasionally)
Drug Influence: antibiotics (penicillin, tetracyclines); antiseptics (phenol compounds, phenazopyridine [Pyridium]), barbiturates, hypnotics, phenothiazines (chlorpromazine [Thorazine]), procaine, sulfonamides

Procedure

Qualitative (screening test)
■ Collect a random sample of 30 mL or more of fresh urine during or immediately after an acute attack of porphyria. The patient has acute abdominal pain.
■ Protect the specimen from light.

Quantitative (24 hour)
■ Collect the urine in a dark container. If it is collected in a clear container, protect it from light and refrigerate. The container should have an acidic preservative. Delta amino levulinic acid (ALA), which forms porphobilinogen, is not stable unless the urine is acidic. Urine should be collected immediately after the patient has an acute attack.
■ Have the patient void, discard the urine, and then save all urine for 24 hours.
■ Label the specimen with the date and the exact time the test started and ended.
■ Encourage the patient to take fluids. There is no food restriction.

■ Factors Affecting Laboratory Results

■ Exposure of the urine sample to light
■ Drugs (*See Drug Influence above.*)
■ Contamination of the urine with toilet paper or feces

NURSING IMPLICATIONS WITH RATIONALE

Patient Teaching

■ Explain the procedure to the patient and family and tell them not to throw away any urine. Tell them that urine should not be exposed to light and should be refrigerated.
■ Inform the patient that he or she should not contaminate the urine with toilet paper or stools.

Elevated Level

■ Recognize that this test is usually done during an acute attack (acute abdominal pain) to detect porphyria.

- Observe and report urine color prior to an acute attack. The urine color could be amber to burgundy.
- Observe for signs and symptoms of an acute porphyria attack, such as severe abdominal pain (colicky), mental disturbances, and neuropathy. Respiratory distress could occur.

Patient Teaching

- Instruct the patient with porphyria to stay away from bright sunlight. Skin photosensitivity is a common problem, and skin lesions could result. Suggest that the patient use sun screen on exposed skin areas and wear protective clothing.
- Instruct the patient not to take barbiturates, alcohol, or estrogens without the physician's permission. These agents can precipitate an acute attack of porphyria.

PORPHYRINS—COPROPORPHYRINS, UROPORPHYRINS (URINE)

Reference Values

Coproporphyrins: Adult: Random: 3–20 μg/dL; Quantitative: 50–160 μg/24 h. *Child:* 0–80 μg/24 h

Uroporphyrins: Adult: Random: negative. Quantitative: <30 μg/24 h. *Child:* 10–30 μg/24 h

Description

Porphyrins are used in the synthesis of hemoglobin and of any hemoproteins that are carriers of oxygen. The porphyrins are eliminated from the body in feces and urine, mainly as coproporphyrin I and III and as uroporphyrins. Normal excretion of coproporphyrins is minimal, but the amount excreted rises during liver damage, lead poisoning, and congenital porphyria (an inherent error of metabolism).

There is an increase in urine porphobilinogen with disorders of porphyrin metabolism. Porphobilinogen is one of the precursors of porphyrins (formed in the liver).[3,8,10,12,14]

Clinical Problems

Elevated Level: lead toxicity, cirrhosis of the liver, acute intermittent porphyria, viral hepatitis, infectious mononucleosis, porphyria variegata, porphyria cutanea tarda, acquired hemolytic anemia (autoimmune). *Drug Influence:* antibiotic (tetracyclines, penicillin), antiseptics (ethoxazene [Diaphenyl], phenazopyridine [Pyridium]), sulfonamides (sulfamethoxazole [Gantanol], sulfisoxazole [Gantrisine]), barbiturates and hypnotics, phenothiazines such as chlorpromazine (Thorazine), procaine

Procedure

- Collect urine in a dark container containing the preservative sodium carbonate. If a large, clear container is used, protect it from light and refrigerate it.
- Have the patient void, discard the urine, and then save all urine for 24 hours.
- Label the specimen with the exact date and time the test started and ended (eg, 7/24/93, 7:00 A.M. to 7/25/93, 7:01 AM).
- There is no food or fluid restriction.

■ **Factors Affecting Laboratory Results**

- Exposure of the urine to light
- Drugs (*See Drug Influence.*)
- Contamination of the urine with toilet paper and feces

NURSING IMPLICATIONS WITH RATIONALE

Patient Teaching

- Explain the procedure to the patient. Inform the patient and family that all urine must be saved for 24 hours. Emphasize that the urine should *not* be exposed to light.
- Inform the patient not to contaminate the urine with toilet paper or feces.

Elevated Level

- Recognize clinical problems and drugs related to elevated porphyrin levels. Liver disease and lead poisoning cause an excessive amount of coproporphyrin III to be excreted.
- Observe the color of a urine specimen exposed to light. A pinkish or red color should be reported.

POTASSIUM (K) (SERUM)

Reference Values

Adult: 3.5–5.0 mEq/L; 3.5–5.0 mmol/L (SI units)

Child: Infant: 3.6–5.8 mEq/L. *Child:* 3.5–5.5 mEq/L

Description

Potassium is the electrolyte found most abundantly in intracellular fluids (cells). The serum potassium has a narrow range, and cardiac arrest could occur if serum level is less than 2.5 mEq/L or greater than 7.0 mEq/L.

Eighty to 90% of the body potassium is excreted by the kidneys. When there is tissue breakdown, potassium leaves the cells and enters the extracellular fluid (interstitial and intravascular fluids). With adequate kidney functions, the potassium in the intravascular fluid (plasma/blood vessels) will be excreted, and with excessive potassium excretion, a serum potassium deficit (hypokalemia) occurs. However, if the kidneys are excreting less than 600 mL of urine daily, potassium will accumulate in the intravascular fluid and serum potassium excess (hyperkalemia) will occur.

The body does not conserve potassium, and the kidneys excrete an average of 40 mEq/L daily (the range is 25 to 120 mEq/L/24 h), even with a low dietary potassium intake. The daily potassium requirement is 3 to 4 g, or 40 to 60 mEq/L.[9,13,23,24]

Clinical Problems

Decreased Level: vomiting/diarrhea, dehydration, malnutrition/starvation, crash diet, stress (trauma, injury, or surgery), gastric suction, intestinal fistulas, diabetic acidosis, burns, renal tubular disorders, hyperaldosteronism, excessive ingestion of licorice, excessive ingestion of glucose, alkalosis (metabolic). *Drug Influence:* potassium-wasting diuretics (furosemide [Lasix], thiazides [Hydrodiuril], ethacrynic acid [Edecrin]), steroids (cortisone, estrogen) antibiotics (gentamicin, amphotericin, polymyxin B) bicarbonate, insulin, laxatives, lithium carbonate, sodium polystyrene sulfonate-(Kayexalate), salicylates (aspirin)

Increased Level: oliguria and anuria, acute renal failure, IV potassium in fluids, Addison's disease (adrenocortical hormone), crushed injury and burns (with kidney shutdown), acidosis (metabolic or lactic). *Drug Influence:* potassium-sparing diuretics, spironolactone (Aldactone), triamterene (Dyrenium), antibiotics (penicillin G potassium, cephaloridine (Loridin), heparin, epinephrine, histamine, isoniazid

Procedure

- Collect 5 to 10 mL of venous blood in a red-top tube. Avoid hemolysis.
- Avoid leaving the tourniquet on for >2 minutes if possible.
- Food, fluid, and drug restrictions are not necessary.

- Factors Affecting Laboratory Results

  - The hydration status of the patient can cause false potassium test values. Overhydration can cause a false serum-potassium deficit through hemodilution. Dehydration can cause a serum potassium excess through hemoconcentration. After the patient is hydrated, his or her serum potassium level may be normal or slightly low.
  - The use of a tourniquet can cause an increase in the serum potassium level.
  - Hemolysis of the specimen (blood) can result in high serum-potassium level.
  - Drugs (*See Drug Influence.*)

NURSING IMPLICATIONS WITH RATIONALE

- Compare serum potassium levels with urine potassium levels. When serum potassium level is decreased, urine potassium level is frequently increased and vice versa.

Decreased Level

- Observe for signs and symptoms of hypokalemia, such as vertigo (dizziness), hypotension, arrhythmias, nausea, vomiting, diarrhea, abdominal distention, decreased peristalsis, muscle weakness, and leg cramps.
- Record intake and output. Polyuria can cause an excessive loss of potassium. Potassium is not conserved well in the body, and the kidney excretes potassium regardless of potassium intake.
- Report serum potassium levels below 3.5 mEq/L. If the potassium level is 3.0 to 3.5 mEq/L, it will take 100 to 200 mEq/L of potassium chloride (KCl) to raise the potassium level 1 mEq/L. If the potassium level is 2.9 mEq/L or less, it will take 200 to 400 mEq/L of KCl to raise the level 1 mEq/L.
- Determine the patient's hydration status when hypokalemia is present. Overhydration can dilute the serum potassium level.
- Recognize behavioral changes as a sign of hypokalemia. Low potassium levels can cause confusion, irritability, and mental depression. The serum potassium level should be checked in the presence of any behavioral changes.
- Report ECG changes. A prolonged and depressed ST segment and a flat or inverted T-wave is indicative of hypokalemia.
- Dilute oral potassium supplements in at least 4 oz of water or juice. Potassium is a corrosive agent and is most irritating to the gastric mucosa.
- Monitor the serum potassium level in patients receiving potassium-wasting diuretics and steroids. Examples of potassium-wasting diuretics are Hydrodiuril, Lasix, and Edecrin. Cortisone steroids (such as prednisone) cause sodium retention and potassium excretion.
- Assess for signs and symptoms of digitalis toxicity when the patient is receiving a digitalis preparation and a potassium-wasting diuretic or steroid. A lower serum-potassium level enhances the action of digitalis. Signs and symptoms of digitalis toxicity are nausea and vomiting, anorexia, bradycardia, arrhythmia, and visual disturbances.
- Monitor serum chloride, serum magnesium, and serum protein test results when hypokalemia is present. Correcting a potassium deficit with potassium only is not effective if chloride, magnesium, and protein levels are also low.
- Administer IV KCl in a liter of parenteral fluids. Never give an IV or bolus push of KCl, since cardiac arrest can occur. Parenteral KCl can only be administered intravenously when it is diluted (20 to 40 mEq per liter) and should never be given subcutaneously or intramuscularly. Concentrated IV KCl is irritating to the heart muscle and to the veins, causing phlebitis.
- Check the IV site when the patient is receiving KCl in IV fluids. Infiltrated potassium is most irritating to the subcutaneous tissues (fatty tissues) and can cause tissue sloughing.
- Measure GI fluid loss from suctioning, vomiting, or diarrhea for appropriate potassium and other electrolyte replacement. Potassium, sodium, hydrogen, and chloride are most plentiful in the gastrointestinal tract.
- Irrigate GI tubes with normal saline solution to prevent electrolyte loss.

Patient Teaching

- Instruct the patient and family to eat foods high in potassium (fruits, dry fruits, vegetables, meats, nuts, coffee, tea, cocoa, and Coca Cola). The daily potassium requirement is 3 to 4 g, or 40 to 60 mEq/L.
- Teach patients to eat foods rich in potassium when they are taking drugs and foods (ie, cortisone, potassium-wasting diuretics, laxatives, lithium carbonate, salicylates, insulin, glucose, and licorice) that decrease body potassium.

Increased Level

- Observe for signs and symptoms of hyperkalemia, or serum potassium excess (slow pulse rate [bradycardia], abdominal cramps, oliguria or anuria, tingling, and twitching or numbness of the extremities).
- Assess urine output to determine renal function. Urine output should be at least 25 mL/h, or 600 mL daily, and a urine output of less than 600 mL/day could cause hyperkalemia.
- Report serum potassium levels greater than 5.0 mEq/L. High serum-potassium levels can cause cardiac arrest.
- Regulate the rate of IV fluids so that no more than 10 mEq KCl/L are administered per hour. Rapid administration of KCl intravenously can result in hyperkalemia.
- Check the age of whole blood before administering it to a patient with hyperkalemia. Blood 2 weeks old or older has an elevated serum potassium level.
- Assess the patient's serum potassium level every 6 to 8 hours when it is elevated (>6.5 mEq/L) and during treatment for hyperkalemia. The serum potassium level can change frequently during treatment.
- Monitor the ECG for QRS spread and peaked T-waves (signs of hyperkalemia). The pulse may be rapid, but if hyperkalemia persists, bradycardia or slow pulse can occur.
- Restrict potassium intake when the serum potassium level is greater than 6.0 mEq/L.
- Monitor patients receiving various medical treatments for hyperkalemia for signs and symptoms of continuous hyperkalemia or developing hypokalemia. The various medical treatments are as follows: (1) IV sodium bicarbonate increases the pH, causing potassium to shift back into the cells; (2) IV glucose and insulin can also cause potassium to shift back into the cells and are usually effective for 6 hours; (3) calcium gluconate decreases the myocardial irritability resulting from hyperkalemia but does not decrease the serum potassium level; (4) sodium polystyrene sulfonate (Kayexalate) is a drug used as ion (resin) exchange, sodium for potassium. It can be administered orally or rectally and is considered the most effective method for treating hyperkalemia.
- Notify the physician if the patient is receiving a digitalis preparation when calcium gluconate is given. An elevated serum calcium level enhances the action of digitalis, causing digitalis toxicity.
- Observe for signs and symptoms of hypokalemia when administering Kayexalate for a prolonged period of time (2 or more days).

POTASSIUM (K) (URINE)

Reference Values

Adult: Broad Range: 25–100 mEq/24 h. *Average Range:* 40–80 mEq/24 h, 40–80 mmoL/24 h (SI units)

Description

Eighty to 90% of the body's potassium is excreted in the urine. A 24-hour urine potassium level is a valuable indicator of serum potassium status. A decrease in urinary potassium can indicate hyperkalemia (elevated serum potassium), and an increase in urinary potassium can indicate hypokalemia (low serum potassium) or may result from an increased potassium intake. If the kidneys are not functioning properly and there is decreased urine output (oliguria), the potassium excreted in the urine will be decreased and the serum potassium level will be elevated.[8,10,13,24]

Clinical Problems

Decreased Level: elevated serum potassium level, acute renal failure, diarrhea. *Drug Influence:* potassium-sparing diuretics (eg, Aldactone)

Elevated Level: decreased serum potassium level, dehydration/starvation, chronic renal failure, diabetic acidosis, vomiting and gastric suction, increased adrenal cortical hormone or Cushing's disease, salicylate toxicity. *Drug Influence:* potassium-wasting diuretics (eg, Hydrodiuril, Lasix), prednisone

Procedure

- The 24-hour urine specimen should be kept on ice or refrigerated.
- There is no food or fluid restriction.
- Potassium supplements given as salt replacement should be eliminated for 48 hours.

■ **Factors Affecting Laboratory Results**

- Failure to refrigerate the urine container affects test results.
- Fecal material and toilet paper contaminate urine specimen.
- Vomiting or gastric suctioning can cause hypokalemia due to potassium loss from the GI tract, and the accompanying metabolic alkalosis can cause an increase in urinary potassium loss. With a high urinary potassium excretion, the hypokalemic state could become more severe.

NURSING IMPLICATIONS WITH RATIONALE

Decreased Level

- Explain to the patient that the purpose of the test is to determine whether the kidneys are excreting an adequate amount of potassium or whether the body is retaining it.

- Instruct the patient to save all of his or her urine for 24 hours and to place it in the container, which should be on ice or refrigerated.
- Observe for signs and symptoms of hyperkalemia. When urinary potassium excretion is decreased, the serum potassium level may be increased. Signs and symptoms of hyperkalemia are oliguria, abdominal cramps, bradycardia, and tingling, twitching, or numbness in the extremities. Check the arterial pH or the serum CO_2 levels. If metabolic acidosis is present (decreased pH and serum CO_2), the serum potassium may be elevated and the urinary potassium may be decreased. Potassium is frequently retained in the body during metabolic acidosis.

   Metabolic acidosis: ↓ pH, ↓ serum CO_2 → ↑ Serum K, ↓ urinary K.

Elevated Level

- Explain to the patient that an increase in potassium intake or the use of diuretics (potassium wasting) will result in an excess urinary potassium excretion.
- Observe for signs and symptoms of hypokalemia. When urinary potassium excretion is increased, the serum potassium level is frequently decreased. Signs and symptoms of hypokalemia are vertigo (dizziness), hypotension, arrhythmia, muscle weakness, and decreased peristalsis.
- Determine arterial pH or serum CO_2 levels. If metabolic alkalosis is present (elevated pH and serum CO_2), the serum potassium level may be low and the urine potassium may be increased. Hydrogen and potassium are excreted together in the urine and alkalosis results. Vomiting and gastric suction can cause metabolic alkalosis.

   Metabolic alkalosis: ↑ pH, ↑ serum CO_2 → ↓ Serum K, ↑ urinary K.

PREGNANEDIOL (URINE)

Reference Values

Adult: *Male:* 0.1–1.5 mg/24 h. *Female:* 0.5–1.5 mg/24 h (proliferative phase), 2–7 mg/24 h (luteal phase), 0.1–1.0 mg/24 h (postmenopausal)

PREGNANCY	
Gestation weeks	**mg/24 h**
10–19	5–25
20–28	15–42
28–32	25–49

Child: 0.4–1.0 mg/24 h

Description

Pregnanediol is the major metabolite of progesterone produced by the ovary during the secretory phase of the menstrual cycle (second half) and by the placenta. Progesterone is responsible for uterine changes after ovulation and for maintaining pregnancy after fertilization. A steady rise in urinary pregnanediol levels occurs during pregnancy, and a decrease in these levels indicates placental dysfunction (not fetal) and the possibility of an abortion. Progesterone therapy would be indicated when urine pregnanediol is decreased.

Urinary pregnanediol levels may be used to determine menstrual disturbances and are used to verify ovulation in those who have not been able to become pregnant. The pregnanediol levels rise rapidly after ovulation, and they can be used as an indicator of ovulation time. This test should not be mistaken for the pregnanetriol test.[5,6,8,10,12,13]

Clinical Problems

Decreased Level: amenorrhea (menstrual disorder), ovarian hypofunction, threatened abortion, pregnancy complicated by intrauterine death, benign neoplasms of the ovary and breast, lutein cell tumor of the ovary, preeclampsia

Elevated Level: pregnancy, ovarian cyst, choriocarcinoma of the ovary, adrenal cortex hyperplasia

Procedure

- Collect urine over a 24-hour period in a large container bottle with preservative, and keep it refrigerated.
- Label the bottle with the patient's name and the dates and exact times of collection (eg, 4/10/93, 8:00 AM to 4/11/93, 8:00 AM).
- Record on the laboratory slip the date of the last menstrual period.
- Take the urine bottle to the laboratory immediately after the urine collection has been completed.
- There is no food or fluid restriction.
- The urine may also be used to determine estradiol (E_3) levels in conjunction with the pregnanediol levels.

■ Factors Affecting Laboratory Results

- Toilet paper and feces in the urine
- An unrefrigerated urine collection that has not been analyzed for several days

---

NURSING IMPLICATIONS WITH RATIONALE

- Ask when the patient had her last period; this should be recorded on the laboratory slip.

Patient Teaching

- Explain to the patient the procedure for collecting urine. Explain that all urine should be saved and placed in the labeled container in the refrigerator.
- Instruct the patient not to put toilet paper or feces in the urine.

Decreased Level

- Recognize clinical problems that may cause a decreased pregnanediol level, such as menstrual disorder (amenorrhea), threatened abortion, and complicated pregnancy.
- Obtain a history of menstrual changes (menstruation patterns—frequency, length of period, flow, and discomfort).
- Obtain a history of pregnancy complications or problems. Record when the patient had her last menstrual period and whether bleeding is present (how long has it occurred, how much bleeding, and is it continuous?).
- Give support to the patient and family by listening, spending time with them, and answering questions, if possible. Supportive care can reduce anxiety.
- Monitor the urine pregnanediol levels if several tests have been ordered over a period of days or weeks. The levels can indicate progesterone production and whether progesterone therapy is needed.

Elevated Level

- Recognize clinical problems that can cause an elevated pregnanediol level, such as pregnancy and an ovarian cyst. Pregnanediol level should increase during pregnancy. After 18 to 24 weeks, the level should be 13 to 22 mg/24 h, and after 28 to 32 weeks, the level should be 27 to 47 mg/ 24 h. In the last 2 weeks of pregnancy, the urine pregnanediol level decreases.

PREGNANETRIOL (URINE)

Reference Values

Adult: Male: 0.4–2.4 mg/24 h. *Female:* 0.5–2.0 mg/24 h
Child: Infant: 0–0.2 mg/24 h. *Child:* 0–1.0 mg/24 h

Description

Pregnanetriol (17-hydroxyprogesterone) comes from adrenal corticoid synthesis. It should not be mistaken for pregnanediol because it is not a derivative of progesterone. The pregnanetriol test is useful in diagnosing congenital adrenocortical hyperplasia.[5,8,10]

Clinical Problems

Decreased Level: anterior pituitary hypofunction

Elevated Level: adrenogenital syndrome, congenital adrenocortical hyperplasia, adrenocortical hyperfunction, malignant neoplasm of the adrenal gland

Procedure

- Collect urine for 24 hours in a large, refrigerated container. No preservative is needed.
- Label the bottle with the patient's name, dates, and exact times of collection (eg, 2/3/93, 8:00 AM to 2/4/93, 8:02 AM).
- There is no food or fluid restriction.

■ Factors Affecting Laboratory Results

  ■ None known

NURSING IMPLICATIONS WITH RATIONALE

- Monitor urine pregnanetriol levels with cortisone replacement.

Patient Teaching

- Instruct the patient and family to save all urine for 24 hours, to keep the urine refrigerated, and not to put toilet paper or feces in the urine.

PROCAINAMIDE HYDROCHLORIDE (SERUM)
(Pronestyl, Procan, Procamide)

Reference Values

Therapeutic Range: Adult: 4–10 μg/mL, 5–30 μg/mL for sum of procainamide + NAPA. *Child:* not done

Toxic Level: Adults: >10 μg/mL, >30 μg/mL sum of procainamide + NAPA

Description

Procainamide (Pronestyl, Procan), an antiarrhythmic agent, is used to treat cardiac arrhythmias. It acts by prolonging refractory period of the heart, reducing conduction velocity, and decreasing myocardial excitability. This drug is absorbed readily from the GI tract and is metabolized by the liver to active metabolites.

Procainamide can be administered orally, intramuscularly, and intravenously; the commonest method is oral administration. Peak level occurs 1½ hours after oral administration. Steady state is about 24 hours after ingestion with good renal function. Half-life for procainamide is about 3 to 4 hours and for the metabolite *N*-acetylprocainamide (NAPA) about 6 to 8 hours. Approximately 50% of the drug is excreted unchanged in the urine.

Common side effects of this drug are nausea, vomiting, bitter taste, hypotension, bradycardia. Lupus erythematosuslike syndrome occurs in about 30% to 40% of patients on long-term procainamide therapy (1 year or more).[2,3,8]

Clinical Problems

Elevated Level: overdose of procainamide, renal disease, liver disease. *Drug Influence:* acetazolamide (Diamox), cimetidine (Tagamet), sodium bicarbonate. Increased hypotensive effect with methyldopa (Aldomet), reserpine (Serpasil).

Procedure

- Collect 3 to 5 mL of venous blood in a red-top tube.
- Record dose, route, and last time drug was administered on the laboratory requisition slip.
- Obtain blood samples during peak level, 1 to 2 hours after oral administration, or ½ hour after IV administration.
- Trough level (before next dose) may be requested.
- There is no food or fluid restriction.

■ Factors Affecting Laboratory Results

- Drugs (*see Drug Influence*) could elevate serum procainamide level.

NURSING IMPLICATIONS WITH RATIONALE

- Report patient with a history of renal disease to physician. The procainamide dose might need to be adjusted.
- Monitor the serum procainamide level frequently, since one serum sample is not enough for evaluating therapy.
- Monitor IV procainamide; it should not exceed 25 to 50 mg/min.
- Administer oral dosage 1 hour before or 2 hours after meals with a glass of water to increase absorption.
- Assess vital signs frequently during oral and parenteral drug therapy. Report if pulse rate and BP decrease substantially from base line levels. Fever may occur during the first few days of therapy. Report temperature elevation.

Elevated Level

- Observe for signs and symptoms of side effects and procainamide overdose, such as anorexia, nausea, vomiting, bitter taste, dizziness, mental changes, muscle and joint pain, rash, hypotension, and bradycardia.
- Observe for signs and symptoms of lupus erythematosuslike syndrome, (skin rash, erythema, fever, polyarthralgias, pleuritic pain). These symptoms are reversible.

PROGESTERONE (SERUM)

Reference Values[1,5,6]

Adult: Female: Follicular Phase: 0.1–1.5 ng/mL, 20–150 ng/dL; Luteal Phase: 2–28 ng/mL, 250–2800 ng/dL; Postmenopausal: <1.0 ng/mL, <100 ng/dL. *Pregnancy:* First trimester: 9–50 ng/mL; Second trimester: 18–150 ng/mL; Third Trimester: 60–260 ng/mL. *Male:* <1.0 ng/mL, <100 ng/dL

Description

Progesterone, a hormone produced primarily by the corpus luteum of the ovaries and a small amount by the adrenal cortex, peaks during the luteal phase of the menstrual cycle for 4 to 5 days and during pregnancy. It prepares the endometrium for implantation of the fertilized egg. Only a small amount of progesterone is detected in the blood, since most is metabolized in the liver to pregnanediol, a progesterone metabolite.

Serum progesterone is useful in evaluating infertility problems, in confirming ovulation, and in assessing placental functions in pregnancy. A urine pregnanediol might be ordered to verify serum progesterone results.[1,3,6,9]

Clinical Problems

Decreased Levels: gonadal dysfunction, luteum deficiency, threatened abortion, toxemia of pregnancy, placental failure, fetal death

Elevated Levels: ovulation, pregnancy, ovarian cysts, tumors of the ovary or adrenal gland. *Drug Influence:* ACTH, progesterone preparations

Procedure

- Collect 7 mL of venous blood in a red-top (preferred) or green-top tube. Avoid hemolysis. Invert the green-top tube several times to mix with the anticoagulant in the tube.
- There is no food or fluid restriction.
- Note on the laboratory slip the phase of the patient's menstrual cycle or weeks of gestation if pregnant.

- Factors Affecting Laboratory Results

- Hemolysis from rough handling of the blood sample
- Progesterone and estrogen therapy

NURSING IMPLICATIONS WITH RATIONALE

- Obtain a history from the patient of her menstrual phase or weeks or months of gestation. Record findings.

Patient Teaching

- Inform the patient that the blood test may be repeated or that a urine test may be ordered. Repeated tests at different times are usually for information concerning progesterone secretion.
- Listen to the patient's concerns and fears. If unable to answer patient's questions, direct to appropriate health professionals.

PROLACTIN (PRL) SERUM
Lactogenic Hormone, Lactogen

Reference Values

Female: Follicular phase: 0–23 ng/mL; Luteal Phase: 0–40 ng/mL; Postmenopausal: <12 ng/mL. *Pregnancy:* First trimester: <80 ng/mL; Second Trimester: <160 ng/mL; Third Trimester: <400 ng/mL. *Male:* 0–20 ng/mL

Description

Prolactin, a hormone secreted by the anterior pituitary gland, is necessary in developing the mammary glands for lactation and for stimulating and maintaining lactation postpartum. If the mother does not breast-feed, serum prolactin falls to normal range. Impotence in the male might be attributed to excess prolactin secretion that suppresses gonad function.

Serum prolactin, >300 ng/mL in nonpregnant and nonlactating females as well as males, might indicate a pituitary adenoma (tumor).[1,3,6,7,9,10,20]

Clinical Problems

Decreased Level: postpartum pituitary infarction. *Drug Influence:* levodopa, ergot derivatives, apomorphine

Elevated Level: pituitary tumor, amenorrhea, galactorrhea, ectopic prolactin-secreting tumors of the lung, primary hypothyroidism, hypothalamic disorder, endometriosis, polycystic ovary, Addison's disease, stress, coitus, sleep, exercise, renal disease *Drug Influence:* phenothiazines, tricyclic antidepressants, amphetamine, morphine, methyldopa (Aldomet), haloperidol (Haldol), estrogens, procainamide derivatives, reserpine (Serpasil), isoniazid (INH), alcohol, cimetidine (Tagamet), verapamil, antihistamines, monoamine oxidase inhibitors (MAO)

Procedure

- Collect 7 mL in a red-top or a lavender-top tube. Avoid hemolysis. Blood should not be drawn until patient has been awake for 1 to 2 hours because serum prolactin elevates during sleep.
- Fasting specimen is preferred.

- List on the laboratory slip drugs that the patient is taking that might cause false-positive results.

■ Factors Affecting Laboratory Results.

- Drugs that can cause false-positive or negative laboratory test results (*See drug influence.*)
- Exercise, stress, pain, surgical trauma, sleep

NURSING IMPLICATIONS WITH RATIONALE

- Check with physician if drugs that could affect test results should be withheld until after the test.

Patient Teaching

- Inform the patient that blood sample would be drawn after patient is awake for at least 1 hour, preferably 2 hours. Sleep might cause false-positive results.
- Inform the patient that test results might take several days.
- Instruct the patient to avoid stress before the test if possible. If stress is present, report to physician and record on laboratory slip. Stress might cause false-positive results.
- Listen to patient's concerns.

PROPRANOLOL HYDROCHLORIDE (BLOOD, SERUM, OR PLASMA)
(Inderal, Detensol, Novopranol)

Reference Values

Therapeutic Range: *Adult:* 50–100 ng/mL, 193–386 nmol/L (*SI units*). *Child:* not done

Toxic Level: *Adult:* >150 ng/mL

Description

Propranolol (Inderal) is a β-adrenergic blocking agent used in the treatment of angina pectoris, cardiac arrhythmias, hypertension, and in some cases migraine headaches (prophylactically only). This drug blocks the cardiac effects of β_1-adrenergic stimulation, causing decreased heart rate and force of heart contraction. Propranolol also blocks the bronchodilator effect of catecholamines, causing bronchoconstriction. In hypertensive patients it will lower both supine and standing BPs by blocking sympathetic flow and suppressing renin activity.

    Almost all of oral propranolol is absorbed through the GI tract and is metabolized in the liver to a large number of metabolites. Ninety to 95% is bound to plasma protein and is excreted in urine as free and conjugated propranolol and as active metabolites. The half-life of plasma propranolol is 3 to 4 hours. Peak plasma level for the oral dosage form is 1 to 1½ hours and for an IV dose in 15 minutes. Propranolol crosses the placental and blood-brain barriers.

Careful monitoring for signs and symptoms of side effects of propranolol is necessary to prevent the three commonest symptoms: bradycardia, hypotension, and bronchoconstriction. This drug is contraindicated for patients with asthma and low BP.[2,3,6,9]

Clinical Problems

Elevated level: overdose of propranolol (Inderal), liver and renal diseases.
Drug Influence: quinidine, cimetidine (Tagamet)

Procedure

- Collect 5 to 7 mL of venous blood in a red-top tube.
- Record the dose, route, and last-administered dose on the laboratory requisition slip.
- There is no food or fluid restriction.

■ Factors Affecting Laboratory Results

- Spuriously low values have been reported with the use of certain blood collection tubes.

NURSING IMPLICATIONS WITH RATIONALE

- Record dose, route, and last time the drug was given on the requisition slip.
- Check serum propranolol level, and report any nontherapeutic level to physician.
- Take apical pulse and BP before administering propranolol. If pulse rate and BP are lower than the base-line levels, notify physician before administering the drug.
- Check daily intake and output and patient's weight. Propranolol can cause sodium retention.
- Recognize that digitalis glycoside (eg, digoxin) taken with propranolol could cause a bradycardic effect.

Elevated Level

- Observe for signs and symptoms of drug side effects (ie, decreased pulse rate or bradycardia, decreased BP or hypotension, vertigo, syncope, dyspnea, bronchospasm, nausea, diarrhea, dry eyes, and dry skin).

251

Patient Teaching

- Instruct the patient on how to take a radial pulse. Inform the patient to notify the physician if the pulse rate is lower than the base-line level or if the pulse becomes irregular.
- Explain to the patient that propranolol should never be abruptly discontinued. Propranolol is tapered to lower doses over 1 to 2 weeks to prevent withdrawal syndrome (ie, severe headaches, palpitation, and rebound hypertension).
- Inform the patient that before general anesthesia for planned surgery is considered or given, the surgeon and anesthetist should be notified if the patient is taking propranolol.

PROTEIN (TOTAL) (SERUM)

Reference Values

Adult: 6.0–8.0 g/dL

Child: Premature: 4.2–7.6 g/dL. *Newborn:* 4.6–7.4 g/dL. *Infant:* 6.0–6.7 g/dL. *Child:* 6.2–8.0 g/dL

Description

The total protein is composed mostly of albumin and globulins (*see Protein Electrophoresis*). The use of the total serum protein test is limited unless the serum albumin, A/G ratio, or protein electrophoresis tests are also performed.

The protein level needs to be known to determine the significance of its components. With certain disease entities (ie, collagen diseases, cancer, and infections), the total serum protein levels may be normal when the protein fractions are either decreased or elevated.[1,3,10,13]

Clinical Problems

Decreased Level: prolonged malnutrition, starvation, low-protein diet, malabsorption syndrome, cancer of the GI tract, ulcerative colitis, Hodgkin's disease, severe liver disease, chronic renal failure, severe burns, water intoxication

Elevated level: dehydration (hemoconcentration), vomiting, diarrhea, multiple myeloma, respiratory distress syndrome, sarcoidosis

Procedure

- Collect 5 to 7 mL of venous blood in a red-top tube. Avoid hemolysis.
- There is no food or fluid restriction. A high-fat diet should not be given for 24 hours before the test. Check with your laboratory.

- ### Factors Affecting Laboratory Results

  - A high-fat diet before the test

NURSING IMPLICATIONS WITH RATIONALE

Patient Teaching

■ Instruct the patient to avoid eating foods high in fat content for 24 hours before the test.

Decreased Level

■ Assess the patient's dietary intake. If the deficit is due to poor nutrition, encourage the patient to increase protein intake (eggs, cheese, meats, beans).
■ Plan a well-balanced diet with the patient. Collaborate with the dietitian and/or have the dietitian see the patient.

Elevated Level

■ Recognize clinical problems associated with a serum protein excess. Hemoconcentration caused by dehydration is a frequent cause of total serum protein excess.
■ Assess the patient for signs and symptoms of dehydration, such as extreme thirst, poor skin turgor, dry mucous membranes, tachycardia, and increased respirations.
■ Check urinary output. The serum protein level may be increased (it also could be decreased) with kidney dysfunction. If kidney dysfunction is due to dehydration, vomiting or diarrhea, the serum protein level will most likely be elevated.
■ Monitor fluid replacement (intravenously or orally). The serum protein level should return to normal when the patient is adequately hydrated. Care should be taken to prevent overhydration when forcing fluids.

PROTEIN (URINE)

Reference Values

Random Specimen: *Negative:* 0–5 mg/dL. *Positive:* 6–2000 mg/dL (trace to +2)

24-Hour Specimen: 15–150 mg/24 h

Description

Proteinuria is usually caused by renal disease due to glomerular damage and/or impaired renal tubular reabsorption. With a random urine specimen, protein can be detected using a reagent strip or dipstick, such as Combstix. Normally albumin is measured with the dipstick, since it is sensitive to reagent strip. A positive urine specimen (proteinuria) suggests that a 24-hour urine specimen be obtained for quantitative analysis of protein.

The amount of proteinuria in 24 hours is an indicator of the severity of renal involvement. Minimal proteinuria (<500 mg or 0.5 g/24 h) may be associated with chronic pyelonephritis; moderate proteinuria (500 to 4000 mg or 0.5 to 4 g/24 h) may be associated with acute or chronic glomerulonephritis or toxic nephropathies (ie, use of aminoglycosides [gentamicin]; and marked proteinuria (>4000 mg or >4 g/24 h) may be associated with nephrotic syndrome.

Emotions and physiologic stress may cause transient proteinuria. Newborns may have an increased proteinuria during the first 3 days of life.[3,9,12]

Clinical Problems

Decreased Level: diluted urine. *Drug Influence:* sulfosalicylic acid

Elevated Level: Heavy Proteinuria: acute or chronic glomerulonephritis, nephrotic syndrome, lupus nephritis, amyloid disease. *Moderate Proteinuria:* drug toxicities (aminoglycosides), cardiac disease, acute infectious disease, multiple myeloma, chemical toxicities. *Mild Proteinuria:* chronic pyelonephritis, polycystic kidney disease, renal tubular disease. *Drug Influence:* penicillin, gentamicin, sulfonamides, cephalosporins, contrast media, tolbutamide (Orinase), acetazolamide (Diamox), sodium bicarbonate

Procedure

- There is no food or fluid restriction.
- List drugs patient is taking that could affect test results.

Random Urine Specimen
- Collect clean-caught or midstream urine specimen.
- Place the reagent strip/dipstick (eg, Combistix) in the urine specimen.
- Match the results from the dipstick with the color chart on the bottle.

24-Hour Specimen (Quantitative Analysis Test)
- Have patient void prior to test and discard urine. Then save all urine for 24 hours in a urine collection container.
- Keep urine specimen bottle refrigerated or on ice.
- Label the urine bottle with patient's name, date, exact time of collection (eg, 7/12/93, 8:01 AM to 7/13/93, 8:02 AM).

- Factors Affecting Laboratory Results

  - Drugs (*See Drug Influence.*)
  - Diluted urine
  - Toilet paper or stool in the urine

NURSING IMPLICATIONS WITH RATIONALE

- Explain the test procedure to the patient (*see Procedure*). Emphasize the importance of following the test procedure for accurate results.
- Record on the laboratory slip all drugs that the patient is taking and the date and time of last dose. The physician may withhold drugs for 24 hours prior to test.
- Assess for signs and symptoms of renal dysfunction, such as fatigue, decreased urine output, peripheral edema, increased serum creatinine.
- Answer the patient's questions or refer the questions to the appropriate health professionals.

PROTEIN ELECTROPHORESIS (SERUM)

Reference Values

Adult

	WEIGHT (g/dL)	PERCENTAGE OF TOTAL PROTEIN
Albumin	3.5–5.0	52–68
Globulin	1.5–3.5	32–48
Alpha-1 (α_1)	0.1–0.4	2–5
Alpha-2 (α_2)	0.4–1.0	7–13
Beta (β)	0.5–1.1	8–14
Gamma (γ)	0.5–1.7	12–22

Child

	ALBUMIN (g/dL)	GLOBULINS (g/dL)			
		α_1	α_2	β	γ
Premature	3.0–4.2	0.1–0.5	0.3–0.7	0.3–1.2	0.3–1.4
Newborn	3.5–5.4	0.1–0.3	0.3–0.5	0.2–0.6	0.2–1.2
Infant	4.4–5.4	0.2–0.4	0.5–0.8	0.5–0.9	0.3–0.8
Child	4.0–5.8	0.1–0.4	0.4–1.0	0.5–1.0	0.3–1.0

Description

Serum proteins are made up of albumin and globulins. Albumin is the smallest of the protein molecules, but it makes up the largest percentage of the total protein value. Changes in the albumin level will affect the total protein value. Albumin plays an important role in maintaining serum colloid osmotic pressure. The globulin molecules are about 2.5 times as large as albumin molecules, but they are not as effective in maintaining osmotic pressure as albumin molecules are.

Serum protein electrophoresis is a process that separates various protein fractions into albumin, alpha-1 globulin, alpha-2 globulin, beta globulin, and gamma globulin. The gamma globulins are the body's antibodies, which contribute to immunity.[1,3,4,8,10,12,13]

Clinical Problems

PROTEIN FRACTION	DECREASED LEVEL	ELEVATED LEVEL
Albumin	Chronic liver disease	Dehydration
	Malnutrition	Exercise
	Starvation	
	Malabsorption syndrome	
	Advanced malignancy	
	Leukemia	
	Congestive heart failure	
	Toxemia of pregnancy	
	Nephrotic syndrome	
	Chronic renal failure	
	Burns (severe)	
	Systemic lupus erythematosus (SLE)	
Globulin		
α_1	Emphysema due to α_1-antitrypsin deficiency	Pregnancy
		Neoplasm
		Acute and chronic infection
		Tissue necrosis
α_2	Hemolytic anemia	Acute infection
	Severe liver disease	Injury, trauma
		Burns (severe)
		Extensive neoplasms
		Obstructive jaundice
		Rheumatic fever
		Rheumatoid arthritis
		Acute myocardial infarction
		Nephrotic syndrome
β	Hypocholesterolemia	Hypothyroidism
		Biliary cirrhosis
		Kidney nephrosis
		Diabetes mellitus
		Cushing's disease
		Malignant hypertension
γ	Nephrotic syndrome	Collagen disease
	Lymphocytic leukemia	Rheumatoid arthritis
	Lymphosarcoma	Lupus erythematosus
	Hypogammaglobulinemia or agammaglobulinemia	Hodgkin's disease
		Malignant lymphoma
		Chronic lymphocytic leukemia
		Multiple myeloma
		Liver disease

**ELECTROPHORETIC
PATTERNS**

Pattern I	↓ albumin ↑ α_2-globulin	Acute stressful situation Acute infections Myocardial infarction Severe burns Surgery

Pattern II	↓ (slightly) albumin
	
	↑ (slightly) α_2-globulin
	↑ (slightly) γ globulin
		Chronic infection and
		   inflammation
		Cirrhosis
		Collagen disease
		   (rheumatoid)

Pattern III	↓ (moderately) albumin ↑ γ globulin ↑ or normal β	Collagen disease (lupus) Subacute bacterial endocarditis Sarcoidosis

Procedure

- Collect 5 to 10 mL of venous blood in a red-top tube. Avoid hemolysis.
- There is no food or fluid restriction.

- Factors Affecting Laboratory Results

  - Hemolysis of the blood sample.

NURSING IMPLICATIONS WITH RATIONALE

- Check the albumin level from the protein electrophoresis results. Many clinical problems are the result of a serum albumin deficit.
- Assess for peripheral edema in the lower extremities when the albumin level is decreased. Albumin is the major protein compound responsible for plasma colloid osmotic pressure. With a decreased albumin level, fluid seeps out of the blood vessels into the tissue spaces. Cirrhosis of the liver and congestive heart failure are clinical problems that can cause an albumin deficit and edema.
- Encourage the patient to increase protein intake. Malnutrition and cirrhosis of the liver are associated with a poor-protein diet. Suggest foods high in protein (ie, beans, eggs, meats, and milk).
- Assess urinary output. Renal and collagen (lupus) diseases occur with abnormal protein fractions. Urine output should be 25 mL/h or 600 mL/ 24 h.
- Check for albumin/protein in the urine.

PROTHROMBIN TIME (PT) (PLASMA)
Pro-Time

Reference Values

Adult: 11–15 seconds (depending on the method and reagents used) or 70%–100%. *For Anticoagulant Therapy:* 2–2.5 times the control in seconds or 20%–30%

Child: same as adult

Description

Prothrombin (factor II of the coagulation factors) is synthesized by the liver and is an inactive precursor in the clotting process. (*see Factor Assay*). Prothrombin is converted to thrombin by the action of thromboplastin, which is needed to form a blood clot.

The PT test measures the clotting ability of factors I (fibrinogen), II (prothrombin), V, VII, and X. Alterations of factors V and VII will prolong the PT for about 2 seconds, or 10% of normal. In liver disease the PT is usually prolonged, since the liver cells cannot synthesize prothrombin.

The major use of the PT test is to monitor oral anticoagulant therapy (ie, with bishydroxycoumarin [dicumarol] and warfarin sodium [Coumadin]).[1,3,9,10,13]

Clinical problems

Decreased Level: thrombophlebitis, myocardial infarction, pulmonary embolism. *Drug Influence:* barbiturates, digitalis preparations, diuretics, diphenhydramine (Benadryl), oral contraceptives, rifampin, metaproterenol (Alupent, Metaprel), vitamin K

Increased Level: liver diseases (cirrhosis of the liver, hepatitis, liver abscess, cancer of the liver), afibrinogenemia, factor II deficiency, factor V deficiency, factor VII deficiency, factor X deficiency, fibrin degradation products (FDP), leukemias, congestive heart failure, erythroblastosis fetalis (hemolytic disease of the newborn). *Drug Influence:* antibiotics (penicillin, streptomycin, carbenicillin, chloramphenicol [Chloromycetin], kanamycin [Kantrex], neomycin, tetracyclines), anticoagulants, oral (dicumarol, warfarin), chlorpromazine (Thorazine), chlordiazepoxide (Librium), diphenylhydantoin (Dilantin), heparin, methyldopa (Aldomet), mithramycin, reserpine (Serpasil), phenylbutazone (Butazolidin), quinidine, salicylates (aspirin), sulfonamides

Procedure

- The test (collection) tube should contain an anticoagulant, either sodium oxalate or sodium citrate.
- Collect 7 to 10 mL of venous blood in a black-top tube (sodium oxalate). The blood must be tested within 1 hour after it has been drawn. The tube should be filled to its capacity. Some black-top tubes contain sodium citrate, so check with the laboratory.

or

- Collect 7 to 10 mL of venous blood in a blue-top tube (sodium citrate). The blood should be tested within 2 hours to prevent inactivation of some of the factors. The tube should be filled to its capacity.

■ Deliver the blood sample to the laboratory packed in ice. If the blood clots before testing, a new blood sample should be taken.

■ Control values are given with the patient's PT values. Control values may change from day to day; this is an indication of the minor variables in the testing conditions.

■ There is no food or fluid restriction.

■ List on the laboratory slip drugs patient is taking that could affect test results.

■ Factors Affecting Laboratory Results

■ A clotted blood sample will cause an inaccurate result.

■ A high-fat diet (decreased PT) and alcohol (increased PT) may cause an endogenous change of PT production.

■ Leaving a blood sample at room temperature for several hours (1 to 4 hours) may affect results.

NURSING IMPLICATIONS WITH RATIONALE

■ Explain to the patient that the purpose of the test is to determine how fast the blood clots. If the purpose of the test is to monitor anticoagulant therapy, inform the patient that blood will be drawn daily or at specified times.

■ Hold medications (if possible) that may affect the PT test results until after the test. If such medications *are* given, list the names of the drugs on the laboratory slip and when the last dose was given.

■ Take the blood sample immediately to the laboratory for testing. There should be an anticoagulant in the tube, and the blood should fill the tube.

Increased Level

■ Monitor the PT when the patient is receiving anticoagulant therapy. The desired PT with anticoagulant therapy is 2 to 2.5 times the control PT in seconds. The PT may be slightly lower when treating cardiac patients—18 to 24 seconds. In patients with a thrombus, the desired PT range is 26 to 40 seconds. When the PT is above 40 seconds, bleeding may occur.

■ Inform the physician of the patient's PT daily or as ordered. The physician may want the anticoagulant held (drug adjustment) until the current PT has been received. The results are usually called to the floor by the laboratory personnel.

■ Observe the patient for signs and symptoms of bleeding (purpura [skin] hematuria [Hemastix test], hematemesis, nosebleeds). Report observations to the physician and record them in the patient's chart.

■ Administer vitamin K intramuscularly as ordered when the PT is over 40 seconds or when there is bleeding. IM injections can cause hematomas at the injection site when anticoagulants are used.

Patient Teaching

- Instruct the patient not to self-medicate when receiving anticoagulant therapy. OTC drugs may either increase or decrease the effects of the anticoagulants (drug interaction) and the results of the PT test.
- Instruct the patient to take the prescribed anticoagulants as ordered by the physician. Missed doses could affect the PT test.
- Inform the patient not to consume alcohol, over a period of time since it can affect liver function and cause a prolonged prothrombin time.
- *(See Partial Thromboplastin Time, Activated Partial Thromboplastin Time.)*

QUINIDINE (SERUM)

Reference Values

Therapeutic Range: Adult: 2–5 μg/mL, 6.2–15.4 μmol/L (SI units). *Child:* not done

Toxic Level: Adult: >6 μg/mL, >18.5 μmol/L (SI units)

Description

Quinidine, one of the first antiarrhythmic agents, is used for treating supraventricular and ventricular cardiac arrhythmias. It acts by decreasing the excitability of the heart and increasing the refractory period. Today quinidine is not the drug of choice, since it causes many side effects (ie, GI upset, severe cardiac problems [bradycardia, congestive heart failure, heart block, circulatory collapse], hypersensitivity reactions [urticaria, rash], and central nervous system disturbances). Daily dosage of quinidine should be regulated according to the serum therapeutic range.

Half-life of quinidine is 6 to 8 hours. Quinidine is metabolized by the liver, and 20% is excreted unchanged through the kidneys. Sixty to 80% is bound to plasma protein.

Care should be taken when digoxin and quinidine are coadministered. Quinidine can increase serum digoxin level 2½ times its expected level. As a result of taking the two drugs, digitalis toxicity could appear 3 to 7 days after quinidine therapy was started. Both serum digoxin and quinidine levels should be monitored.[2–6]

Clinical Problems

Decreased Level: Drug Influence: barbiturates, phenytoin (Dilantin), rifampin

Elevated Level: overdose of quinidine, renal disease, severe heart failure and liver disease. *Drug Influence:* acetazolamide (Diamox), antacids, thiazides

Procedure

- Collect 3 to 5 mL of venous blood in a red-top tube. Some laboratories may request that a heparinized plasma specimen be collected (ie, green-top tube).

- Collect the specimen during the peak (2 hours after dose) and/or trough (before the next dose) levels to determine the therapeutic range for the patient.
- Record the dose, route, and last-administered dose on the laboratory requisition slip.
- There is no food or fluid restriction.

■ Factors Affecting Laboratory Results

- Certain drugs might elevate or decrease quinidine concentration in the body (*see Drug Influence*).
- Certain blood collection tubes may cause small decreases in serum levels.

NURSING IMPLICATIONS WITH RATIONALE

- Record dose, route, and last-administered dose on the requisition slip. Record drugs patient is taking that might affect test result.
- Take apical pulse and BP before administering dose. Report pulse and BP changes from base-line levels to the physician.

Patient Teaching

- Instruct the patient on how to take a radial pulse before discharge. Tell patient to report significant change of pulse rate from base-line level to the physician.
- Inform patient to take quinidine with food to avoid or to decrease GI effects.

Elevated Level

- Observe for side effects of quinidine (bradycardia, hypotension, dizziness, nausea, vomiting, diarrhea, skin eruptions).
- Observe for signs and symptoms of digitalis toxicity with patients taking a digitalis preparation concurrently with quinidine.

RAPID PLASMA REAGIN (RPR) (SERUM)

Reference Values

Adult: nonreactive
Child: nonreactive

Description

(*See Description for VDRL*).

The RPR test is a rapid screening test for syphilis. A nontreponemal antibody test like VDRL, the RPR test detects reagin antibodies in the serum and is more sensitive but less specific than VDRL. Frequently it is used on donor's blood as a syphilis detection test. As with other nonspecific reagin tests, false positives can occur as the result of acute and chronic diseases. A positive RPR should be verified by VDRL and/or FTA-ABS tests.[3,10,13]

Clinical Problems

Reactive (positive): syphilis. *False Positive:* tuberculosis, pneumonia, infectious mononucleosis, chickenpox, smallpox vaccination (recent), rheumatoid arthritis, lupus erythematosus, hepatitis, pregnancy.

Procedure

■ Follow the directions on the RPR kit.

■ Factors Affecting Laboratory Results

■ False positive results caused by acute and chronic diseases (*See Clinical Problems for VDRL.*)

NURSING IMPLICATIONS WITH RATIONALE

Reactive (positive)

■ Explain to patient that further testing will be done to verify test results.
■ If repeat result is positive, sexual contacts need to be notified to seek treatment.

RED BLOOD CELL INDICES (MCV, MCH, MCHC, RDW) (BLOOD)
Erythrocyte Indices

Reference Values

	ADULT	NEWBORN	CHILD
RBC count (million/μL $\times 10^{12}$/L [SI units])	Male: 4.6–6.0 Female: 4.0–5.0 4.6–6.0 $\times 10^{12}$L	4.8–7.2 4.8–7.2 $\times 10^{12}$L	3.8–5.5 3.8–5.5 $\times 10^{12}$L
MCV (cuμ [conventional]) or fl [SI units])	80–98	96–108	82–92
MCH (pg [conventional and SI units])	27–31	32–34	27–31
MCHC (% or g/dL [conventional] or SI units)	32%–36% 0.32–0.36	32%–33% 0.32–0.33	32%–36% 0.32–0.36
RDW (coulter S)	11.5–14.5		

Description

RBC indices include the RBC count, RBC size (MCV: mean corpuscular volume), weight (MCH: mean corpuscular hemoglobin), hemoglobin concentration (MCHC: mean corpuscular hemoglobin concentration), and size differences (RDW: RBC distribution width). Other names for RBC indices are erythrocyte indices and corpuscular indices. To identify the types of anemias, the physician depends on the following RBC indices:

■ *MCV:* MCV indicates the size of RBC: microcytic(small size), normocytic (normal size), and macrocytic(large size). A decreased MCV, or microcyte, might be indicative of iron deficiency anemia and thalassemia. An example of an increased MCV, or macrocyte, is pernicious anemia and folic acid anemia. MCV value can be calculated if the RBC count and hematocrit (Hct) are known.

$$MCV = \frac{Hct \times 10}{RBC\ count}$$

■ *MCH:* MCH indicates the weight of hemoglobin in the RBC regardless of the size. In macrocytic anemias, the MCH is elevated, and it is decreased in hypochromic anemia. The MCH is derived by dividing the RBC count into 10 times the hemoglobin (Hb) value.

$$MCH = \frac{Hb \times 10}{RBC\ count}$$

■ *MCHC:* MCHC indicates the hemoglobin concentration per unit volume of RBCs. A decreased MCHC can indicate a hypochromic anemia. The MCHC can be calculated from MCH and MCV or from hemoglobin and hematocrit.

$$MCHC = \frac{MCH \times 100}{MCV} \quad OR \quad MCHC = \frac{Hb \times 100}{Hct}$$

■ *RDW:* The RBC distribution width (RDW) is the size (width) differences of RBCs. RDW is the measurement of the width of the size distribution curve on a histogram. It is useful in predicting anemias early, before MCV changes and before signs and symptoms occur. An elevated RDW indicates iron deficiency, folic acid deficiency, and vitamin B_{12} deficiency anemias. RDW and MCV are used to differentiate among various RBC disorders (*see Anemias: RDW and MCV Values*).

ANEMIAS: RDW AND MCV VALUES[1,6,8,12,13]

RBC Disorder	RDW	MCV
Early factor deficiency (iron, folate, vitamin B_{12})	High	Normal
Iron deficiency anemia	High	Low
Folic-acid deficiency anemia	High	High
Vitamin B_{12} deficiency (pernicious anemia)	High	High
Hemolysis (RBC fragmentation)	High	Low
Hemolysis (autoimmune) anemia	High	High
Sickle cell anemia	High	Normal
Sickle cell trait	High	Normal

Clinical Problems

INDICES	decreased level	ELEVATED LEVEL
RBC count	Hemorrhage (blood loss) Anemias Chronic infections Leukemias Multiple myeloma Excessive intravenous fluids Chronic renal failure Pregnancy Overhydration	Polycythemia vera Hemoconcentration/dehydration High altitude Cor pulmonale Cardiovascular disease

MCV	Microcytic anemia: iron deficiency
	Malignancy
	Rheumatoid arthritis
	Hemoglobinopathies
	  Thalassemia
	  Sickle cell anemia
	  Hemoglobin C
	Lead poisoning
	Radiation
		Macrocytic anemia: aplastic,
		  hemolytic, pernicious
		Chronic liver disease
		Hypothyroidism (myxedema)
		Drug influence
		  Vitamin B_{12} deficiency
		  Anticonvulsants
		  Antimetabolics

MCH MCHC	Microcytic, hypochromic anemia Hypochromic anemia Iron deficiency anemia Thalassemia	Macrocytic anemias
RDW		Iron deficiency anemia Folic acid deficiency anemia Pernicious anemia Homozygous hemoglobinopathies (S, C, H)

Procedure

- Collect 7 to 10 mL of venous blood in a lavender-top tube. Avoid hemolysis. Avoid leaving the tourniquet on too long.
- There is no food or fluid restriction.
- Usually a particle counter is used that will provide all CBC results along with all the indices.

- Factors Affecting Laboratory Results

  - Drugs (*See Clinical Problems.*)

NURSING IMPLICATIONS WITH RATIONALE

Decreased Level

- Relate a decreased RBC count, MCV, MCH, and MCHC to clinical problems.
- Assess for the cause(s) of a decreased RBC count. Check for blood loss, and

---

obtain a history of anemias, renal insufficiency, chronic infection, or leukemia. Determine whether the patient is overhydrated.

■ Observe for signs and symptoms of advanced iron-deficiency anemia (fatigue, pallor, dyspnea on exertion, tachycardia, and headache). Chronic symptoms include cracked corners of the mouth, smooth tongue, dysphagia, and numbness and tingling of the extremities. With mild iron deficiency the patient is usually asymptomatic.

Patient Teaching

■ Instruct the patient to follow the physician's orders (medical regimen), such as iron supplement therapy and a diet rich in iron.
■ Instruct the patient to eat foods rich in iron (ie, liver, red meats, green vegetables, and iron-fortified bread).
■ Explain to the patient who is taking iron supplements that the stools usually appear dark in color (tarry appearance). Tell the patient to take an iron medication with meals. Milk and antacids can interfere with iron absorption.

Elevated Level

■ Relate an elevated RBC count, MCV, MCH, MCHC and RDW to clinical problems and drugs.
■ Assess for signs and symptoms of hemoconcentration. Dehydration, shock, and severe diarrhea are some of the causes of hemoconcentration that can elevate the RBC count.

RENIN (PLASMA)

Reference Values

Adult: Thirty Minutes Supine: 0.2–2.3 ng/mL; *Upright:* 1.3–4.0 ng/mL; *Restricted Salt Diet:* 4.1–7.7 ng/mL

Child: not usually done

Description

Renin is an enzyme secreted by the kidneys. This enzyme activates the renin-angiotensin system, which causes vasoconstriction and the release of aldosterone (a hormone from the adrenal medulla that causes sodium and water retention). Vasoconstriction and aldosterone can cause hypertension.

Increased plasma renin levels can occur as a result of hypovolemia and kidney disorders. In addition, postural change (from a recumbent to an upright position) and a decreased sodium (salt) intake will stimulate renin secretion. Plasma renin levels are usually higher from 8:00 AM to noon and lower from noon to 6:00 PM.

Clinical Problems

Decreased Level: essential hypertension, Cushing's syndrome, diabetes mellitus, hypothyroidism, high-sodium diet. *Drug Influence:* antihypertensives (methyldopa [Aldomet], guanethidine [Ismelin]), propranolol (Inderal); levodopa

Elevated Level: hypertension (malignant, renovascular), hyperaldosteronism, cancer of the kidney, acute renal failure, Addison's disease, cirrhosis, chronic obstructive lung disease, manic-depressive disorder, pregnancy (first trimester), preeclampsia and eclampsia, hyperthyroidism, hypokalemia, low-sodium diet. *Drug Influence:* estrogens, diuretics, antihypertensives (hydralazine [Apresoline], diazoxide [Hyperstat], nitroprusside), oral contraceptives

Procedure

■ Check with the laboratory and physician to determine whether the plasma renin test is to include urine aldosterone and/or urine sodium tests.

Plasma Renin
■ Keep the tube and/or syringe cold in an ice bath before collection.
■ The tourniquet should be released before the blood is drawn.
■ Note on the laboratory slip if the patient is in a supine or upright position.
■ A normal or low-salt diet may be indicated.
■ Collect 5 to 7 mL of venous blood in a lavender-top tube.
■ The blood sample should be placed in an ice bath; after centrifugation, the plasma is separated, frozen immediately to preserve renin activity, and sent to a special laboratory.

■ Factors Affecting Laboratory Results

■ Drugs (*See Drug Influence.*)

NURSING IMPLICATIONS WITH RATIONALE

■ Check with the laboratory on procedural changes or modifications.

Elevated Level

■ Monitor the patient's BP every 4 to 6 hours or as ordered.
■ Assess kidney function by recording urinary output. If urinary output is less than 25 mL/h or 600 mL/day, renal insufficiency should be suspected.

RETICULOCYTE COUNT (BLOOD)

Reference Values

Adult: 0.5%–1.5% of all RBCs, 25,000–75,000 μL

$$\text{Reticulocyte count} = \text{reticulocytes (\%)} \times \text{RBC count}$$

Child: *Newborn:* 2.5%–6.5% of all RBCs. *Infant:* 0.5%–3.5% of all RBCs. *Child:* 0.5–2.0% of all RBCs

Description

The reticulocyte count is an indicator of bone marrow activity and is used for diagnosing anemias. Reticulocytes are immature, nonnucleated RBCs that are formed in the bone marrow and passed into circulation. Normally there is a small number of reticulocytes in circulation; however, an increased number (count) indicates RBC production acceleration. An increased count could be due to hemorrhage or hemolysis or to treatment of iron deficiency, vitamin B_{12} deficiency, or folic acid deficiency anemia. This test is also done to check on persons working with radioactive material or receiving radiotherapy. A persistently low count could be suggestive of bone marrow hypofunction or aplastic anemia.

Giving a percentage is not always the most accurate way of reporting the reticulocyte count, especially when the total RBC (erythrocyte) count is *not* within normal range. Both the RBC count and the reticulocyte count should be reported.[1,7,10,13]

Clinical Problems

Decreased Level: anemias (pernicious, folic acid deficiency, aplastic) radiation therapy, effects of x-ray irradiation, adrenocortical hypofunction, anterior pituitary hypofunction, cirrhosis of the liver (alcohol suppresses reticulocytes)

Elevated Level: anemias (hemolytic, sickle cell), thalassemia major, chronic hemorrhage, posthemorrhage (3 to 4 days), treatment for anemias (iron deficiency, vitamin B_{12}, folic acid), leukemias, erythroblastosis fetalis (hemolytic disease of the newborn), hemoglobin C and D diseases, pregnancy

Procedure

■ Venous or capillary blood could be used for the reticulocyte count test.

Venous Blood
■ Collect 5 to 7 mL of venous blood in a lavender-top tube.
■ There is no food or fluid restriction.

Capillary Blood
■ Cleanse the finger and puncture the skin with a sterile lancet.
■ Wipe the first drop of blood away. Collect the blood by using a micropipette. The blood is mixed in equal proportions with methylene blue solution. The reticulocytes stain blue.
■ There is no food or fluid restriction.

■ Factors Affecting Laboratory Results

■ The use of the wrong colored-top tube for venous blood. The tube should contain anticoagulant (EDTA).

NURSING IMPLICATIONS WITH RATIONALE

Decreased Level

■ Recognize clinical problems related to a decreased reticulocyte count, such as pernicious and aplastic anemias.
■ Obtain a history regarding radiation exposure—x-ray and others.

Elevated Level

■ Monitor the reticulocyte count when the patient is being treated for pernicious anemia or folic acid anemia. There is usually an increase in reticulocytes.

RHEUMATOID FACTOR (RF), RHEUMATOID ARTHRITIS (RA) FACTOR, RA LATEX FIXATION (SERUM)

Reference Values

Adult: <1:20 titer; 1:20–1:80 positive for rheumatoid arthritis and other conditions; >1:80 positive for rheumatoid arthritis

Child: not usually done

Elderly: slightly increased

Description

The rheumatoid factor (RF) or rheumatoid arthritis (RA) factor test is a screening test used to detect antibodies (IgM, IgG, or IgA) found in the serum of patients with rheumatoid arthritis. RF occurs in 53% to 94% (average 76%) of patients with rheumatoid arthritis, and if the test is negative, it should be repeated.

The RF tests can be positive in many of the collagen diseases. The RF tests should not be used for monitoring follow-up or treatment stages of RA, since RF tests often remain positive when clinical remissions have been achieved. It also takes approximately 6 months for a significant elevation of titer. For diagnosing and evaluating RA, the ANA and the C-reactive protein agglutination tests are frequently used.[3,8–10,12,13]

Clinical Problems

Elevated Level: rheumatoid arthritis, lupus erythematosus, dermatomyositis, scleroderma, infectious mononucleosis, tuberculosis, leukemia, sarcoidosis, cirrhosis of the liver, hepatitis, syphilis, chronic infections, old age

Procedure

■ Collect 5 to 10 mL of venous blood in a red-top tube.
■ There is no food or fluid restriction.

■ **Factors Affecting Laboratory Results**

- A positive RF test result frequently remains positive regardless of clinical improvement.
- The RF test result can be positive in various clinical problems (ie, collagen diseases, cancer, and liver cirrhosis).
- The older adult may have an increased RF titer without the disease.
- Due to the variability in the sensitivity and specificity of these screening tests, positive results must be interpreted in corroboration with the patient's clinical status.

NURSING IMPLICATIONS WITH RATIONALE

Elevated Level

- Relate an increased RF titer to clinical problems. A titer greater than 1:80 is most likely due to RA. Titers between 1:20 and 1:80 could be due to lupus, scleroderma, or liver cirrhosis.
- Consider the age of the patient when the RF is slightly increased. There can be a slight titer increase in the older adult without clinical symptoms of RA. With juvenile rheumatoid arthritis, only 10% of the children have a positive RF titer.
- Assess for pain in the small joints of the hands and feet (especially the proximal interphalangeal), which could be indicative of an early stage of rheumatoid arthritis.

Rh TYPING (BLOOD)

Reference Values

Adult: Rh + (positive), Rh − (negative)

Child: same as adult

Description

Rh typing is performed when typing donors'/recipients' blood and for cross-matching blood for transfusion. Rh factor (also known as Rh antigen) was first discovered by Landsteiner and Weiner in 1941; it was named Rh because of the use of rhesus monkeys in the research. Rh positive (most common Rh factor) indicates the presence of antigen on RBCs; Rh negative indicates an absence of the antigen.

An Rh-negative woman carrying a fetus with an Rh-positive blood group can cause Rh-positive antigens from the fetus to seep into the mother's blood, causing Rh antibody formation. If the mother develops a high anti-Rh antibody titer, the child can be born with a condition called erythroblastosis fetalis (hemolysis of the RBCs). To prevent Rh antibodies, the Rh-negative woman is given

Rho(D) immune globulin, such as Rho-GAM, within 3 days after delivery with the first child or after a miscarriage to neutralize any anti-Rh antibodies.[3,9,10]

Clinical Problems

Elevated Anti-Rh Antibodies Infant: erythroblastosis fetalis

Procedure

- Collect 5 mL of venous blood in a red-top tube or 7 to 10 mL in a lavender-top tube.
- There is no food or fluid restriction.
- Blood testing for Rh factor (antigen) should be done with care to avoid false-positive and false-negative results.

■ Factors Affecting Laboratory Results

  ■ None known

NURSING IMPLICATIONS WITH RATIONALE

- Obtain a history of previous blood transfusions the patient has received. If the patient is a pregnant woman, determine whether she has been pregnant before and whether the child (children) was (were) born jaundiced.
- Ask the patients if they know their Rh factor. Compare the tested Rh factor with the patient's stated Rh factor. This could prevent administering incorrect blood.
- Inform the pregnant woman with Rh-negative factor that her blood will be tested at intervals during her pregnancy to find out whether antibodies are produced. The Rh-negative woman usually receives RhoGAM (Rh immune globulin) after delivery to prevent anti-Rh antibody production.

RUBELLA ANTIBODY DETECTION (SERUM)
Hemagglutination Inhibition Test (HI or HAI) for Rubella (German Measles)

Reference Values

Adult: susceptibility to Rubella: <1.8 titer. *Past Rubella Exposure:* 1.10–1.32 titer. *Immunity:* 1.32–1.64 titer. *Definite immunity:* 1.64 titer and higher

Description

Rubella (German measles) is a mild viral disease of short duration causing a fever and a transient rash. If it occurs in a woman in early pregnancy who is not immune from previous rubella infection and has not received rubella vaccination, the disease can produce serious deformities in her unborn child, especially if exposed during the first 2 months of gestation. Women should be immune to rubella (vaccinated) before marriage and definitely before pregnancy.

The rubella virus produces antibodies (natural immunity) against future rubella infections, but the exact antibody titer in the blood is unknown. Hemagglutination inhibition (HI or HAI) measures rubella antibody titers and is considered sensitive and reliable. If the antibody titer is 1.64 or higher, protection against rubella infection is assured.

Clinical indications for the HAI antibody (screening) test are as follows.

1. To determine the rubella antibody titer of a woman of child-bearing age if she has previously had the rubella infection. She will need the rubella vaccine if her titer is less than 1.8 (some physicians state less than 1.20, others 1.32 or less)
2. To determine the rubella antibody titer at the first antepartum visit
3. To check pregnant women (during their first trimester of pregnancy) at the time of rubella exposure and again in 3 to 4 weeks
4. To check personnel who work in obstetrics in the hosptial, clinic, or physician's office
5. To diagnose a recent rubella infection in pregnant women (first trimester of pregnancy). The HAI test is done 3 days following the onset of the rash and is repeated 2 to 3 weeks later. A fourfold increase with the second HAI test usually indicates that the rash was due to rubella. A therapeutic abortion might be considered [1,9,10,13]

Clinical Problems

Decreased Level (<1.8): susceptible to rubella (German measles)

Elevated Level (>1.64): definite immunity (resistance) to rubella

Procedure

■ Collect 3 to 5 mL of venous blood in a red-top tube.
■ There is no food or fluid restriction.

■ Factors Affecting Laboratory Results

■ None known

NURSING IMPLICATIONS WITH RATIONALE

Patient Teaching

■ Explain to the patient the HAI antibody titer for rubella susceptibility is <1.8 and for rubella immunity is 1.64 and greater. The antibody titer to protect the unborn child differs among experts and physicians. Some of them feel 1.20 gives adequate immunity, while others think it should be greater than 1.32. All agree that a 1.64 or higher dilution is a definite immunity titer.
■ Teach young female adults and families about the need to have their blood checked for rubella immunity (against German measles). This test should be done before pregnancy, and if the titer is less than 1.8, they should receive the rubella vaccine. Some states require a rubella test before a marriage license is issued.

- Instruct pregnant women who are susceptible to German measles to avoid exposure to the disease if at all possible. If they have been exposed to German measles or develop a rash, they should notify the obstetrician immediately so that HAI antibody titer testing can be done. Exposure to German measles does not mean that the person will develop the disease, but it does mean that the antibody titer must be monitored. Emphasize the importance of calling the physician when exposed to German measles.
- Explain to interested persons some of the fetal abnormalities (congenital heart disease, deafness, mental retardation) that can occur if a woman develops German measles during the first 3 months of pregnancy.

SALICYLATE (SERUM)

Reference Values

Adult: *Normal:* negative. *Therapeutic:* 5 mg (headache); 15–30 mg/dL (rheumatoid arthritis). *Mild Toxic:* >30 mg/dL. *Severe Toxic:* >50 mg/dL. *Lethal:* >60 mg/dL

Elderly: *Mild Toxic:* >25 mg/dL

Child: *Toxic:* >25 mg/dL

Description

Salicylate levels are measured to check the therapeutic level, as in the treatment of rheumatic fever, and to check the levels caused by an accidental or deliberate overdose. Blood salicylate reaches its peak in 2 to 3 hours, and the blood level can be elevated for as long as 18 hours.

An overdose of aspirin will cause respiratory alkalosis, and if not corrected, metabolic acidosis will occur due to cellular breakdown and increase in organic acids. Prolonged use of salicylates (aspirins) can cause bleeding tendencies, since it inhibits platelet aggregation. It may be toxic in children because of Reye's syndrome.[2,4,9,10,12]

Clinical Problems

Elevated Level: overdose or large, continuous doses of acetylsalicyclic acid (aspirin, ASA), drugs containing aspirin

Procedure

- Collect 5 mL of venous blood in a red-top or a green-top tube.
- There is no food or fluid restriction.
- A urine test may also be done as a screening test.

- Factors Affecting Laboratory Results

  - None reported

NURSING IMPLICATIONS WITH RATIONALE

- Observe for signs and symptoms of early aspirin overdose (ie, hyperventilation, flushed skin, and ringing in the ears).
- Obtain a history from the child or parent concerning the approximate number of aspirins taken. A toxic dose for a small child is 3.33 grains/kg, or 200 mg/kg. For a child weighing 15 kg (33 lb), the toxic dose would be 10 adult aspirins (5 grains each). Salicylates are not the choice agent for children with virus because of the possibility of developing Reye's syndrome.
- Recognize that acid-base imbalance is common with salicylate toxicity. Respiratory alkalosis usually occurs first, followed by metabolic acidosis. Symptoms of toxicity usually occur 6 hours following aspirin ingestion. Most of the aspirin has already been absorbed by that time.

Patient Teaching

- Instruct the patient who takes aspirins constantly that before any surgery the surgeon should be informed of the number of aspirins taken daily. Explain that aspirins will prolong bleeding time.

SCHILLING TEST
(See Vitamin B$_{12}$.)

SEMEN EXAMINATION

Reference Values

Semen Examination: Volume: 1.5–5.0 mL. *Count:* 60–150 million/mL. *Mobility:* 3 hours >60%. *Normal forms:* >70%. *Appearance:* translucent, turbid, viscous. *Viscosity:* liquid after 30 minutes

Antisperm Antibody test: Adult: negative to 1:32

Description

Semen examination is used as one of the tests to determine the cause of infertility. The sperm count; volume of fluid; percent of normal, mature spermatozoa (sperms); and percent of actively mobile spermatozoa are studied when analyzing the semen content. Conception has been reported even when the sperm count has been as low as 10 million/mL.

Sperm count is frequently used to monitor the effectiveness of sterilization after a vasectomy (severing of the vas deferens). The sperm count is checked

273

periodically. In cases of rape, a forensic or medicolegal analysis is done to detect semen in vaginal secretions or on clothes.

The three methods used to collect semen are masturbation, coitus interruptus, and intercourse using a condom. Sexual abstinence is usually required for 3 days before the test. Masturbation is the usual method for obtaining a semen specimen; however, for religious reasons intercourse with a condom is sometimes preferred. With coitus interruptus, only a partial semen specimen may be obtained. A semen specimen may be collected at home or in the physician's office.

The *antisperm antibody test* could be ordered to identify a possible cause of infertility. Autoantibodies to sperm might result from a blocking of the efferent ducts in the testes.[1,3,9,12,13]

Clinical Problems

Decreased Level: vasectomy; infertility (0–2 million/mL). *Drug Influence:* antineoplastic agents, estrogen

Procedure

- Abstinence from intercourse for 3 days before collecting semen.
- Collect semen by:

    1. Masturbation—collect in a clean container.
    2. Coitus interruptus—collect in a clean glass container.
    3. Intercourse with a clean, washed condom—place the condom in a clean container.

- Keep the semen specimen from chilling, and take it immediately to the laboratory. It should be tested within 2 hours after collection—the sooner, the better.
- Alcoholic beverages should be avoided for several days (at least 24 hours) before the test. There is no other fluid or food restriction.

- Factors Affecting Laboratory Results

    - Recent intercourse (within 3 days) could have an effect on the sperm count.

NURSING IMPLICATIONS WITH RATIONALE

- Explain to the patient the purpose of the test. He will most likely know the reason for semen collection and examination, which is either to determine the cause of infertility or to determine the effectiveness of sterilization following vasectomy.
- Check with the physician on what he or she has told the patient. Be able to supplement the physician's explanation to the patient, with the physician's approval.
- Be available to discuss methods of semen collection with the patient and his spouse/partner (ie, masturbation, coitus interruptus, and intercourse with a condom). This can be most embarrassing for the man and woman. Some persons prefer to discuss the test in detail with the nurse rather than with the physician. Religious beliefs need to be considered.

- Be supportive of the patient and his spouse. Be a good listener and give them time to express their concerns.
- Answer their questions. If you are unable to respond, refer the question to the appropriate person (ie, the physician, a clergyman).
- Avoid giving your moral convictions about the test or the surgical procedure (vasectomy).

SERUM GLUTAMIC OXALOACETIC TRANSAMINASE (SGOT)
(See Aspartate Aminotransferase.)

SERUM GLUTAMIC PYRUVIC TRANSAMINASE (SGPT)
(See Alanine Aminotransferase.)

SICKLE CELL (SCREENING) TEST (BLOOD)

Reference Values
Adult: 0
Child: 0

Description
(See Hemoglobin Electrophoresis.)

Hemoglobin S (sickle cell), an abnormal hemoglobin, causes RBCs (erythrocytes) to form a crescent shape when deprived of oxygen. With adequate oxygen, the red cells with hemoglobin S will maintain a normal shape.

If a sickle cell screening test is positive for hemoglobin S, hemoglobin electrophoresis should be ordered to differentiate between sickle cell anemia caused by hemoglobin S/S and sickle cell trait caused by hemoglobin A/S. If the patient's hemoglobin level is less than 10 g/dL or the hematocrit is less than 30%, test results could be falsely negative.[1,9,10,12,13]

Clinical Problems
Positive Results: sickle cell anemia, sickle cell trait

Procedure

- Collect 5 to 7 mL of venous blood in a lavender-top tube.
- If a commercial-test kit (Sickledex) is used, follow the directions given on the kit.

- There is no food or fluid restriction.
- Note on the laboratory slip if blood transfusion was given 3 to 4 months before the screening test. If so, inaccurate results could result.

■ Factors Affecting Laboratory Results

- A blood transfusion given within 3 to 4 months could cause inaccurate results.
- Hemoglobin less than 10 g/dL or hematocrit less than 30% could cause false-negative test results.
- Reagents from the test kit may deteriorate and may no longer be active test agents.
- The test result could be falsely negative in an infant less than 6 months old.

NURSING IMPLICATIONS WITH RATIONALE

- Explain to the patient and/or family that the purpose of the test is to determine the presence of sickle cells (hemoglobin S).

Positive Test Results

- Observe for signs and symptoms of sickle cell anemia. Early symptoms are fatigue and weakness. Chronic symptoms are dyspnea on exertion, swollen joints, "aching bones," and chest pains.

Patient Teaching

- Instruct the patient to avoid people with infections and colds. Persons with sickle cell anemia are susceptible to infections.
- Encourage the patient to seek genetic counseling if he or she has sickle cell anemia or the sickle cell trait.
- Instruct the patient with sickle cell anemia to minimize strenuous activity and to avoid high altitudes and extreme cold. Encourage the patient to take rest periods.

SODIUM (Na) (SERUM)

Reference Values

Adult: 135–145 mEq/L, 135–145 mmol/L (SI units)

Child: Infant: 134–150 mEq/L. *Child:* 135–145 mEq/L

Description

Sodium (Na) is the major cation in the extracellular fluid (ECF), and it has a water-retaining effect. When there is excess sodium in the ECF, more water will be reabsorbed from the kidneys.

Sodium has many functions. It helps to maintain body fluids, is responsible for conduction of neuromuscular impulses via the sodium pump (sodium shifts into cells as potassium shifts out for cellular activity), it is involved in enzyme activity, and it regulates acid-base balance by combining with chloride or bicarbonate ions.

The body needs approximately 2 to 4 g of sodium daily. The American people daily consume approximately 6 to 12 g (90 to 240 mEq/L) of sodium in the form of salt (NaCl). A teaspoon of salt contains 2.3 g of sodium.

The names for sodium imbalances are hyponatremia (serum sodium deficit) and hypernatremia (serum sodium excess). When the serum sodium level is 125 mEq/L, sodium replacement with normal saline (0.9% NaCl) should be considered, and if the serum sodium level is 115 mEq/L or lower, concentrated saline solutions (3% or 5% NaCl) might be ordered. When rapidly replacing sodium loss, assessment for overhydration is important.[9,10,12,23,24,42]

Clinical Problems

Decreased Level: vomiting, diarrhea, gastric suction, excessive perspiration, continuous IV D5W, syndrome of inappropriate antidiuretic hormone (SIADH, due to surgery, trauma, pain, narcotics), low-sodium diet, burns, inflammatory reactions, tissue injury (fluid and sodium shift to the third space); psychogenic polydipsia, salt-wasting renal disease. *Drug Influence:* potent diuretics (furosemide [Lasix], ethacrynic acid [Edecrin], thiazides, mannitol)

Elevated Level: dehydration, severe vomiting and diarrhea (water loss is greater than sodium loss), congestive heart failure, Cushing's disease, hepatic failure, high-sodium diet. *Drug Influence:* cough medicines, cortisone preparations, antibiotics, laxatives, methyldopa (Aldomet), hydralazine (Apresoline), reserpine (Serpasil)

Procedure

- Collect 5 to 10 mL of venous blood in a red- or green-top tube.
- There are no restrictions on food and fluid. If the patient has eaten large quantities of foods high in salt content in the last 24 to 48 hours, this should be noted on the laboratory slip and the physician should be notified. Sodium is rarely requested alone but is rather given as part of the serum electrolytes (ie, Na, K, Cl, CO_2).

- Factors Affecting Laboratory Results

  - A diet high in sodium
  - Drugs—potent diuretics, cortisone preparations, various antihypertensive agents, cough medicines

---

NURSING IMPLICATIONS WITH RATIONALE

Decreased Level

- Assess for signs and symptoms of hyponatremia (ie, apprehension, anxiety, muscular twitching, muscular weakness, headaches, tachycardia, and hypotension).

- Recognize that hyponatremia after surgery is the result of SIADH. There is usually an excess secretion of ADH for a day or two after surgery, which causes water reabsorption from the kidney and sodium dilution.
- Report to the physician if the patient has received D5W infusions for more than 2 days. Hyponatremia and water intoxication could occur. IV fluids with dextrose and one third or one half normal saline solution (0.33% to 0.45%) are frequently ordered.
- Monitor the medical regimen for correcting hyponatremia (ie, water restriction, normal saline [0.9% percent] solution to correct a serum sodium level of 120 to 130 mEq/L, and 3% or 5% saline to correct a serum sodium level of less than 115 mEq/L).
- Observe for signs and symptoms of overhydration when the patient is receiving 3% or 5% percent saline intravenously. Symptoms of overhydration are a constant, irritated cough; dyspnea; neck-and hand-vein engorgement; and chest rales.
- Check the specific gravity of urine. A specific gravity of less than 1.010 could indicate hyponatremia.
- Check serum sodium and other laboratory results and report serum electrolyte changes. An extremely low serum sodium level requires that the test be repeated.
- Irrigate nasogastric tubes and wound sites with normal saline instead of sterile water.
- Take vital signs to determine cardiac status during hyponatremia.
- Compare the serum sodium level with the urine sodium level. A low or normal serum sodium and a low urine sodium could indicate sodium retention or a decrease in sodium intake.

Patient Teaching

- Encourage the patient to avoid drinking only plain water. Suggest fluids with solutes (ie, broth and juices).

Elevated Level

- Observe for signs and symptoms of hypernatremia (ie, restlessness; thirst; flushed skin; dry, sticky mucous membranes; a rough, dry tongue; and tachycardia).
- Check for body fluid loss by keeping an accurate intake and output record and weighing the patient daily. A liter of fluid will add on approximately 2.5 lb of body weight.
- Check the specific gravity of the urine. A specific gravity over 1.030 could indicate hypernatremia.
- Report to the physician if the patient is receiving IV fluids containing normal saline (0.9% NaCl). A liter of normal saline contains 155 mEq of sodium. The body needs 40 to 70 mEq/L of sodium daily, though the average daily intake for adults is 90 to 240 mEq/L. The maximum daily tolerance of sodium is 400 mEq/L, and if the patient receives 3 L of normal saline, he or she will receive 465 mEq/L.

- Observe for edema and overhydration resulting from an elevated serum-sodium level. Signs and symptoms of overhydration are a constant, irritated cough; dyspnea; neck-and hand-vein engorgement; and chest rales.

Patient Teaching

- Encourage the patient to drink 8 to 10 glasses of water, unless this is contraindicated (for instance, with a history of congestive heart failure).
- Instruct the patient to avoid foods that are high in sodium (ie, corned beef, bacon, ham, tuna fish, cheese, celery, catsup, pickles, olives, and potato chips). Avoid using salt when cooking or at mealtime.

SODIUM (Na) (URINE)

Reference Values

Adult: 40–220 mEq/L/24 h

Child: similar to adult

Description

Sodium excretion varies according to the sodium intake, aldosterone secretion, urine volume, and disease entities, such as chronic renal failure, adrenal gland dysfunction (Addison's disease and Cushing's syndrome), cirrhosis of the liver, and congestive heart failure.

When the urine sodium level is less than 40 mEq/24 h, the decreased sodium excretion could be due to sodium retention or decreased sodium intake. The body could be retaining sodium even with a low serum sodium level.

The urine sodium level should be monitored when edema is present and the serum sodium level is low or normal.[10,12,24]

Clinical Problems

Decreased Level: Cushing's syndrome, congestive heart failure, hepatic failure, renal failure, Chronic obstructive lung disease (COLD), low sodium (salt) intake. *Drug Influence:* cortisone preparations.

Elevated Level: Addison's disease, dehydration, essential hypertension, diabetes mellitus, anterior pituitary hypofunction, high sodium intake. *Drug Influence:* potent diuretics (furosemide [Lasix], ethacrynic acid [Edecrin])

Procedure

- Collect a 24-hour urine sample and place it in a large specimen container. Label the container with the exact times the urine collection started and ended. First-voided specimen should be discarded.
- The urine specimen should be refrigerated or placed in a container of ice.
- There is no food or fluid restriction.

■ Factors Affecting Laboratory Results

- A diet high or low in sodium content
- Drugs such as cortisone and potent diuretics
- Renal dysfunction
- Discarded urine

NURSING IMPLICATIONS WITH RATIONALE

Patient Teaching

■ Explain the procedure for collecting the 24-hour urine. Inform the patient that all voidings (urine) should be placed in the large container. Have patients inform their families of the procedure. Tell the patient not to put toilet paper or feces in the urine.

Decreased Level

■ Compare the serum sodium level with the urine sodium level. A low or normal serum sodium and a low urine sodium could indicate sodium retention or a decrease in sodium intake.

Elevated Level

■ Report to the physician if the patient is receiving several liters of normal saline solution intravenously (*see Sodium [Serum]*).

Patient Teaching

■ Instruct the patient to avoid eating foods high in sodium if the cause is due to high-sodium intake.

TESTOSTERONE (SERUM OR PLASMA)

Reference Values

Adult: *Male:* 0.3–1.0 μg/dL, 300–1000 ng/dL. *Female:* 0.03–0.1 μg/dL, 30–100 ng/dL

Child: *Male:* 12–14 Years Old: >0.1 μg/dL, >100 ng/dL

Description

Testosterone, a male sex hormone, is produced by the testes and adrenal glands in the male and by the ovaries and adrenal glands in the female. It is useful in diagnosing male sexual precocity before the age of 10 years and male infertility.

In males, the highest serum testosterone levels occur in the morning. Serum testosterone is low in both primary and secondary hypogonadism.[7,9,12,13]

Clinical Problems

Decreased Level: testicular hypofunction. Klinefelter's syndrome (primary hypogonadism), alcoholism, anterior pituitary hypofunction, estrogen therapy, hypopituitarism

Elevated Level: male sexual precocity, adrenal hyperplasia or tumor, neoplasm or hyperplasia of ovaries, adrenogenital syndrome in women, polycystic ovaries in females

Procedure

- Collect 7 to 10 mL of venous blood in a red- or green-top tube. Avoid hemolysis.
- There is no food or fluid restriction.

- Factors Affecting Laboratory Results

  - None known

NURSING IMPLICATIONS WITH RATIONALE

Decreased Level

- Determine whether the patient is complying with medical treatment for testicular hypofunction or hypogonadism. Discuss the side effects of testosterone.
- Be supportive of the male patient and his family concerning physical changes caused by hormonal deficiency.

Elevated Level

- Observe for signs and symptoms of excess testosterone secretion (ie, hirsutism, masculine voice, and increased muscle mass [especially in women]). Report findings to the physician and record on the chart.

THEOPHYLLINE (SERUM)
Aminophylline, Theo-Dur, Theolaire, Slo-Phyllin, Elixophyllin, Sustaire

Reference Values

Therapeutic Range: Adult: 5–20 μg/mL, 28–112 μmol/L (SI units). *Elderly:* 5–18 μg/mL. *Child:* Premature Infants: 7–14 μg/mL; Neonate: 3–12 μg/mL; Child: same as adult

Toxic Level: Adult: >20 μg/mL, >112 μmol/L (SI units). *Elderly:* Same as adult. *Child:* Premature Infants: >14 μg/mL; Neonate: >13 μg/mL; Child: same as adult

Description

Theophylline, a xanthine derivative, relaxes smooth muscle of the bronchi and pulmonary blood vessels; reduces pulmonary hypertension; stimulates the CNS; stimulates myocardium, resulting in an increase in the force of contraction and cardiac output; increases renal blood flow, causing diuresis; and relaxes smooth muscles of the GI tract. Usually theophylline products are given to control asthmatic attacks and to treat acute attack. Oral theophylline preparations are well absorbed from the gastrointestinal tract.

Ninety percent of theophylline is metabolized in the liver, with about 60% bound to plasma protein and 40% free. Ten percent of the drug is excreted unchanged in the urine. The half-life of theophylline is 5 to 10 hours in a nonsmoker, 3½ to 5 hours in a smoker, and 3½ hours in children. Peak blood levels after an orally administered dose of theophylline occurs in 1 to 2 hours.

Persons with heart failure or liver disease or who are either very young or elderly could develop theophylline toxicity quickly. Serum theophylline levels in these persons should be monitored frequently.

Early signs and symptoms of theophylline toxicity are anorexia, nausea, vomiting, abdominal discomfort, nervousness, jitters, tachycardia, and cardiac arrhythmias. If severe theophylline toxicity occurs (>30 μg/mL), cardiac arrhythmias, seizures, respiratory arrest, and/or cardiac arrest might result.[2–4,6,7]

Clinical Problems

Decreased Level: smoking. *Drug Influence:* phenytoin (Dilantin)

Elevated Level: theophylline overdose, congestive heart failure, liver disease, lung disease, renal disease. *Drug Influence:* antibiotics (erythromycin, lincomycin), allopurinol, barbiturates, caffeine, cimetidine (Tagamet), furosemide (Lasix), ephedrine, propranolol (Inderal), sulfonamides, theobromine, other xanthines, flu vaccine

Procedure

- Collect 5 mL of venous blood in a red-top tube. Avoid hemolysis.
- Record the name of the drug, dose, route, and last-dose administered on the laboratory requisition slip. Test might be ordered for peak levels or for trough levels (before next dose).
- The patient should not drink coffee, tea, or colas, or eat chocolates 8 hours prior to the test.
- Note on the laboratory requisition slip drugs the patient is taking that could affect test results.
- Do not shake the collecting tube of blood specimen. This could decrease the serum theophylline level.

■ Factors Affecting Laboratory Results

■ Drugs (*see Drug Influence*), food and fluids, such as chocolate, coffee, tea, and colas, could increase serum theophylline level.
■ Shaking the collecting tube vigorously could cause a false-negative test result.

NURSING IMPLICATIONS WITH RATIONALE

■ Explain to the patient that the purpose of the test is to monitor therapeutic theophylline level.
■ Check theophylline level and report nontherapeutic levels to the physician immediately.
■ Record name of the drug, dose, route, and last time drug was given on the requisition slip.
■ Record the time the blood sample was drawn on the requisition slip. This informs the laboratory personnel and the physician of the theophylline level time (peak or trough before the next dose).

Decreased Level

■ Recognize that smoking causes a short half-life and promotes a faster theophylline clearance. The drug phenytoin (Dilantin) has been reported to decrease the theophylline half-life.
■ Report to the physician if the patient is a smoker because a larger dose of theophylline might be needed.

Elevated Level

■ Recognize that liver, lung, and renal diseases and certain drugs might cause an elevated serum theophylline level (*see Drug Influence above*).
■ Observe for signs and symptoms of theophylline toxicity (ie, anorexia, nausea, vomiting, abdominal discomfort, nervousness, irritability, tachycardia, and cardiac arrhythmias).
■ Monitor pulse rate and report signs of tachycardia and skipped beats.
■ Monitor intake and output. Report if patient's output has greatly increased because of diuresis.

Patient Teaching

■ Instruct the patient not to drink or eat coffee, teas, colas, and chocolate within 8 hours of the test.

THYROGLOBULIN ANTIBODIES
(See Thyroid Antibodies.)

THYROID ANTIBODIES (TA) (SERUM)
Thyroglobulin Antibodies or Thyroid Hemagglutination Test

Reference Values
Adult: negative to 1:20, tanned red cell (TRC) results under 100
Child: similar to adult but usually not done

Description
A thyroid autoimmune disease usually produces thyroid antibodies (thyroglobulin antibodies). These autoantibodies (against the body's own tissue) combine with thyroglobulin from the thyroid gland and cause inflammatory lesions of the gland.

A serum titer evaluation is ordered to detect the presence of thyroid antibodies. With Hashimoto's thyroiditis, the titer is high, 1:5000. The titer can also be elevated with carcinoma of the thyroid, rheumatoid-collagen diseases, and thyrotoxicosis. A positive thyroid antibodies (TA) test does not always confirm the diagnosis of Hashimoto's thyroiditis, unless the titer is extremely high.[8–10,12]

Clinical Problems
Elevated Titer: Hashimoto's thyroiditis, carcinoma of the thyroid gland, pernicious anemia, lupus erythematosus, rheumatoid arthritis, thyrotoxicosis (Graves' disease)

Procedure
- Collect 5 mL of venous blood in a red-top tube.
- The tanned red cell (TRC) test is more sensitive for detecting thyroid autoimmune disease (such as Hashimoto's thyroiditis) than the TA test. It is useful for detecting microsomal antigen.
- There is no food or fluid restriction.

- ### Factors Affecting Laboratory Results
  - Sex (thyroid disease is commoner in women than in men).

NURSING IMPLICATIONS WITH RATIONALE

Elevated Titer Level

- Check serum thyroglobin antibody titer results and relate them to clinical problems. The test is usually ordered to diagnose Hashimoto's thyroiditis; however, the titer level can be elevated in other clinical conditions (*see Clinical Problems*).
- Obtain a family history of thyroid disease. Determine whether the patient has had a viral infection in the last few weeks or months. It is believed that viral infections can trigger autoimmune disease.

THYROID-STIMULATING HORMONE (TSH) (SERUM)

Reference Values

Adult: 2–5.4 μIU/mL, <10 μU/mL, <10^{-3}IU/L (SI units), <3 ng/mL

Newborn: <25 μIU/mL by the third day

Description

The anterior pituitary gland (anterior hypophysis) secretes thyroid-stimulating hormone (TSH) in response to thyroid-releasing hormone (TRH) from the hypothalamus. TSH stimulates the secretion of thyroxine (T_4) produced in the thyroid gland. The secretion of TSH is dependent on the negative feedback system—a decreased T_4 level promotes the release of TRH, which stimulates TSH secretion. An elevated T_4 level suppresses TRH release, which suppresses TSH secretion.

TSH and T_4 levels are frequently measured to differentiate pituitary from thyroid dysfunctions. A decreased T_4 level and a normal or elevated TSH level can indicate a thyroid disorder. A decreased T_4 level with a decreased TSH level can indicate a pituitary disorder.[9,10,13,43]

Clinical Problems

Decreased Level: secondary hypothyroidism (pituitary gland involvement), anterior pituitary hypofunction, Klinefelter's syndrome. *Drug Influence:* aspirin, steroid, dopamine, heparin

Elevated Level: primary hypothyroidism (thyroid gland involvement with a decreased T_4); thyroiditis (Hashimoto's disease, autoimmune disease); cirrhosis of the liver. *Drug Influence:* antithyroid therapy

Procedure

- Collect 5 mL of venous blood in a red-top or green-top tube. Avoid hemolysis.
- There is no food or fluid restriction. Avoid shellfish for several days prior to the test.

■ Factors Affecting Laboratory Results

- None known

NURSING IMPLICATIONS WITH RATIONALE

- Recognize the cause of hypothyroidism by comparing the TSH level with the T_4 level. Decreased TSH and T_4 levels could be due to anterior pituitary dysfunction causing secondary hypothyroidism. A normal or elevated TSH and a decreased T_4 could be due to thyroid dysfunction.
- Observe for signs and symptoms of myxedema (hypothyroidism; ie, anorexia; fatigue; weight gain; dry and flaky skin, puffy face, hands, and feet; abdominal distention; bradycardia; infertility, and ataxia).

- Monitor vital signs before and during treatment for hypothyroidism. Report immediately if tachycardia occurs.
- Refer to the patient's triiodothyronine (T_3), T_4, and thyroglobulin results to observe correlations with the TSH result.

THYROXINE (T_4) (SERUM)

Reference Values

Adult: Reported as Serum Thyroxine: T_4 by column: 4.5–11.5 µg/dL; T_4 (RIA): 5–12 µg/dL; Free T_4: 1.0–2.3 ng/dl. *Reported as Thyroxine Iodine:* T_4 by column: 3.2–7.2 µg/dL

Child: Newborn: 11–23 µg/dL. *1 to 4 Months Old:* 7.5–16.5 µg/dL. *4 to 12 Months Old:* 5.5–14.5 µg/dL. *1 to 6 Years Old:* 5.5–13.5 µg/dL. *6 to 10 Years Old:* 5–12.5 µg/dL

Description

Thyroxine (T_4) is the major hormone secreted by the thyroid gland and is at least 25 times more concentrated than triiodothyronine (T_3). The serum T_4 levels are commonly used to measure thyroid hormone concentration and the function of the thyroid gland. The use of protein-bound iodine (PBI) is considered obsolete, and this test is seldom performed.

In some institutions the T_4 test is required for all newborns (as is the PKU test) to detect a decreased thyroxine secretion, which could lead to irreversible mental retardation.[1,3,9–12,43]

Clinical Problems

Decreased level: hypothyroidism (cretinism, myxedema), protein malnutrition, anterior pituitary hypofunction, strenuous exercise. *Drug Influence:* cortisone, chlorpromazine (Thorazine), phenytoin (Dilantin), heparin, lithium, sulfonamides, reserpine (Serpasil), testosterone, tolbutamide (Orinase)

Elevated Level: hyperthyroidism, acute thyroiditis, viral hepatitis, myasthenia gravis, pregnancy, preeclampsia. *Drug Influence:* oral contraceptives, estrogens, clofibrate

Procedure

- Various methods are used for measuring T_4.
- Thyroid medication will interfere with the T_4 by column method. Check with your laboratory for an alternate procedure.
- Collect 5 mL of venous blood in a red-top tube. Avoid hemolysis.
- There is no food or fluid restriction.
- Note on the laboratory slip drugs patient is taking that could affect test results.

■ Factors Affecting Laboratory Results

■ Drugs: (*See Drug Influence.*)

NURSING IMPLICATIONS WITH RATIONALE

Decreased Level

■ Observe for signs and symptoms of hypothyroidism (ie, fatigue, forgetfulness, weight gain, dry skin with poor turgor, dry and thin hair, bradycardia, decreased peripheral circulation, depressed libido, infertility, and constipation).

Elevated Level

■ Observe for signs and symptoms of hyperthyroidism (ie, nervousness, tremors, emotional instability, increased appetite, weight loss, palpitations, tachycardia, diarrhea, decreased fertility, and exophthalmos).
■ Monitor the pulse rate. Tachycardia is common and if severe could cause heart failure and cardiac arrest.

TORCH SCREEN TEST
TORCH Battery, TORCH Titer

Reference Values

Maternal: IgG titer antibodies: negative. *IgM titer antibodies:* negative

Infant: same as maternal; infant should be under 2 months of age

Description

TORCH stands for toxoplasmosis, rubella, cytomegalovirus (CMV), and herpes simplex. It is a screen test to detect the presence of these organisms in the mother and infant. During pregnancy, TORCH infections can cross the placenta and could result in mild or severe congenital malformation, abortion, or stillbirth. The severe effect from these organisms occurs during the first trimester of pregnancy. Prenatally the TORCH screening test is performed only when a TORCH infection is suspected, such as rubella infection.

TORCH screening test is more frequently performed when congenital infection in the infant is suspected. The IgG titers are compared with both mother's and infant's serum. If the IgG titer level is higher in the infant than mother and the IgM titer is present in the infant, congenital TORCH infection is likely. This test might be repeated in several weeks. Individual testing might be necessary along with clinical information to identify the TORCH infection; rubella and CMV are the commonest.[3,6,9]

Clinical Problems

Positive IgG, IgM Titers: toxoplasmosis, rubella, CMV, herpes simplex

Procedure

- Collect 7 mL of venous blood in a red-top tube.
- There is no food or fluid restriction.
- TORCH kits: Follow directions on the kit.

■ Factors Affecting Laboratory Results

■ None known

NURSING IMPLICATIONS WITH RATIONALE

- Obtain a history from the patient about any previous infection.

Patient Teaching

- Inform the patient that if a positive test result occurs, more testing will be needed.

TRICYCLIC ANTIDEPRESSANTS (TCA OR TAD) SERUM

Reference Values[1–4,6,9,26]

Adult

DRUG	THERAPEUTIC RANGE	PEAK TIME	TOXIC LEVEL
Amitriptyline (Elavil)	125–200 ng/mL	2–12 hours	>500 ng/mL
Desipramine (Norpramin)	125–300 ng/mL	4–6 hours	>500 ng/mL
Doxepin (Sinequan)	150–250 ng/mL	2–4 hours	>500 ng/mL
Imipramine (Tofranil)	150–300 ng/mL	1–2 hours (PO) 30 min (IM)	>500 ng/mL
Nortriptyline (Aventyl)	50–150 ng/mL	8 hours	>200 ng/mL
Protriptyline (Vivactil)	70–170 ng/mL	8–12 hours	>200 ng/mL
Amoxapire (Asendin)	200–400 ng/mL	1½ hours	>500 ng/mL
Maprotiline (Ludiomil)	200–300 ng/mL	12 hours	>500 ng/mL

Description

Tricyclic antidepressants (TCAs) are useful in treating clinical depression and bipolar disorders. Laboratory measurements for TCAs are used to monitor the therapeutic range, to adjust drug dosages, and to detect toxic levels due to overdose (unintentional or intentional). Peak times should be noted when the patient is obtaining maximum effects. The average time at which these drugs reach their steady state varies from days to 1 to 2 weeks. The serious toxic effect of these drugs is cardiotoxicity, which includes depressed myocardial contractility, decreased heart rate, and decreased coronary blood flow.[1,3,6,9,26]

Clinical Problems

Decreased Level: Drug Influence: barbiturates, alcohol

Elevated Level: overdose of TCAs. *Drug Influence:* steroids, antipsychotics (neuroleptics)

Procedure

■ Collect 7 mL of venous blood in a red-top tube.
■ There is no food or fluid restriction.

■ Factors Affecting Laboratory Results

■ Drugs—Barbiturates and alcohol can lower the serum TCAs, and steroids and antipsychotics can elevate serum level.

NURSING IMPLICATIONS WITH RATIONALE

■ Obtain a history from the patient concerning daily drug dosing, having blood samples taken at regular intervals and keeping doctor's appointments.
■ Record and report noncompliance to drug regimen, if appropriate.

Patient Teaching

■ Instruct the patient to follow the prescribed drug dosage. Explain to the patient that if prescribed dose is not taken (undosing), therapeutic effects will not be obtained and depressed feelings might remain. Explain that with overdosing, serious cardiotoxicity might result.
■ Encourage the patient to express feelings about drug regimen. Listen to patient's concern.
■ Explain to the patient that when the dose is increased, it may take 7 to 10 days for a clinical change because the half-life (t ½) is long with most of these agents.
■ Explain to the patient that when discontinuing the medication, the drug dosage should be tapered to avoid extrapyramidal side effects (EPS).

TRIGLYCERIDES (SERUM)

Reference Values

Adult: *12–29 years:* 10–140 mg/dL. *30–39 years:* 20–150 mg/dL. *40–49 years:* 30–160 mg/dL *>50 years:* 40–190 mg/dL. 0.44–2.09 mmol/L (SI units)

Child: *Infant:* 5–40 mg/dL. *Child:* 5–11 years: 10–135 mg/dL

Description

Triglycerides, a blood lipid formed by esterification of glycerol and three fatty acids, are carried by the serum lipoproteins. The intestine processes the triglycerides from dietary fatty acids (exogenous), and they are transported in the blood stream as chylomicrons (tiny fat droplets covered by protein), which gives the serum a milky or creamy appearance after a meal rich in fats. The liver is also responsible for manufacturing triglycerides, but these do not travel as chylomicrons. The majority of triglycerides is stored as lipids in the adipose tissue. A function of triglycerides is to provide energy to the heart and skeletal muscles.

Triglycerides are a major contributor to arterial diseases and are frequently compared with cholesterol by the lipoprotein electrophoresis. As the concentration of triglycerides increases, so will the very low-density lipoproteins (VLDL) increase, leading to hyperlipoproteinemia. Alcohol intake can cause a transient elevation of serum triglyceride level.[3,7,9,10,12]

Clinical Problems

Decreased Level: congenital β-lipoproteinemia, hyperthyroidism, hyperparathyroidism, protein malnutrition, exercise. *Drug Influence:* ascorbic acid, clofibrate (Atromid-S), phenformin, metformin

Elevated Level: hyperlipoproteinemia, acute myocardial infarction, hypertension, cerebral thrombosis, hypothyroidism, nephrotic syndrome, arteriosclerosis, Laënnec's or alcoholic cirrhosis, uncontrolled diabetes mellitus, pancreatitis, Down's syndrome, stress, high-carbohydrate diet, pregnancy. *Drug Influence:* estrogen, oral contraceptives

Procedure

- Collect 5 to 7 mL of venous blood in a red-top tube.
- The patient should be NPO (food, drink, or medications) after 6 PM the night before the test, except for water. Medications should be held until after blood is drawn. The patient should be on a normal diet for several days before the test. No alcohol is allowed for 24 hours prior to the test.
- Note on the laboratory slip if the patient's weight has increased or decreased in the last 2 weeks.

- Factors Affecting Laboratory Results

  - A high-carbohydrate diet and alcohol can elevate the serum triglycerides level.

NURSING IMPLICATIONS WITH RATIONALE

Elevated Level

- Relate clinical problems and drugs to increased serum triglycerides levels. When triglycerides and/or cholesterol are elevated, a lipoprotein electrophoresis is frequently ordered.
- Check the serum cholesterol level. At times only one of the body's lipids will be elevated. If the cholesterol level is elevated, suggest which foods should be avoided (*see Cholesterol*). Consult with the dietetics department.
- Check to see if a lipoprotein electrophoresis has been ordered. This is frequently done when the triglycerides are elevated.

Patient Teaching

- Instruct the patient that he or she is not to eat food or to drink anything except water for 12 to 14 hours before the test. Patient should avoid alcoholic intake for 24 hours. Medications may be withheld until after the test. Check with the physician and laboratory.
- Instruct the patient with a high serum triglycerides level to avoid eating excessive amounts of sugars and carbohydrates as well as dietary fats. The patient should be encouraged to eat fruit.

TRIIODOTHYRONINE (T₃) (SERUM)
T₃ RIA

Reference Values

Adult: 80–200 ng/dL

Child: Newborn: 90–170 ng/dL. *Age 6 to 12 years:* 115–190 ng/dL

Description

Triiodothyronine (T₃), one of the thyroid hormones, is present in small amounts in blood and is more short acting and more potent than thyroxine (T₄). Both T₃ and T₄ have similar actions in the body. Serum T₃ is secreted in response to thyroid-stimulating hormone (TSH) from the pituitary gland and thyroid-releasing hormone (TRH) from the hypothalamus and is measured directly by radioimmunoassay (RIA).

Serum T₃ RIA measures both bound and free T₃. It is effective for diagnosing hyperthyroidism, especially T₃ thyrotoxicosis, in which T₃ is increased and T₄ is in normal range. It is not as reliable for diagnosing hypothyroidism, since T₃ remains in normal range. T₃ RIA and T₃ update are two different tests.[3,6,9,12,43]

Clinical Problems

Decreased Level (<80 ng/dL): malnutrition, severe acute illness and trauma. *Drug Influence:* propylthiouracil, methylthiouracil, methimazole (Tapazole), lithium, phenytoin (Dilantin), propranolol (Inderal), reserpine (Serpasil), salicylates (aspirin), steroids, sulfonamides

Elevated Level (>200 ng/dL): T_3 thyrotoxicosis, Hashimoto's thyroiditis, toxic adenoma. *Drug Influence:* estrogen, progestins, methadone, liothyronine (T_3)

Procedure

- Collect 5 to 10 mL of venous blood in a red-top tube. Avoid hemolysis.
- Send blood sample to the laboratory as soon as possible.
- Drugs that affect laboratory results should be withheld 24 hours with the physician's approval. If the drugs are taken prior to the test, they should be listed on the laboratory slip.

■ Factors Affecting Laboratory Results

- Drugs (*See Drug Influence.*)
- Hemolysis of blood specimen from rough handling.

NURSING IMPLICATIONS WITH RATIONALE

- List on the laboratory slip any drugs the patient is taking that could cause false-negative or false-positive results.

Elevated Level

- Observe for signs and symptoms of hyperthyroidism (ie, nervousness, tremors, emotional instability, increased appetite, weight loss, palpitations, tachycardia, diarrhea, decreased fertility, and exophthalmos [eyeballs protruding])
- Monitor pulse rate. Tachycardia is common and, if severe, could cause heart failure.

TRIIODOTHYRONINE RESIN UPTAKE (T_3 RU) (SERUM)
T_3 Uptake

Reference Values

Adult: 25–35 relative percentage uptake

Description

Triiodothyronine (T_3) resin uptake is an indirect measure of free thyronine (T_4), whereas serum T_3 RIA is a direct measurement of T_3. This is an in vitro test in which the patient's blood is mixed with radioactive T_3 and synthetic resin material in a test tube. The radioactive T_3 will bind at available thyroid-binding globulin(protein) sites. The unbound radioactive T_3 is added to resin for T_3 uptake. In hyperthyroidism there are few binding sites left, so more T_3 is taken up by the resin, thus causing a high T_3 resin uptake. In hypothyroidism there is less T_3 resin uptake.

This test can be performed when patients receive drugs, diagnostic agents (contrast media), and food containing iodine. Usually this test is not affected by inorganic or organic iodine, but it is affected by radioactive iodine, which interferes with the test reagents.

T_3 RU is one of the thyroid tests but should not be the only test used to determine thyroid dysfunction.[3,6,9,12,43]

Clinical Problems

Decreased Level: hypothyroidism (cretinism, myxedema), pregnancy, menstruation, thyroiditis (Hashimoto's), Acute hepatitis *Drug Influence:* ACTH,* corticosteroids,* estrogen, oral contraceptives, antithyroid agents (methimazole, propylthiouracil), thiazides, chlordiazepoxide (Librium), sulfonylureas (eg, tolbutamide [Orinase])

Elevated Level: hyperthyroidism, protein malnutrition, malignancies (breast) and metastatic carcinoma, myasthenia gravis, nephrotic syndrome, uremia, threatened abortion. *Drug Influence:* ACTH,* corticosteroids,* anticoagulants (oral), heparin, phenytoin (Dilantin), phenylbutazone (Butazolidin), salicylates (high doses of aspirin compounds), thyroid agents

Procedure

- Collect 5 to 7 mL of venous blood in a red-top tube. Avoid hemolysis.
- There is no food or fluid restriction.
- Note on the laboratory slip drugs patient is taking that could affect test results.

■ Factors Affecting Laboratory Results

- Drugs (*See Drug Influence.*)
- Previous administration of radioactive iodine or other radioactive substances could cause inaccurate results.

NURSING IMPLICATIONS WITH RATIONALE

- List on the laboratory slip any drugs the patient is taking that could cause a false-negative or false-positive result. Also note any radioactive substance the patient has taken.
- Check results of the T_4 test.

---

*May cause decreased or elevated T_3 uptake levels.

Decreased Level

■ Observe for signs and symptoms of hypothyroidism (ie, fatigue, forgetfulness, weight gain, dry skin with poor turgor, dry and thin hair, bradycardia, decreased peripheral circulation, depressed libido, infertility, and constipation).

Elevated Level

■ Observe for signs and symptoms of hyperthyroidism (ie, nervousness, tremors, emotional instability, increased appetite, weight loss, palpitations, tachycardia, diarrhea, decreased fertility, and exophthalmos [eyeballs protruding]).
■ Monitor the pulse rate. Tachycardia is common and, if severe, could cause heart failure and cardiac arrest.

TYPE AND CROSSMATCH
(See Rh Typing and Crossmatching.)

URIC ACID (SERUM)

Reference Values

Adult: Male: 3.5–8.0 mg/dL. *Female:* 2.8–6.8 mg/dL (normal range may differ slightly among laboratories)
Child: 2.5–5.5 mg/dL
Elderly: 3.5–8.5 mg/dL

Description

Uric acid is a by-product of purine metabolism. An elevated urine and serum uric acid (hyperuricemia) depend on renal function, purine metabolism rate, and dietary intake of purine foods. Excess quantities of uric acid are excreted in the urine. Uric acid can crystallize in the urinary tract in acidic urine; therefore effective renal function and alkaline urine are necessary with hyperuricemia. The commonest problem associated with hyperuricemia is gout. Uric acid levels frequently change day by day, thus several uric acid levels may be repeated several days or weeks.

Patients/clients with elevated serum uric acid should avoid foods high in purine.[1,3,6,7,9,10]

Clinical Problems

Decreased Level: Wilson's disease, proximal renal tubular acidosis, folic acid deficiency anemia, burn, pregnancy. *Drug Influence:* allopurinol, azathioprine (Imuran), coumadin, probenecid (Benemid), sulfinpyrazone (Anturane)

Elevated Level: gout, alcoholism, leukemias (lymphocytic, myelocytic, mono-cytic), metastatic cancer, multiple myeloma, severe eclampsia, hyperlipopro-teinemia, diabetic mellitus (severe), congestive heart failure, glomerulone-phritis, renal failure, stress, lead poisoning, x-ray exposure (excessive), strenuous exercise, high-protein weight reduction diet, hemolytic anemia, lym-phoma. *Drug Influence:* ascorbic acid, diuretics (acetazolamide [Diamox], thiazides [chlorothiazide], furosemide [Lasix]) levodopa, methyldopa (Aldomet), 6-mercaptopurine, phenothiazines, salicylates (prolonged use), theophylline

Procedure

- Collect 5 to 7 mL of venous blood in a red-top tube. Avoid hemloysis.
- There is no food or drink restriction; however, in many cases, high-purine foods, such as meats (liver, kidney, brain, heart, and sweetbreads), scallops, and sardines, are restricted for 24 hours before the test.
- List drugs the patient is taking that could affect test results on the labora-tory slip.

- ## Factors Affecting Laboratory Results

  - Excessive stress and fasting could cause an elevated serum uric acid level.
  - Foods high in purine (*See Nursing Implications.*)
  - Drugs (*See Drug Influence.*)

NURSING IMPLICATIONS WITH RATIONALE

- Check with the physician and/or laboratory to determine whether foods high in purine should be restricted.

Elevated Level

- Recognize clinical problems and drugs related to hyperuricemia. Gout is a problem commonly associated with a high serum uric acid.
- Request the dietitian to visit the patient to discuss food preference and to plan a low-purine diet.
- Observe for signs and symptoms of gout (ie, tophi of the ear lobe and joints, joint pain, and edema in the "big" toe). An elevated uric acid level leads to urate deposits in the tissues and in the synovial fluid of joints.
- Monitor the pH of the urine and the amount of the urinary output. The urine pH should be kept alkaline to prevent the formation of uric acid stones in the kidney. A decreased urine output (<600 mL/24 h) with an elevated serum uric acid could indicate kidney disease.
- Check serum urea and serum creatinine levels if the serum uric acid level

---

is elevated and the urinary output is decreased. If the serum urea, creatinine, and uric acid are elevated and the urine output is decreased, kidney dysfunction should definitely be suspected. It could be secondary to another clinical problem.

Patient Teaching

■ Instruct the patient to avoid eating foods that have moderate or high amounts of purines. Examples are as follows.

HIGH (100–1000 mg PURINE NITROGEN/100 g FOOD)	MODERATE (9–100 mg PURINE NITROGEN/100 g FOOD)
Brains	Meat
Heart	Poultry
Kidney	Fish
Liver	Shellfish
Sweetbreads	Asparagus
Roe	Beans
Sardines	Mushrooms
Scallops	Peas
Mackerel	Spinach
Anchovies	
Broth	
Consommé	
Mincemeat	

■ Instruct the patient to decrease alcoholic intake. Ethanol causes renal retention of urate.

URIC ACID (URINE—24 HOUR)

Reference Values
Adult: 250–750 mg/24 h (low-purine diet), 250–750 mg/24 h (normal diet)
Child: similar to adult

Description
(*See Uric Acid* [*Serum*])

Uric acid is the end-product of purine metabolism, which takes place in the bone marrow, muscles, and liver. Excess quantities of uric acid are excreted in the urine, unless there is renal dysfunction caused by obstruction of renal flow.

The main purpose of this 24-hour urine test is to detect and/or to confirm the diagnoses of gout or kidney disease.[1,10,12]

Clinical Problems

Decreased Level: renal diseases (chronic glomerulonephritis, urinary obstruction, uremia), eclampsia (toxemia of pregnancy), lead toxicity. *Drug Influence:* allopurinol, acetazolamide (Diamox), salicylates (prolonged low doses), triamterene

Elevated Level: gout, high-purine diet, leukemias (lymphocytic, myelocytic), polycythemia vera, Fanconi's syndrome, neurologic disorders (cerebral hemorrhage, cerebral thrombosis, brain infarction, cerebral embolism, encephalomyelitis), psychiatric disorders (manic-depressive disease, paranoid states, depressive neurosis), ulcerative colitis, viral hepatitis, x-ray therapy, febrile illnesses. *Drug Influence:* bishydroxycoumarin, corticosteroids, cytotoxic agents (treatment for cancer), probenecid (Benemid), salicylates (high doses)

Procedure

- Collect a 24-hour sample in a large container and refrigerate. A preservative in the container may be necessary. Check with the laboratory on the need for preservative.
- Label the container with the patient's name and the dates and times of urine collection (e.g., 9/23/93, 7:11 AM to 9/24/93, 7:11 AM).
- A diet low or high in purines may be ordered before and/or during the time of urine collection.
- There is no drink restriction.

- Factors Affecting Laboratory Results

  - Drugs (*See Drug Influence above.*)
  - A high- or low-purine diet
  - Excessive x-ray exposure
  - Febrile illnesses

NURSING IMPLICATIONS WITH RATIONALE

- Monitor urinary output. Poor urine output could indicate inadequate fluid intake or poor kidney function.
- Compare the serum uric acid level with the urine acid level. An elevated serum uric acid level (hyperuricemia) and a decreased urine uric acid level can indicate kidney dysfunction. Increased serum and urine uric acid levels are frequently seen in gout, so it is important to obtain both the urine and serum values.
- Check the urine pH, especially if hyperuremia is present. Uric stones can occur when the urine pH is low (acidic). Alkaline urine helps to prevent stones in the urinary tract.

Patient Teaching

- Explain to the patient the purpose of and procedure for the test. Explain to the patient and family that all urine should be saved for 24 hours. Tell the patient not to put feces or toilet paper in the urine.

■ Instruct the patient as to which foods to avoid before and during the test, as ordered by the physician.

URINALYSIS (ROUTINE)
(Color, Appearance, Odor, Foam, pH, Specific Gravity, Protein, Glucose, Ketones, RBC, WBC, and Casts)

Reference Values

	ADULT	NEWBORN	CHILD
Color	Light straw to dark amber		Light straw to dark yellow
Appearance	Clear	Clear	Clear
Odor	Aromatic		Aromatic
Foam	White (small amount)		White (small amount)
pH	4.5–8.0 Average is 6	5–7	4.5–8
Specific gravity (SG)	1.005–1.030 (1.015–1.024, normal fluid intake)	1.001–1.020	1.005–1.030
Protein	(2–8 mg/100 mL— negative reagent strip test		
Glucose	Negative		Negative
Ketones	Negative		Negative
Microscopic examination			
RBC	1–2 per low power field		Rare
WBC	3–4		0–4
Casts	Occasional hyaline		Rare

Description

Urinalysis is a physical, chemical, and microscopic analysis of the urine. Routine urine tests were performed as early as 1821. Until recently urine was manually tested for individual constituents, but now multiple-reagent strips are used for quick chemical screening.

Urinalysis is useful for diagnosing renal disease or urinary tract infection and for detecting metabolic disease not related to the kidneys. Many routine urinalyses are done in the physician's office as well as in the hospital or in a private laboratory. The color, appearance, odor, and foam of the urine are examined, and the pH, protein, glucose ketones, and bilirubin are tested with the reagent strips. Specific gravity is measured with a urinometer, and a microscopic examination of the urinary sediment is performed to detect RBCs, WBCs, casts, crystals, and bacteria.[1,5,7,9,10,12–14]

Clinical Problems

PROPERTY OR CONSTITUENT	CLINICAL CONDITIONS/ PROBLEMS	COMMENTS
Color		
Colorless (very pale)	Large fluid intake Diabetes insipidus Chronic kidney disease Alcohol ingestion Nervousness	A pale color usually indicates diluted urine, and dark yellow or amber indicates concentrated urine.

Red or red-brown	Hemoglobinuria
	Porphyrins
	Menstrual contamination
	Drug influence
	  Sulfisoxazole with
	    phenazopyridine
	    (Azogantrisin)
	  Phenytoin (Dilantin)
	  Cascara
	  Chlorpromazine (Thorazine)
	  Docusate Ca (Doxidan)
	  Phenolphthalein (Ex-Lax)
	Foods
	  Beets
	  Rhubarb
	  Food color
		Drugs and foods will change the color of the urine.

Orange	Restricted fluid intake
	Concentrated urine
	Excess sweating
	Fever
	Drug influence
	  Amidopyrine
	  Furazolidone (Furoxone)
	  Nitrofurantoin
	  Phenazopyridine
	    (Pyridium)
	  Sulfonamides
	Foods and others
	  Carrots (carotene)
	  Rhubarb
	  Food color
	  Bilirubin	

Blue or green	*Pseudomonas* toxemia
	Drug influence
	  Amitriptyline (Elavil)
	  Methylene blue
	  Methocarbamol (Robaxin)
	  Vitamin B complex
	  Yeast concentrate	

Brown or black	Lysol poisoning Melanin Bilirubin	

(continued)

PROPERTY OR CONSTITUENT	CLINICAL CONDITIONS/ PROBLEMS	COMMENTS
	Methemoglobin	
	Porphyrin	
	Drug influence	
	Cascara	
	Chloroquine (Aralen)	
	Iron injectable compounds	
Appearance		
Hazy, cloudy	Bacteria	
	Pus, tissue	
	RBCs	
	WBCs	
	Phosphates	
	Prostatic fluid	
	Spermatozoa	
	Urates, uric acid	
Milky	Fat	
	Pyuria	
Odor		
Ammonia	Urea breakdown by bacteria	
Foul or putrid	Bacteria (UTI)	
Mousey	Phenylketonuria	
Sweet or fruity	Diabetic acidosis (ketoacidosis)	
	Starvation	
Foam		
Yellow—large	Severe cirrhosis of the liver	
amounts	Bilirubin or bile pigment	
pH		
<4.5	Metabolic acidosis	
	Respiratory acidosis	
	Starvation	
	Diarrhea	
	Diet high in meat protein and/ or cranberries	
	Drug influence	
	Ammonium chloride	
	Methenamine mandelate (mandelic acid)	
>8.0	Bacteriuria	
	Urinary tract infection due to *Pseudomonas* or *Proteus*	
	Drug influence	
	Antibiotics	
	Kanamycin	
	Neomycin	
	Streptomycin	
	Sulfonamides	
	Excess salicylates (aspirin)	
	Sodium bicarbonate	
	Acetazolamide (Diamox)	
	Potassium citrate	

PROPERTY OR CONSTITUENT	CLINICAL CONDITIONS/ PROBLEMS	COMMENTS
	Diet	
	High in citrus fruits	
	High in vegetables	
Specific gravity (SG)		
<1.005	Diabetes insipidus	Low, fixed SG can indicate kid-
	Excess fluid intake	ney disease because of in-
	Overhydration	ability to concentrate urine.
	Renal disease	
	Glomerulonephritis	
	Pyelonephritis	
	Polycystic disease	
	Severe potassium deficit	
>1.026	Decreased fluid intake	
	Fever	
	Administration of IV	
	dextran, albumin	
	Diabetes mellitus	
	Vomiting, diarrhea	
	Dehydration	
	X-ray contrast media	
Protein		
>8 mg/dL or	Proteinuria	Proteinuria is a sensitive indi-
>80 mg/24 h	Mild, transitory	cator of kidney dysfunction.
	Protein	
	Exercise	
	Severe stress	
	Cold baths	
	Fever	
	Acute infectious diseases	
	Renal disease	
	Glomerulonephritis	
	Nephrotic syndrome	
	Polycystic kidney	
	Lupus erythematosus	
	Leukemia	
	Multiple myeloma	
	Cardiac disease	
	Toxemia of pregnancy	
	Septicemia	
	Materials	
	Arsenic	
	Mercury	
	Lead	
	Carbon tetrachloride	
	Drug influence	
	Barbiturates	
	Neomycin	
	Massive doses of penicillin	
	Sulfonamides	
<2 mg/dL	Very diluted urine	

(continued)

PROPERTY OR CONSTITUENT	CLINICAL CONDITIONS/ PROBLEMS	COMMENTS
Glucose		

>15 mg/dL (random) or +4	Diabetes mellitus
	CNS disorders
	  Stroke (CVA)
	  Meningitis
	Cushing's syndrome
	Anesthesia
	Glucose infusions
	Severe stress
	Infections
	Drug influence
	  (false positive results)
	Ascorbic acid
	Aspirin
	Cephalothin (Keflin)
	Streptomycin
	Epinephrine
		The renal threshold for blood glucose is 160–180 mg/dL.
		
		Tes-tape should be used in place of Clinitest when the patient is receiving drugs.

Ketones Positive +1 to +3	*See Ketone Bodies, Acetone* Ketoacidosis Starvation A diet high in protein and low in carbohydrates	Acetest or Ketostix should be tested when Clinitest or Tes-tape is tested.

Microscopic Examination of Urinary Sediment
RBCs:
  RBCs and RBC
  casts
>2 per low power field
	Trauma to the kidney
	
	Renal disease
	  Pyelonephritis
	  Glomerulonephritis
	  Hydronephrosis
	Renal calculi
	Cystitis
	Lupus nephritis
	  (collagen disease)
	Aspirins (excess)
	Anticoagulants
	Sulfonamides
	Menstrual contamination	

WBCs:
  WBC and WBC
  casts >4 per low power field
	Urinary tract infection
	Fever
	Strenuous exercise
	Lupus nephritis
	Renal diseases
		If WBC are present in the urine, a urine culture should be done.

Casts:	Fever Renal disease Heart failure	

Procedure

- Collect a freshly voided urine specimen, approximately 50 mL or more, in a clean, dry container and take it to the laboratory within 30 minutes. An early morning urine specimen collected before breakfast is preferred. The urine specimen could be refrigerated for 6 to 8 hours.
- A clean-caught or midstream urine specimen could be requested if WBC are in the urine or if bacteria are suspected.
- There is no food or fluid restriction unless the urinalysis is to be done in the early morning.

- Factors Affecting Laboratory Results

  - A urine specimen that has been sitting for an hour or longer without refrigeration
  - Drugs and foods (*See Clinical Problems.*)
  - Feces or toilet paper in the urine

NURSING IMPLICATIONS WITH RATIONALE

- Assist the patient with the urine collection as needed.
- Obtain a history of any drugs the patient is currently taking. Such drugs as cascara, Azo gantrisin, nitrofurantoin, Thorazine, sulfonamides, Elavil, Ex-Lax, Pyridium, and others cause a discoloration of the urine. These should be noted on the laboratory slip.
- Assess the fluid status of the patient. Urine should be concentrated if the urine specimen is obtained in the morning or if the patient has a decreased fluid intake or is dehydrated. An increase in fluid intake will dilute the urine contents.
- Obtain a history of an excess amount of a certain food (eg, carrots, rhubarb, beets) that can cause a change in the urine color or of foods (eg, excess amounts of meat, cranberry juice) that could lower the urine pH (acidic).

Patient Teaching

- Explain to the patient the procedure for collecting the urine. Inform the hospitalized patient that an early morning urine specimen taken before breakfast is needed. Instruct the patient that approximately one third or one half of a small container or urine is needed. Have the patient void in a clean, dry container or a clean urinal or bedpan that can be poured into the container. Inform the patient not to put feces or toilet paper in the urine. The urine specimen should be taken to the laboratory within 30 minutes or refrigerated.
- Instruct the patient at home to place the fresh morning urine specimen in the refrigerator. The urine specimen, however, should be taken to the laboratory within an hour. Urine is an excellent medium for the growth of bacteria, and the bacterial growth begins approximately one-half hour

after collection. Refrigeration may help to retard growth for a short period of time.

■ Explain to the patient the procedure for a clean-catch or midstream urine collection (*see Cultures*). This procedure may be requested when culture of the urine is needed as well as for urinalysis.

UROBILINOGEN (URINE)

Reference Values

Adult: Random: 0.3–3.5 mg/dL. *2-Hour Specimen:* 0.3–1.0 Ehrlich units. *24-Hour Specimen:* 0.05–2.5 mg/24 h, 0.5–4.0 Ehrlich units/24 h, 0.09–4.23 μmol/24 h (SI units)

Child: similar to adult

Description

Bile, which is formed mostly from conjugated bilirubin, reaches the duodenum, where the intestinal bacteria change the bilirubin to urobilinogen. Most of the urobilinogen is lost in the feces; a large amount goes back to the liver through the blood stream, where it is reprocessed to bile; and approximately 1 percent is excreted by the kidneys in the urine.

The urobilinogen test is one of the most sensitive tests for determining liver damage, hemolytic disease, and severe infections. In early hepatitis, mild liver cell damage, or mild toxic injury, the urine urobilinogen level will increase despite an unchanged serum bilirubin level. The urobilinogen level will frequently decrease with severe liver damage, since less bile will be produced. The urobilinogen test might be performed with the urinalysis.[9,10,12,13]

Clinical Problems

Decreased Level: biliary obstruction, severe liver disease, cancer of the pancreas, severe inflammatory disease, cholelithiasis, severe diarrhea. *Drug Influence:* antibiotics (decreasing gut bacteria), ammonium chloride, ascorbic acid (vitamin C)

Elevated Level (>3.5 mg/dL [adult, random]): infectious hepatitis, toxic hepatitis, cirrhosis of the liver (early and recovery stages), hemolytic anemia, pernicious anemia, erythroblastosis fetalis, sickle cell anemia, infectious mononucleosis. *Drug Influence:* sulfonamides, phenothiazines, acetazolamide (Diamox), cascara, phenazopyridine (Pyridium), methenamine mandelate (Mandelamine), procaine, sodium bicarbonate

Procedure

■ There is no food or fluid restriction.

Single Specimen
- The single urine specimen should be fresh and should be tested immediately. This may be done as part of the routine urinalysis. A reagent color dipstick is dipped in the urine and is compared to a color chart, in Ehrlich units.

2-Hour Urine Specimen
- Collect 2-hour specimen between 1 and 3 PM or between 2 PM and 4 PM, since urobilinogen peaks in the afternoon. Urine should be kept refrigerated or in a dark container. Urine should be tested within one-half hour, since urine urobilinogen oxidizes to urobilin (orange substance).
- Label the container and laboratory slip with the exact time the urine was collected.

24-Hour Urine Specimen
- Discard the first urine specimen and then start urine collection.
- Collect 24-hour urine specimen, place in a large container, and keep refrigerated. A preservative may be added to the container. Keep urine collection from the light.
- Label the container with the patient's name, date, and time of urine collection.
- Withhold patient's medications that affect test results for 24 hours or until after the test, with the physician's permission. If drugs are given, list the drugs on the laboratory slip.

- Factors Affecting Laboratory Results

  - Antibiotics decrease the bacterial flora in the intestine
  - Certain drugs increase the urine urobilinogen level (*See Drug Influence.*)
  - pH changes (strongly acidic urine) could cause a decreased urobilinogen level, and strongly alkaline urine could cause an elevated level. Urine sitting for ½ hour or longer may become alkaline.
  - The urobilinogen level is highest in the afternoon and evening. The 2-hour urine specimen is frequently collected in the afternoon.

NURSING IMPLICATIONS WITH RATIONALE

- Explain to the patient the procedure for collecting a 2-hour urine specimen or a 24-hour urine specimen. The bladder should be emptied before starting the 2-hour or 24-hour urine test. Inform the patient that all urine must be saved during the specified time.
- Keep the collected urine from light in a urine container with a preservative. Refrigerate.
- Label the container and laboratory slip with the exact times urine collection begins and ends (after the last voiding).

Decreased Level

- Relate clinical problems and drugs to decreased urine urobilinogen. Most antibiotics will reduce the bacterial flora in the intestines, thus decreasing the formation of urobilinogen.

Elevated Level

- Check for an elevated urobilinogen level in freshly voided urine with a reagent color dipstick. Record the results of the single test. Note if the patient is receiving drugs that could elevate the urobilinogen level.
- Assess for signs and symptoms of jaundice (yellow sclera, skin on the forearm is yellow).

VANILLYLMANDELIC ACID (VMA) (URINE)

Reference Values

Adult: 1.5–7.5 mg/24 h, 7.6–37.9 μ/24 h (SI units)

Child: adolescent: 1–5 mg/24 h

Description

VMA is the major by-product of catecholamines (epinephrine and norepinephrine). An elevated level of VMA excretion might indicate severe hypertension, tumors of the adrenal medulla (pheochromocytoma in the adult and neuroblastoma and ganglioneuroblastoma in the child). Other methods should be used to verify positive VMA results, such as urine catecholamine.

The VMA test is a simple screening method. However, many foods (bananas, tea, coffee, chocolate, carbonated drinks, etc) and drugs (aspirin, sulfonamides, some cough medicines, and others) produce false-positive results.[10,12,13]

Clinical Problems

Decreased: uremia. *Drug Influence:* clofibrate; antihypertensives (guanethidine [Ismelin], methyldopa [Aldomet], reserpine [Serpasil]), monamine (MAO) inhibitors

Elevated level: pheochromocytoma, neuroblastoma, ganglioblastoma, myasthenia gravis, muscular dystrophy (progressive), physical and mental stress. *Foods:* fruits (banana), fruit juices, chocolate, tea, coffee, carbonated drinks (except ginger ale), vanilla and vanilla products, candy, mints, jelly, cheese, gelatins, and cough drops. *Drug Influence:* salicylates (aspirin), sulfonamides, penicillin, chlorpromazine (Thorazine), isoproterenol (Isuprel), levodopa, lithium carbonate, nitroglycerin, glyceryl guaiacolate, methenamine (Mandelamine), methocarbamol (Robaxin)

Procedure

- No drugs should be taken for 3 days before the test, *if possible,* especially those listed under *Drug Influence.*
- Insert 10 mL of concentrated hydrochloric acid (HCl) in a large bottle. Some laboratories do not require that a preservative be added to the bottle.
- Label the bottle and laboratory slip with the patient's name, dates, and times

the urine collection started and ended. Keep the bottle refrigerated during the 24-hour collection time.

■ Those foods listed under *Clinical Problems* above should be omitted from the diet for 3 days before the test. Other foods and fluid are not restricted.

■ Factors Affecting Laboratory Results

■ Drugs (*See Drug Influence.*)
■ Food (*See Clinical Problems.*)
■ Strenuous exercise will elevate VMA levels.
■ Stress will elevate VMA levels.

NURSING IMPLICATIONS WITH RATIONALE

■ Monitor vital signs, especially BP. Maintain a BP chart.

Patient Teaching

■ Explain to the patient and family that all urine excreted over the 24-hour period must be saved and kept refrigerated. Inform the patient not to put toilet paper or feces in the urine.
■ Instruct the patient not to eat the foods listed under *Clinical problems* above for 3 days before the test. Write the restricted foods on a piece of paper for the patient's reference.
■ Explain to the patient that he or she should eat well-balanced meals. Starvation or severe lack of food could increase the VMA levels.
■ Encourage the patient to avoid emotional stress and physical activity. Stress and activity increase VMA levels. Encourage the patient to rest during the test.

VDRL (VENEREAL DISEASE RESEARCH LABORATORY) (SERUM)
VDRL Screening Test

Reference Values

Adult: nonreactive
Child: nonreactive

Description

Syphilis, a venereal disease caused by the spirochete *Treponema pallidum,* is usually transmitted through sexual contact. There are stages of syphilis (primary, secondary, and tertiary) that left untreated, could lead to death.

■ *Primary Stage: Duration After Contact:* 3 to 6 weeks. A chancre develops approximately 3 weeks after contact. Spirochetes in the exudate of the chancre lesion (sore) may be visualized with dark-field microscopy. Chancres are generally found in genital areas and in the mouth or on the lips.

■ *Secondary Stage: Duration After Contact:* 2 weeks to 6 months. Secondary lesions are highly contagious and at times may be visualized on dark-field microscopy. The lesions are usually red papular or "snail track" ulcers and may be seen anywhere on the body, especially in the palms of the hands and the soles of the feet. A relapse may occur in 2 to 4 years; this is called latent syphilis. The patient may have a low fever.

■ *Tertiary Stage: Duration After Contact:* 4 to 20 years. This is referred to as late syphilis. Untreated syphilis (tertiary stage) normally does not have clinical signs; however, it does affect the person's cardiovascular system and CNS. The person may develop cardiac valvular disease, aneurysms, general paresis, blindness, slurred speech, delusions, and "insanity."

Two groups of blood tests are used to identify the spirochete *T pallidum:* the nontreponemal antibody test (VDRL and RPR) and the treponemal antibody test (FTA-ABS, TPI).

The VDRL test is useful for detecting primary syphilis 1 to 3 weeks after the presence of a primary lesion and for detecting secondary syphilis.

T pallidum stimulates the development of nonspecific reaginic antibodies in the serum. If these antibodies are present and react with a lipid antigen (cardiolipin), the VDRL test is positive or reactive. A titer about 1:32 can indicate the secondary stage. With tertiary stage syphilis, the VDRL test is not sensitive and may fail to react or may produce variable titers.

The results of the VDRL test may be negative in the early infectious phase of syphilis or could produce biologic false positives (BFP) because of other acute or chronic diseases. If the VDRL test is negative, weekly VDRL tests may be indicated. RPR (rapid plasma reagin) may be used first as a screening test for syphilis.[1,8,10,12,18]

Clinical Problems

Nonreactive (negative): *False Negatives:* early primary stage of syphilis, tertiary stage of syphilis

Reactive (positive): syphilis—*T pallidum* organism. *False Positives* (*return to nonreactive within 6 months*): tuberculosis, pneumonia, infectious mononucleosis, chicken pox, smallpox vaccination (recent), subacute bacterial endocarditis, leprosy. *False Positives* (*chronic; persist longer than 6 months*): malaria, Hashimoto's thyroiditis, rheumatoid arthritis, progressive systemic sclerosis, systemic lupus erythematosus, hepatitis

Procedure

■ Collect 5 mL of venous blood in a red-top tube. Avoid hemolysis.
■ There is no food or fluid restriction; however, some laboratories require NPO, so check with the laboratory. Alcohol should not be consumed for 24 hours before the VDRL test.

■ Factors Affecting Laboratory Results

■ Hemolysis of the blood sample could affect test result.
■ Alcoholic intake decreases the test reaction.

NURSING IMPLICATIONS WITH RATIONALE

■ Instruct the patient not to drink alcohol for 24 hours prior to the test. If the patient has consumed alcohol, the test may be postponed for 24 hours.
■ Obtain a history of any acute or chronic disease. Related BFP may occur with certain diseases (*see Clinical Problems*).
■ List present acute and/or chronic diseases in the patient's chart and on the laboratory slip and notify the physician.
■ Interpretation of tests for syphilis requires skill and experience.

Nonreactive (negative)

■ Relate a nonreactive VDRL test result to false-negative causes if the history and symptoms are suggestive of syphilis. Test should be repeated weekly for several weeks. Nonreactive (negative) results can occur in the early primary stage of syphilis.

Reactive (positive)

■ Relate a reactive VDRL test result to a positive indication of syphilis or a possible false positive due to acute or chronic diseases (*see Clinical Problems*). If the history is suggestive of syphilis but an acute or chronic disease is present, the FTA-ABS or TPI test may be performed.
■ Check with the patient about receiving treatment for syphilis. If primary syphilis persists for weeks before treatment, the VDRL test could remain positive for up to 6 months after treatment. The test results after treatment for secondary syphilis could remain positive for 12 to 18 months. The history of treatment (where, when, how long, and what drugs) is extremely important. The health department should be notified when there is a positive test result.
■ Be supportive of the patient. Be willing to listen, and do not make a judgment concerning the patient's life-style.
■ Elicit from the patient his or her contacts (friends) so that they can be properly tested and treated. Explain the importance of preventing the transmission of the disease.
■ Refer the patient to a veneral disease clinic if one is available (with the physician's permission). Many clinics have case workers and a good follow-up care program.
■ Emphasize the importance of follow-up care. Frequently patients are checked every 3 months for 2 years as a preventive measure for detecting a relapse (syphilis).
■ Observe for signs and symptoms of tertiary (late) syphilis (*see Descrip-*

tion). These signs and symptoms should be documented and reported. The VDRL test is usually negative with tertiary syphilis.

VITAMIN B$_{12}$ (SERUM)

Reference Values

Adult: 200–900 pg/mL

Description

Vitamin B$_{12}$ is essential for RBC maturation and for GI and neurologic function. The extrinsic factor of vitamin B$_{12}$ is obtained from foods and is absorbed in the small intestines when the intrinsic factor is present. The intrinsic factor is produced by the gastric mucosa, and when this factor is missing, pernicious anemia, a megaloblastic anemia, develops.[3,6,9,13]

Clinical Problems

Decreased level: pernicious anemia, malabsorption syndrome, liver diseases, hypothyroidism(myxedema), pancreatic insufficiency, sprue, Crohn's disease, gastrectomy. *Drug Influence:* neomycin, metformin, anticonvulsants, ethanol

Elevated Level: acute hepatitis, acute and chronic myelocytic leukemia, polycythemia vera. *Drug Influence:* oral contraceptives

Procedure

- Collect 5 to 7 mL of venous blood in a red-top tube. Avoid hemolysis.
- There is no food or fluid restriction.

- Factors Affecting Laboratory Results

  - Drugs (*See Drug influences.*)
  - Hemolysis of the blood specimen

NURSING IMPLICATIONS WITH RATIONALE

- Assess for signs and symptoms of pernicious anemia, such as, pallor; fatigue; dyspnea; sore mouth; smooth, beefy-red tongue; indigestion; tingling, numbness in the hands and feet; and behavioral changes.

Patient Teaching

- Instruct the patient to eat foods high in vitamin B$_{12}$, such as milk, eggs, meat, and liver. Contact the dietitian to assist the patient in meal planning. Intramuscular vitamin B$_{12}$ may be ordered.

WHITE BLOOD CELLS (WBC) TOTAL (BLOOD)
Leukocytes

Reference Values

Adult: Total WBC count: 4500–10,000 μL (mm^3)

Child: Newborn: 9000–30,000 μL. *2 years:* 6000–17,000 μL

Description

(*See WBC Differential.*)

WBCs, or leukocytes, are divided into two groups: the polymorphonuclear leukocytes (neutrophils, eosinophils, and basophils) and the mononuclear leukocytes (monocytes and lymhocytes). Leukocytes are a part of the body's defense system; they respond immediately to foreign invaders by going to the site of involvement. An increase in WBCs is called leukocytosis, and a decrease in WBCs is called leukopenia.[1,5,10,12,23]

Clinical Problems

Decreased Level: hematopoietic diseases (aplastic anemia, pernicious anemia, hypersplenism, Gaucher's disease), viral infections, malaria, agranulocytosis, alcoholism, systemic lupus erythematosus (SLE), rheumatoid arthritis. *Drug Influence:* antibiotics (pencillins, cephalothins, chloramphenicol), acetaminophen (Tylenol), sulfonamides, propylthiouracil, barbiturates, cancer chemotherapy agents, diazepam (Valium), diuretics (furosemide [Lasix], ethacrynic acid [Edecrin]), chlordiazepoxide (Librium), oral hypoglycemic agents, indomethacin (Indocin), methyldopa (Aldomet), rifampin, phenothiazine

Elevated Level: acute infection (pneumonia, meningitis, appendicitis, colitis, peritonitis, pancreatitis, pyelonephritis, tuberculosis, tonsillitis, diverticulitis, septicemia, rheumatic fever), tissue necrosis (myocardial infarction, cirrhosis of the liver, burns, cancer of the organs, emphysema, peptic ulcer), leukemias, collagen diseases, hemolytic and sickle cell anemias, parasitic diseases, stress (surgery, fever, long-lasting emotional upset). *Drug Influence:* aspirin, heparin, digitalis, epinephrine, lithium, histamine, antibiotics (ampicillin, erythromycin, kanamycin, methicillin, tetracyclines, vancomycin, streptomycin), gold compounds, procainamide (Pronestyl), triamterene (Dyrenium), allopurinol, potassium iodide, hydantoin derivatives, sulfonamides (long acting)

Procedure

Venous Blood

■ Collect 7 mL of venous blood in a lavender-top tube. Avoid hemolysis.
■ There is no food or fluid restriction.

Capillary Blood

■ Collect blood from a finger puncture with a micropipette.
■ Dilute immediately with the proper reagent.

■ Factors Affecting Laboratory Results

  ■ Drugs that can increase and decrease the WBC count. (*See Drug Influence.*)
  ■ The time the blood sample was taken. The WBC count is lower in the morning than in the afternoon.
  ■ The age of the individual. Children can have a high WBC count, especially during the first 5 years of life.

NURSING IMPLICATIONS WITH RATIONALE

■ Check the vital signs and note if the temperature and pulse rate are increased. Also check for signs and symptoms of inflammation and infection, such as redness, heat, swelling, drainage at tissue site.
■ Notify the physician of changes in the patient's condition, such as fever, increased pulse and respiration rate, and leukocytosis.

Patient Teaching

■ Instruct the patient to check the side effects of patent medicines, such as cold medications, which could cause agranulocytosis, severe leukopenia. With agranulocytosis, the major defense system is lost, and the patient is susceptible to severe or long-lasting infection.
■ Instruct patients with leukopenia to avoid persons with any contagious condition. Their body resistances are reduced, and they are prime candidates for severe colds or infections.

WHITE BLOOD CELL DIFFERENTIAL (BLOOD)
Differential WBC

Reference Values

	DIFFERENTIAL WBC VALUES		
	ADULT		CHILD
WBC TYPE	**%**	**μL (mm^3)**	**Same as adult except**
Neutrophils (total)	50–70	2500–7000	*Newborn:* 61%. *1-year-old:* 32%
Segments	50–65	2500–6500	
Bands	0–5	0–500	
Eosinophils	1–3	100–300	
Basophils	0.4–1.0	40–100	
Monocytes	4–6	200–600	*1 to 12 years:* 4%–9%
Lymphocytes	25–35	1700–3500	*Newborn:* 34%. *1 year:* 60%
			6 years: 42%. *12 years:* 38%

Description

(See White Blood Cells [WBCs].)

Differential WBC count, part of the CBC, is composed of five types of WBC (leukocytes): neutrophils, eosinophils, basophils, monocytes, and lymphocytes. The differential WBC count is expressed as cubic millimeters (mm^3, μL) and percent of the total number of WBC. Neutrophils and lymphocytes make up 80% to 90% of the total WBC. Differential WBC count provides more specific information related to infections and disease process.

■ *Neutrophils:* Neutrophils are the most numerous circulating WBC, and they respond more rapidly to the inflammatory and tissue injury sites than other types of WBC. During an *acute* infection, the neutrophils are the body's first line of defense. The segments are mature neutrophils, and the bands are immature ones that multiply quickly during an acute infection.

■ *Eosinophils:* Eosinophils increase during allergic and parasitic conditions. With an increase in steroids, either produced by the adrenal glands during stress or administered orally or by injection, eosinophils decrease in number.

■ *Basophils:* Basophils increase during the healing process. With an increase in steroids, the basophil count will decrease.

■ *Monocytes:* Monocytes are the second line of defense against bacterial infections and foreign substances. They are stronger than neutrophils and can ingest larger particles of debris. Monocytes respond late during the acute phase of infection and inflammatory process, and they continue to function during the chronic phase of phagocytes.

■ *Lymphocytes:* Increased lymphocytes (lymphocytosis) occur in chronic and viral infections. Severe lymphocytosis is commonly caused by chronic lymphocytic leukemia. Lymphocytes play a major role in the immune response system as B lymphocytes and T lymphocytes. Like eosinophils, lymphocytes decrease in number during excess adrenocortical hormone secretion or steroid therapy.[5,8–10,23]

Clinical Problems

Decreased Level

Neutrophils: viral diseases, leukemias (lymphocytic and monocytic), agranulocytosis, aplastic and iron deficiency anemias. *Drug Influence:* antibiotic therapy, immunosuppressive agents. *Eosinophils:* Stress: burns, shock; adrenocortical hyperfunction. *Drug Influence:* cortisone, ACTH. *Basophils:* stress, hypersensitivity reaction, pregnancy, hyperthyroidism. *Monocytes:* lymphocytic leukemia, aplastic anemia. *Lymphocytes:* cancer, leukemia, adrenocortical hyperfunction, agranulocytosis, aplastic anemia, multiple sclerosis, renal failure, nephrotic syndrome, systemic lupus erythematosus (SLE)

Elevated Level

Neutrophils: acute infections (localized and systemic), inflammatory diseases (rheumatoid arthritis, gout, pneumonia), tissue damage (acute myocardial infarction, burns, crushed injury, surgery), Hodgkin's disease, myelocytic leukemia, hemolytic disease of newborns, acute cholecystitis, acute appendicitis, acute pancreatitis. *Drug Influence:* epinephrine, digitalis, heparin, sulfonamides, lithium, cortisone, ACTH. *Eosinophils:* allergies, parasitic disease, cancer (bone, ovary testes, brain), phlebitis, thrombophlebitis, asthma, emphysema, renal disease (renal failure, nephrotic syndrome). *Basophils:* inflammatory process, leukemia, healing stage of infection or inflammation, acquired hemolytic anemia. *Monocytes:* viral diseases (infectious mononucleosis, mumps, herpes zoster), parasitic diseases (Rocky Mountain spotted fever, toxoplasmosis, brucellosis), monocytic leukemia, cancer (esophagus, stomach, colon, liver, bone, prostate, uterus, brain, bladder), anemias (sickle cell, hemolytic), collagen diseases (SLE), rheumatoid arthritis, ulcerative colitis. *Lymphocytes:* lymphocytic leukemia, viral infections (infectious mononucleosis, hepatitis, mumps, rubella, viral pneumonia, pertussis), chronic infections, Hodgkin's disease, multiple myeloma, adrenocortical hypofunction

Procedure

- Collect 7 mL of venous blood in a lavender-top tube. Avoid hemolysis.
- There is no food or fluid restriction.
- If eosinophils value is needed, record the time that the blood sample was drawn. If drawn in the afternoon or evening, the count could be slightly higher.

- **Factors Affecting Laboratory Results**

  - Steroids could decrease eosinophil and lymphocyte values.
  - Certain drugs can increase or decrease blood values (*See Drug Influence.*)

NURSING IMPLICATIONS

- Check the WBC count and the differential WBC count. Elevated neutrophils may be indicative of an acute infection. Elevated eosinophils may be a sign of allergy. Increased basophils can be caused by the healing process. Increased monocytes occur during a bacterial infection, and increased lymphocytes occur in chronic or viral infections.
- Assess the patient for signs and symptoms of an infection, such as elevated temperature, increased pulse rate, edema, redness, and exudate (wound drainage).
- Assess the patient for signs and symptoms of allergies, such as tearing, "runny nose," rash, and more severe reactions.
- Assess for signs and symptoms of healing, such as ability to increase movement at the injured site, and decreased edema and exudate.

Patient Teaching

- Instruct the patient to report any signs and symptoms of infection, such as the presence of a fever.
- Encourage the patient to rest, take medications such as antibiotics as prescribed, increase fluid intake as appropriate, and monitor temperature.

Laboratory Tests

REFERENCES

1. Byrne, D.J., Saxton, D.F., & Pelikan, P.K. *Laboratory tests* (2nd ed.). Reading, Mass: Addison-Wesley, 1986.
2. Govoni, L.E. & Hayes, J.E. *Drugs and nursing implications* (6th ed.). Norwalk, Conn: Appleton & Lange, 1988.
3. Jacobs, D.S. *Laboratory test handbook* (2nd ed.). St. Louis, Mo: Mosby, 1988.
4. Wiener, M.B., & Pepper, G.A. *Clinical pharmacology and therapeutics in nursing* (2nd ed.). New York: McGraw-Hill, 1985.
5. Brunner, L.S., & Suddarth, D.S. *Textbook of medical-surgical nursing* (6th ed.). Philadelphia, Pa: Lippincott, 1988.
6a. Billet, E.T., & Welch, M. J. (1979). The use of clinical laboratory findings in diagnosing and managing critically ill children. *Critical Care Quarterly, 2* (3), 19–35.
6b. Corbett, J.V. *Laboratory tests and diagnostic procedures with nursing diagnoses* (2nd ed.). Norwalk, Conn: Appleton & Lange, 1987.
7. Wallach, J. *Interpretation of diagnostic tests* (5th ed.). Boston, Ma: Little, Brown, 1986.
8. Widmann, F. *Clinical interpretation of laboratory tests* (9th ed.). Philadelphia, Pa: Davis, 1983.
9. *Diagnostic tests handbook*. Springhouse, Penn: Springhouse Corp, 1987.
10. Fischbach, F. A. *A manual of laboratory diagnostic tests* (3rd ed.). Philadelphia, Pa: Lippincott, 1988.
11. Henry, J.B. *Todd-Sanford-Davidsohn: Clinical diagnosis and management by laboratory methods* (17th ed.). Philadelphia, Pa: Saunders, 1984.
12. Tilkian, S.M., Conover, M.B., & Tilkian, A.G. *Clinical implications of laboratory tests* (4th ed.). St. Louis, Mo: Mosby, 1989.
13. Ravel, R. *Clinical laboratory medicine* (5th ed.). Chicago, Ill: Year Book Medical Publishers, 1989.
14. Linne, J.J., & Lingsrud, K.M. *Basic techniques for medical laboratory* (2nd ed.). New York: McGraw-Hill, 1979.
15. Reeder, S.J. *Maternity nursing* (15th ed.). Philadelphia, Pa: Lippincott, 1983.
16. Whaley, L.F., & Wong, D.L. *Nursing care of infants and children* (3rd ed.). St. Louis, Mo: Mosby, 1987.
17. Coulter, D.L. Valproic acid therapy in childhood epilepsy. *JAMA,* 1980, *244* (8), 785–788.
18. Phipps, W.J., Long, B.C., & Woods, N.F. *Medical-surgical nursing* (3 rd ed.). St. Louis, Mo: Mosby, 1987.
19. McFarland, M.B., & Grant, M.M. *Nursing implications of laboratory tests* (2nd ed.). New York: Wiley, 1988.
20. Kee, J.L. *Handbook of laboratory and diagnostic tests with nursing implications*. Norwalk, Conn: Appleton & Lange, 1990.

21. Tiongson, J.G., & Woods, A.L. Cardiac isoenzymes: Clinical implications and limitations. *Critical Care Quarterly,* 1979, *2* (3), 47–51.
22. Stark, J. BUN/creatinine: Your keys to kidney function. *Nursing'80 ,* 1980, *10* (5), 33–38.
23. Kee, J. L. Clinical implications of laboratory studies in critical care. *Critical Care Quarterly,* 1979, *2* (3), 1–17.
24. Kee, J.L. *Fluids and electrolytes with clinical applications* (4th ed.). New York: Wiley, 1986.
25. Tietz, N. *Clinical guide to laboratory tests.* Philadelphia, Pa: Saunders, 1983.
26. *Drug facts and comparisons.* Philadelphia, PA: Lippincott, 1989.
27. Rossi, L.P., & Antman, E.M. Calcium channel blockers. *American Journal of Nursing,* 1983, *83* (3), 382–387.
28. Cholesterol update. 1988, *1* (6), 7, 8.
29. Watson, J.E. The national cholesterol education program: The role of nursing. *Cardiovascular Nursing,* 1988, *24* (3), 13–17.
30. Abrams, D.I., Parker-Martin, J., & Unger, K.W. AIDS—:Caring for the dying patient. *Patient Care,* 1989, *23* (19), 22–36.
31. Abrams, D.I., Parker-Martin, J., & Unger, K.W. Psychosocial aspects of terminal AIDS. *Patient Care,* 1989, *23* (19), 41–60.
32. Adam, H. Introduction. In H. Adam (Ed.), *Pediatric AIDS* (pp. 2–3). *Report of the twentieth Ross round table on critical approaches to common pediatric problems.* Columbus, Oh: Ross Laboratories, 1989.
33. Bennett, J.A. AIDS: Epidemiologic update. *American Journal of Nursing,* 1985, *85* (9), 968–973.
34. Bennett, J.A. HTLV-III AIDS link. *American Journal of Nursing,* 1985, *85* (10), 1086–1089.
35. Finkbeiner, A. AIDS: Just the facts. *John Hopkins Magazine,* 1985, *27* (6), 22–28.
36. *Human T-Lymphotropic Virus, Type III, Abbott HTLV-III EIA.* Abbott Laboratories, Diagnostic Division, 1985.
37. Perdew, S. *Facts about AIDS: A guide for health care providers.* Philadelphia, Pa: Lippincott, 1990.
38. Population Information Program, Center for Communications Programs. Population reports: AIDS educations—A beginning. *Issues in World Health,* 1989 *17* (3), 1–32), Baltimore, Md: The Johns Hopkins University.
39. Elbaum, N. Detecting and correcting magnesium imbalance. *Nursing'77 ,* 1977, *7,* 34–35.
40a. Grant, M.M., & Winifred, M.K. Assessing a patient's hydration status. *American Journal of Nursing,* 1975, *75* (8), 1306–1311.
40b. Tripp, A. Hyper and hypocalcemia. *American Journal of Nursing,* 1976, *76* (7), 1142–1145.
41. Lancour, J. Two hormones: Regulators and fluid balance. *Nursing skillbook: Monitoring fluid and electrolytes precisely* (2nd ed., pp. 29–39). Horsham, Pa: Intermed Communications, 1983.
42. Schwartz, J.S. Understanding laboratory test results. *Medical Clinics of North America,* 1987, *71* (4), 639–652.
43. Kee, J.L. Implementing the diagnostic workup. In *Endocrine* (pp. 31–45) Springhouse, Pa: Springhouse Corp, 1984.

Part II

Diagnostic Tests

Acid Perfusion
Amniotic Fluid Analysis
Angiography (Angiogram)
Arthrography
Arthroscopy
Barium Enema
Bronchography (Bronchogram)
Bronchoscopy
Cardiac Catheterization
Cholangiography (IV), Percutaneous
  Cholangiography, T-Tube
  Cholangiography
Cholecystography (Oral)
Chorionic Villi Biopsy
Colonoscopy
Colposcopy
Computerized Tomography (CT)
  Scan, Computerized Axial Tomography (CAT)
Cystocopy, Cystography (Cystogram)
Echoencephalography
Electrocardiography
  (Electrocardiogram—ECG or EKG),
  Vectorcardiography
  (Vectorcardiogram—VCG)
Electroencephalography
  (Electroencephalogram—EEG)
Electromyography
  (Electromyogram—EMG)
Endoscopic Retrograde
  Cholangiopancreatography (ERCP)
Esophageal Acidity

Esophageal Manometry
Esophageal Studies
Esophagogastroduodenoscopy,
  Esophagogastroscopy
Fluoroscopy
Gastric Analysis (Basal and Stimulation) Tubeless Gastric Analysis
Gastrointestinal (GI) Series, Upper GI
  Series, Barium Swallow, Small Bowel
  Series, Hypotonic Duodenography
Gastroscopy
Hysterosalpingography
  (Hysterosalpingogram)
Intravenous Pyelography (IVP)
Lymphangiography
  (Lymphangiogram)
Magnetic Resonance Imaging (MRI)
Mammography (Mammogram)
Mediastinoscopy
Myelography (Myelogram)
Nephrotomography
Nuclear Scans (Bone, Brain, Heart,
  Kidney, Liver and Spleen, Lung, and
  Thyroid)
Papanicolaou Smear (Pap Smear)
Positron Emission Tomography (PET)
Proctosigmoidoscopy, Proctoscopy,
  Sigmoidoscopy
Pulmonary Function Tests
Radioactive Iodine (RAI) Uptake Test
Retrograde Pyelography (Retrograde
  Pyelogram)

Sex Chromatin Mass, Buccal Smear, Barr Body Analysis

Skin Tests (Tuberculin, Blastomycosis, Coccidioidomycosis, Histoplasmosis, Trichinosis, and Toxoplasmosis)

Stress/Exercise Testing (Stress Testing), Exercise Electrocardiology (Electrocardiogram—ECG), Exercise Thallium Perfusion Imaging Test (Thallium Stress Test)

Thermography (Breast)

Ultrasonography (Abdominal Aorta, Brain, Doppler—Arteries and Veins, Gallbladder, Heart, Kidney, Liver, Pregnant Uterus, Pancreas, Spleen, and Thyroid)

Venography (Lower Limb)

Ventilation Scan

X-Ray (Chest, Heart, Flat Plate of Abdomen, Kidney, Ureter, Bladder, and Skull)

ACID PERFUSION
(See Esophageal Studies.)

AMNIOTIC FLUID ANALYSIS
Amniocentesis, Amnioscopy

Normal Finding

Clear amniotic fluid, no chromosomal or neural tube abnormalities

Description

Amniotic fluid analysis is useful for detecting chromosomal abnormality, such as Down's syndrome or mongolism (trisomy 21); neural tube defects (spina bifida); sex-linked disorders, such as hemophilia; and for determining fetal maturity. The amniotic fluid is obtained by amniocentesis. This procedure includes an insertion of a needle into the suprapubic area after the fetus has been located and manually elevated and the aspiration of 5 to 15 mL of amniotic fluid. Ultrasound may be used to locate the placenta and fetal positions so that the needle contact can be avoided. Amniocentesis is performed during the 14th to 16th weeks of pregnancy. It usually is not done before the 14th week because of the insufficient amount of amniotic fluid or after the 16th week if a therapeutic abortion might be suggested.

Analyses of the amniotic fluid may also include color, bilirubin (present in the fluid until the 28th week but absent at full term), meconium (present during stress—eg, in breech presentation), creatinine, lecithin/sphingomyelin (L/S) ratio (a decreased ratio can indicate respiratory distress syndrome), glucose, lipids, and alpha-fetoprotein (AFP).

Amnioscopy involves insertion of a fiberoptic lighted instrument (amnioscope) into the cervical canal to visualize the amniotic fluid. The color of the amniotic fluid can indicate fetal hypoxia. This test is normally performed close to full term, since it requires cervical dilation. Because there is a risk of rupturing the amniotic membrane and of intrauterine infection, the test is rarely performed.[1-3]

Clinical Problems

Indications: to detect chromosomal disorders (eg, Down's syndrome), neural tube defects (eg, spina bifida), hemolytic disease due to Rh incompatibility; to determine fetal sex (important for sex-linked disorders—eg, hemophilia), fetal maturity, pulmonary maturity of the fetus (L/S ratio).

Procedure

- Obtain a signed consent form.
- Food and fluids are not restricted.

- Have the patient void before the procedure to prevent puncturing the bladder and aspirating urine.
- Cleanse the suprapubic area with an antiseptic such as, povidone-iodine (Betadine). A local anesthetic is injected at the site for the amniocentesis.
- The placenta and fetus should be located by ultrasound or manually (fetus only). A 22-gauge spinal needle with stylet is inserted through the skin to the amniotic cavity.
- Aspirate 5 to 15 mL of amniotic fluid. Apply a small dressing to the needle insertion site.
- The procedure takes approximately 30 minutes.

- Factors Affecting Diagnostic Results

  - A traumatic amniocentesis tap may produce blood in the amniotic fluid.

NURSING IMPLICATIONS WITH RATIONALE

- Recognize when amniocentesis for amniotic fluid analysis is indicated (ie, with a familial history of sex-linked, genetic, or chromosomal disorders; with a history of previous miscarriages; and in advanced maternal age [more than 35 years old]). It is not a screening test.
- Be sure that the patient urinates before the test and that the consent form is signed.
- Be supportive of the woman and her spouse. Be a good listener. Allow them time to ask questions and to express any concerns. Refer questions you cannot answer to the appropriate health professionals.

Patient Teaching

- Inform the patient that normal results, do not guarantee a normal infant, nor do they always predict sex correctly. The physician should tell the woman of potential risks, such as premature labor, spontaneous abortion, infection, and fetal or placental bleeding from the needle. These complications rarely occur, but the woman should be told of the risk factors.
- Instruct the patient to notify the physician immediately of any of the following: bleeding or leaking fluid from the vagina, abdominal pain or cramping, chills and fever, or lack of fetal movement.
- Encourage the woman and her spouse to seek genetic counseling, especially if chromosomal abnormality has been determined. Usually the final decision about terminating a pregnancy rests on the pregnant woman and her spouse.

ANGIOGRAPHY (ANGIOGRAM)

Arteriography: Cardiac (See Cardiac Catheterization.), Cerebral Angiography, Pulmonary Angiography, and Renal Angiography

Normal Finding

Normal structure and potency of the blood vessels

Description

The terms angiography (examination of the blood vessels) and arteriography (examination of the arteries) are used interchangeably. A catheter is inserted into either the femoral, brachial, or carotid artery, and a contrast dye is injected to allow visualization of the blood vessels. Normally the patient feels a warm, flushed sensation as the dye is injected. Angiographies are useful for evaluating patency of blood vessels and for identifying abnormal vascularization resulting from neoplasms (tumors). This test may be indicated when CT or radionuclide scanning suggests vascular abnormalities.

Cerebral Angiography: Any of the three arteries (femoral, brachial, or carotid) can be used. The dye will outline the carotid artery, vertebral artery, large blood vessels of the circle of Willis, and small cerebral arterial branches.

Pulmonary Angiography: The catheter is inserted into the brachial artery (in the arm) or the femoral artery and is threaded to the pulmonary artery. The dye is injected for visualizing pulmonary vessels. During the test the patient should be monitored for cardiac arrhythmias.

Renal Angiography: The catheter is inserted into the femoral artery and is passed upward through the iliac artery and the aorta to the renal artery. This test permits visualization of the renal vessels and the parenchyma. An aortogram is sometimes made with real angiography to detect any vessel abnormality and to show the relationship of the renal arteries to the aorta.[1,2,4,5]

Clinical Problems

TYPE OF ANGIOGRAPHY	INDICATIONS
Cerebral	To detect cerebrovascular aneurysm; cerebral thrombosis; hematomas; tumors from increased vascularization; cerebral plaques or spasm; cerebral fistula
	To determine cerebral blood flow, cause of increased intracranial pressure ($\uparrow$ ICP)
Pulmonary	To detect pulmonary embolism; tumors; aneurysms; congenital defects; vascular changes associated with emphysema, blebs, and bullae; heart abnormality
	To evaluate pulmonary circulation
Renal	To detect renal artery stenosis; renal thrombus or embolus; space-occupying lesions (ie, tumors, cysts); aneurysms
	To determine the causative facor of hypertension, cause of renal failure
	To evaluate renal circulation

Procedure

- A consent form should be signed by the patient or a designated family member.
- The patient should be NPO for 8 to 12 hours before the angiogram. Anticoagulants (heparin) are usually discontinued.
- Record vital signs. Have patient void before the test.
- Dentures and metallic objects should be removed before the test.
- The injection site should be shaved.
- Premedications (ie, a sedative or narcotic analgesic), if ordered, are administered an hour before the test. If the patient has a history of severe allergic reactions to various substances or drugs, the physician may order steroids or antihistamines before and after the procedure as a prophylactic measure.
- Intravenous (IV) fluids may be started before the procedure so that emergency drugs, if needed, may be administered.
- The patient lies in a supine position on an x-ray table. A local anesthetic is administered to the injection incisional site.
- The test takes approximately 1 to 2 hours.

Renal: A laxative or cleansing enema is usually ordered the evening before the test.

Pulmonary: ECG (EKG) electrodes are attached to the patient's chest for cardiac monitoring (tracings of heart activity) during the angiography. Pulmonary pressures are recorded, and blood samples are obtained before the contrast dye is injected.

- Factors Affecting Diagnostic Results

  - Feces and gas can distort or decrease the visualization of the kidneys.
  - Barium sulfate from a recent barium study can interfere with the test results.
  - Movement during the filming can distort the x-ray picture.

NURSING IMPLICATIONS WITH RATIONALE

Pre-Test

- Obtain a patient history of hypersensitivity to iodine, seafood, or contrast dye from other x-ray procedures (eg, intravenous pyelography [IVP]). The physician should also know if the patient is highly sensitive to other substances. Skin testing could be done before the test, or prophylactic medications (ie, steroids, antihistamines) may be given prior to and/or following the test.
- Record base-line vital signs.
- Give a laxative or cleansing enema, if ordered. Explain to the patient that it will cleanse the lower intestinal tract, allowing better visualization.
- Have the patient void, wear a gown, and remove dentures.
- Administer premedications (sedative and narcotic analgesic) as ordered. Check that the consent form has been signed before giving premedica-

tions. The patient should be in bed with the bed sides up after the pre-medications are given.

■ Encourage the patient to ask questions. This test can be frightening to patients, and they will need time to express any concerns.

■ Assess for vasovagal reaction (common complication; ie, decreased pulse rate and blood pressure [BP], cold and clammy skin). Give IV fluids and atropine IV. This reaction lasts about 15 to 20 minutes.

Patient Teaching

■ Explain the procedure to the patient (*see Description and Procedure*). Inform the patient that the radiologist, surgeon, or physician will inject a contrast dye into an artery at the groin, elbow, or neck. The area will be numbed, and a catheter will be inserted and threaded with the guidance of fluoroscopy to the appropriate site.

■ Inform the patient that when the dye is injected he or she will most likely feel a warm, flushed sensation that should last for a minute or two. Explain to the patient that the test should not cause pain but can cause some periodic discomfort during the procedure.

Post-test

■ Apply pressure on the injection site for 5 to 10 minutes or longer until bleeding has stopped. Check the injection site for bleeding when taking vital signs.

■ Monitor vital signs as ordered, such as every 15 minutes for the first hour, every 30 minutes for the next 2 hours, and then every hour for the next 4 hours, or until stable. The temperature should be taken every 4 hours for 24 to 48 hours or as ordered.

■ Enforce bed rest for 12 to 24 hours or as ordered. Activities should be restricted for a day.

■ Assess the injection site for swelling and for hematoma.

■ Check peripheral pulses in the extremities (ie, dorsalis pedis, femoral, and radial). Absence or weakness in pulse volume should be reported immediately.

■ Note the temperature and color of the extremity. Report changes (eg, color—pale) to the physician immediately. Arterial occlusion to the extremity could occur.

■ Apply cold compresses or an ice pack to the injection site for edema or pain, if ordered.

■ Monitor ECG tracings, urine output, and IV fluids. IV fluids and cardiac monitoring may be discontinued after the angiography.

■ Inform the patient that coughing usually is not abnormal following a pulmonary angiography.

■ Assess for dysphagia and for respiratory distress if the carotid artery was used for cerebral angiography.

■ Assess for weakness or numbness in an extremity, confusion, or slurred speech following a cerebral angiography. These could be symptoms of transient ischemic attack (TIA), known as "small strokes."

■ Observe for a delayed allergic reaction to the contrast dye (ie, tachycardia, dyspnea, skin rash, urticaria [hives], decreasing systolic BP, and decreased urine output).

■ Be supportive of the patient and his or her family. Answer questions, and explain your nursing implications.

ARTHROGRAPHY

Normal Finding

Knee: normal medial meniscus

Shoulder: bicipital tendon sheath, normal joint capsule, and intact subscapular bursa

Description

Arthrography is an x-ray examination of a joint using air, contrast media, or both in the joint space. The purposes are to detect abnormalities of the cartilage and/or ligaments (eg, tears) and to visualize structures of the joint capsule.

This procedure is performed when patients complain of persistent knee or shoulder pain or discomfort. Usually it is performed on an outpatient basis.

Arthrography is not indicated if the patient is having acute arthritic attack, joint infection, or is pregnant.[2,6–9]

Clinical Problems

Indications: to detect osteochondritis dissecans, osteochondral fractures, cartilage abnormalities, synovial abnormalities, tears of the ligaments, and joint capsule abnormalities. *Shoulder:* adhesive capsulitis, tears of rotator cuff, bicipital tenosynovitis or tears.

Procedure

■ Prepare the knee or shoulder area using aseptic technique.
■ Local anesthetic is administered to puncture site.
■ A needle is inserted into the joint space (eg, knee), and synovial fluid is aspirated for synovial fluid analysis.
■ Air and/or contrast medium is injected into the joint space, and x-rays are taken.
■ The knee may be bandaged.
■ Food and fluids are not restricted.

■ **Factors Affecting Diagnostic Results**

■ None known

NURSING IMPLICATIONS WITH RATIONALE

- Explain the procedure to the patient to allay anxiety and fear and to increase the patient's cooperation.
- Obtain a patient history of allergies to seafood, iodine, and contrast dye. An antihistamine, diphenhydramine (Benadryl), may be given orally or intravenously if there is a history of iodine or seafood hypersensitiveness.
- Provide ongoing assessment before, during, and after the procedure, including vital signs, discomfort, and others.

Patient Teaching

- Inform the patient that changes in body positions may be asked for during the procedure. At other times, the patient is to remain still.
- Inform the patient that he or she will not be asleep during the arthrography and may ask questions prior, during and after the test procedure.

Post-test

- Apply an ace bandage to leg, including the knee, if indicated to decrease swelling and pain.

Patient Teaching

- Instruct the patient to rest the joint for the time specified by the physician, usually 12 hours.
- Inform the patient that a crepitant noise may be heard with joint movement. This should stop in a few days; however, if noise persists, the physician should be contacted.
- Instruct the patient to apply ice (bag with cover) to the affected joint to decrease swelling if noted. An analgesic for pain and/or discomfort may be ordered or suggested.

ARTHROSCOPY

Normal Finding

Normal lining of the synovial membrane. Cartilage is smooth and white, and ligaments and tendons are intact.

Description

Arthroscopy is an endoscopic examination of the interior aspect of a joint (usually the knee) using a fiberoptic endoscope. Normally an *arthrography* is performed prior to arthroscopy.

Arthroscopy may be used to diagnose meniscal, patellar, extrasynovial, and synovial diseases; to perform joint surgery; and to monitor disease process or the effects of medical or surgical therapeutic regimen. Frequently biopsy or surgery is performed during the test procedure. For a surgical procedure, spinal or general anesthesia is used and for visualization of the interior joint space, a local anesthetic. Arthroscopy is contraindicated if a wound or severe skin infection is present or if the patient has severe fibrous ankylosis.[2,6,8,9]

Clinical Problems

Indications: to detect meniscal disease with torn lateral or medial meniscus, patellar disease, chondromalacia, patellar fracture, osteochondritis dissecans, osteochondromatosis, torn ligaments, Baker's cyst, synovitis, and rheumatoid and degenerative arthritis

Procedure

- Obtain a signed consent form.
- There is no food or fluid restriction for local anesthetic. NPO after midnight for spinal and general anesthesia.
- Local, spinal, or general anesthesia is used, depending on the purpose and procedure for the test.
- Ace bandage and/or tourniquet may be applied to decreased blood volume in the leg.
- The arthroscope is inserted into the interior joint for visualization, for draining fluid from the joint, for biopsy, and/or for surgery.
- Dressing is applied to the incision site of the affected joint.

- Factors Affecting Diagnostic Results

- Septic technique used during test procedure could cause pain and discomfort and could further complicate the joint disease.

NURSING IMPLICATIONS WITH RATIONALE

- Check on the type of anesthesia to be used. If general or spinal anesthesia is ordered, inform the patient to remain NPO after midnight prior to the test.
- Assess the involved area for possible skin lesion or infection.
- Determine the patient's anxiety level, and be available to answer questions. Be prepared to repeat information if the level of anxiety or fear is determined to be high.
- Use aseptic technique throughout the procedure. Sepsis can cause severe complication to the joint and tissues.

Post-test

- Assess the patient before, during, and after procedure, including vital signs, bleeding, swelling. Report abnormal findings to the physician.
- Apply ice (bag with cover) to the area as indicated.

- Administer analgesic for pain or discomfort as ordered.
- Answer the patient's and family members' questions. If unable to, refer the questions to the appropriate health professionals.

Patient Teaching

- Instruct the patient to avoid excessive use of joint for 2 to 3 days or as ordered. Walking should be minimized.

BARIUM ENEMA
Lower Gastrointestinal Test, X-Ray Examination of the Colon

Normal Finding

Adult: normal filling, normal structure of the large colon

Description

The barium enema test is an x-ray examination of the large intestine (colon) to detect the presence of polyps, an intestinal mass, diverticuli, an intestinal stricture/obstruction, or ulcerations. Barium sulfate (single contrast) or barium sulfate and air (double contrast or air contrast) is administered slowly through a rectal tube into the large colon. The filling process is monitored by fluoroscopy, and then x-rays are taken. The colon must be free of fecal material so that the barium will outline the large intestine to detect any disorders. The double-contrast technique (barium and air) is useful for identifying polyps.

The barium enema test is indicated for patients complaining of lower abdominal pain and cramps; blood, mucus, or pus in the stool; changes in bowel habits; and changes in stool formation. The test can be performed in a hospital, in a clinic, or at a private laboratory.[1,2,10]

Clinical Problems

Abnormal Findings: carcinoma (tumor or lesion), inflammatory disease (ulcerative colitis, granulomatous colitis, diverticulitis), diverticulae, fistulas, polyps, intussusception

Procedure

In most institutions the procedures for the barium enema are similar; however, they usually differ to some degree. Some institutions request that the patient maintain a low-residue diet (tender meats, eggs, bread, clear soup, pureed bland vegetables and fruits, potatoes, and boiled milk) for 2 to 3 days before the test. Abdominal x-rays, ultrasound studies, radionuclide scans, and proctosigmoidoscopy, should be done *before* the barium enema. It is important that the colon is free of fecal material.

Prepreparation
- Oral medications should not be given for 24 hours before the test, unless indicated by the physician. Narcotics and barbiturates could interfere with fecal elimination before and after the test.
- The patient should be on a clear, liquid diet for 18 to 24 hours before the test. This would include broth, ginger ale, cola, black coffee or tea with sugar only, gelatin, and syrup from canned fruit. Some institutions permit a white chicken sandwich (*no* butter, lettuce, or mayonnaise) or hard boiled eggs and gelatin for lunch and dinner, then NPO after dinner.
- Encourage the patient to increase water and clear liquid intake 24 hours before the test to maintain adequate hydration.
- Prescribe laxatives (castor oil or magnesium citrate) to be taken the day before the test in the late afternoon or early evening (4PM to 8 PM).
- A cleansing enema or laxative suppository such as bisacodyl (Dulcolax) may be given the evening before the test.
- Saline enemas (maximum three enemas) should be given early in the morning (6 AM) until the returned solution is clear. Some private laboratories have clients use bisacodyl suppositories in the morning instead of the enemas.
- Black coffee or tea is permitted 1 hour before the test. Some institutions permit dry toast.

Postpreparation
- The patient should expel the barium in the bathroom or bedpan immediately after the test.
- Fluid intake should be increased for hydration and prevent constipation due to retained barium.
- A laxative, such as milk of magnesia or magnesium citrate, or an oil retention enema should be given to remove the barium from the colon. A laxative may need to be repeated the following day after the test.

■ Factors Affecting Diagnostic Results

- Inadequate bowel preparation with fecal material remaining in the colon could affect results.
- The use of barium sulfate in upper gastrointestinal (GI) and small bowel studies 2 to 3 days before the barium enema test could affect the results.

NURSING IMPLICATIONS WITH RATIONALE

- Review the written procedure for that institution. Explain the procedure to the patient. Procedures do differ from one institution to another. Usually the preparations for a barium enema have similarities (clear liquids, increased fluid intake, laxatives, and cleansing enemas). Fecal material in the large intestine (bowel or colon) should be completely eliminated.
- List the procedure step by step for the patient. Most private laboratories and hospitals have written preparation slips. The procedure may be sent to the patient at home.

■ Emphasize the importance of following dietary restrictions and of bowel preparation. Adequate pre-preparation is essential or the test may need to be repeated.

■ Notify the physician if the patient has severe abdominal cramps and pain prior to the test. The barium enema test should not be performed if the patient has severe ulcerative colitis, suspected perforation, or tachycardia.

Patient Teaching

■ Explain to the patient that he or she will be lying on a tilting x-ray table for positioning purposes to increase the barium flow into the colon. Explain that a technician will be with him or her and will explain each step of the procedure.

■ Inform the patient that the test takes approximately ½ to 1 hour to complete. Tell the patient to take deep breaths through the mouth, which helps to decrease tension and to promote relaxation.

■ Administer a laxative or cleansing enema after the test. Instruct the patient to check the color of the stools for 2 to 3 days. Stools may be light in color because of the barium sulfate. Absence of stool should be reported. Retention of barium sulfate after the test could cause obstruction and/or fecal impaction.

BRONCHOGRAPHY (BRONCHOGRAM)

Normal Finding

Normal tracheobronchial structure

Description

Bronchography is an x-ray test to visualize the trachea, bronchi, and the entire bronchial tree after a radiopaque iodine contrast liquid is injected through a catheter into the tracheobronchial space. The bronchi are coated with the contrast dye, and a series of x-rays is then taken. Bronchography may be done in conjunction with bronchoscopy.

Bronchography is contraindicated during pregnancy. This test should also not be done if the patient is hypersensitive to anesthetics, iodine, or x-ray dyes.[1,2,4,11]

Clinical Problems

Indications: to detect bronchial obstruction (ie, foreign bodies, tumors; cysts or cavities; bronchiectasis)

Procedure

■ Obtain a signed consent form.
■ NPO for 6 to 8 hours before the test.

- Oral hygiene should be given the night before the test and in the morning. This will decrease the number of bacteria that could be introduced into the lungs.
- Postural drainage is performed for 3 days before the test. This procedure aids in the removal of bronchial mucus and secretions. An expectorant (ie, potassium iodide) may be ordered for 1 to 3 days before the test to loosen secretions and could detect an allergy to iodine.
- A sedative and atropine are usually given 1 hour before the test. The sedative/tranquilizer is to promote relaxation; atropine is to reduce secretions during the test.
- A topical anesthetic is sprayed into the pharynx and trachea. A catheter is passed through the nose into the trachea, and a local anesthetic and iodized contrast liquid are injected through the catheter.
- The patient is usually asked to change body positions so that the contrast dye can reach most areas of the bronchial tree.
- Following the bronchography procedure, the patient may receive nebulization and should perform postural drainage to remove contrast dye. Food and fluids are restricted until the gag (cough) reflex is present.

■ Factors Affecting Diagnostic Results

- Secretions in the tracheobronchial tree can prevent the contrast dye from coating the bronchial walls.

NURSING IMPLICATIONS WITH RATIONALE

- Obtain a signed consent form. Check that the consent form is signed before pre-medication is given.
- Explain the procedure of the test. Generally patients are extremely apprehensive about this test and are fearful that they may be unable to breathe. Reassure the patient that the airway will not be blocked. Inform the patient that he or she may have a sore throat after the test as the result of catheter irritation.
- Obtain a history of hypersensitivity to anesthetics, iodine, and x-ray dyes. Usually the patient will receive an expectorant several days before the test to loosen secretions.
- Record vital signs.

Patient Teaching

- Instruct the patient how to perform postural drainage (over the side of the bed or in the Trendelenberg's position for 15 to 20 minutes three times a day). It is important that chest secretions be removed prior to the test to ensure good visualization of the bronchial tree.
- Encourage the patient to relax, and teach relaxation techniques.
- Instruct the patient to practice good oral hygiene the night before and the morning of the test. Check the oral hygiene procedure. Dentures should be removed before the test.

- Answer the patient's questions, and refer questions you cannot answer to other appropriate health professionals. Permit the patient time to express his or her concerns.

Post-test

- Assess for signs and symptoms of laryngeal edema (ie, dyspnea, hoarseness apprehension). This could be caused by a traumatic insertion of the catheter.
- Assess for allergic reaction to the anesthetic and iodized contrast dye (ie, apprehension, flushing, rash, urticaria [hives], dyspnea, tachycardia, and/or hypotension).
- Check the gag reflex to see that it has returned before offering food and fluids. Have the patient swallow and cough, or tickle the posterior pharynx with a cotton swab; if gag reflex is present, offer ice chips or sips of water before food.
- Monitor vital signs. The temperature may be slightly elevated for 1 or 2 days after the test.
- Check breath signs. If rhonchi and fever are present, notify the physician and record on the patient's chart.
- Have the patient perform postural drainage post-test. This procedure helps with the removal of the contrast dye. Physiologic damage will not occur if some of the dye remains in the lung for a period of time.
- Offer throat lozenges or an ordered medication for sore throat.
- Be supportive of the patient and family. Be available to answer their questions.

BRONCHOSCOPY

Normal Finding

Normal structure and lining of the larynx, trachea, and bronchi

Description

Bronchoscopy is the direct inspection of the larynx, trachea, and bronchi through a standard metal bronchoscope or a flexible fiberoptic bronchoscope called a bronchofibroscope. The flexible fiberoptic bronchoscope has a lens and light at its distal end, and because of its smallness in width and its flexibility, it allows for visualization of the segmental and subsegmental bronchi.

Through the bronchoscope, a catheter brush, biopsy forceps, or biopsy needle can be passed to obtain secretions and tissues for cytologic examination. The two main purposes of bronchoscopy are visualization and specimen collection in the tracheobronchial tree. Other purposes include removal of the secretions and laser of the lesions.[1,2,4,9]

Clinical Problems

Indications: to detect tracheobronchial lesion (ie, a tumor), bleeding site; to remove foreign bodies, secretions (liquid and tissue) for cytologic and bacteriologic examinations, mucus plugs; to improve tracheobronchial drainage

Procedure

- A consent form for bronchoscopy should be signed by the patient or an appropriate family member.
- The patient should be NPO for 6 hours before the bronchoscopy and preferably for 8 to 12 hours.
- The patient should remove dentures, contact lenses, jewelry.
- Obtain a history of hypersensitivity to analgesics, anesthetics, and antibiotics.
- Check vital signs and record.
- Administer premedications.
- Record vital signs, premedications, and when the patient voided on the preoperative check list and the patient's chart.
- The patient will be lying on a table in the supine or semi-Fowler's position with head hyperextended, or he or she will be seated in a chair. Local anesthetic will be sprayed in the patient's throat and nose, and the bronchoscope will be inserted through the patient's nose or mouth by the physician. It is frequently inserted through the mouth when using the rigid scope and is inserted through the nose when using the fiberoptic scope.
- Specimen containers should be labeled, and specimens should be taken immediately to the laboratory. The procedure takes about 1 hour.

- Factors Affecting Diagnostic Results

  - Improper labeling of the specimen.
  - Failure to take specimens immediately to the laboratory.

NURSING IMPLICATIONS WITH RATIONALE

- Explain the procedure to the patient. Explanation is important to help allay the patient's anxiety.
- Check that the consent form is signed and that the patient has voided before administering premedications. One of the drugs usually administered is atropine, which causes dryness of the mouth.
- Check that dentures, contact lenses, and jewelry have been removed.
- Obtain vital signs (VS), and prepare a VS flow chart. Record admission and pre-test vital signs, which will serve as base-line VS.
- Advise the patient that the procedure takes about 1 hour.

Patient Teaching

- Instruct the patient to relax before and during the test. The premedications will aid in increasing relaxation and decreasing anxiety. Tell the patient the physician will inform him or her of how the procedure is progressing. Bronchoscopy usually is performed under local anesthesia but could be performed under general anesthesia. The patient should be told whether he or she will receive a local or a general anesthetic.

■ Inform the patient that the drugs will make him or her feel sleepy and the mouth feel dry. The patient should remain in bed, and the bed sides should be up after premedications are given.

■ Instruct the patient to practice breathing in and out through the nose with the mouth opened. This is important if the bronchoscope is inserted through the mouth.

■ Encourage the patient to ask questions and give him or her time to express concerns. Inform the patient that there may be some discomfort but that the spray will help to decrease it. Inform the patient that he or she will receive adequate air exchange. Oxygen can be given through the side arm of the bronchoscope or rigid scope and by mask for fiberoptic scope.

■ Inform the patient that there may be hoarseness and/or a sore throat after the test.

Post-test

■ Recognize the complications that can follow bronchoscopy (ie, laryngeal edema, bronchospasm, pneumothorax, cardiac arrhythmias, and bleeding from the biopsy site).

■ Check VS until stable and as indicated.

■ Elevate the head of the bed (semi-Fowler's position). If the patient is unconscious, turn him or her on the side with the head of the bed slightly elevated.

■ Assess for signs and symptoms of respiratory difficulty (ie, dyspnea, wheezing, apprehension, and decreased breath sounds). Notify the physician at once.

■ Check for hemoptysis (coughing up excessive bloody secretions), and notify the physician. Inform the patient that some blood-tinged mucus may be coughed up and that this is not abnormal. It usually occurs following a biopsy or after a traumatic insertion of the bronchoscope.

■ Assess the gag (cough) reflex before giving food and liquids. Ask the patient to swallow or cough. It normally takes 2 to 8 hours before the gag reflex returns. Offer ice chips and sips of water before offering food.

■ Offer the patient lozenges or prescribed medication for mild throat irritation after the gag reflex is present.

■ Be supportive of the patient. Touch the patient's hand or arm for reassurance, as necessary.

Patient Teaching

■ Instruct the patient not to smoke for 6 to 8 hours. Smoking may cause the patient to cough and start bleeding, especially after a biopsy.

■ Inform the patient that collection of postbronchoscopic secretions may be required for cytologic testing.

CARDIAC CATHETERIZATION
Cardiac Angiography (Angiocardiography), Coronary Arteriography

Normal Finding
Patency of coronary arteries; normal heart size, structure, valves; normal heart and pulmonary pressures

Description
The first cardiac catheterization was performed in 1844 on a horse. It was not until 1929 that the first right-cardiac catheterization was performed on a human—the young Dr Werner Forssmann catheterized himself. During the 1930s and 1940s there were a number of right-cardiac catheterizations done, but the first left-cardiac catheterization was not performed until the early 1950s. In the late 1960s and during the 1970s the procedure and equipment for cardiac catheterization were greatly improved.

Cardiac catheterization is a procedure in which a long catheter is inserted into a vein or artery of the arm or leg. This catheter is threaded to the heart chambers and/or coronary arteries with the guidance of fluoroscopy. Contrast dye is injected for visualizing the heart structures. During injection of the dye, cineangiography is used for filming heart activity. The terms *angiocardiography* and *coronary arteriography* are used interchangeably with the term *cardiac catheterization;* however, with coronary arteriography, dye is injected directly into the coronary arteries, and with angiocardiography, dye is injected into heart, coronary, and/or pulmonary vessels.

With right-cardiac catheterization, the catheter is inserted into the femoral vein or an antecubital vein and threaded through the inferior vena cava into the right atrium to the pulmonary artery. Right atrium, right ventricle, and pulmonary artery pressures are measured, and blood samples from the right side of the heart can be obtained. While the dye is being injected, the functions of the tricuspid and pulmonary valves can be observed.

For left-cardiac catheterization, the catheter is inserted into the brachial or femoral artery and is advanced retrograde through the aorta to the coronary arteries and/or left ventricle. Dye is injected. The patency of the coronary arteries and/or functions of the aortic and mitral valves and the left ventricle can be observed. This procedure is indicated before heart surgery.

The frequency of complications arising from cardiac catheterizations have decreased to less than 2%. The complications that can occur, although rare, are myocardial infarction, arrhythmias, cardiac tamponade, pulmonary embolism, and cerebral embolism (CVA).[1,2,4,11,12]

Clinical Problems
Abnormal Findings: Right-sided Cardiac Catheterization: tricuspid stenosis, pulmonary stenosis, pulmonary hypertension, septal defects. *Left-sided Cardiac Catheterization:* coronary artery disease, partial or complete coronary occlusion, mitral stenosis, mitral regurgitation, aortic regurgitation, left ventricular hypertrophy, ventricle aneurysm

Procedure

- Obtain a signed consent form. Check that the physician has discussed possible risk factors before the consent form is signed.
- Food and fluids are restricted for 6 to 8 hours before the test, according to the hospital's policy. Some institutions permit clear liquids until 4 hours before the test.
- Antihistamines (eg, diphenhydramine [Benadryl]) may be ordered the evening before and the morning of the test if an allergic reaction is suspected, such as to iodine products.
- Medications are restricted for 6 to 8 hours before the test unless otherwise ordered by the physician. Oral anticoagulants are discontinued, or the dosage is reduced to prevent excessive bleeding. Heparin may be ordered to prevent thrombi.
- The injection site of the arm or groin is shaved and cleansed with antiseptics.
- The weight and height of the patient should be recorded. These are used to calculate the amount of dye needed (ie, 1 mL/kg of body weight).
- The patient should void before receiving the premedications. Dentures should be removed unless this is not indicated.
- Record base-line VS. Note the volume intensity of pulses. VS should be monitored during the test.
- Premedications may be given ½ to 1 hour before the cardiac catheterization.
- The patient is positioned on a padded table that tilts. Skin anesthetic is given at the site of catheter insertion. Patient lies still during insertion of the catheter and filming.
- A D5W infusion is started at a keep-vein-open (KVO) rate for administering emergency drugs, if needed.
- ECG leads are applied to the chest skin surface to monitor heart activity.
- A local skin anesthetic is injected at the catheter insertion site. A cutdown to locate the vessel may be needed. The patient will feel a hot, flushing sensation for several seconds or a minute as the dye is injected.
- Coughing and deep breathing are frequently requested. Coughing can decrease nausea and dizziness and possible arrhythmia.
- The procedure takes 1½ to 3 hours.

- Factors Affecting Diagnostic Results

  - Insufficient amount of contrast dye could affect results.
  - Movement by the patient could cause complications and interfere with the filming.

NURSING IMPLICATIONS WITH RATIONALE

- Explain to the patient that the purpose of the test is to check the coronary arteries for blockage or to check for heart valve defects. This test is almost always done before heart surgery, mostly to determine if heart surgery is necessary.
- Explain the procedure to the patient. The cardiologist or cardiac surgeon should explain the risk factors to the patient.

- Obtain a patient history of allergic reactions to seafood, iodine, or iodine contrast dye used in other x-ray tests (eg, IVP). A skin test may be performed to determine the severity of the allergy. An antihistamine (eg, diphenhydramine [Benadryl]) may be given the day before and/or the day of the test as a prophylactic measure.
- Record base-line VS, and monitor the VS during the procedure.
- Have the patient void, and remove dentures before the test. Check that the catheter insertion site has been prepped (shaved and cleansed with an antiseptic).
- Encourage the patient to ask questions, and allow the patient and family time to express any concerns. Refer questions you cannot answer to the cardiologist or other health professionals.
- Administer premedications ½ to 1 hour before the test. Make sure that the patient has voided and that the consent form has been signed before giving the premedications.

Patient Teaching

- Inform the patient that he or she will be in a special cardiac catheterization room. Give information about the padded table, the ECG leads to monitor heart activity, the IV fluids, which will run slowly, the local skin anesthetic, and instructions that he or she may receive (such as to cough and to breath deeply).
- Inform the patient that there should be no pain, except some discomfort at the catheter insertion site and from lying on the back. Instruct the patient to ask any questions he or she may have during the test. Tell the patient to tell the physician of any chest pain or difficulty in breathing during the procedure. The patient's ECG and VS are monitored.
- Tell the patient that a hot, flushing sensation may be felt for a minute or two because of the dye. The reason for this is a brief vasodilation caused by the dye.
- Tell the patient that the test takes approximately 1½ to 3 hours.

Post-test

- Monitor VS (BP, pulse, respirations) every 15 minutes the first hour, every 30 minutes until stable, or as ordered. Temperatures are monitored for several days.
- Observe the catheter insertion site for bleeding or hematoma. Change dressings as needed.
- Check peripheral pulses below the insertion site; if the femoral artery was used, then check the popliteal and dorsalis pedis pulses; if the brachial artery was used, then check the radial pulse. Note the strength of the pulse beat.
- Assess the patient's skin color and temperature.
- Be supportive of the patient and family. Answer questions, or refer them to the appropriate health professionals. Communicate with the patient about the nursing care being given.
- Administer narcotic analgesics or analgesics as ordered for discomfort. Give antibiotics, if ordered.

Patient Teaching

- Instruct the patient that he or she is to remain on bed rest for 8 to 12 hours. The patient can turn from side to side, but the bed should not be elevated for 6 hours if the femoral artery was used for the cardiac catheterization. The leg should be extended. If the brachial artery was used, the head of the bed can be slightly elevated; however, the arm should be immobilized for 3 hours.
- Encourage fluid intake after the test, unless contraindicated (eg, in the case of congestive heart failure).

CHOLANGIOGRAPHY (IV), PERCUTANEOUS CHOLANGIOGRAPHY, T-TUBE CHOLANGIOGRAPHY

Normal Finding

Patent biliary ducts (absence of stones and strictures)

Description

Intravenous (IV) cholangiography examines the biliary ducts (hepatic ducts within the liver, the common hepatic duct, the cystic duct, and the common bile duct) by radiographic and tomographic visualization. Often the gall bladder is not well visualized. The contrast substance, an iodine preparation such as iodipamide meglumine (Cholografin), is injected intravenously. Approximately 15 minutes later x-rays are taken. IV cholangiography is a tedious and time-consuming test, and reactions are commoner with the IV contrast substance than with the oral agents.

Percutaneous cholangiography is indicated when biliary obstruction is suspected. The contrast substance is directly instilled into the biliary tree. The process is visualized by fluoroscopy, and spot films are taken.

T-tube cholangiography, also known as postoperative cholangiography, may be done 7 to 8 hours after a cholecystectomy to explore the common bile duct for patency of the duct and to see if any gallstones are left. During the operation, a T-shaped tube is placed in the common bile duct to promote drainage. The contrast substance is injected into the T-tube. A stone or two could be missed during a cholecystectomy, causing occlusion of the duct.[1,2,5,11]

Clinical Problems

TEST	INDICATIONS
IV cholangiography	To detect stricture, stones, or tumor in the biliary system
Percutaneous cholangiography	To detect obstruction of the biliary system, caused from stones, cancer of the pancreas
T-tube cholangiography	To detect obstruction of the common bile duct from stones or stricture; fistula

Procedure

IV Cholangiography
■ Obtain a signed consent form for IV cholangiography.
■ NPO for 8 hours before the test. Some radiologists encourage fat-free liquids before the test to prevent renal toxicity caused by the injected dye.
■ A laxative (ie, citrate of magnesium or caster oil) may be given the night before the test, and a cleansing enema may be given in the morning. Keeping the GI tract clear can prevent shadows in the x-ray films. Check with the radiology department for the exact preparation needed.
■ A contrast agent, iodipamide meglumine (Cholografin) is injected intravenously while the patient is lying on a tilting x-ray table. X-rays are taken every 15 to 30 minutes until the common bile duct is visualized.

Percutaneous Cholangiography
■ Obtain a signed consent form for percutaneous cholangiography.
■ NPO for 8 hours before the test.
■ A laxative the night before and cleansing enema the morning of the test may be ordered.
■ Preoperative medications usually include sedatives/tranquilizers. An antibiotic may be ordered for 24 to 72 hours before the test for prophylactic purposes.
■ The patient is placed on a tilting x-ray table that rotates. The upper right quadrant of the abdomen is cleansed and draped. A local (skin) anesthetic is given.
■ The patient should exhale and hold his or her breath while a needle is inserted with the guidance of fluoroscopy into the biliary tree. Bile is withdrawn, and the contrast substance is then injected. Spot films are taken.
■ A sterile dressing is applied to the puncture site.

T-tube Cholangiography
■ Obtain a signed consent form for T-tube cholangiography.
■ NPO for 8 hours before the test.
■ A cleansing enema may be ordered in the morning before the test.
■ The patient lies on an x-ray table, and a contrast agent, such as sodium diatrizoate (Hypaque), is injected into the T-tube and an x-ray is taken. The final x-ray is taken 15 minutes later.
■ The T-tube may be removed after the procedure or it may be left in place.

■ **Factors Affecting Diagnostic Results**

■ Obesity, gas, or fecal material in the intestines can affect the clarity of the x-ray.

NURSING IMPLICATIONS WITH RATIONALE

■ Explain to the patient the purpose and procedure for the IV cholangiography, percutaneous cholangiography, or T-tube cholangiography. Check with your institution to see if procedures differ, and make modifications in your explanation to the patient. List the procedure step by step for the patient, as requested. This can decrease high levels of anxiety.

- Obtain a patient history of allergies to seafood, iodine, or x-ray dye. Report a history of allergies to these substances to the physician, and record in the patient's chart.
- Permit the patient to ventilate his or her concerns. Answer questions, if possible. Refer questions you cannot answer to the physician or radiologist.
- Check that the consent form has been signed by the patient before giving a sedative and before the test.
- Administer the pre-test orders (ie, laxatives, sedatives, etc).
- Inform the patient having IV cholangiography that the test may take several hours (up to 4 hours).
- Observe for signs and symptoms of allergic reaction to contrast agents (ie, nausea; vomiting; flushing; rash; urticaria [hives]; hypotension; slurred, thick speech; and dyspnea).
- Check the infusion site for signs of phlebitis (ie, pain, redness, swelling). Apply warm compresses to the infusion site if symptoms are present, as ordered.
- Check vital signs as ordered following the percutaneous cholangiography.

Patient Teaching

- Instruct the patient to remain in bed for 6 hours following percutaneous cholangiography.

CHOLECYSTOGRAPHY (ORAL)
Gallbladder Radiography, Gallbladder (GB) Series

Normal Finding
Normal size and structure of gallbladder. No gallstones

Description
Oral cholecystography is an x-ray test used to visualize gallstones in the gallbladder. There are two types of gallstones: radiopaque, usually composed of calcium carbonate, and radiolucent, composed of cholesterol or bile pigment. The radiolucent stones are the commonest ones and can be visualized using contrast material (radiopaque dye) absorbed by the gallbladder. It takes 12 to 14 hours for the dye to be concentrated in the gallbladder. Nonfunctioning liver cells can hamper the excretion of the radiopaque dye.

Failure to visualize the gallbladder could be due to hypermotility of the bowel (diarrhea), liver disease, obstruction of the cystic duct, and inadequate patient preparation (ie, a high-fat diet the night before will cause the gallbladder to empty, thus losing the dye). If the gallbladder cannot be visualized using an oral-contrast substance, the IV cholangiography may be ordered.

Immediately after the oral cholecystography test, the patient may be given a fat-stimulus meal. Fluoroscopic examination and x-rays are taken to observe the ability of the gallbladder to empty the dye. If GI x-rays are ordered, the gallbladder x-ray should be obtained first, because barium could interfere with the test results.[1,2,5,10,11]

Clinical Problems

Abnormal Findings: cholelithiasis (gallstones), neoplasms (tumors) of the gallbladder, cholecystitis (inflammation of the gallbladder, with or without stones), obstruction of the cystic duct

Procedure

- The patient should have a fat-free diet 24 hours before the x-ray. Some x-ray departments suggest a high-fat meal at noon to empty the gallbladder and then a low-fat meal in the evening. After the dinner meal the night before the test, the patient should be NPO except for sips of water.
- Two hours after the dinner meal, radiopaque tablets are administered according to the directions on the folder. There are various commercial contrast agents (ie, iopanoic acid [Telepaque], calcium or sodium spodate [Oragrafin], iodoalphionic acid [Priodax], and iodipamide meglumine [Cholografin]). The patient should take the tablets or capsules (6 tablets of iopanoic acid) 5 minutes apart with a full glass of water (240 mL total).
- No laxatives should be taken until after the x-ray tests. Some x-ray departments request a saline enema the morning of the test to clear the GI tract so that fecal material does not interfere with the gallbladder test.
- A high-fat meal (cream, butter, eggs) or synthetic fat-containing substances (Bilevac) may be given in the x-ray department after the fasting x-rays are taken. Post–fatty-meal films will be taken at intervals to determine how fast the gallbladder expels the dye.
- The fasting x-ray tests (stage I) takes from 45 minutes to 1 hour, and the post-fatty meal tests (stage II) take another hour or two.

- Factors Affecting Diagnostic Results

  - Inadequate patient preparation (ie, a high-fat meal the night before, not taking all the tablets)
  - GI series, barium enema, thyroid scan, I-131 uptake before the cholecystography test
  - Diarrhea or vomiting, which can inhibit absorption of the contrast substance
  - Liver disease

NURSING IMPLICATIONS WITH RATIONALE

- Explain the test purpose and procedure to the patient. Check your x-ray department's procedure for changes, and modify the procedure if needed. Some institutions send a written procedure to patients who are not hospitalized.
- Obtain a history of allergies the patient may have to seafood, iodine, or x-ray dye.

- Observe for signs and symptoms of jaundice (ie, yellow sclera of the eyes, yellow skin, and a serum bilirubin level greater than 3 mg/dL).
- Administer the radiopaque tablets every 5 minutes with a full glass of water 2 hours after the dinner meal. Patients may take the tablets on their own, but they may need to be reminded.
- Observe for signs and symptoms of allergic reaction to the radiopaque tablets (ie, elevated temperature, rash, urticaria [hives], hypotension, thick speech, or dyspnea).
- Report vomiting and diarrhea prior to the test to the physician. The tablets may not be absorbed because of hypermotility. The test is then cancelled.
- Report to the physician and/or the x-ray department if the patient is scheduled for a barium enema, GI series, thyroid scan, or I-131 uptake before the GB series. These tests should be done after the GB series to prevent test interference.

Patient Teaching

- Inform the patient that the evening meal before the test should be fat free. If there are foods high in fat on the tray (ie, whole milk, cream, butter, sauces, fatty meats, etc), the patient should not eat them. In some institutions coffee or tea with sugar is given in the morning.
- Explain to the patient that it is not uncommon for the test to be repeated and that he or she should not be alarmed. If the test is repeated, the patient should remain on a low-fat diet, and the radiopaque tablets should be taken again as directed.
- Inform the patient that the test does not hurt. Check to determine if there are two stages of the test; the first stage takes approximately 45 minutes to 1 hour. If the second stage is ordered, the patient will receive a high-fat meal or fat-containing agent, and then more x-ray pictures will be taken.

CHORIONIC VILLI BIOPSY (CVB)

Normal Findings

Normal fetal cells

Description

Chorionic villi sampling can detect early fetal abnormalities. Fetal cells are obtained by suction from fingerlike projections around the embryonic membrane, which eventually becomes the placenta. The test is performed between the eighth and tenth weeks of pregnancy. After the tenth week, maternal cells begin to grow over the villi.

The advantages of CVB over amniocentesis is that CVB may be performed earlier, and results can be obtained in a few days and not weeks. CVB can diagnose many chromosomal and biochemical fetal disorders. The disadvantage is that CVB cannot determine neural-tubal defects and pulmonary maturity.[2,11]

Clinical Problems

Indications: to detect chromosomal disorders, hemoglobinopathies such as sickle cell anemia, lysosomal storage disorders such as Tay-Sachs disease

Procedure

- Consent form should be signed.
- There is no food or fluid restriction.
- Place patient in lithotomy position.
- Ultrasound is used to verify the placement of the catheter at the villi. Suction is applied, and tissue is removed from the villi.
- Test takes approximately 30 minutes.

■ Factors Affecting Diagnostic Results

- Performing test after 10 weeks of gestation.

NURSING IMPLICATIONS WITH RATIONALE

- Obtain a history of last menstrual period (LMP) from patient and a history of family genetic disorders.
- Assess for signs of spontaneous abortion resulting from procedure, such as cramping, bleeding.
- Assess for infection resulting from procedure, such as chills, fever.
- Be supportive of patient and family. Be a good listener.

Patient Teaching

- Explain to the patient that she will be in a lithotomy position and that ultrasound is used during the procedure.
- Instruct the patient to report if excessive bleeding or severe cramping occurs after the procedure.

COLONOSCOPY

Normal Finding

Normal mucosa of the large intestine; absence of pathology

Description

Colonoscopy is an inspection of the large intestine (colon) using a long, flexible fiberscope (colonoscope). This instrument is inserted anally and is advanced through the rectum, the sigmoid colon, and the large intestine to the cecum. Occasionally fluoroscopy may be used to guide the colonoscope through the intestine and to locate the tip of the colonoscope when it does not advance.

This test is useful for evaluating suspicious lesions in the large colon (ie, tumor mass, polyps, and inflammatory tissue). Biopsy of the tissue or polyp can be obtained. Biopsy forceps or cytologic brush is passed through the scope to obtain the tissue specimen. Polyps can be removed with the use of an electrocautery snare.

Colonoscopy should not be done on pregnant women near term, following an acute myocardial infarction, after recent abdominal surgery, in acute diverticulitis, in severe (active) ulcerative colitis, or a confused/uncooperative patient. Occasionally colon perforation is caused by the fiberscope; however, this is rare. Bleeding may be a side effect of the biopsy or polypectomy.[2,4,11]

Clinical Problems

Indications: to detect the origin of lower-intestinal bleeding, diverticular disease, or benign or malignant lesions (ie, polyps or tumors); to diagnose and to follow up ulcerative colitis; to screen and to follow up patients with "high-risk colons"

Procedure

- Obtain a signed consent form.
- Specific laboratory tests (hemoglobin, hematocrit, PT, PTT, and platelet count) should be done within the 2 days before the test.
- Iron medication should be withheld at least 4 days before the procedure.
- A sedative/tranquilizer may be ordered prior to the test to promote relaxation. A narcotic analgesic may be titrated IV during the procedure.
- Glucagon or IV anticholinergics may be given to decrease bowel spasms.
- Barium sulfate from other diagnostic studies can decrease visualization; therefore the study should not be attempted within 10 days to 2 weeks of a barium study.
- Avoid using soapsuds enemas. These can irritate intestine.
- Patient should be accompanied by someone who can drive him or her home following the test.
- The procedure takes from ½ to 1½ hours.

Preparation A (Use of GoLytely/Colyte Solution)
- Two days prior to test, have patient take magnesium citrate at 4 PM.

Day before Test
- Patient should prepare GoLytely or Colyte solution according to instructions, and refrigerate solution.
- Patient should have regular lunch.
- Patient should have liquid dinner (ie, broth, gelatine, etc).
- Patient should drink GoLytely/Colyte as instructed at 7 PM to 10 PM.

Morning of Test:
- Patient may drink 8 oz of clear liquid (black coffee, tea, water, clear juice) up to 1 hour before test.

Preparation B (72-hour clear liquid/enemas):
- Patient should maintain clear liquid diet 3 days before test.
- Patient should follow 48-hour Fleet Prep Kit No. 2.

■ Factors Affecting Diagnostic Results
- A soapsuds enema can cause intestinal irritation.
- Barium sulfate from other diagnostic studies can decrease visualization; therefore the study should not be attempted within 10 days to 2 weeks of a barium study.

NURSING IMPLICATIONS WITH RATIONALE

Pre-test

- Explain the procedure of the test. The patient lies in Sims position on left side. A lubricated colonoscope is inserted. Air may be insufflated for better visualization. X-rays are taken.
- Record base-line vital signs and pertinent laboratory values.
- Report anxiety and fears to the physician conducting the procedure.

Post-test

- Monitor vital signs every ½ hour for 2 hours or until stable.
- Assess for anal bleeding, abdominal distention, severe pain, severe abdominal cramps, and fever, and report any of these signs or symptoms to the physician *immediately.*

Patient Teaching

- Instruct patient to breathe deeply and slowly through the mouth during the insertion of the colonscope.
- Instruct the patient to rest for 2 to 6 hours following the procedure.

COLPOSCOPY

Normal Finding

Normal appearance of the vagina and cervical structures

Description

Colposcopy is the examination of the vagina and cervix using a binocular instrument (colposcope) that has a magnifying lens and a light. This test is for identifying precancerous lesions of the cervix and can be performed in the gynecologist's office or in the hospital. After a positive Papanicolaou (Pap) smear or a suspicious cervical lesion, colposcopy is indicated for examining the vagina and cervix more thoroughly. A typical epithelium, leukoplakia vulvae, and irregular blood vessels can be identified with this procedure, and photographs and a biopsy specimen can be obtained.

Since this test has become more popular, there has been a decreased need for conization (surgical removal of a cone of tissue from the cervical os). Colposcopy is also useful for monitoring women whose mothers received diethylstilbestrol during pregnancy; these women are prone to develop precancerous and cancerous lesions of the vagina and cervix. Colposcopy is used to monitor female patients who have had cervical lesions removed.[2,4,5,11]

Clinical Problems

Indications: to identify vaginal and cervical lesions, abnormal cervical tissue after a postive Pap smear, irregular blood vessels, leukoplakia vulvae; to monitor previous treatment for dysplasia and cervical lesions, vaginal and cervical tissue changes for women whose mothers took diethylstilbestrol during pregnancy

Procedure

- Obtain a signed consent form.
- Food and fluids are not restricted.
- The patient's clothes should be removed, and the patient should wear a gown and be properly draped.
- The patient assumes a lithotomy position (legs in stirrups). A speculum is inserted into the vagina, and a long, dry cotton swab applicator is used to clear away any cervical secretions. Another long cotton-swab applicator with saline may be used to swab the cervix for visualizing vascular patterns.
- Acetic acid (3%) is applied to the vagina and cervix. This produces color changes in the cervical epithelium and helps in detecting abnormal changes.
- A biopsy specimen of suspicious tissues and photographs may be taken. Pressure should be applied to control bleeding at the biopsy site, or cautery may be used.
- A vaginal tampon may be worn after the procedure.
- The test takes approximately 15 to 20 minutes.

- Factors Affecting Diagnostic Results

- Mucus, cervical secretions, creams, and medications can decrease visualization.

NURSING IMPLICATIONS WITH RATIONALE

- Explain the purpose and procedure to the patient.
- Encourage the patient to ask questions and to express any concerns or fears. Reducing anxiety is important for the patient and for the test. Remain with the patient during the procedure.
- Place the biopsy tissue into a bottle containing a preservative and place the cells, if obtained, on a slide and spray them with a fixative solution.

Patient Teaching

- Inform the patient that she should not experience pain but that there may be some discomfort with the insertion of the speculum or when the biopsy specimen is taken.
- Tell the patient that the test takes 15 to 20 minutes.

Post-test
Patient Teaching

- Inform the patient that she may have some bleeding for a few hours because of the biopsy. Tell the patient that she can use tampons and that if bleeding becomes heavy and it is not her menstrual period, she should call the gynecologist.
- Instruct the patient not to have intercourse for a week until the biopsy side is healed or as ordered by the physician.
- Inform the patient that the doctor will notify her of the results, and tell her to call if she has not heard from the office in a week.

COMPUTERIZED TOMOGRAPHY (CT) SCAN, COMPUTERIZED AXIAL TOMOGRAPHY (CAT)
CAT Scan, Computerized Transaxial Tomography (CTT), EMI Scan

Normal Finding
Normal tissue; no pathologic findings

Description
The computerized tomography (CT) scan was developed in England in 1972 by the Electric Music Industries, Ltd and was originally called the EMI scan. Other names for the CT scan are computerized axial tomography, or CAT scan; computerized transaxial (transverse) tomography, or CTT scan; and computer-assisted transaxial tomography, or CATT scan. The preferred term is computerized tomography, or CT scan.

The CT scanner produces a narrow x-ray beam that examines body sections from many different angles. It produces a series of cross-sectional images in sequence that build up a three-dimensional picture of the organ or structure. The traditional x-ray takes a flat or frontal picture, which gives a two-dimensional view. The CT scanner is about 100 times more sensitive than the x-ray machine. Although it is a costly diagnostic test, CT scanning is popular because it can diagnose an early stage of disease.

The CT scan can be performed with or without iodine contrast media (dye). It is not an invasive test unless contrast dye is used. The contrast dye causes a greater tissue absorption and is referred to as contrast enhancement. This enhancement enables small tumors to be seen.

CT is capable of scanning the head, abdomen (stomach, small and large intestines, liver, spleen, pancreas, bile duct, kidney, and adrenals), pelvis (bladder, reproductive organs, and small and large bowel within pelvis), and chest (lung, heart, mediastinal structure). Magnetic resonance imaging (MRI), a noninvasive test, has *not* replaced CT scans.[2,13,14]

Clinical Problems

CT TYPE	ABNORMAL FINDINGS
Head	Cerebral lesions: hematomas, tumors, cysts, abscess, infarction, edema, atrophy, hydrocephalus
Abdomen:	
Liver	Hepatic lesions: cysts, abscess, tumors, hematomas, cirrhosis with ascites
Biliary	Obstruction due to calculi
Pancreatic	Acute and chronic pancreatitis; pancreatic lesions: tumor, abscess, pseudocysts
Kidney	Renal lesions: tumors, calculi, cysts, congenital anomalies; perirenal hematomas and abscesses
Adrenal	Adrenal tumors
Chest and thoracic	Chest lesions: tumors, cysts, abscesses; aortic aneurysm; enlarged lymph nodes in mediastinum; pleural effusion
Spine	Tumors, paraspinal cysts, vascular malformation, congenital spinal anomalies (eg, spina bifida, herniated intervertebral disk)

Procedure

General Preparation for all Scans
■ Obtain a signed consent form.
■ For AM scheduling: NPO 8 hours before test. For PM scheduling: NPO after a full liquid breadfast. Small sips of water may be taken 2 hours before test. NPO may not be necessary if contrast dye is *not* used.
■ Medications can be taken until 2 hours before the test.
■ If contrast media (dye) is ordered and the patient is allergic to iodine products, steroids or antihistamines may be given several days before the scan or may be given IV during the CT scan.
■ IV infusion or heparin lock inserted may be required prior to test.
■ CT scanning usually takes 30 minutes to 1½ hours.

Head CT
■ Remove hairpins, clips, and jewelry (earrings) before the test.
■ A mild sedative or analgesic may be ordered for restless patients or for those who have aches and pains of the neck or back.
■ Head is positioned in a cradle, and a wide, rubberized strap is applied snugly around the head to keep it immobilized during test.

Abdominal and Pelvic CT
■ Abdominal x-ray (KUB) may be requested before CT scan.
■ Laboratory reports of serum creatinine and BUN should be available.
■ GI tract must be free from barium. An enema may be ordered.
■ For abdominal scan, give the oral contrast media (15 oz) 1 hour before scan.

Half of the oral solution may be given 1 hour before and the remaining solution ½ hour before scan.

■ For pelvic scan, give the oral contrast media (15 oz) between 8 PM and 10 PM the evening before the scan. Additional oral contrast media is usually given the morning of the scan.

Chest CT

■ A chest x-ray may be requested before a chest scan.
■ IV contrast media is frequently given in left arm.

Spine CT

■ NPO is not indicated, since contrast media is usually not ordered.
■ Spine x-rays taken prior to scan should be available.

■ Factors Affecting Diagnostic Results

■ Barium sulfate can obscure visualization of the abdominal organs. Barium studies should be performed 4 days before the CT or after the CT.
■ Excessive flatus can cause patient discomfort and may cause an inaccurate reading.
■ Movement can cause artifacts.

NURSING IMPLICATIONS WITH RATIONALE

Pre-test

■ Explain the procedure to the patient. The CT scanner is circular, with a doughnutlike opening. The patient is strapped to a special table, with the scanner revolving around the body area that is to be examined. Clicking noises will be heard from the scanner. The radiologist or specialized technician is stationed in a control room and can observe and communicate with the patient at all times through an intercom system. The test is not painful.
■ Inform the patient that holding breath may be requested several times during an abdominal scan.
■ Inform the patient that the CT of the head takes 30 minutes without contrast media and 1 to 1½ hours with use of contrast. For body CT, the test takes 1½ hours.
■ Obtain a history of allergies to seafood, iodine, and contrast dye from other x-ray tests. Contrast enhancement is not always done with CT, especially for head, chest, and spinal CT scanning.
■ Advise the patient that if contrast dye is injected IV, a warm, flushed sensation may be felt in the face or body. A salty or metallic taste may be experienced. Nausea is not uncommon. These sensations usually last for 1 or 2 minutes.
■ Observe for signs and symptoms of a severe allergic reaction to the dye (ie, dyspnea, palpitations, tachycardia, hypotension, itching, and urticaria). Emergency drugs should be available.

Post-test

- Observe for delayed allergic reaction to the contrast dye (ie, skin rash, urticaria, headache, and vomiting). An oral antihistamine may be ordered for mild reactions.
- Be supportive of the patient and family. The use of CT scan can be frightening. The major risk involved is an allergic reaction to the dye.

Patient Teaching

- Instruct the patient to resume his or her usual level of activity and diet, unless otherwise indicated.

CYSTOSCOPY, CYSTOGRAPHY (CYSTOGRAM)

Normal Finding

Normal structure of the urethra, bladder, prostatic urethra, and ureter orifices

Description

Cystoscopy is the direct visualization of the bladder wall and urethra with the use of cystoscope (a tubular lighted telescopic lens). Usually this diagnostic test is performed by a urologist. Small renal calculi can be removed from the ureter, bladder, or urethra with this procedure, and a tissue biopsy can be obtained. In addition, a *retrograde pyelography* (injection of contrast dye through the catheter into the ureters and renal pelvis) may be performed during the cystoscopy.

Cystoscopy is performed in a cystoscopy room of a hospital or in a urologist's office under general or local anesthesia. Premedications are administered an hour prior to the test.

Cystography is the instillation of a contrast dye into the bladder via a catheter. This procedure can detect a rupture in the bladder, a neurogenic bladder, fistulas, and tumors. The test is useful when x-rays are needed and a cystoscopy or retrograde pyelography is contraindicated.[1,2,4,11]

Clinical Problems

Indications: to determine the cause of hematuria or the cause of urinary tract infection; to detect renal calculi (stones), tumors, or prostatic hyperplasia; to remove renal stones

Procedure

- Obtain a signed consent form.
- The patient can have a full liquid breakfast the morning of the test if local anesthetic is used. Several glasses of water may be ordered. If the patient is to have general anesthesia, NPO for 8 hours before cystoscopy.
- Record base-line vital signs

- A narcotic analgesic (meperidine, morphine) may be ordered an hour before the cystoscopy. The procedure is done under local or general anesthesia.
- The patient is placed in a lithotomy position (feet or legs in stirrups). A local anesthetic is injected into the urethra. Water may be instilled to enhance better visualization. Urine specimen may be obtained.
- The cystoscopy takes approximately 30 minutes to 1 hour.

■ Factors Affecting Diagnostic Results

- None reported

NURSING IMPLICATIONS WITH RATIONALE

Pre-test

- Obtain history concerning the presence of cystitis, prostatitis, which could result in sepsis.
- Explain the procedure to the patient. Answer questions, refer questions you cannot answer to the urologist.
- Check with the urologist about the form of anesthesia the patient will receive—local or general. Inform the patient that a local anesthetic will be injected into the urethra several minutes before the cystoscope is inserted.
- Check that the consent form has been signed before administering the premedications. Normally the drugs are given 1 hour before the test.
- Check with patient concerning hypersensitivity to anesthetics.
- Assess urinary patterns, such as amount, color, odor, specific gravity of the urine.
- Take base-line vital signs.
- Inform the patient that there may be some pressure or burning discomfort during and/or following the test.

Post-test

- Recognize the complications that can occur as the result of a cystoscopy, such as hemorrhaging, perforation of the bladder, urinary retention, and infection.
- Monitor vital signs (VS). Compare with baseline VS. VS may be ordered every half hour until stable.
- Monitor the urinary output for 48 hours following a cystoscopy. If urine output is less than 200 mL in 8 hours, encourage fluid intake. Anuria could indicate urinary retention due to blood clots or urethral stricture. Report findings to the urologist. An indwelling catheter may be ordered.
- Report and record gross hematuria. Inform the patient that blood-tinged urine is not uncommon after a cystoscopic examination.
- Observe for signs and symptoms of an infection (ie, fever, chills, an increased pulse rate, and pain). Antibiotics may be given before and after the test as a prophylactic measure.
- Apply heat to the lower abdomen to relieve pain and muscle spasm as ordered.

Patient Teaching

- Advise the patient to avoid alcoholic beverages for 2 days after the test.
- Inform the patient that a slight burning sensation when voiding for a day or two is considered normal. Usually the urologist leaves an order for an analgesic.

ECHOENCEPHALOGRAPHY
(See Ultrasonography)

ELECTROCARDIOGRAPHY (ELECTROCARDIOGRAM—ECG or EKG), VECTORCARDIOGRAPHY (VECTORCARDIOGRAM—VCG)

Normal Finding

Normal electrocardiogram deflections (P, PR, QRS, ST, and T)

Description

An electrocardiogram (ECG or EKG) records the electrical impulses of the heart by the means of electrodes and a galvanometer (ECG machine). These electrodes are placed on the legs, arms, and chest. Combinations of two electrodes are called bipolar leads (ie, lead I is the combination of both arm electrodes, lead II is the combination of the right-arm and left-leg electrodes, and lead III is the combination of the left-arm and left-leg electrodes). The unipolar leads are AVF, AVL, and AVR; the A means augmented, V is the voltage, and F is left foot, L is left arm, and R is right arm. There are at least six unipolar chest or precordial leads. A standard ECG consists of 12 leads: six limb leads (I, II, III, AVF, AVL, AVR) and six chest (precordial) leads (V_1, V_2, V_3, V_4, V_5, V_6).

With each cardiac cycle or heartbeat, the sinoatrial node (SA or sinus node) sends an electrical impulse through the atrium, causing atrial contraction or atrial depolarization. The SA node is called the pacemaker, since it controls the heart beat. The impulse is then transmitted to the atrioventricular (AV) node and the bundle of His and travels down the ventricles, causing ventricular contraction or ventricular depolarization. When the atria and the ventricles relax, repolarization and recovery occurs.

The electrical activity that the ECG records is in the form of waves and complexes: P wave (atrial depolarization); QRS complex (ventricular depolarization); and ST segment, T wave, and U wave (ventricular repolarization). An abnormal ECG indicates a disturbance in the electrical activity of the myocardium. A person could have heart disease and have a normal ECG as long as the cardiac problem did not affect the transmission of electrical impulses.

P wave (atrial contraction): the normal time is 0.12 seconds or three small blocks. An enlarged P wave deflection could indicate atrial enlargement, which could be the result of mitral stenosis. An absent or altered P wave could suggest that the electrical impulse did not come from the SA node.

PR interval (from the P wave to the onset of the Q wave): the normal time interval is 0.2 seconds or five small blocks. An increased interval could imply a conduction delay in the AV node. It could be the result of rheumatic fever or arteriosclerotic heart disease. A short interval could indicate Wolff-Parkinson-White syndrome.

QRS complex (ventricular contraction): the normal time is less than 0.12 seconds or three small blocks. An enlarged Q wave may imply an old myocardial infarction. An enlarged R-wave deflection could indicate ventricular hypertrophy (enlargement). An increased time duration may indicate a bundle-branch block.

ST segment (beginning ventricular repolarization): a depressed ST segment indicates myocardial ischemia (decreased supply of oxygen to the myocardium). An elevated ST segment can indicate acute myocardial infarction or pericarditis. A prolonged ST segment may imply hypocalcemia or hypokalemia. A short ST segment may be due to hypercalcemia.

T wave (ventricular repolarization): a flat or inverted T wave can indicate myocardial ischemia, myocardial infarction, or hypokalemia. A tall, peaked T wave (>10 mm or 10 small blocks in precordial leads, or >5mm or 5 small blocks in limb leads) can indicate hyperkalemia.

Vectorcardiogram (VCG): the VCG records electrical impulses from the cardiac cycle, making it similar to the ECG. However, it shows a three-dimensional view (frontal, horizontal, and sagittal planes) of the heart, whereas the ECG shows a two-dimensional view (frontal and horizontal planes). The VCG is considered more sensitive than the ECG for diagnosing a myocardial infarction. It is useful for assessing ventricular hypertrophy in adults and children.[1,2,4,11,15]

Clinical Problems

Indications: to detect cardiac arrhythmias, cardiac hypertrophies, myocardial ischemia, electrolyte imbalances (potassium, calcium, and magnesium), myocardial infarction, pericarditis; to determine the effects of drugs (ie, digitalis, quinidine, etc); to monitor ECG changes during the stress/exercise test and the recovery phase after a myocardial infarction.

Procedure

- Food, drinks, and medications are not restricted, unless otherwise indicated.
- Clothing should be removed to the waist, and the female patient should wear a gown.
- Nylon stockings should be removed, and trouser bottoms should be raised.
- The patient should lie in a supine position.
- The skin surface should be prepared. Excess hair should be shaved from the chest, if necessary.
- Electrodes with electropaste or pads are strapped to the four extremities. The

color-coded lead wires are inserted into the correct electrodes. Chest electrodes are applied. The lead selector is turned to record the 12 standard leads unless the ECG machine automatically records the lead strips.

■ The ECG takes approximately 15 minutes.

■ Factors Affecting Diagnostic Results

■ Body movement and electromagnetic interference during the ECG recording could distort the tracing.

NURSING IMPLICATIONS WITH RATIONALE

■ Record the list of medications the patient is taking. The physician may want to compare ECG readings to check for improvement and changes; therefore knowing the drugs the patient is taking at the time of the ECG would be helpful.

■ Instruct the patient to relax and to breathe normally during the ECG procedure. Tell the patient to avoid tightening the muscles, grasping bed rails or other objects, and talking during the ECG tracing.

■ Tell the patient that the ECG should not cause pain or any great discomfort.

■ Inform the patient to tell you if he or she is having chest pain during the ECG tracing. Mark the ECG paper at the time the patient is having chest pain.

■ Allow the patient time to ask questions. Refer questions you cannot answer to the physician or cardiologist.

■ Inform the patient that the ECG takes about 15 minutes.

■ Remove the electropaste or jelly, if used, from the electrode sites when ECG is completed. Assist the patient with dressing, if necessary.

ELECTROENCEPHALOGRAPHY (ELECTROENCEPHALOGRAM—EEG)

Normal Finding
Adult and Child: normal tracing, regular short waves

Description
The EEG test measures the electrical impulses produced by brain cells. Electrodes, applied to the scalp surface at predetermined measured positions, record brain-wave activity on moving paper. EEG tracings can detect patterns characteristic of some diseases (ie, seizure disorders, neoplasms, cerebral vascular accidents, head trauma, and infections of the nervous system). At times, recorded brain waves may be normal when there is pathology.

Another use for the EEG is to determine cerebral breath. If the EEG recording gives a flat or straight line for many hours, this usually indicates severe hypoxia and brain death. The cardiovascular functions are usually being maintained through the use of life-support systems (eg, a respirator, oxygen, and IVs). The neurologist interprets the EEG readings and gives suggestions.[1,2,11]

Clinical Problems

Abnormal Tracing: epilepsy, seizures (grand mal, petit mal, psychomotor), brain neoplasms (tumors), brain abscesses, head injury, intracranial hemorrhage, encephalitis, unconsciousness, coma, "brain dead"

Procedure

The procedure may be performed while the patient is (1) awake (2) drowsy, (3) asleep, (4) undergoing stimuli (hyperventilation or rhythmic flashes of bright light), or (5) a combination of any of these.

Pre-test

■ Shampoo the hair the night before. Instruct the patient not to use oil or hair spray on the hair.

■ The decision concerning withdrawal of medications before the EEG is made by the physician. Sleeping pills and other sedatives may not be given the night before the test because they can affect the EEG recording.

■ Food and drinks are not restricted except *no* coffee, tea, cola, and alcohol before the test.

■ The EEG tracing is usually obtained with the patient lying down; however, the patient could be seated in a reclining chair.

■ For a sleep recording, keep the patient awake 2 to 3 hours later the night before the test and wake the patient up at 6 AM. A sedative such as chloral hydrate may be ordered.

■ The EEG test takes approximately 1½ to 2 hours. Flat electrodes will be applied to the scalp.

Post-test

■ Remove the collodion or paste from the patient's head. Acetone may be used to remove the paste.

■ The patient should resume normal activity unless he or she has been sedated.

■ Factors Affecting Diagnostic Results

■ Drugs (ie, sedatives, barbiturates, anticonvulsants, and tranquilizers) can affect test results.

■ Alcohol could decrease cerebral impulses.

■ Oily hair or the use of hair spray can affect test results.

NURSING IMPLICATIONS WITH RATIONALE

■ Explain the procedure to the patient, step by step. List the important steps on paper for the patient if needed.

■ Inform the patient that he or she will *not* get an electric shock from the machine (electroencephalograph) and that the machine does not determine the patient's intelligence and cannot read the patient's mind. Many patients are apprehensive and fearful of this test.

■ Encourage the patient to eat a meal before the test. Hypoglycemia should be prevented because it can affect normal brain activity. Coffee, tea, cola, and any other stimulants should be avoided. Alcohol is a depressant and can affect the test result.

■ Inform the patient that the test does not produce pain.

■ Report to the physician if the patient is taking medications that could change the EEG result.

■ Check with the physician and/or EEG department in regard to the type or types of recordings ordered (ie, awake, sleep, stimuli). Advise the patient to be calm and to relax during the test. If rest and stimuli (flashing lights) recordings are ordered, inform the patient that there will be a brief time when there are flashing lights. Prepare the patient, but do not increase the patient's apprehension, if possible.

■ Be supportive of the patient. Answer questions and permit the patient to express concerns.

■ Report to the physician and inform the EEG laboratory if the patient is extremely anxious, restless, or upset.

■ Inform the patient that the test takes 1½ to 2 hours. The room is quiet where the EEG recording is made and is conducive to rest and sleep.

■ Observe for seizures and describe the seizure activity—the movements and how long they last. Have a tongue blade by the bedside at all times. Chart all seizure activity and the time of its occurrence, because it is very important for the technologist and electroencephalographer to know this.

Patient Teaching

■ Instruct the patient after the test, that normal activity can be resumed.

ELECTROMYOGRAPHY (ELECTROMYOGRAM—EMG)

Normal Finding

At Rest: minimal electrical activity

Voluntary Muscle Contraction: markedly increased electrical activity

Description

EMG measures electrical activity of skeletal muscles at rest and during voluntary muscle contraction. A needle electrode is inserted into the skeletal muscle to pick up electrical activity, which can be heard over a loudspeaker, viewed on an oscilloscope, and recorded on graphic paper all at the same time. Normally there is no electrical activity when the muscle is at rest; however, in motor disorders abnormal patterns can occur. With voluntary muscle contraction there is a loud popping sound and increased electrical activity (wave) is recorded.

The test is useful in diagnosing neuromuscular disorders. The EMG can be used to differentiate between myopathy and neuropathy.[1,2,4,11]

Clinical Problems

Abnormal Findings: muscle disorders (muscular dystrophy), neuromuscular disorders (peripheral neuropathy [ie, diabetes mellitus, alcoholism], myasthenia gravis, myotonia), central neuronal degeneration (amyotrophic lateral sclerosis [ALS], anterior poliomyelitis)

Procedure

- A consent form should be signed.
- Food and drinks are not restricted, with the exceptions of *no* coffee, tea, colas, or other caffeine drinks, and *no* smoking for at least 3 hours before the EMG.
- Medications such as muscle relaxants, anticholinergics, and cholinergics should be withheld before the test with the approval of the physician. If the patient needs the specific medication, the time for the test should be rearranged.
- The patient lies on a table or stretcher or sits in a chair in a room free of noise. The EMG takes 1 hour but could take longer if a group of muscles is to be tested.
- Needle electrodes are inserted in selected or affected muscles. If the patient experiences pain, the needle should be removed and reinserted.
- If serum enzyme tests are ordered (ie, SGOT, CPK, LDH), the samples should be drawn before the EMG or 5 to 10 days after the test.

- Factors Affecting Diagnostic Results

  - Pain could cause false results.
  - Age of the patient: electrical activity may be decreased in some elderly persons.
  - Drugs: muscle relaxants, anticholinergics, and cholinergics could affect the results.
  - Fluids that contain caffeine can affect results.

NURSING IMPLICATIONS WITH RATIONALE

- Explain the procedure to the patient. Inform the patient that the test will not cause electrocution; however, there may be a slight temporary discomfort when the needle electrodes are inserted. If pain persists for several minutes, the patient should tell the technician.
- Ask the physician about withholding patient medications that could affect EMG results. If the patient takes drugs that could interfere with test results prior to the test, the drugs should be listed on the request slip and recorded in the chart.
- Check the physician's order for a serum enzyme request. Blood needed for serum enzyme determinations (ie, AST [SGOT], CPK, LDH) should be drawn before the EMG test.

Patient Teaching

■ Instruct the patient to follow the technician's instructions (ie, to relax the specified muscle(s) and to contract the muscle(s) when requested). An analgesic may be ordered before and after the test.

■ Inform the patient that the EMG test usually takes 1 hour, but it could take longer.

ENDOSCOPIC RETROGRADE CHOLANGIOPANCREATOGRAPHY (ERCP)

Normal Finding

Normal biliary and pancreatic ducts

Description

ERCP is an endoscopic and x-ray examination of the biliary pancreatic ducts after contrast medium is injected into the duodenal papilla. The purpose for this procedure is to identify the cause of the biliary obstruction, which could be due to structure, cyst, stones, or tumor. Jaundice is usually present.

ERCP is performed following abdominal ultrasound, CT, liver scanning, and/or biliary tract x-ray studies to confirm or diagnose hepatobiliary or pancreatic disorder.[2,9,11]

Clinical Problems

Indications: to detect biliary stones, stricture, cyst, or tumor; primary cholangitis; cirrhosis; pancreatic stones, stricture, cysts or pseudocysts, or tumor; chronic pancreatitis; pancreatic fibrosis; or duodenal papilla tumors

Procedure

■ Food and drinks are restricted for at least 8 hours before the test.
■ The consent form should be signed prior to premedication.
■ Obtain base-line vital signs. Have the patient void.
■ Premedicate with mild narcotic or sedative. Atropine may be given prior to or after insertion of the endoscope. Atropine relaxes GI motility and will cause dryness of mouth.
■ Local anesthetic is sprayed in back of throat (pharynx) to decrease the gag reflex prior to the insertion of the fiberoptic endoscope.
■ Secretin may be given intravenously to paralyze the duodenum. Contrast medium is injected after the endoscope is at the duodenal papilla and the catheter is in the pancreatic duct.[2,8,9]

■ Factors Affecting Diagnostic Results

   ■ None known

NURSING IMPLICATIONS WITH RATIONALE

- Obtain a patient history of allergies to seafood, iodine, and contrast dye. Report allergic findings.
- Determine whether anxiety level may interfere with patient's ability to absorb information concerning the procedure.
- Check that the consent form has been signed prior to premedications.
- Explain to the patient that when the contrast medium is injected, there usually is a transient flushing sensation.
- Be supportive of the patient prior to and during the test procedure.
- Monitor the vital signs during the test and compare to base-line vital signs. Increase in pulse rate could be due to atropine. Rupture within the GI tract caused by endoscope perforation could cause shock.

Patient Teaching

- Inform the patient that the endoscope will not obstruct breathing.
- Inform the patient that atropine will make the mouth dry and the tongue feel large or swollen.
- Inform the patient that the test takes approximately 1 hour and that lying still on the x-ray table is important.

Post-test

- Monitor vital signs. A rise in temperature might indicate infection (bacteremia or septicemia). Check respirations for respiratory distress resulting from anesthetic spray and/or the endoscope.
- Check skin color. Increased or decreased jaundice is an indicator of disease process or result of therapy.
- Check the gag reflex before offering food or drink.
- Check signs and symptoms of urinary retention caused by atropine.

Patient Teaching

- Suggest warm saline gargle and/or lozenges to decrease throat discomfort.
- Explain to the patient that he or she may have a sore throat for a few days after the test. This is due to the endoscope.

ESOPHAGEAL ACIDITY
(See Esophageal Studies.)

ESOPHAGEAL MANOMETRY
(See Esophageal Studies.)

ESOPHAGEAL STUDIES
Esophageal Acidity, Esophageal Manometry, Acid Perfusion (Bernstein Test)

Normal Finding

Esophagus secretions of pH 5 to 6.

Description

Esophageal studies may be performed to determine cause of pyrosis (heart-burn) and dysphagia (difficulty in swallowing). Most esophageal problems result from a reflux of gastric juices into the lower part of the esophagus because of inadequate closure of the cardioesophageal (low esophageal) sphincter.

Gastric secretions are highly acidic with a pH of 1.0 to 2.5, whereas the pH in the esophagus is 5.0 to 6.0. Backflow of gastric juices causes esophageal irritation or esophagitis.

Esophageal acidity, esophageal manometry, and acid perfusion (Bernstein test) are three common studies performed.

Esophageal Acidity: A pH electrode attached to a catheter is passed into the lower esophagus to measure esophageal acidity. Measurement of pH in the esophagus is taken. If there is no acid reflux, 0.1% (HCl) is instilled into the stomach. Analysis of esophageal acidity is repeated. A pH <2.0 indicates acid reflux, which is most likely caused by an incompetent lower esophageal sphincter.

Esophageal Manometry: This procedure measures esophageal sphincter pressure and records peristaltic contractions (duration and sequence). It detects esophageal motility disorder (eg, achalasia). The base-line cardioesophageal sphincter pressure is approximately 20 mm Hg. In achalasia, the base-line sphincter pressure could be as high as 50 mm Hg, and the relaxation pressure could be around 24 mm Hg. This indicates that peristalsis is weak and that food and fluid cannot pass into the stomach until the weight of the contents is increased. For spasms of the esophagus, the sphincter is normal and peristalsis has irregular motility and force.

Acid Perfusion (Bernstein test): this test is useful to distinguish between gastric acid reflux causing "heartburn" or esophagitis, and cardiac involvement (ie, angina, myocardial infarction). Saline and HCl 0.1% are dripped through tubing, one at a time, into the esophagus. If the patient complains of symptoms of esophagitis (ie, epigastric discomfort, heartburn after ½ hour of IV HCl drip), then the cause is acid reflux. Additional GI studies, such as barium swallow and esophagogastroduodenoscopy are needed to confirm the suspected diagnosis.[1,2,16]

Clinical Problems

Esophageal Acidity: incompetent lower esophageal sphincter, chronic reflux esophagitis

Esophageal Manometry: spasm of esophagus, achalasia, esophageal scleroderma

Acid Perfusion (Bernstein test): esophagitis, epigastric pain or discomfort

Procedure

- Food and drinks are restricted 8 to 12 hours prior to the test. Avoid alcohol intake 24 hours before the test.
- Place patient in high Fowler's position.
- Monitor pulse during test procedure to detect arrhythmias from catheter insertion.
- Withhold antacids and autonomic nervous system agents (ie, anticholinergics, cholinergics, and adrenergic blockers, glucocorticoids, and cimetidine) for 24 hours before the test as indicated, or note on the laboratory slip the last time administered and dosage.

Esophageal Acidity

- Catheter with pH electrode is inserted into the esophagus through the patient's mouth.
- The patient is asked to stimulate acid reflux by performing Valsalva's maneuver or lifting the legs.
- If there is no acid reflux, then 300 mL of HCl 0.1% is administered over 3 minutes, and the Valsalva's maneuver or lifting the legs is repeated.

Esophageal Manometry

- A manometric catheter with a pressure transducer is inserted through the mouth into the esophagus.
- Esophageal sphincter pressure is measured before and after swallowing.
- Peristaltic contractions are recorded.

Acid Perfusion (Bernstein test)

- A catheter is passed through the nose into the esophagus.
- Saline solution is dripped (6 to 10 mL/min) through the catheter.
- The patient is told to indicate when pain occurs.
- HCl 0.1% is dripped through the catheter for ½ hour.
- The patient is told to indicate when pain occurs.
- As soon as pain or discomfort is reported, the HCl line is turned off, and saline solution is started until symptoms have subsided.

■ **Factors Affecting Diagnostic Results**

- Antacids, anticholinergics, and cimetidine may increase pH, thus reducing acidity and causing false test results.
- Cholinergics, adrenergic blockers, alcohol, or corticosteroids may decrease pH, thus increasing acidity and relaxing the lower esophageal sphincter.

NURSING IMPLICATIONS WITH RATIONALE

- Explain the test procedure(s) to the patient (*see Procedure*). Answer the patient's questions, or refer the questions to appropriate health professionals.
- Assess communications for verbal-nonverbal expressions of anxiety and fear about tests and/or the potential or actual problem.
- Monitor pulse and BP during procedure. Base-line vital signs should be recorded. Report irregularity of pulse rate immediately to the physician. Check for signs of respiratory distress during catheter insertion.

Patient Teaching

- Inform the patient that food and drinks are restricted for 8 to 12 hours before the test. Avoid alcoholic beverage for 24 hours prior to test.
- Explain to the patient that certain drugs taken (ie, antacids, anticholinergics, adrenergic blockers, cholinergics, cimetidine) may be withheld for 24 hours. If these drugs are not withheld, the drug name, dose, and last time drug was taken should be recorded on the laboratory slip.
- Instruct the patient to sit in high Fowler's position for insertion of the catheter.

Patient Teaching
Esophageal Acidity

- Inform the patient that a catheter (with electrode) will be swallowed and the pH of the esophagus secretions will be recorded.
- Tell the patient to perform the Valsalva's maneuver (bear down and hold breath) or to lift legs to stimulate gastric acid reflux. The patient needs to follow directions.
- Instruct the patient to inform the physician of any pain or discomfort during the test.

Patient Teaching
Esophageal Manometry

- Inform the patient that a manometric catheter is to be swallowed. The esophageal pressure and peristaltic contractions are recorded.
- Tell the patient that drinking ice water may be requested. Check with the physician first.

Patient Teaching
Acid Perfusion (Bernstein test)

- Inform the patient that a catheter is inserted through the nose into the esophagus.
- Tell the patient there will be two IV solutions and that only one will be dripping into the catheter at a time.
- Instruct the patient to inform the physician immediately when pain or discomfort occurs during the procedure.

ESOPHAGOGASTRODUODENOSCOPY, ESOPHAGOGASTROSCOPY
Gastroscopy, Esophagoscopy, Duodenoscopy, Endoscopy

Normal Finding

Normal mucous membranes of the esophagus, stomach, and duodenum; absence of pathology

Description

Esophagogastroscopy includes gastroscopy and esophagoscopy. If duodenoscopy is included with the endoscopic examination, the term is esophagogastroduodenoscopy. A flexible fiberoptic endoscope is used for direct visualization of the internal structures of the esophagus, stomach, and duodenum. Biopsy forceps or a cytology brush can also be inserted through a channel of the endoscope. Suction can be applied for the removal of secretions and foreign bodies.

This test is performed under local anesthesia in a gastroscopic room of the hospital or in the clinic, usually by a gastroenterologist. This procedure can be done on an emergency basis for removal of foreign objects (a bone, a pin, etc) and for diagnostic purposes. The major complications that can occur from esophagogastroduodenoscopy are perforation and hemorrhage.[2,8,9,11]

Clinical Problems

Esophageal: esophagitis, hiatal hernia, esophageal stenoses, achalasia, esophageal neoplasms (benign or malignant tumors), esophageal varices, Mallory-Weiss tear

Gastric: gastritis, gastric neoplasm (benign or malignant), gastric ulcer (acute or chronic), gastric varices

Duodenal (small intestine): duodenitis, diverticula, duodenal ulcer, neoplasm (benign or malignant)

Procedure

- A consent form should be signed.
- NPO for 8 to 12 hours before the test. When this procedure is used during an emergency and NPO cannot be enforced, the patient's stomach is lavaged (suctioned) to prevent aspiration.
- Patient may take prescribed medications at 6 AM on the day of the test. Check with laboratory or physician for any changes.
- A sedative/tranquilizer, a narcotic analgesic, and atropine are given an hour before the test, or they can be titrated intravenously immediately prior to the procedure and during the procedure as needed.
- A local anesthetic may be used.
- Dentures, jewelry, and clothing should be removed from the neck to the waist.
- Record base-line vital signs. The patient should void before the procedure.
- Specimen containers should be labeled with the patient's name, the date, and the type of tissue.

- Emergency drugs and equipment should be available for hypersensitivity to medications (premedications and anesthetic) and for severe laryngospasms.
- The test takes approximately 1 hour or less.
- The patient should not drive self home following the test because of sedative.

■ Factors Affecting Diagnostic Results

- Barium from a recent GI series can decrease visualization of the mucosa. This test should not be performed within 2 days after a GI series. An x-ray film of the abdomen can be taken to see if barium is in the stomach or duodenum.

NURSING IMPLICATIONS WITH RATIONALE

- Recognize that a gastroscopy test for visualizing the esophageal, gastric, and duodenal mucosa is actually an esophagogastroduodenoscopy. These names are frequently used interchangeably.
- Explain the procedure to the patient. Inform the patient that the instrument is flexible; the procedure will be done under local anesthesia (the throat will be sprayed); premedications will be given before the test; dentures and jewelry should be removed; and food and drinks will be restricted for 8 to 12 hours before the test.
- Check that the patient's dentures, eyeglasses, and jewelry are removed. Give the patient a hospital gown.
- Have the patient void. Take vital signs.
- Check that a consent form has been signed before giving the patient premedications. Once the sedative and the narcotic analgesic are given, the patient should remain in bed with the bed sides up. Tell him or her that these medications will cause drowsiness.
- Explain to the patient that he or she may feel some pressure with the insertion of the endoscope and may feel some fullness in the stomach when air is injected for better visualization of the stomach and intestine areas.
- Be a good listener. Allow the patient time to ask questions and to express concerns or fears. Refer questions you cannot answer to the gastroenterologist or physician.

Post-test

- Keep the patient NPO for 2 to 4 hours after the test, as ordered. Check the gag reflex before offering food and fluids by asking the patient to swallow and by touching the posterior pharynx with a cotton swab or tongue blade, if the throat was sprayed with an anesthetic.
- Monitor vital signs (BP, pulse, respirations) as ordered.
- Give the patient throat lozenges or analgesics for throat discomfort. Inform the patient that he or she may have flatus or "burp-up gas," which is normal. This is caused by the instillation of air during the procedure for visualization purposes.
- Observe the patient for possible complications (eg, perforation in the GI

tract from the endoscope). Symptoms could include pain (epigastric, abdominal, back pain), dyspnea, fever, tachycardia, and subcutaneous emphysema in the neck.
■ Be supportive of the patient and family.

FLUOROSCOPY
Fluoroscopic Examination

Normal Finding

Normal size, structure, and physiologic function of the organ(s) being examined (chest, heart, intestines)

Description

The fluoroscopic examination allows the radiologist and physician to view in motion the physiologic function of organs on a fluorescent screen. Usually the patient is between the x-ray tube and the fluorescent screen. The x-ray beam penetrates the patient and then strikes the screen. Unfortunately, the patient can receive substantially more radiation than he would receive from standard radiography. Today fluoroscopy is used with many diagnostic tests for visualization and for guidance.

During cardiac catheterization, the fluoroscopic procedure is essential for visualizing the coronary arteries. The moving images can be recorded on videotape and can be a valuable aid to diagnosis.

During fluoroscopic examination, the room is dark for contrast and visualization purposes. If the radiologist and assistant remain in the room, aprons should be worn.[2,5,10,11]

Clinical Problems

TEST AREA	INDICATIONS
Thorax	To visualize lung expansion, diaphragm movement or paralysis, bronchiolar obstruction
Abdomen	To detect bowel obstruction (stricture or tumor), filling defects, active bleeding and ulceration (peptic ulcer), Meckel's diverticulum, intra-abdominal hernias
Heart	To detect coronary occlusion (partial or total)

Procedure

Thorax

■ Food and drinks are usually not restricted.
■ Jewelry should be removed. A patient gown should be worn.
■ The patient should breathe deeply and cough as instructed.

Abdomen
- NPO after midnight.
- A patient gown should be worn.
- The patient swallows a chalky substance, barium sulfate.
- Food and fluids are permitted after the examination.
- A laxative is usually ordered after the test or that evening.

Heart
- NPO after midnight.
- Follow the procedure for cardiac catheterization (*See Cardiac Catheterization*).

■ Factors Affecting Diagnostic Results

- Jewelry and metal objects
- Nausea and vomiting
- Medications: narcotics, barbiturates

NURSING IMPLICATIONS WITH RATIONALE

- Explain the procedure to the patient.
- Inform the patient that the fluoroscopic examination should *not* cause discomfort.
- Discuss the patient's anxiety and fears. Refer questions you cannot answer to other appropriate health professionals.
- Explain to the patient that the chest fluoroscopy should take approximately 10 minutes and the abdominal fluoroscopy 30 minutes to 1 hour.
- Determine if the patient is pregnant or if pregnancy is suspected. Report findings immediately to the physician. Fluoroscopy should not be done during pregnancy.
- Inform the patient that the radiologist or x-ray personnel will give step-by-step instructions during the procedure. Tell the patient to ask questions if he or she has any.
- Determine if the patient has had extensive x-rays in the last few years or during his or her lifetime. Excessive radiation can be cumulative. Notify the physician of previous prolonged exposure to radiation.

GASTRIC ANALYSIS (BASAL AND STIMULATION WITH TUBE), TUBELESS GASTRIC ANALYSIS

Normal Finding
Fasting: 1.0–5.0 mEq/L/h
Stimulation: 10–25 mEq/L/h
Tubeless: detectable dye in the urine

Description

The gastric analysis test examines the acidity of the gastric secretions in the basal state (without stimulation) and the maximal secretory ability (with stimulation; ie, with histamine phosphate, betazole hydrochloride [Histalog], pentagastrin). An increased amount of free hydrochloric acid (HCl) could indicate a peptic ulcer (stomach or duodenal), and an absence of free HCl (achlorhydria) could indicate gastric atrophy (possibly caused by gastric malignancy) or pernicious anemia. In addition, gastric contents can be collected for cytologic examination.

Gastric analysis by tube (basal and stimulation) and tubeless gastric analysis (urine examination after a resin dye and stimulant are administered) are the methods used for evaluating gastric secretions.

Basal Gastric Analysis (tube): Gastric secretions are aspirated through a nasogastric tube after a period of fasting. Specimens are obtained to evaluate the basal acidity of the gastric content first and the gastric stimulation test follows.

Stimulation Gastric Analysis (tube). The stimulation test is usually a continuation of the basal gastric analysis. After samples of gastric secretions are obtained, a gastric stimulant (ie, Histalog or pentagastrin) is administered, and gastric contents are aspirated every 15 to 20 minutes until several samples are obtained.

Tubeless Gastric Analysis: This test is for screening purposes to detect the presence or absence of HCl; however, it will *not* indicate the amount of free acid in the stomach. A gastric stimulant (caffeine, Histalog) is given, and an hour later a resin dye (Azuresin, Diagnex Blue) is taken orally by the patient. The free HCl releases the dye from the resin base; the dye is absorbed by the GI tract and is excreted in the urine. Absence of the dye in the urine 2 hours later is indicative of gastric achlorhydria. This test method saves the patient the discomfort of being intubated with a nasogastric tube; however, it does lack accuracy.

There is controversy over the usefulness of gastric acid secretory tests; however, they are still used to document gastric acid hypersecretions (eg, Zollinger-Ellison syndrome and hypergastrinemia).[1,2,4,8,16]

Clinical Problems

Decreased Level: pernicious anemia, gastric malignancy (atrophy), atrophic gastritis

Elevated Level: peptic ulcer (duodenal), Zollinger-Ellison syndrome

Procedure

Basal Gastric Analysis (tube)

- The patient should be NPO for 8 to 12 hours prior to the test. Smoking should be restricted for 8 hours.
- Certain groups of drugs (ie, anticholinergics, cholinergics, adrenergic blockers, antacids, steroids) and alcohol and coffee should be restricted for at least 24 hours before the test. It should be noted on the request slip if the drugs cannot be withheld.

- Base-line vital signs should be recorded.
- Loose dentures should be removed.
- A lubricated nasogastric tube is inserted through the nose or mouth.
- A residual gastric specimen and four additional specimens taken 15 minutes apart should be aspirated and labeled with the patient's name, the time, and a specimen number. The nasogastric tube may be attached to low intermittent suction.

Stimulation Test: A continuation of the basal gastric analysis

- A gastric stimulant is administered (ie, betazole hydrochloride [Histalog] or histamine phosphate intramuscularly; pentagastrin subcutaneously.
- Several gastric specimens are obtained over a period of 1 to 2 hours (histamine four 15-minute specimens in 1 hour and Histalog eight 15-minutes specimens in 2 hours). Specimens should be labeled with the patient's name, the date, the time, and specimen numbers.
- Vital signs should be monitored. Emergency drugs such as epinephrine (adrenalin) should be available.
- The test usually takes 2½ hours for both parts (basal and stimulation).

Tubeless Gastric Analysis

- The patient should be NPO for 8 to 12 hours before the test.
- The morning urine specimen is discarded.
- Certain drugs are withheld for 48 hours before the test (ie, antacids, electrolyte preparations (potassium, calcium, sodium, magnesium), quinidine, quinine, iron, vitamin B complex with physician's permission.
- Give the patient caffeine sodium benzoate 500 mg in a glass of water.
- Collect a urine specimen 1 hour later. This is the control urine specimen.
- Give the patient the resin dye agent (Azuresin or Diagnex Blue) in a glass of water.
- Collect a urine specimen 2 hours later. The urine may be colored blue or blue-green for several days. Absence of color in the urine usually indicates absence of HCl in the stomach.

■ Factors Affecting Diagnostic Results

- Incorrect labeling of specimens could affect test results.
- Drugs—Antacids, anticholinergics, and cimetidine could decrease HCl levels; adrenergic blockers, cholinergics, steroids, and alcohol could elevate HCl levels; antacids, electrolyte and iron preparations, vitamin B complex, and quinidine could falsely elevate the Diagnex Blue level.
- Stress, smoking, and sensory stimulation could increase HCl secretion.

NURSING IMPLICATIONS WITH RATIONALE

- Explain the purpose and procedure of the tube or tubeless gastric analysis test to the patient. Check with the physician before you give your explanation to find out whether he or she will perform both parts—both basal and stimulation gastric analysis (*see Procedure*). List the steps of the test on paper for the patient, if needed.

- Tell the patient how the nasogastric tube is inserted (ie, the tube is lubricated and passes through the nose or mouth) and that he or she will be asked to swallow or will be given sips of water as the tube is passed into the stomach. The end of the tube may be attached to low intermittent suction.
- Notify the physician if the patient is receiving the following categories of drugs: antacids, antispasmodics, anticholinergics, adrenergic blockers, cholinergics, and steroids. Drugs from the above groups and a few others should be withheld for 24 to 48 hours before the gastric analysis. Drugs that cannot be withheld should be listed on the request slip.
- Monitor vital signs. Observe for possible side effects from use of stimulants (ie, dizziness, flushing, tachycardia, headache, and a lower systolic BP).
- Label the specimens (gastric or urine) with the patient's name, the date, the time, and the specimen number.
- Be supportive of the patient. Encourage the patient to express his or her concerns or fears. Answer questions to refer them to the physician or to other appropriate health professionals.

GASTROINTESTINAL (GI) SERIES, UPPER GI SERIES, BARIUM SWALLOW, SMALL BOWEL SERIES, HYPOTONIC DUODENOGRAPHY

Normal Finding

Normal structure of the esophagus, stomach, and small intestine, and normal peristalsis

Description

Upper GI and small-bowel series are fluoroscopic and x-ray examinations of the esophagus, stomach, and small intestine. Oral barium meal (barium sulfate) or a water-soluble contrast agent, Gastrografin (meglumine diatrizoate), is swallowed. By means of fluoroscopy, the barium is observed as it passes through the digestive tract, and spot films are taken. Inflammation, ulcerations, and tumors of the stomach and duodenum can be detected through this procedure.

Upper GI series are performed in hospitals or in private laboratories. A preparation sheet is given or sent to the patient prior to the test.

If increased peristalsis, a spastic duodenal bulb, or a space-occupying lesion is observed or suspected in the duodenal area during the GI series, a *hypotonic duodenography* procedure can be performed by giving glucagon, atropine, or propantheline (Probanthine) to slow down the action of the small intestine. Preparations for the hypotonic duodenography are similar to those for the upper GI series. Because of the anticholinergic effect of the drug, the patient should be observed closely for urinary retention.[2,4,5,10,11]

Clinical Problems

Abnormal Findings: hiatal hernia; esophageal varices; esophageal or small-bowel strictures; gastric or duodenal ulcer; gastritis or gastroenteritis; gastric polyps; benign or malignant tumor of the esophagus, stomach, or duodenum; diverticula of the stomach and duodenum; pyloric stenosis; malabsorption syndrome; volvulus of the stomach; foreign bodies

Procedure

- NPO (food and fluids) and no smoking for 8 to 12 hours before the test. A low-residue diet may be ordered for the 2 and 3 days before the test.
- Withhold medications 8 hours before the test unless otherwise indicated. Narcotics and anticholinergic drugs are withheld for 24 hours to avoid intestinal immobility.
- Laxatives may be ordered the evening before the test.
- The patient swallows a chalk-flavored (chocolate, strawberry) barium meal or meglumine diatrizoate (Gastrografin) in the calculated amount (16 to 20 oz).
- Spot films are taken during the fluoroscopic examination. The procedure takes approximately 1 to 2 hours but could take 4 to 6 hours if the test is to include the bowel series. A 24-hour x-ray film (post-GI series) may be requested.
- A laxative is usually ordered after the completion of the test to get the barium out of the GI tract.

- Factors Affecting Diagnostic Results

  - Barium in the GI tract from a recent barium study
  - Retention of foods and liquids, which would decrease visualization
  - Excessive air in the stomach and small intestine

NURSING IMPLICATIONS WITH RATIONALE

- Explain the procedure to the patient concerning diet and medication restrictions; no smoking; the length of time required to complete the procedure; and the post-test laxative, if ordered (*see Procedure*).
- Inform the patient that all of the chalk-flavored liquid must be swallowed. Tell the patient the tests should not cause pain or any significant discomfort.
- Encourage the patient to ask questions or to express any concerns. Refer questions you cannot answer to other appropriate health professionals.
- Record vital signs. Note in the chart any epigastric pain or discomfort.

Post-test

- Check with the radiology department that the upper GI series and/or small bowel studies are completed before giving the late breakfast or late lunch. Usually the x-ray department will send a slip with the patient stating that the test is finished or a 24-hour x-ray film will be needed.
- Administer the ordered laxative (eg, milk of magnesia) after the test.

Patient Teaching

■ Inform the patient that the stools should be light in color for the next several days. Instruct the patient to notify the physician if he or she does not have a bowel movement in 2 to 3 days. Barium can cause fecal impaction.

GASTROSCOPY
(See Esophagogastroduodenoscopy.)

HYSTEROSALPINGOGRAPHY (HYSTEROSALPINGOGRAM)

Normal Finding

Normal structure of the uterus and patent fallopian tubes

Description

Hysterosalpingography is a fluoroscopy and x-ray examination of the uterus and fallopian tubes. A contrast substance, either oil-base Ethiodol or Lipiodol or water-soluble Salpix, is injected into the cervical canal. It flows through the uterus and into the fallopian tubes and spills into the abdominal area for visualizing the uterus, the fallopian tubes, and the body of the uterus. Usually both a radiologist and a physician (gynecologist) perform the procedure.

The hysterosalpingogram should be done on the seventh to the ninth day after the menstrual cycle. The patient should not be pregnant or have active bleeding, or an acute infection; if any of these conditions exists, the test should be canceled.

There may be some abdominal cramping, and sometimes there are chills and transient dizziness as the contrast substance spills into the abdominal area. Normally the spillage is not harmful and is expected.

The amount of radiation exposure is high because of the fluoroscopic examination. Today ultrasonography is replacing hysterosalpingography, except that the latter test is more effective in determining tubal patency.[2,5,9,11]

Clinical Problems

Indications: to identify uterine masses (ie, fibroids, tumor), uterine fistulas, cause of bleeding (eg, traumatic injury); to identify fallopian tubal occlusion (ie, adhesions, stricture), extrauterine pregnancy; to evaluate repeated fetal losses

Procedure

■ A consent form for hysterosalpingography should be signed by the patient.
■ Food and drinks are not restricted.
■ A cleansing enema and douche may be ordered prior to the test.

- A mild sedative (eg, diazepam [Valium]) may be ordered prior to the test.
- The patient lies on an examining table in the lithotomy position. The gynecologist, physician, or radiologist inserts the speculum into the vaginal canal, and the contrast substance is injected into the cervix under fluoroscopic control. X-rays are taken throughout the 15- to 30-minute procedure.

- Factors Affecting Diagnostic Results

  - Tubal spasm may cause tubal stricture, which could give the appearance of a partial or complete tubal obstruction in a normal fallopian tube.

NURSING IMPLICATIONS WITH RATIONALE

- Explain to the patient that the purpose of the test is to visualize the uterus and tubes for any abnormalities or to determine the patency of the fallopian tubes.
- Explain the procedure to the patient. The procedure may slightly differ in your institution, so check before explaining to the patient.
- Check to see that the consent form is signed. Ask the patient when she had her last menstrual period. Record the information. If pregnancy is suspected, the procedure should not be done.
- Administer pre-test orders—enema, douche, or sedative. If the patient comes from home, check that she has prepared herself as ordered.
- Inform the patient that the test takes about 15 to 30 minutes.
- Encourage the patient to ask questions and to express concerns. Be a good listener. Refer questions and concerns you cannot handle adequately to other appropriate health professionals.
- Check for signs and symptoms of infection following the test, such as fever, increased pulse rate, and pain. Notify the physician.

Patient Teaching

- Inform the patient that she may experience some abdominal cramping and some dizziness. Explain that this is normal but that if there is continuous and severe cramping, she should tell the examiners.
- Inform the patient that there may be some bloody discharge for several days following the test. If it is continuous, then after 3 to 4 days she should notify her physician.
- Instruct patient to call the physician if a high fever is present.

INTRAVENOUS PYELOGRAPHY (IVP)
Intravenous Pyelogram, Excretory Urography

Normal Finding

Normal size, structure, and functions of the kidneys, ureters, and bladder

Description

Intravenous pyelography (IVP) is more properly called *excretory urography,* since it visualizes the entire urinary tract and not just the kidney pelvis. A radiopaque substance (sodium diatrizoate or meglumine diatrizoate [Renografin-60]) is injected intravenously and a series of x-rays are taken at specific times. The test usually takes 30 to 45 minutes.

Excretory urography is useful for locating stones and tumors and for diagnosing kidney diseases (ie, polycystic kidney, renovascular hypertension). A few patients may be hypersensitive to the radiopaque iodine dye, especially if they have a history of allergy to many substances. Emergency drugs (epinephrine, vasopressors, etc), a tracheostomy set, a suction machine, and oxygen should be available for treating anaphylactoid reaction if it should occur.[1,2,4,11]

Clinical Problems

Abnormal Findings: renal calculi, neoplasm (tumor) of the kidney or bladder, kidney diseases (polycystic kidney, hydronephrosis, renovascular hypertension)

Procedure

- A consent form for IVP should be signed by the patient or an appropriate member of the family.
- The patient should be NPO for 8 to 12 hours before the test. In the morning the patient may be slightly dehydrated; however, this will help the kidney to concentrate the dye.
- A laxative is ordered the night before, and a cleansing enema(s) is ordered the morning of the test. These preparations may vary, so check with the radiology department for exact preparations.
- An antihistamine or a steroid may be given prior to the test to patients who are hypersensitive to iodine, seafood, and contrast dye used in other diagnostic tests as well as for those who have histories of asthma and severe allergies.
- Base-line vital signs should be recorded.
- The patient lies in the supine position on an x-ray table. X-rays are taken 3, 5, 10, 15, and 20 minutes after the dye is injected.
- Emergency drugs and equipment should be available at all times.
- The test takes approximately 30 to 45 minutes. A delay in visualizing the kidneys could indicate kidney dysfunction.
- The patient voids at the end of the test and another x-ray is taken to visualize the residual dye in the bladder.

- Factors Affecting Diagnostic Results

  - Feces, gas, and barium in the intestinal tract can decrease visualization of the kidney, ureters, and bladder.

NURSING IMPLICATIONS WITH RATIONALE

- Explain to the patient that the purpose of the test is to detect any kidney disorder or to observe the size, shape, and structure of the kidney, ureters, and bladder.

- Explain the procedure to the patient. As a reminder, the procedural steps could be listed for the patient.
- Obtain a patient history of known allergies. Notify the physician if the patient is allergic to seafood, iodine preparations, or contrast dye. As a precaution, the physician may order an antihistamine or a steroid drug if the patient has an allergic reaction to drugs. A skin test may be performed to determine how hypersensitive the patient is to the radiopaque contrast dye.
- Check the BUN. If BUN levels are greater than 40 mg/dL, notify the physician. Normally the test would not be done.
- Encourage the patient to ask questions and to express any concerns before and during the procedure to the nurse, radiologist, and technician.

Patient Teaching

- Instruct the patient that he or she is not to eat or drink after dinner. Mild dehydration usually occurs. This could be harmful to patients with poor renal output, especially the aged and the debilitated. Sips of water or a glass of water may be indicated to avoid complications.
- Inform the patient that he or she may feel a transient flushing or burning sensation and a salty or metallic taste during or following the IV injection of the contrast dye.

Post-test

- Monitor vital signs and urinary output.
- Observe report, and record possible delayed reactions to the contrast dye (ie, dyspnea, rashes, flushing, urticaria [hives], tachycardia, and others).
- Check the site where the dye was injected. Usually it is in the antecubital fossa vein. For pain, warmth, redness at the injection site, apply warm compresses, with the physician's permission.
- Administer oral antihistamines or steroids as ordered for treating dye reactions.

LYMPHANGIOGRAPHY (LYMPHANGIOGRAM)
Lymphography

Normal Finding

Normal lymphatic vessels and lymph nodes

Description

Lymphangiography is an x-ray examination of the lymphatic vessels and lymph nodes. A radiopaque iodine contrast oil substance (eg, Ethiodol) is injected into the lymphatic vessels of each foot; the dye can also be injected into the hands to visualize axillary and supraclavicular nodes. Fluoroscopy is used with x-ray filming to check on lymphatic filling of the contrast dye and to determine when the infusion of the contrast dye should be stopped. The infusion rate is controlled by a lymphangiographic pump, and approximately 1½ hours are required for dye to reach the level of the third and fourth lumbar vertebrae.

This test is useful to identify malignant lymphoma (Hodgkin's disease) and metastasis to the lymph nodes. Lymphangiograms are also used for staging malignant lymphoma, from stage I (a single lymph node area of involvement) to stage IV (diffuse extranodal involvement). Other tests, such as ultrasonography, computerized tomography, and/or biopsy may be used to confirm the diagnosis and to stage lymphoma involvement.

Lymphangiography is usually contraindicated if the patient is hypersensitive to iodine or has severe chronic lung disease, cardiac disease, or advanced liver or kidney disease. Persons with possible allergies to iodine and/or contrast dye used in other diagnostic tests (eg, IVP) should receive antihistamines or steroids before the test, and emergency drugs should be available during the test. Lipid pneumonia may occur if the contrast dye flows into the thoracic duct and sets up microemboli in the lungs. The small emboli that can occur will gradually disappear after several weeks or months.[2,5,11]

Clinical Problems

Indications: to identify malignant lymphoma (Hodgkin's disease), metastasis to the lymph nodes, the cause of lymphedema (primary [decreased number of lymphatic vessels] or secondary [tumor or surgical removal]); to assist with the staging of malignant lymphoma

Procedure

- A consent form should be signed by the patient.
- Food and drinks are not restricted.
- Antihistamines and a sedative may be ordered prior to the test.
- Contrast dye (blue) is injected intradermally between several toes of each foot, staining the lymphatic vessels of the feet in 15 to 20 minutes. This is for visualization of the lymphatic vessels.
- A local skin anesthetic is injected, and small incisions are made on the dorsum of each foot.
- A 30-gauge lymphangiographic needle with polyethylene tubing is inserted carefully into the identified lymphatic vessel. The contrast dye is slowly infused with the aid of the infusion pump over a period of 1½ hours until it reaches the third and fourth lumbar vertebrae. The patient should remain still during the procedure. X-rays are taken of the lymphatics in the leg, pelvic, abdominal, and chest areas. The entire test takes 2½ to 3 hours.
- Twenty-four hours later, a second set of films is taken to visualize the lymph nodes. X-ray filming usually takes 30 minutes. The contrast dye remains in the lymph nodes for 6 months to a year; thus repeated x-rays can be taken to determine the disease process and the response to treatment.

■ Factors Affecting Diagnostic Results

  ■ None known

NURSING IMPLICATIONS WITH RATIONALE

■ Explain the purpose and procedure to the patient. Be available to answer questions, and be supportive of the patient and family.
■ Check that the consent form was signed by the patient before giving the sedative for the test.
■ Obtain a patient history of allergies to seafood, iodine preparations, or contrast dye used in another x-ray test.
■ Record base-line vital signs, and have the patient void before the test.

Patient Teaching

■ Instruct the patient that he or she should remain still during the test, as instructed. Inform the patient that there may be some discomfort with the injection of the local skin anesthetic into each foot. The sedative is given to promote relaxation and to decrease movement during the test.
■ Inform the patient that the blue contrast dye discolors the urine and stool for several days and could cause the skin to have a bluish tinge for 24 to 48 hours.
■ Inform the patient that the test takes 2½ to 3 hours and that he or she will be told to return the next day for additional x-rays. Tell the patient that the procedure will *not* be repeated the next day; only x-rays will be taken.

Post-test

■ Keep the patient on bed rest for 24 hours or as ordered.
■ Monitor vital signs until stable and as indicated.
■ Observe for dyspnea, pain, and hypotension, which could be due to microemboli from the spillage of the contrast dye.
■ Assess the incisional site for signs of an infection (ie, redness, oozing, and swelling). Report and record findings. The dressing is usually not changed for the first 48 hours.
■ Check for leg edema. Elevate lower extremities as indicated.

MAGNETIC RESONANCE IMAGING (MRI)
Nuclear Magnetic Resonance (NMR) Imaging

Normal Findings:

Normal tissue, structure and blood flow

Description*

Magnetic resonance imaging (MRI) produces pictures of the body similar to CT scans. Cell nuclei in the body react as little magnets in the presence of a strong external magnetic field. MRI uses a strong magnetic field in conjunction with radio-frequency waves to transmit the signals from cells to a computer that produces pictures, or cross-sectional images, of the body.

Since MRI was first introduced in 1983 for tissue visualization, the imaging quality has greatly improved. MRI does not use ionizing radiation, thus it is free of the hazards found in x-rays.

The clinical applications of MRI are rapidly expanding. MRI is sensitive in detecting edema, hemorrhage, blood flow, infarcts, tumors, and infection and in defining internal organ structure; many of these clinical problems would be difficult to distinguish by x-ray and CT. Bone does not hamper its ability to visualize tissue. Pacemakers, ferrous aneurysm clips, jewelry, watches, and hair clips may affect the magnetic field. MRI is difficult to use to evaluate critically ill patients on life-support systems because of the magnetic field. Nonferrous metals usually pose no danger in MR imaging, although they may produce artifacts that degrade the images.

MRI and CT can be used for similar tissue studies. MRI does use contrast media in certain circumstances, but the IV contrast for MRI is chemically unrelated to the iodinated contrast used in CT and conventional radiography. Presently the only commercially available intravascular contrast for MRI is Gadolinium-DTPA.[2,14,17–20,21]

Clinical Problems

Indications: to detect tumors, blood clots, cysts, edema, hemorrhage, abscesses, infarctions, aneurysm, demyelinating disease (multiple sclerosis), dementia, muscular disease, skeletal abnormalities, congenital heart disease, intervertebral disc abnormalities, causes of spinal cord compression

Procedure

- Obtain a signed consent form.
- Remove all jewelry, including watches, glasses, hairpins, and any metal objects. Magnetic field can damage watches. Those with pacemakers are not candidates for MRI; some with metal prosthetics, especially heart valves, and those with nerve stimulating devices may not be candidates for MRI.
- Occupational history is important. Metal in body, such as shrapnel or flecks of ferrous metal in eye, may cause critical injury, such as retinal hemorrhage.
- Patient must lie absolutely still on a narrow table with a cylinder-type scanner around the body area being scanned.
- There is no food or fluid restriction.
- Procedure takes approximately 45 minutes to 1½ hours.

Blood Flow: Extremities
- The limb to be examined is rested in a cradlelike support. Reference sites to

---

*John L. McCormack, MD, Neuroradiologist, MRI Department, Medical Center of Delaware, Christiana Hospital, Newark, Delaware, 19718.

be imaged are marked on the leg or arm, and the extremity is moved into a flow cylinder.
- Procedure takes approximately 15 minutes for arms and 15 minutes for legs.

■ Factors Affecting Diagnostic Results
- Movement during the procedure will distort the imaging.
- Ferrous metal in the body could cause critical injury to the patient.
- Metal, whether ferrous or nonferrous, may produce artifacts that degrade the images if in close proximity to the area being scanned.

NURSING IMPLICATIONS WITH RATIONALE

- Elicit any problems with claustrophobia. Relaxation techniques or a sedative might be used.
- Alert the physician if patient is on an IV controller or pump. MRI can disrupt IV flow.

Patient Teaching

- Explain the procedure. Inform the patient that various noises from the scanner will be heard. Ear plugs are available. Inform the patient that the MRI personnel will be in another room but can communicate via an intercom system.
- Explain to the patient that there is no exposure to radiation. The contrast media that might be used is not iodinated contrast.
- Instruct the patient to remove watches, hairpins, and jewelry. Magnetic field can damage a watch.
- Caution patients with cardiac pacemakers not to approach the MR unit.

MAMMOGRAPHY (MAMMOGRAM)

Normal Finding
Normal ducts and glandular tissue; no abnormal masses

Description
Mammography is an x-ray examination of the breast to detect cysts or tumors. Benign cysts are seen on the mammogram as well-outlined, clear lesions and tend to be bilateral, whereas malignant tumors are irregular and poorly defined and tend to be unilateral. A breast mass (neoplasm) cannot be clinically palpable until it is 1 cm in size, so it may take 5 years or longer to grow and be detectable. A mammogram can detect a breast lesion approximately 2 years before it is palpable.

There is much controversy on how often a woman should receive a mammogram and whether this x-ray test should be only for symptomatic women having a palpable mass, nipple discharge, skin thickening of the breast, or a markedly asymmetric breast, rather than for those who are asymptomatic.

The American Cancer Society and the American College of Radiologists have suggested that women between 35 and 40 years of age have a mammogram every 2 years and that women over 50 years have an annual mammogram. Radiation received is very low dose.

The mammogram can detect approximately 90% of breast malignancies; however, the test carries a 10% false-positive rate. A positive test should be confirmed by biopsy, ultrasonography (ultrasound technique), or diaphanography (transillumination technique).[2,4,5,8,11]

Clinical Problems

Indications: to detect a palpable breast mass (cyst or tumor); to examine the breast periodically, as indicated by the physician

Procedure

- Food and fluids are not restricted.
- The patient removes clothes and jewelry from the neck to the waist and wears a paper or cloth gown that opens in the front. Powder and ointment on the breast should be removed to avoid false-positive result.
- The patient is seated, and each breast (one at a time) rests on a x-ray cassette table. As the breast is compressed, the patient will be asked to hold her breath while the x-ray is taken. Two x-rays are taken of each breast.
- The procedure usually takes 15 to 30 minutes.

■ Factors Affecting Diagnostic Results

- Previous breast surgery can affect the reading of the x-ray film.
- Jewelry, metals, ointment, and powder could cause false-positive results.

NURSING IMPLICATIONS WITH RATIONALE

- Explain the procedure to the patient. Explain that the test will not hurt but may cause a little discomfort when the breast is compressed during the x-ray.
- Inform the patient that the test takes 15 to 30 minutes; however, the patient will be asked to wait until the x-rays are developed and readable. Inform the patient not to be alarmed if an additional x-ray is needed.
- Ascertain whether the patient is pregnant or is suspected of being pregnant. A mammogram is contraindicated during pregnancy.
- Ask the patient to identify the lump in the breast if one is present.
- Be supportive of the patient. Allow the patient time to express her fears and concerns. Notify the physician of her concerns, especially if they cause her great anxiety.
- Answer the patient's questions when possible or refer the question(s) to her physician or to the radiologist.

Patient Teaching

- Instruct the patient not to use ointment, powder, or deodorant on the breast or under the arms on the day of the mammogram.
- Instruct the patient to perform a self-examination of the breast after each menstrual period. Demonstrate breast examination, if necessary.

MEDIASTINOSCOPY

Normal Finding

Normal mediastinal structure and lymph nodes; absence of disease process

Description

This is a surgical procedure in which a mediastinoscope is inserted through a small incision at the suprasternal notch. The purpose is to visualize mediastinal structure and lymph nodes and to obtain lymph node biopsy. These mediastinal lymph nodes receive lymphatic drainage from the lungs. They are examined to detect lymphoma (eg, Hodgkin's disease, sarcoidosis, lung metastasis, and for staging of lung cancer).

Mediastinoscopy is an invasive procedure and usually is performed when x-rays, sputum cytology, and lung scans (CT and nuclear) have not confirmed a diagnosis. Complications from this test may include perforation of the trachea, esophagus, aorta, or other blood vessels; pneumothorax; laryngeal nerve damage; and infection.[2,5,8]

Clinical Problems

Indications: to detect lymphoma (eg, Hodgkin's disease), sarcoidosis, lung metastasis to mediastinal lymph nodes, granulomatous infection, mediastinal tuberculosis

Procedure

- Food and drinks are restricted 8 to 12 hours prior to the test.
- Consent should be signed before premedication by the patient or by the designated family member.
- Obtain base-line vital signs and have patient void prior to the surgical procedure.
- Complete a preoperative checklist.

■ Factors Affecting Diagnostic Results

  ■ None known

NURSING IMPLICATIONS WITH RATIONALE

- Explain the procedure to the patient. It is a surgical procedure and the patient will receive general anesthesia. Ask the patient if he or she is allergic to any anesthetic. Explain that this test procedure will take approximately 1 hour.
- Check that the consent form is signed before the patient is premedicated for surgery.
- Record base-line vital signs. Check to be sure that the preoperative checklist is completed.
- Encourage the patient to express concerns about the mediastinoscopy. Answer questions; refer questions you cannot answer to appropriate health professionals.
- Be available to family members and provide time for them to express concerns and ask questions.

Post-test

- Monitor vital signs until stable and as indicated. Report changes (ie, increase in pulse rate [tachycardia], increase in respirations and dyspnea, decrease in BP).
- Check breath sounds. Report absence of breath sounds if noted.
- Check dressing for bright blood or increased blood on dressing.
- Report if crepitus is detected at chest or neck area. This could be due to air leaking into the subcutaneous tissue as the result of perforated lung.
- Be supportive to patient and family members. Provide comfort measures as needed (ie, position change, medication).

MYELOGRAPHY (MYELOGRAM)

Normal Finding

Normal spinal subarachnoid space; no obstructions

Description

Myelography is a fluoroscopic and radiologic examination of the spinal subarachnoid space (spinal canal) using air or a radiopaque contrast agent (oil and water soluble). With patients who are hypersensitive to iodine and seafood, air is the contrast agent used. This procedure is performed in an x-ray department by a radiologist, a neurologist, and/or a neurosurgeon. After the contrast dye is injected into the lumbar area, the fluoroscopic table is tilted until the suspected problem area can be visualized, and spot films are taken.

If the contrast agent is an oil (ie, Pantopaque or isophendylate), then the contrast agent must be removed at the end of the test. Because oil is heavier than spinal fluid, it does not mix and tends to sink to the lower part of the spinal canal. Water-soluble contrast agents (eg, metrizoate sodium [Amipaque]) do not have to be removed; however, after the procedure the patient should remain in a high Fowler's position (60-degree elevation of the head) for 8 hours.

The myelogram is usually performed to detect spinal lesions (ie, intervertebral disks, tumors, or cysts). This procedure is contraindicated if increased intracranial pressure is suspected.[1,2,4,5,11]

Clinical Problems

Indications: to identify herniated intervertebral disks, metastatic tumors, cysts, astrocytomas and ependymomas (within the spinal cord), neurofibromas and meningiomas (within the subarachnoid space); to detect spinal nerve root injury, arachnoiditis

Procedure

- A consent form should be signed.
- The patient should be NPO for 4 to 8 hours before the test. If the myelogram is scheduled for the afternoon, then the patient may have a light breakfast or clear liquids in the morning, as ordered.
- A cleansing enema may be ordered the night before or early in the morning of the test to remove feces and gas for improving visualization.
- Premedications include a sedative and/or narcotic analgesic and usually atropine. The drugs are prescribed by the physician.
- The patient is placed in the prone position on a fluoroscopic table and is secured to the table with the use of several straps. A spinal puncture is performed, and contrast dye is injected. As the dye enters the spinal canal, the table is tilted.
- After the test the radiopaque oil is removed, and the patient should remain flat for 6 to 8 hours. If a water-soluble radiopaque agent was used, then the patient's head should be elevated at 60 degrees for 8 hours.
- The myelogram takes approximately 1 hour.

- Factors Affecting Diagnostic Results

  - Gas or fecal material in the GI tract

NURSING IMPLICATIONS WITH RATIONALE

- Explain the procedure to the patient. Inform the patient that he or she will most likely lie on the abdomen and will be strapped to a table. The physician will tilt the table as the dye circulates in the spinal canal.
- Inform the patient that he or she may have a transient burning sensation and/or a flushed, warm feeling as the dye is injected; the sensation may last for a short time afterwards.
- Instruct the patient to let the physician know of any discomfort (ie, pain down the legs). The test takes about 1 hour.

- Obtain a patient history of allergies to iodine, seafood, and radiopaque dye used in other x-ray tests. Inform the physician, since air or oxygen may then be used as the contrast agent instead of the dye. A skin test may be performed.
- Follow the prescribed pre-test regimen (ie, NPO, a cleansing enema, and premedications [sedative or narcotic analgesic]). Check that the consent form has been signed before giving a sedative or narcotic.
- Allow the patient the time to ask questions and to express concerns or fears. Refer questions you cannot answer to the physician or to other health professionals.
- Recognize conditions in which myelography would be contraindicated (ie, multiple sclerosis [could cause an exacerbation] and increased intracranial pressure [↑ ICP]). The radiologist and/or neurosurgeon should be notified if they are unaware of the patient's condition.
- Record base-line vital signs.

Post-test

- Monitor vital signs until stable and as indicated.
- Instruct the patient to lie in the prone and/or supine position for 6 to 8 hours, as ordered. If the patient received a water-soluble contrast agent or if all the contrast oil was not removed, the head of the bed should be elevated at a 60-degree angle for 8 hours or longer.
- Monitor urinary output. The patient should void in 8 hours.
- Encourage the patient to increase fluid intake. The fluids will help restore the cerebrospinal fluid loss. Increased fluid intake may decrease a post–lumbar-puncture headache, which could be due to a loss of spinal fluid.
- Observe for signs and symptoms of chemical or bacterial meningitis (ie, severe headache, fever, stiff neck, irritability, photophobia, and convulsions).

Patient Teaching

- Instruct the patient about prevention measures for avoiding back injury (ie, principles of good body mechanics, such as flexing the knees and keeping the back straight when lifting).

NEPHROTOMOGRAPHY

Normal Finding

Normal size and shape of kidney; no abnormality noted in kidney tissue

Description

Nephrotomography visualizes the kidney in detail by combining the use of tomography and IVP. Tomography is a radiographic examination in which each sequence of x-ray film represents a slice of a single layer of tissue. Flat-plate x-ray cannot give detailed visualization of tissue from various angles and depth as can tomography. Contrast medium is injected prior to the tomographic examination. The purpose of this test is to differentiate between solid renal tumor and renal cyst. The thickness of the mass and its interior are recorded on film.[2,8,9]

Clinical Problems

Indications: to detect solid renal tumors, renal cysts, renal sinus-related lesions, adrenal tumors, renal trauma, renal areas of nonperfusion

Procedure

- Food and fluids are restricted for 8 hours before the test.
- A consent form should be signed.
- Check that the patient is not allergic to contrast medium used in other x-ray tests, iodine, or seafood. Notify the physician if the patient has allergies to these substances.
- During the test changes in positions to prone, supine, and lateral might be requested. The x-ray tube moves rapidly during the test procedure.
- Contrast medium is injected intravenously (by infusion or bolus), and tomographic filming takes place while the dye is perfusing the kidney and while kidney is excreting dye.

- Factors Affecting Diagnostic Results

  - Recent use of barium sulfate for GI series and barium enema might decrease detailed visualization of the kidney.

NURSING IMPLICATIONS WITH RATIONALE

- Explain the procedure to the patient (*see Procedure*). Inform the patient that the test takes approximately 1 hour and that there should be no discomfort except for lying on the x-ray table.
- Obtain base-line vital signs prior to the test.
- Check patient's history for allergy to contrast dye, iodine, or seafood. The physician should be notified of any past allergic reaction or sensitivity to the above substances.

Patient Teaching

- Inform the patient that several x-rays are taken first, then dye is injected, and more x-rays are taken.
- Tell the patient that a flush may be felt as the dye is injected. The contrast medium can be given as an infusion or as a bolus injection.
- Inform the patient that changing body positions, such as back to side, may be requested by the radiologist.
- Allow time for patient to express concern about the test and unknown findings. Answer the patient's questions or refer the questions to appropriate health professionals.

Post-test

- Monitor vital signs and urine output. Changes in pulse rate (tachycardia) should be reported immediately to the physician.
- Observe for allergic reaction to contrast medium (ie, rash, itching, dysphagia, or urticaria [hives]).

NUCLEAR SCANS (BONE, BRAIN, HEART, KIDNEY, LIVER AND SPLEEN, LUNG, AND THYROID)
Radioisotope Scans, Radionuclide Imaging

Normal Finding

Adult: normal; no observed pathology

Description

Nuclear medicine is the clinical field concerned with the diagnostic and therapeutic uses of radioactive materials or isotopes (one or more atoms of the same chemical element but with different atomic weights). A radioactive isotope is an unstable isotope that decays or disintegrates, emitting radiation or energy. In many institutions radioisotopes are referred to as radionuclides. Radioactive materials are concentrated by certain organs of the body, and their distribution in normal tissue differs from the distribution in diseased tissue.

Examples of radionuclides or radiopharmaceuticals used for studying the function, anatomy, and morphology of the organs are technitium (Tc)-99m–labeled phosphate, sulfur colloid, aggregated normal serum albumin, Tc-99m-glucoheptonate, iodine (I)-125, I-123, thallium (Tl)-201, and xenon (Xe)-133.

Scintillation (gamma) camera detectors are used for imaging, and the results usually are recorded on x-ray film. Equal or uniform gray distribution is normal, but darker areas can be referred to as hot spots (hyperfunction) and lighter areas as cold spots (hypofunction).[2,7,22–25]

Clinical Problems

ORGAN	INDICATIONS
Bone	To detect early bone disease (ie, osteomyelitis); carcinoma metastasis to the bone; bone response to therapeutic regimens (ie, radiation therapy, chemotherapy (antineoplastic agent)
	To determine unexplained bone pain
	To detect fractures and abnormal healing of fractures; degenerative bone disorders
Brain	To detect an intracranial mass (ie, tumors [malignant or benign], abscess, cancer metastasis to the brain, head trauma [subdural hematoma], cerebral vascular accident [stroke] after the third or fourth week, aneurysms)

ORGAN	INDICATIONS
Heart (cardiac)	To identify cardiac hypertrophy (cardiomegaly) To quantify cardiac output (ejection fraction) To detect myocardial infarction; ischemic heart disease, congestive heart failure (CHF), and aneurysm
Kidney (renal)	To detect parenchymal renal disease (ie, tumor, cysts, glomerulonephritis), obstruction of the urinary tract To assess the function of renal transplantation
Liver and spleen	To detect tumors, cysts, or abscesses of the liver or spleen; hepatic metastasis; splenic infarct To assess liver response to therapeutic regimens (ie, radiation therapy, chemotherapy) To identify hepatomegaly and splenomegaly To identify liver position and shape
Lung	To detect pulmonary emboli; tumors; pulmonary diseases with perfusion changes (ie, emphysema, bronchitis, pneumonia) To assess arterial perfusion changes secondary to cardiac disease
Thyroid	To detect thyroid mass (ie, tumors); diseases of the thyroid gland (ie, Graves', Hashimoto's thyroiditis) To determine the size, structure, and position of the thyroid gland To evaluate thyroid function resulting from hyperthyroidism and hypothyroidism[1,2,13]

Procedure

The radionuclide (radioisotope) is administered orally or intravenously. The interval from the time the radioactive substance is given to the time of the imaging can differ according to the radionuclide and organ in question. Scintillation camera detects the radiation that comes from the organ. Normally masses such as tumors absorb more of the radioactive substance than does normal tissue.

For diagnostic purposes the dose of radionuclide is low (<30 mCi) and should have little effect on the patient's visitors, other patients, and nursing and medical personnel. Usually food and drinks are not restricted.

The procedures for the organ scans are listed according to the radionuclides used, the method of administration, the waiting period after injection, the food and drinks allowed, and other instructions.

1. Bone.
   a. Radionuclides: Tc-99m–labeled phosphate compounds (Tc-99m diphosphonate, pyrophosphate, medronate sodium)
   b. Administration: Intravenously
   c. Waiting period after injection: Waiting periods can differ according to the radionuclides used (eg, for Tc-99m the period is 2 to 3 hours [3 hours for an edematous person]).
   d. Food and drinks: No restrictions; for Tc-99m, water is encouraged during the waiting period (at least 6 glasses).
   e. Other instructions: The patient should void before the imaging begins. Imaging usually takes ½ to 1 hour to complete. A sedative may be ordered if the patient has difficulty lying quietly during imaging.

2. Brain: For cerebral blood-dynamic study or static imaging flow.
   a. Radionuclides Tc-99m-glucoheptonate Tc-99m-O_4, Tc-99m-DTPA (Tc-99m diethylenetriamine penta-acetic acid).
   b. Administration: Inttravenously
   c. Waiting period after injection: Tc-99m-O_4, 1 to 3 hours; Tc-99m-DTPA, 45 minutes to 1 hour. Frequently a few photo scans are taken before the waiting period is over.
   d. Food and drinks: No restrictions
   e. Other instructions: When Tc-99m-O_4 is used, the patient may be given 10 drops of Lugol's solution the night before or at least 1 hour before the injection or potassium perchlorate, 200 mg to 1 g, 1 to 3 hours before the scheduled scan. These drugs block the uptake of Tc-99m-O_4 in the salivary glands, thyroid, and choroid plexus. With Tc-99m-DTPA, blocking agents are not necessary. The patient should remain still during the imaging (for ½ to 1 hour).

3. Heart (Cardiac).
   a. Radionuclides: Tc-99m-pyrophosphate or Tc-99m-pertechnetate for MI 2 to 6 days after suspected MI; Tl-201 testing for ischemic heart disease. Tl-201 testing can be done as part of the stress test. Tc-99m–labeled RBCs or albumin is used for ejection fraction studies.
   b. Administration: Intravenously
   c. Waiting period after injection: Tc-99m, 30 minutes to 1 hour, Tl-201, 10 to 15 minutes. After the patient reaches maximum heart stress on the treadmill, IV Tl-201 is given.
   d. Food and drinks: For thallium and stress ejection fraction studies, patients should be NPO from midnight until the study.
   e. Other instructions: The patient should lie quietly for 15 to 30 minutes during the imaging for an MI and for 1 hour during the imaging for ischemic heart disease.

4. Kidney: For renal blood-flow (renogram) studies and imaging.
   a. Radionuclides: Tc-99m compounds: Tc-99m-pertechnetate, Tc-99m DTPA, Tc-99m-DSML, Tc-99m-glucoheptonate; I-131 hippuran: Usually I-131 hippuran for perfusion studies and Tc-99m-DTPA for renal disorders
   b. Administration: Intravenously
   c. Waiting period after injection:
      (1) Renal perfusion study: Imaging is done immediately after I-131 hippuran is given intravenously. Renogram curves are plotted.
      (2) Kidney disorders: 3 to 30 minutes after Tc-99m-DTPA is injected
   d. Food and drinks: No restrictions. The patient should be well hydrated. He or she should drink at least 2 to 3 glasses of water 30 minutes before the scheduled scan. Dehydration could cause abnormal results in normal patients.
   e. Other instructions: The patient should void before the scan. If the patient has had an IVP or a renogram the scan should be delayed 24 hours. Lugol's solution, 10 drops, may be ordered if I-131 hippuran is given. The patient should lie quietly for 30 minutes to 1 hour during imaging.

5. Liver and spleen.
   a. Radionuclides: Tc-99m compounds: Tc-99-sulfur colloid, Tc-99m-Sn phytate; colloid of indium, In-113m
   b. Administration: Intravenously
   c. Waiting period after injections: Tc-99-sulfur colloid, 15 minutes. A spleen scan can be done at the same time.
   d. Food and drinks: No restriction. Some institutions may require the patient to be NPO after midnight.
   e. Other instructions: The patient should lie quietly for 30 minutes to 1 hour during the imaging. The patient may be asked to turn from side to side and onto his or her abdomen during imaging. Patient may have to return at a specified time.
6. Lung.
   a. Radionuclides: Tc-99m compounds: Tc-99m-MAA (macroaggregated albumin), Tc-99m-HAM (human albumin microspheres); ^{133}Xe ventilation (inhaled)
   b. Administration: Intravenously or inhaled
   c. Waiting period after injection: Tc-99m compounds, 5 minutes after the injection of the radionuclide
   d. Food and drinks: No restrictions
   e. Other instructions: A chest radiograph is usually ordered for comparison with the nuclear medicine study. The patient should lie quietly for 30 minutes during the imaging.
7. Thyroid.
   a. Radionuclides: I-131 sodium iodide, I-123, I-125, Tc-99m-pertechnetate.
   b. Administration: I-123, I-125, I-131 (oral: liquid or capsule), Tc-99m-pertechnetate (intravenously)
   c. Waiting period after injection: I-123, I-125, I-131—24 hours. I-123 is the radionuclide most commonly used because it has a shorter half-life. Tc-99m-pertechnetate, 30 minutes
   d. Food and drinks: No breakfast and NPO for 2 hours following oral iodine.
   e. Other instructions: Three days before the scan (imaging), iodine preparations, thyroid hormones, phenothiazines, corticosteroids, aspirin, sodium nitroprusside, cough syrups containing iodides, and multivitamins are usually discontinued with the physician's permission. Seafoods and iodized salt should be avoided. If the drugs cannot be withheld for 3 days, the drugs should be listed on the nuclear medicine request slip. The patient should lie quietly for 30 minutes during the imaging procedure.[1,2,13]

■ **Factors Affecting Diagnostic Results**

■ Antihypertensives may affect results.
■ Two radionuclides administered in 1 day may interfere with each other.
■ Movement by the patient may distort the image.
■ A distended bladder could decrease visibility of the pelvic (bone) area.
■ Diet and drugs containing iodine could interfere with the results of the thyroid scan (*see Procedure for the thyroid*).

■ Too short or too long a waiting period after injection of the radionuclide could affect the results.
■ Dehydration prior to imaging could affect the results.

NURSING IMPLICATIONS WITH RATIONALE

■ Explain to the patient the procedure for the ordered study. Procedures will differ according to the type of study (*see Procedure*). In most cases, food and drinks are not restricted. For the bone scan (Tc-99m), water is encouraged during the waiting period. For the renal scan the patient should be well hydrated before the scheduled scan. Blocking agents (ie, Lugol's solution and potassium perchlorate) are usually ordered before studies that use radioiodine, except for the thyroid scan.
■ Obtain a signed consent form, if required.
■ Obtain a brief health history in regard to recent exposure to radioisotopes (radionuclides), allergies that could cause an adverse reaction, being pregnant, breastfeeding, and drugs.
■ Adhere to the instructions from the nuclear medicine laboratory concerning the patient and the radionuclide procedure. The patient should arrive on time. This is especially true if he or she has received the injection. The waiting periods for each study have specified times.
■ Be supportive of the patient and family. Answer questions, if possible, and refer questions you cannot answer to appropriate personnel.
■ Advise the patient to ask questions and to communicate any concerns. Be available when the patient wishes to discuss concerns and fears.
■ Report to the physician if the patient is extremely apprehensive. The physician may wish to see the patient and/or order a sedative.
■ Notify the dietitian and/or dietary department not to send foods high in iodine content for 3 days to the patient who is to receive a thyroid scan, unless otherwise indicated. This also includes iodized salt. Instruct the patient not to eat foods rich in iodine (ie, seafood, table salt).
■ List restricted drugs containing iodine that the patient is taking on the nuclear medicine slip (*see Procedure for the thyroid*). This is important if the radionuclide is iodine.

Patient Teaching

■ Explain to the patient that the dose of radiation he or she will receive from radionuclide imaging is usually less than the amount of radiation he or she would receive from diagnostic x-rays.
■ Inform the patient that the injected radionuclide should not affect the family, visitors, other patients, or hospital staff members. The radioactive substance usually leaves the body in 6 to 24 hours. The dose of radionuclide is very low.
■ Inform the patient that there could be a waiting period after the injection of the radioactive substance. Some of the tissues take longer than others to concentrate the substance.

- Instruct the patient to void before the study. Voiding will diminish bladder activity and increase visibility.
- Explain to the patient that the detection equipment will be moved over a section or sections of the body; however, there should not be any discomfort from the imaging equipment.
- Inform the patient that he or she may be asked to change body positions during the test. Other than that, he or she should lie still during the procedure.
- Inform the patient that the imaging may take 30 minutes to 1 hour, depending on which organ is being studied. The patient should be informed that he or she may need to return for additional imaging at specified intervals.
- Instruct the patient to remove jewelry or any metal object in the area of the study.
- Inform the patient that the personnel in nuclear medicine will give step-by-step directions concerning the procedure. Tell the patient to "speak up" if he or she does not understand.
- Inform the patient that heart (cardiac) imaging may be done during the stress test as part of the testing for ischemic heart disease.

PAPANICOLAOU SMEAR (PAP SMEAR)
Cytology Test for Cervical Cancer

Normal Finding
No abnormal or atypical cells

Description
The Pap (Papanicolaou) smear became nationally known and used in the early 1950s for detecting cervical cancer and precancerous tissues. Dr George Papanicolaou developed the cytology test in 1928 after spending 18 years in research. Today he is referred to as the father of modern cytology. As the result of his work, there are many cytology studies done on body tissues and secretions.

Because malignant tissue changes usually take many years, yearly examination of exfoliative cervical cells (cells that have sloughed off) allows detection of early, precancerous conditions. It is suggested that women from the age of 18 to 40 years have yearly Pap smears and that women from the age of 40 years on have either twice-a-year or yearly smears. How often the Pap smear test should be performed is determined by the patient's physician.

The Pap smear (cytology) results are reported on a five-point scale:

- Grade (Class) I   Absence of atypical or abnormal cells
- Grade (Class) II   Atypical cells, but no evidence of malignancy
- Grade (Class) III Suggestive of but not conclusive for malignancy
- Grade (Class) IV   Strongly suggestive of malignancy
- Grade (Class) V   Conclusive for malignancy

For suggestive or positive Pap smears, colposcopy and/or a cervical biopsy are frequently ordered to confirm the test results. Atypical cells can occur due to cervicitis and excessive or prolonged use of hormones.[6,11,26]

Clinical Problems

Indications: to detect precancerous and cancerous cells of the cervix, and cervicitis; to identify viral, fungal, and parasitic conditions; to assess the effects of sex hormonal replacement and the response to the chemotherapy and radiation therapy.

Procedure

- Food and drinks are not restricted.
- The patient should not douche, insert vaginal medications, or have sexual intercourse for at least 24 hours (preferably 48 hours) before the test. The test should be done between menstrual periods.
- The patient is generally asked to remove all clothes, since the breasts are examined after the Pap smear is taken. A paper or cloth gown is worn.
- Instruct the patient to lie on the examining table in the lithotomy position (heels in the stirrups).
- A speculum is inserted into the vagina. The speculum may be lubricated with warm running water.
- A curved spatula (Pap stick) is used to scrape the cervix. The obtained specimen is transferred onto a slide and is immersed immediately in a fixative solution or sprayed with a commercial fixation spray. Label the slide with the patient's name and date.
- The Pap smear procedure takes approximately 10 minutes.

- Factors Affecting Diagnostic Results

  - Allowing cells to dry on the slide before using the fixative solution or spray.
  - Douching, use of vaginal suppositories, or sexual intercourse within the 24 hours before the test.
  - Menstruation can interfere with the test results.
  - Drugs (ie, digitalis preparations, tetracycline, female hormones) could change cellular structure.
  - Lubricating jelly on the speculum can interfere with test results.

NURSING IMPLICATIONS WITH RATIONALE

- Explain the procedure to the patient. Emphasize to the patient that she should not douche, insert vaginal suppositories, or have sexual intercourse for at least 24 hours (some say 48 hours) before the Pap smear. Douching could wash away the cervical cells.
- Obtain a patient history regarding menstruation and any menstrual problems (ie, the last menstrual period, bleeding flow, vaginal discharge, itching, and whether she is taking hormones or oral contraceptives).
- Answer the patient's questions, and refer questions you cannot answer to

---

the physician. Try to alleviate the patient's anxiety, if at all possible. Be a good listener.

■ Inform the patient that a manual examination of the vagina, lower abdomen, rectum, and breast may or will follow the Pap smear.

■ Label the slide with the patient's name and the date. The laboratory slip should include the patient's age and the specimen site(s).

Patient Teaching

■ Explain to the patient that the test should be done yearly or twice a year, as determined by her physician. High-risk patients (with a familial history of cervical cancer or a previous grade II test) and women over 40 years old usually have the Pap smear taken twice a year.

■ Inform the patient that test results should be back in 3 to 5 days. Physicians differ in reporting test results; some send cards to the patient stating that the Pap smear is normal, while other physicians will send cards only if the test is abnormal.

POSITRON EMISSION TOMOGRAPHY (PET)
Emission-Computed Tomography (ECT) Scans; Emission CT Scans

Normal Findings
Normal brain and heart activities and blood flow

Description
Positron emission tomography (PET), a relatively noninvasive test, measures areas of positron-emitting isotope concentration. The patient receives a substance tagged with a radionuclide (ie, radioactive glucose, rubidium-82, oxygen-15, nitrogen-13). Tomographic slices from cross-sections of tissue are detected and visually displayed by computer. PET is most effective in determining blood flow to the brain and heart. Radiation from PET is a quarter of that received by CT.[2,9,26–28]

Clinical Problems
To study the effects of hypoperfusion to brain and heart, stroke, epilepsy, migraine, Parkinson's disease, dementia, Alzheimer's disease, acute myocardial infarction (AMI) for first 72 hours—the size of the infarct and myocardial viability

Procedure
■ Obtain a signed consent form.
■ Start two IVs, one for radioactive substance and the second to draw blood gas samples.

■ A blindfold may be used to keep the patient from being distracted, since alertness is necessary.

■ No coffee, alcohol, tobacco is allowed for 24 hours before the test.

■ No sedatives are given, since patient needs to follow instructions.

■ Empty the bladder 1 to 2 hours before the test.

■ Test takes 45 minutes to 1½ hours.

■ Factors Affecting Diagnostic Results

■ Anxiety could interfere with test results.

■ Sedatives given might prevent patient from following directions

---

NURSING IMPLICATIONS WITH RATIONALE

Pre-test

■ Inform patient that instructions given during test should be followed.

■ Assess IV site.

■ Listen to patient's concerns.

Post-test

■ Avoid postural hypotension by slowly moving the patient to upright position.

Patient Teaching

■ Explain to the patient that the radiation from the test is short lived and that the test is considered to be a relatively noninvasive test.

■ Encourage patient to remain relaxed and to avoid stress. Patient should not sleep but should remain quiet and still.

■ Instruct patient to take fluids post-test to get rid of radioactive substance.

PROCTOSIGMOIDOSCOPY, PROCTOSCOPY, SIGMOIDOSCOPY

Normal Finding

Normal mucosa and structure of the rectum and sigmoid colon

Description

Proctosigmoidoscopy is the term for proctoscopy (an examination of the anus and rectum) and sigmoidoscopy (an examination of the anus, rectum, and sigmoid colon). There are three types of instruments used: (1) a 7-cm rigid proctoscope or anoscope, (2) a 25- to 30-cm rigid sigmoidoscope, (3) a 60-cm flexible sigmoidoscope used to visualize the descending colon. A proctosigmoid-oscopy can be performed in the hospital, in a clinic, or in the physician's office.

With this procedure the rectum and distal sigmoid colon can be visualized, and specimens can be obtained by a biopsy forceps or a snare, cytology brush, or culture swab. This test is usually indicated when there are changes in bowel habits, chronic constipation, or bright blood or mucus in the stool; or it can be done as part of an annual physical examination in patients over 40 years old.[1,2,4,11]

Clinical Problems

Abnormal Findings: hemorrhoids; rectal and sigmoid colon polyps; fistulas, fissures; rectal abscesses; neoplasms (benign or malignant); ulcerative or granulomatous colitis; infection and/or inflammation of the rectosigmoid area.

Procedure

- A consent form should be signed.
- The patient is allowed a light dinner the night before the test and a light breakfast or NPO for 8 hours prior to the test. Usually heavy meals, vegetables, and fruits are prohibited within 24 hours of the test.
- The patient may take prescribed medications by 6 AM the morning of the test with the physician's permission.
- No barium studies should be performed within 3 days of the test.
- A saline or warm tap water enema(s) or hypertonic salt enema(s) (Fleet enema) is given the morning of the test. If enemas are contraindicated, then a rectal suppository, such as bisacodyl (Dulcolax), could be given. Fecal material must be evacuated before the examination. Preparation with Golytely could be used. Oral cathartics are seldom used, since they may increase fecal flow from the small intestine during the test.
- The patient should assume either a knee-chest position or Sims' (side-lying) position for the proctosigmoidoscopy. The patient will be properly draped to avoid embarrassment and strapped to table if needed.
- As the lubricated endoscope (proctoscope, sigmoidoscope, or proctosigmoidoscope) is inserted into the rectum, the patient should be instructed to breathe deeply and slowly. Sometimes air is injected into the bowel to improve visualization. The air can cause gas pains. Cotton swabs and suction should be available.
- Specimens can be obtained during the procedure. Tissue specimen(s) should be placed in a bottle containing a preservative or on a slide and sprayed with a fixative solution. The commercial fixative sprays may cause distortion of cells.
- The procedure takes approximately 15 to 30 minutes.

- Factors Affecting Diagnostic Results

- Barium can decrease the visualization, and so barium studies should be performed a week before the test or afterwards.

- Fecal material in the lower colon can decrease visualization.
- Placement of tissue and cell specimens in solutions without preservative solutions can cause false results. Fixative sprays could distort the cells.

NURSING IMPLICATIONS WITH RATIONALE

- Explain to the patient that the purpose of the test is to determine the cause of symptoms (ie, bright blood or mucus in stools, constipation, bowel changes), or tell the patient that it is part of the routine physical examination for preventive health care.
- Explain the procedure to the patient in regard to body position, pretest preparation (enema and diet), and the time required for the procedure.
- Check the chart to determine if the patient has had a barium study within 3 days before the scheduled proctosigmoidoscopy. If so, the physician should be notified.
- Obtain a patient history in regard to being pregnant or having ulcerative colitis. Frequently enemas and suppositories are contraindicated during pregnancy and with ulcerative colitis.
- Record base-line vital signs before the test. Vital signs may be monitored during the examination.
- Allow the patient time to ask questions and express concerns. Refer questions you cannot answer to a physician or to the appropriate health professional.

Patient Teaching

- Inform the patient that the procedure may cause some discomfort but should not cause severe pain. Encourage the patient to breathe deeply and slowly and to relax during the test. Explain that there may be some gas pains if a small amount of air is injected during the procedure for better visualization.

Post-test

- Monitor vital signs as indicated or at least every 30 minutes for the first 2 hours.
- Encourage the patient to rest for several hours after the test if possible. This procedure may be done in a clinic, in a physician's office, or in the hospital. If the test is done on an outpatient basis, the patient should rest for 1 hour before leaving.
- Observe the signs and symptoms of bowel perforation (ie, pain, abdominal distention, and rectal bleeding). This problem rarely occurs. Also observe for shocklike symptoms (ie, paleness, diaphoresis, tachycardia, and later a drop in BP). Report all symptoms immediately to the physician.
- Be supportive of the patient and his or her family.

PULMONARY FUNCTION TESTS
Pulmonary Diagnostic Tests

Normal Findings

Normal values according to patient's age, sex, and height; >80% of the predicted value

Description*

Pulmonary function tests (PFTs) are useful in differentiating between obstructive and restrictive lung diseases and in quantifying the degree (mild, moderate, or severe) of obstructive or restrictive lung disorders. Other purposes for pulmonary tests include establishing base-line test results for comparison with future pulmonary tests; evaluating pulmonary status before surgery determining pulmonary disability for insurance; tracking the progress of lung disease; and assessing the response to therapy.

In pulmonary physiology testing, the lungs are monitored by many complex devices and tests. The most basic device is the spirometer; it is used to measure flows, volumes, and capacities.

A number of pulmonary tests are conducted, since no single measurement can evaluate pulmonary function. The tests frequently used for PFTs are the slow vital-capacity group, lung-volume groups, forced vital capacity, flow-volume loop, diffusion-study group, bronchodilator response studies, exercise studies, and nutritional studies.

Pulmonary Function Tests

1. *Slow vital-capacity (SVC) tests:*

   Tidal volume (TV, V_t): the amount of air inhaled and exhaled during rest or quiet respiration or normal breathing

   Inspiratory capacity (IC): the maximal inspired amount of air from end-expiratory tidal volume in normal breathing

   Expiratory reserve volume (ERV): the maximal amount of air that can be exhaled from end-expiratory tidal volume in normal breathing

   Inspiratory reserve volume (IRV): the maximal amount of air that can be inspired from end-inspiratory tidal volume in normal breathing

   Vital capacity (VC): the maximal amount of air exhaled after a maximal inhalation

$$VC = ERV + IC$$

   Note: These pulmonary measurements are done slowly, without force.

2. *Lung volume studies:*

   Lung volume using gas:

   Lung volumes are special studies that use data generated in the slow vital-capacity test. To obtain lung volumes, a tracer gas such as helium

---

*David C. Sestili, CRTT, RPFT, Manager of the Pulmonary Laboratories, Medical Center of Delaware, Christiana Hospital, Newark, Delaware, 19718.

or nitrogen, is required. Using one of the gases in a small quantity, the person breathes in and out as the tracer gas is equilibrated in the lung; the functional residual capacity (FRC) is calculated from the changes.
Lung volume by plethysmography method:
Lung volumes can be done by total body *plethysmography* or by radiologic techniques. Body plethysmography is a device that resembles an air-tight telephone booth in which the subject sits. This method is more accurate to measure total volume of the lungs than the tracer gas method.
Lung volume measurements: See Fig. 1.
Residual volume (RV): the amount of air that remains in the lungs after maximal expiration

$$RV = FRC - ERV$$

Functional residual capacity (FRC): the amount of air left in the lungs after tidal or normal expiration

$$FRC = ERC + RV$$

In obstructive disorders FRC is increased because of hyperinflation of the lungs due to air trapping. In restrictive disorders FRC and RV can be normal or decreased.
Total lung capacity (TLC): the total amount of air that is in the lungs at maximal inspiration

$$TLC = VC + RV, \text{ or } TLC = FRC + IC$$

3. *Lung volume and capacity:* See fig 1, graphic of lung volume and capacity

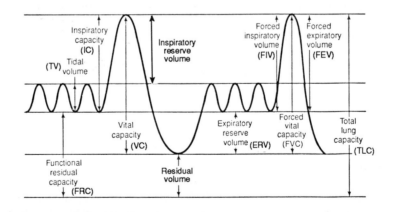

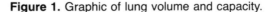

Figure 1. Graphic of lung volume and capacity.

Forced vital capacity (FVC): In obstructive lung disease the FVC is decreased; in restrictive lung disease, the FVC is normal or decreased.

$$FVC = IC + ERV$$

Forced inspiratory volume (FIV): the greatest amount of air inhaled after a maximal expiration

Forced expiratory volume timed (FEV-T): The greatest amount of air exhaled in FEV 0.5 second, 1 second FEV_1, 2 seconds FEV_2, and 3 seconds FEV_3. See Fig 2, graphic of forced expiratory volume timed. FEV_1 is considered the parameter of choice to evaluate asthmatics and other obstructive lung disease and to evaluate the response to bronchodilator therapy. An improvement of greater than 15% after bronchodilator therapy is considered significant and indicates the presence of reversible airway obstruction, such as bronchospasm.

4. *Flow-Volume Loop (FVL):* Another method to visualize forced vital-capacity measurement is by graphing flow versus volume, as seen in Fig 3. Abnormal FVLs in Fig 4 indicate types of pulmonary problems. This test yields the same basic information as the forced vital-capacity (FVC) test but in addition provides the following useful visual information, such as small-airway disease and upper-airway obstruction. Its usefulness in screening people with some types of sleep disorder problems has been recently documented.

Peak expiratory flow (PEF): the highest flow rate achieved at the beginning of the FVC; reported in L/sec

Peak inspiratory flow (PIF): the highest flow rate achieved at the beginning of the forced inspiratory capacity

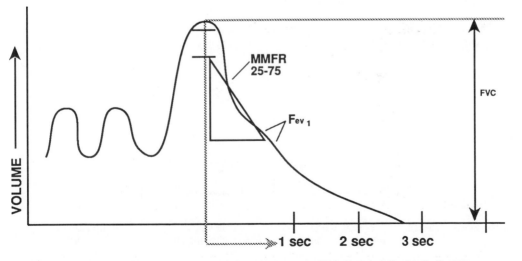

Figure 2. Graphic of forced expiratory volume timed. *(Courtesy of David C. Sestili, CRTT, RPFT.)*

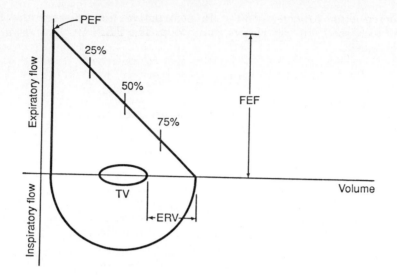

Figure 3. Flow-volume loop (FVL); and forced expiratory flow (FEF). *(Courtesy of David C. Sestili, CRTT; RPFT)*

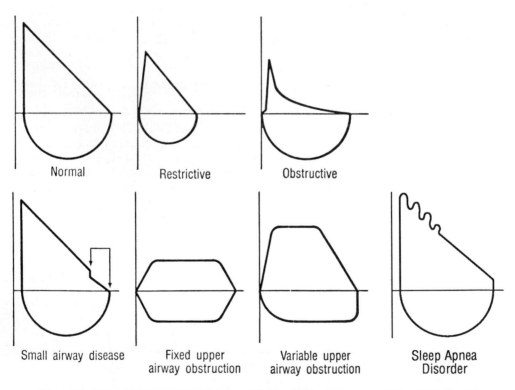

Normal   Restrictive   Obstructive

Small airway disease   Fixed upper airway obstruction   Variable upper airway obstruction   Sleep Apnea Disorder

Figure 4. Abnormal flow volume loops (FVL). (FEF): *(Courtesy of David C. Sestili, CRTT, RPFT)*

Forced expiratory flow (FEF): Figure 3 demonstrates the rate of flow at selected points on the flow-volume loop. The FEF looks at flow at the 25%, 50%, and 75% of the FVC and evaluates flow in various size airways. It can evaluate the effectiveness of bronchodilator therapy. FEF 25% reflects flow through large airways; FEF 50% reflects flow through medium airways; and FEF 75% reflects flow through small airways. Decreased FEF 75% indicates small-airway disease.

5. *Diffusion capacity test:*

   Diffusion tests can be done by a number of techniques. The most commonly used one is the single breath test. This requires the patient to inspire from RV to TLC. The gas inhaled is a mixture of helium 10%, carbon monoxide 0.3%, oxygen 21%, and nitrogen 68.7%. The patient holds his breath for 10 seconds prior to expiration. After the first 750 mL is discarded to wash out dead-space gas, an alveolar sample is collected and analyzed for helium and CO concentration. Results of this reflect the state of the alveolar capillary barrier. Decreased diffusing capacity occurs in disease states such as interstitial fibrosis, interstitial edema, and emphysema. It will also decrease in persons with abnormal hemoglobin, such as anemias, smokers, HbCO.

6. *Bronchial Provocation Studies:*

   Inhalation of pharmacologic and antigenic substances are used to test the sensitivity of the airways toward hyper-reactivity and obstruction. Serial spirometry tests are performed to document the amount or degree of reactivity (usually a drop in FEV_1 greater than 20% of base-line spirometry). A bronchoconstrictor is given first and is then followed by a bronchodilator. A history of symptoms of wheezing or coughing without cause or symptoms related to exposure to industrial substances are indications for this type of test.

7. *Exercise studies:*

   Pulmonary function studies are done at a resting state. Exercise studies allow evaluation during an active state. These tests are performed by having the subject walk on a treadmill or pedal an ergometer to a set protocol to simulate activity at progressive work loads. During the test 12-lead ECGs are taken, and expired gases are analyzed for oxygen consumption and CO_2 production along with tidal volume, respirator rate, BP, oxygen saturation, and arterial blood gases. These tests are used to determine the amount of disability and to evaluate persons with exertional dyspnea.

8. *Nutritional studies:*

   Indirect calorimetry is the measurement of CO_2 production and O_2 consumption. Respiratory quotient (RQ), obtained from the calorimetry, yields the type of substrate used in metabolism (carbohydrate, fat, protein).

   This noninvasive test gives useful information as to the energy expenditure (EE), the amount of calories needed for minimal existence expressed in Kilocalories per 24 hours. Respiratory quotient will give the type of fuel being metabolized. For example, RQ 1.0 is carbohydrates, RQ 0.80 indicates mixed carbohydrates and fats, RQ 0.75 indicates lipids being metabolized.[1,2,7,11,29-32]

Clinical Problems

Obstructive Diseases: emphysema, chronic bronchitis, bronchiectasis, bronchospasm, bronchial secretions, airway inflammation caused by bacterial or viral infections

Restrictive Diseases: pulmonary fibrosis, pneumonia, lung tumors, kyposcoliosis, neuromuscular diseases, chest trauma, obesity, scleroderma, pulmonary edema, surgical removal of lung tissue

Procedure

■ Heavy meal before the test should be discouraged.

■ Avoid smoking 4 to 6 hours before the test.

■ Patient should wear nonrestrictive clothing.

■ Record patient's age, height, and weight, which may be used to predict normal range.

■ Bronchodilators are restricted prior to the test, since they are usually administered in the pulmonary function laboratory with tests. Usually sedatives and narcotics are not given. Other medications are given prior to the test unless indicated by the physician.

■ Postpone procedure if the patient has an active cold or is under the influence of alcohol.

■ Dentures may be left in during testing.

■ The test can be performed in a sitting or standing position. A nose clip is applied and the patient is instructed to breathe in and out through the mouth.

■ Practice sessions on fast-and-deep breathing are given. Normally the test is repeated twice and the best tracing is used. The test may be repeated after using a bronchodilator spray.

Bronchial Provocation Studies

■ The patient inhales varied doses of methacholine chloride, a short-acting bronchoconstrictor, until all doses, approximately five, are administered without a change in FEV_1 or a drop of 20% of baseline FEV_1. The drug is then reversed by administration of a bronchodilator.

■ There should be no exercise, smoking, or caffeine (coffee, cola, or chocolate) consumption for a minumum of 6 hours before testing. Any bronchodilator or antihistamine therapy (PO or inhaled) should be discontinued for at least 48 hours prior to testing.

Nutritional Studies

■ NPO for 12 hours prior and until completion of test.

■ There should be no activity before test. Nutritional studies are usually performed ½ hour after awakening.

■ The patient's exhalation is analyzed for oxygen consumption and CO_2 production. Patients on ventilators, hyperalimentation, or tube feeding can be tested as long as there are no changes in the diet or ventilator settings until the test is completed.

Exercise Studies

■ The patient will be walking on a treadmill or riding a stationary bike. The heart rate and rhythm will be monitored by a 12-lead ECG.

■ The patient will be breathing through a mouthpiece during the test.

- Factors Affecting Diagnostic Results
  - Use of bronchodilators 2 hours before pulmonary function test may produce false-improved pulmonary results.
  - Sedatives and narcotics given before the test could decrease test results.
  - Lack of cooperation by the patient due to not understanding the specific test procedure may affect results.

NURSING IMPLICATIONS WITH RATIONALE

- List on the request slip oral/inhaled bronchodilators and steroids the patient is taking. Record patient's age, height, and weight.
- Record vital signs.
- Assess for signs and symptoms of respiratory distress (ie, breathlessness, dyspnea, tachycardia, severe apprehension, and gray or cyanotic color).
- Be supportive of patient, and answer patient's questions if known.

Patient Teaching

- Instruct the patient to eat a light breakfast, except in nutritional studies; to take medications, except for bronchodilators, sedatives, narcotics, and others as stated by physician orders; to avoid smoking for 4 to 6 hours before test.
- Tell the patient that the test should not be performed if he or she has an active cold or communicable disease unless approved by the physician and the pulmonary function laboratory (PFL) chief.
- Practice breathing patterns for pulmonary function tests with the patient (ie, normal breathing, rapid breathing, and forced deep inspiration and forced deep expiration).

RADIOACTIVE IODINE (RAI) UPTAKE TEST
I-131 Uptake Test, Radioiodine Thyroid Uptake Test

Normal Finding
Adult: 2 hours: 1%–13% (thyroid gland). *6 hours:* 2%–25% (thyroid gland). *24 hours:* 15%–45% (thyroid gland)

Description
The radioactive iodine uptake test is used to determine the metabolic activity of the thyroid gland by measuring the absorption of I-131 or I-123 in the thyroid. The uptake test is one of the tests used in diagnosing hypothyroidism and hyperthyroidism. It is also useful for differentiating between hyperthyroidism

(Graves' disease) and an overactive toxic adenoma. This test tends to be more accurate for diagnosing hyperthyroidism than for diagnosing hypothyroidism.

A calculated dose of I-131 or I-123 (in capsule or liquid form) is given orally. The patient's thyroid is scanned at three different times. The tracer dose has small amount of radioactivity and is considered harmless. The patient's urine output may be checked for radioactive iodine excretion.[2,9,11,23]

Clinical Problems

Decreased Level: hypothyroidism (myxedema). *Drug Influence:* Lugol's solution, vitamins, expectorants (ie, SSKI), antithyroid agents, cortisone preparation, ACTH, aspirin, antihistamines, phenylbutazone (Butazolidin), anticoagulants (ie, warfarin [Coumadin]), thiopental sodium (Pentothal). *Foods:* seafood, cabbage, ionized salt

Elevated Level: hyperthyroidism (Graves' disease), thyroiditis, cirrhosis of the liver. *Drug Influence:* barbiturates, estrogens, lithium carbonate, phenothiazines

Procedure

- The patient should be NPO for 8 hours prior to the test. The patient can eat an hour after the radioiodine capsule or liquid has been taken.
- The amount of radioactivity in the thyroid gland may be measured three times (after 2, 6, and 24 hours).
- The patient should return to the nuclear medicine laboratory at specified times to measure the I-131 uptake level with the scintillation counter.

- Factors Affecting Diagnostic Results

- Certain drugs can affect test results (see Drug influence). Foods containing iodine (seafood, ionized salt) could cause false-negative result.
- Drugs and foods (*see Clinical Problems*).
- Severe diarrhea, intestinal malabsorption, and x-ray contrast media studies may cause a decreased I-131 uptake level, even in normal thyroid glands.
- Rapid diuresis during the test could cause iodine excretion and a low iodine uptake in the thyroid gland.
- Renal failure could cause an increased iodine uptake.

NURSING IMPLICATIONS WITH RATIONALE

- Explain to the patient the purpose and procedure for the test.
- Ask the patient if he or she has allergies to iodine products.
- Inform the patient that a technician from the nuclear medicine laboratory will give the radioactive substance and that he or she must go to the laboratory 2, 6, and 24 hours after taking the iodine preparation. Explain to the patient that the procedure is to determine the percent of I-131 or I-123 uptake, that the test should not be painful, and that the amount of radiation received should be harmless. Emphasize the importance of being on time for each determination.

- List on the request slip for the I-131 uptake test the x-ray studies and drugs the patient has received in the last week that could affect test results. These drugs should, if possible, be discontinued for 3 or more days before the test (*see Drug Influence*).
- Draw blood for T_3 and/or T_4 tests, if ordered, before the patient takes the radioiodine capsule or liquid.
- Answer the patient's questions. Encourage the patient to communicate concerns.
- Observe for signs and symptoms of hyperthyroidism (ie, nervousness, tachycardia, excessive hyperactivity, exophthalmos, mood swings [euphoria to depression], and weight loss). Report these to the physician, and record them in the patient's chart.

Patient Teaching

- Inform the patient that he or she may eat an hour after the radioiodine capsule or liquid has been taken, according to the nuclear medicine laboratory's procedure.
- Instruct the patient to return to the nuclear medicine laboratory at specified times. The testing should be done on time.
- Inform the patient that the radioactive substance should not harm family members, visitors, or other patients, since the dosage is low and gives off very little radiation. Women who are pregnant definitely should not be given this test or any other radioactive tests.

RETROGRADE PYELOGRAPHY (RETROGRADE PYELOGRAM)
Retrograde Ureteropyelography

Normal Finding
Normal size and structure of the bladder, ureters, and kidneys

Description
A retrograde pyelography test may be performed after IVP or in place of IVP. The contrast dye is injected through a catheter into the ureters and the renal pelvis. The visualization of the urinary tract is exceptionally good because the dye is injected directly. Usually this test is done in conjunction with cystoscopy.

Although retrograde pyelograms are not done too frequently today, this test is still performed when there is a suspected nonfunctioning kidney, an unlocated stone, or an allergy to IV contrast dye. Only a small amount of the dye that is injected directly into the ureters will be absorbed through the membranes.[1,2,4,11]

Clinical Problems
Abnormal Findings: renal calculi, neoplasm (tumor), renal stricture, nonfunctioning kidney

Procedure

- A consent form should be signed.
- The patient should be NPO for 8 hours before the retrograde pyelography. The patient should not be dehydrated before the test.
- Laxatives and cleansing enemas may be ordered prior to the test.
- Base-line vital signs should be recorded.
- Sedatives/tranquilizers and narcotic analgesics are given approximately 1 hour before the test.
- The patient is usually placed in the lithotomy position (feet and legs in stirrups).
- Radiopaque contrast dye is injected through a ureteral catheter into the renal pelvis and x-rays are taken. As the catheter is removed, additional x-rays may be taken.
- This procedure is usually done under local or general anesthesia, and the test takes approximately 1 hour.

■ Factors Affecting Diagnostic Results

- Barium in the GI tract could interfere with good visualization. Barium studies should be done after a retrograde pyelogram.

NURSING IMPLICATIONS WITH RATIONALE

- Explain to the patient that the purpose of the test is to identify kidney stones or to determine the cause of his or her kidney problems, or give a similar response related to the symptoms.
- Explain the procedure to the patient. Explain to the patient that he or she will be placed in stirrups. If the patient is having the test done under local anesthesia, tell the patient that he or she will most likely feel pressure and the urge to urinate with insertion of the cystoscope.
- Inform him or her that there should be little to no pain or discomfort. Tell the patient that the test takes about 1 hour.
- Inform the patient that food and drinks are restricted for 8 hours before the test. Some physicians may not restrict water unless the patient is to have general anesthesia. Check for symptoms of dehydration (ie, dry mouth and mucous membranes, poor skin turgor, decreased urine output, and fast pulse and respirations). Report symptoms to the physician and record them on the patient's chart.
- Record base-line vital signs.
- Obtain a patient history of allergies to seafood, iodine, and/or radiopaque dye used in other diagnostic tests.
- Administer laxatives, cleansing enemas, and premedications as prescribed. If the patient is not hospitalized, check that the prescribed orders were completed at home or in another institution. Check that the consent form has been signed before giving premedications.

Post-test

- Monitor vital signs until stable or as ordered.
- Observe for allergic reactions to the contrast dye (ie, skin rash, urticaria [hives], flushing, dyspnea, and tachycardia).
- Monitor urinary output. Report and record gross hematuria. Blood-tinged urine usually is normal. Report to the physician if the patient has not voided in 8 hours or the urinary output is less than 200 mL in 8 hours.
- Give an analgesic for discomfort or pain. Report severe pain to the physician.
- Observe for signs and symptoms of infection (sepsis; ie, fever, chills, abdominal pain, tachycardia, and, later, hypotension).
- Be supportive of the patient and family. Answer the patient's questions, or refer them to the physician or urologist.

SCANS
(See Nuclear Scans.)

SEX CHROMATIN MASS, BUCCAL SMEAR, BARR BODY ANALYSIS

Normal Finding

Barr body in 25% to 50% of the female buccal mucosal cells

Description

The sex chromatin test is a screening method to detect the presence or absence of Barr chromatin body (an inactivated X chromosome in a mass lying at the periphery of the cell nucleus) in the buccal mucosal cells. Buccal smears are used to check for Barr body when chromosomal abnormalities are suspected (eg, Turner's syndrome [absent or <20% Barr body in females] and Klinefelter's syndrome [presence of Barr body in males]). This test is also indicated if amenorrhea or abnormal sexual development is present.

Abnormal findings should be followed up by chromosome analysis (karyotype). The sex chromatin test should not be used for sex determinations.[2,3,8,9,11]

Clinical Problems

Abnormal Findings: Turner's syndrome (female): absence of Barr body, amenorrhea, sterility, underdeveloped breasts; Klinefelter's syndrome (male): presence of Barr body, small penis and testes, sparse facial hair, gynecomastia, sterility

Procedure

- There is no food or fluid restriction.
- The patient should rinse his or her mouth well.

- A wooden or metal spatula is used to scrape the buccal mucosa twice; the first scraping is discarded, and the second is spread over a glass slide. The slide should be sprayed with a fixative solution and sent to the laboratory for identifying a Barr body in the cells. The specimen should be labeled with the patient's name, sex, and age, as well as the date and the specimen site.
- Check that the specimen is not saliva. The smear is stained and examined under a microscope.
- The procedure usually takes 10 to 20 minutes.

■ Factors Affecting Diagnostic Results

  - If the specimen is saliva and not cells, the test result could be inaccurate.
  - Failure to use a preservative spray on the buccal smear specimen will cause cell deterioration.

NURSING IMPLICATIONS WITH RATIONALE

- Explain to the patient and/or parents that the purpose of the test is to determine the cause of abnormal sexual development. Inform them that this is a screening test and that other tests, such as chromosome analysis, may be indicated.
- Explain the procedure to the patient and parents. Inform the patient that the cells from inside the mouth (buccal smear) are used because they are easy to obtain. Tell them that the test has a high percentage of accuracy. The procedure usually takes 10 to 20 minutes; however, the results from the test may take several weeks.
- Inform the patient that there should be a minimal amount of discomfort. Light pressure will be applied when scraping the mucosa.
- Be supportive of the patient and his or her family. Be a good listener. Answer questions or refer them to the appropriate health professionals.
- Record in the chart any abnormal sexual characteristics or problems and note them on the request slip (eg, amenorrhea, gynecomastia).

SKIN TESTS (TUBERCULIN, BLASTOMYCOSIS, COCCIDIOIDOMYCOSIS, HISTOPLASMOSIS, TRICHINOSIS, AND TOXOPLASMOSIS)

Normal Finding

Negative results

Description

Skin testing is useful for determining present or past exposure to an infectious organism: bacterial (tuberculosis), mycotic (blastomycosis, coccidioidomycosis, histoplasmosis), or parasitic (trichinosis and toxoplasmosis). The types of skin tests include scratch, patch, multipuncture, and intradermal. The antigen of the organism is injected intradermally (under the skin), and if the test is positive in 24 to 72 hours, the injection site becomes red, hard, and edematous.

Bacterial Organism and Disease

Tuberculosis: the tuberculin (antigen) skin test indicates whether a person has been infected by the tubercle bacilli. A negative test usually rules out the disease.

The methods for skin testing include:

1. *Mantoux test:* Purified protein derivative tuberculin (PPD) is injected intradermally. PPD has several strengths, but the intermediate strength is usually used unless the patient is known to be hypersensitive to skin tests. The patient should not receive PPD if there has been a previous positive test. The test is read in 48 to 72 hours.
2. *The tine test or Mono-Vacc test:* These are multipuncture tests that use tines impregnated with PPD. This method is used for mass screening. The tine test is read in 48 to 72 hours, and the Mono-Vacc Test is read in 48 to 96 hours.
3. *Vollmer's patch test:* This test resembles a Band-Aid; however, the center piece is impregnated with concentrated old tuberculin (OT). The patch is removed in 48 hours, and the test is read 48 hours later.

Mycotic Organisms and Diseases

Blastomycosis: The organism *Blastomyces dermatitidis* causes blastomycosis. The antigen blastomycin is injected intradermally, and if an erythematic area greater than 5 mm in diameter occurs, the test is positive. The skin test should be read in 48 hours. Positive sputum and tissue specimens will confirm the blastomycin skin test.

Coccidioidomycosis: The coccidioidin skin test is useful for diagnosing coccidioidomycosis, a fungus disease caused by *Coccidioides immitis.* The antigen coccidioidin is injected intradermally, and the skin test should be read in 24 to 72 hours. A patient treated for coccidioidomycosis may remain positive during his or her life-span.

Histoplasmosis: Histoplasmosis is caused by the organism *Histoplasma capsulatum,* which on a lung x-ray resembles tuberculosis. The histoplasmin skin test for histoplasmosis is not always reliable. The antigen is injected intradermally and should be read in 24 to 48 hours. A positive test result occurs when an erythematic area is over 5 mm in diameter. To confirm the skin test results, sputum and tissue specimens should be obtained.

Parasites

Trichinosis: The parasitic organism *Trichinella spiralis* causes trichinosis. This organism is present in uncooked meat, especially pork. Symptoms occur approximately 2 weeks after ingesting the organism; the patient complains of nausea, diarrhea, pain, colic, fever, and swelling of the muscles. The antigen is injected intradermally, and the test should be read in 15 to 20 minutes. A positive test is a blanched wheal with an erythematic area surrounding it.

Toxoplasmosis: *Toxoplasma gondii* is the organism causing toxoplasmosis.

This organism is found in the eye ground and brain tissue of man. It can cause blindness and brain damage. The antigen toxoplasmin is injected intradermally and the test result should be read in 24 to 48 hours. A positive test is an erythematic area over 10 mm in diameter.[1,2,4,11]

Clinical Problems

ANTIGEN SKIN TEST	ORGANISM	DISEASE
Tuberculin	Tubercle bacilli	Tuberculosis
Blastomycin	*Blastomyces dermatitidis*	Blastomycosis
Coccidioidin	*Coccidioides immitis*	Coccidioidomycosis
Histoplasmin	*Histoplasma capsulatum*	Histoplasmosis
Trichinellin	*Trichinella spiralis*	Trichinosis
Toxoplasmin	*Toxoplasma gondii*	Toxoplasmosis

Procedure

- Food and fluids are not restricted.
- Cleanse the inner aspect of the forearm with alcohol and let it dry.
- Inject intradermally 0.1 mL of the antigen into the inner aspect used for the forearm.
- Record the patient's name, the name of the test, the site of the arm of the skin test, the date, and the time it should be read (*see Description for readings of individual tests*).

■ Factors Affecting Diagnostic Results

- Steroids and immunosuppressants given within 4 to 6 weeks can cause false-negative skin test results.
- A skin test performed before the body's incubation period (infectious process) can cause a false-negative result.
- Test results read several days after the designated time can give an inaccurate reading.

NURSING IMPLICATIONS WITH RATIONALE

- Explain to the patient that the purpose of the skin test is to determine the presence of an organism. The organism and the type of skin test should be discussed.
- Explain the procedure to the patient. Tell the patient that a pin prick will be felt as a small needle with a small amount of solution is injected under the skin.
- Obtain a patient history about hypersensitivity to skin tests. Ask the patient if the skin test was performed before and, if so, whether the skin test result was positive or negative. The skin test should only be repeated if it was negative.
- Report if the patient is taking steroids (eg, cortisone) or immunosuppressant drugs in the last 4 to 6 weeks, since false test results could occur.

- Record the patient's abnormal signs and symptoms. Ask the patient about his or her contact with bacterial, fungal, or parasitic organisms, if known.
- Be supportive of the patient and family, and allow them time to express their concerns.

Patient Teaching

- Inform the patient that the result of the skin test must be read during the stated time.
- Inform the patient that a positive skin test does not always indicate active infectious disease. However, the positive test does indicate that the organism is present in the body in either an active or a dormant state. If the results are positive, other studies are performed (ie, x-rays, sputum and tissue cultures, and serum tests).

STRESS/EXERCISE TESTING (STRESS TESTING), EXERCISE ELECTROCARDIOLOGY (ELECTROCARDIOGRAM—ECG), EXERCISE THALLIUM PERFUSION IMAGING TEST (THALLIUM STRESS TEST)

Normal Finding

Normal ECG with little or no ST segment depression with exercise. Normal myocardial perfusion

Description

Stress testing is based on the theory that patients with coronary artery disease will have marked ST segment depression on the ECG when exercising. Depression of the ST segment and depression or inversion of the T wave indicate myocardial ischemia. In 1928 Fiel and Siegel reported on the relationship of exercising and ST segment depression in patients complaining of angina. Master used an exercise test (two-step) in 1929 to demonstrate ischemia but used only pulse and BP to note changes. In 1931 Wood and Wolferth felt exercise was a useful tool for diagnosing coronary disease but that it could be dangerous. Later it was discovered that ST segment depression usually occurred before the onset of pain and was still present for some time after the pain had subsided. Mild ST segment depression after exercise can occur without coronary artery disease.

In 1956 Bruce established guidelines on performing stress testing on a treadmill. Master's Step Test (1955) was also accepted as a method for stress testing. Another method used today is the bicycle ergometer test; however, the treadmill seems to be the choice for testing cardiac status. The body muscles do not seem to tire with the treadmill method as much as leg muscles with the bicycle ergometer. For patients who cannot walk (ie, paraplegics, amputees), an arm ergometer can be used. With the treadmill stress test, the work rate is changed every 3 minutes for 15 minutes by increasing the speed slightly and the degree of incline (grade) by 3% each time (3%, 6%, 9%).

Exercise Thallium Perfusion Test   The radioisotope thallium-201, which accumulates in the myocardial cells, is used during the stress test to determine myocardial perfusion during exercise. With severe narrowing of the coronary arteries, there is less thallium accumulation in the heart muscle. If a coronary vessel is completely occluded, no uptake of thallium will occur at the myocardial area that the vessel supplies.

Patients with coronary artery disease may have normal thallium perfusion scans at rest; however, during exercise, when the heart demands more oxygen, myocardial perfusion decreases. The patient returns in 2 or more hours to take a second scan of the heart at rest. Frequently second scans are done to differentiate between an ischemic area and an infarcted or scar area of the myocardium. This test could be normal even with moderately narrowed coronary arteries and adequate collateral circulation to the heart.

Uses for the stress/exercise test or the exercise thallium perfusion test include screening for coronary artery disease, evaluating myocardial perfusion, evaluating the work capacity of cardiac patients, and developing a cardiac rehabilitation program.[2,9,33,34]

Clinical Problems

Abnormal Finding: Positive: >1 mm ST depression

Indications: to detect coronary artery disease; to evaluate myocardial perfusion, cardiac status for work capability, further diagnostic studies (eg, cardiac catheterization), jogging or an exercise program (especially after the age of 35 years), cardiac rehabilitation programs

Procedure

- A consent form should be signed by the patient.
- The patient should eat a light meal 2 or 3 hours before the test. The patient should not consume alcoholic and caffeine-containing drinks and should avoid smoking for 2 to 3 hours before the test. Milk could cause nausea.
- Medications should be taken, unless otherwise indicated by the physician.
- Comfortable clothes should be worn(ie, shorts or slacks with a belt and sneakers or tennis shoes with socks). Most bedroom slippers are not suitable.
- The chest and/or back are shaved as needed, and the skin is cleansed with alcohol.
- Electrodes are applied to the chest according to the lead selections.
- Base-line ECG, pulse rate, and BP are taken and then are monitored throughout the test.
- The test is stopped if the patient becomes dyspneic, suffers severe fatigue, complains of chest pain, has a rapid increase in pulse rates and/or BP, or develops life-threatening arrhythmias (ie, ventricular tachycardia, premature ventricular contractions [PVCs] over 10 PVC in 1 minute).
- Usually the test is not stopped abruptly unless this is necessary. Vital signs and ECG tracings are recorded at the end of the testing or the recovery stage.

■ The test takes approximately 30 minutes, which includes up to 10 to 15 minutes of exercising.

Treadmill Stress Test: Usually there are five stages. In the first stage the speed is 2 mph at a 3% grade or incline for 3 minutes. In the second stage the speed is 3.3 mph at a 6% grade for another 3 minutes. Normally the speed does not go beyond 3.3 mph. With each stage the grade is increased 3% and the time is increased by 3 minutes, unless fatigue or adverse reactions occur. The power-driven treadmill has support rails to help the patient maintain balance.

Bicycle Ergometer Test: The patient is instructed to pedal the bike against an increased amount of resistance. The bike handlebars are for maintaining balance and should not be gripped tightly for support. The patient should not shower or take a hot bath for 2 hours after testing.

Exercise Thallium Perfusion Test: An IV line is inserted. Exercise time for the stress test is determined. The patient obtains the maximal exercise level, and thallium is injected intravenously 1 minute before the test ends. The patient continues to exercise for 1 to 2 more minutes. A scan taken by scintillator visualizes thallium perfusion of the myocardium.

Patient returns in 2 or more hours for a second scan.

■ Factors Affecting Diagnostic Results

■ Certain drugs (eg, digitalis preparations) can cause a false-positive test result.
■ Leaning on support rails of the treadmill or the handlebars of the bicycle will affect the test results.

NURSING IMPLICATIONS WITH RATIONALE

■ Recognize when the stress/exercise test is contraindicated (ie, with recent myocardial infarction; severe, unstable angina; uncontrolled arrhythmias; congestive heart failure; or recent pulmonary embolism).
■ Explain the procedure to the patient in regard to a light meal 2 to 3 hours prior to test; not smoking, continuing with medications; the clothing and shoes that should be worn; shaving and cleansing the chest area; electrode application; continuous monitoring the ECG, pulse rate, and BP; and not leaning on the rails of the treadmill or the handlebars of the bike.
■ Check that the consent form has been signed.
■ Inform the patient that the electrodes will not hurt; however there may be some itching at the electrode sites.
■ Instruct the patient to inform the cardiologist or technician if he or she experiences chest pain, difficulty in breathing, or severe fatigue. The risk of having a myocardial infarction during the stress test is less than 0.2%.
■ Inform the patient that after 10 to 15 minutes of testing or when the heart rate is at a desired or an elevated rate, the test is stopped. It will be terminated immediately if there are any severe ECG changes (ie, multiple PVCs, ventricular tachycardia).
■ Allow the patient to ask questions. Refer questions you cannot answer to

other appropriate health professionals (ie, a cardiologist, a specialized technician, or a nurse in the stress test laboratory).

■ Instruct the patient to continue the walking exercise at the completion of the test for 3 to 5 minutes to prevent dizziness. The treadmill speed will be decreased. Tell the patient that he or she may be perspiring and may be "out of breath." Profuse diaphoresis, cold and clammy skin, severe dyspnea, and severe tachycardia are not normal.

■ Inform the patient that an ECG and vital signs are taken 5 to 10 minutes after the stress test (recovery stage).

Patient Teaching

■ Encourage the patient to participate in a cardiac/exercise rehabilitation program as advised by the physician/cardiologist. Tell the patient of the health advantages—constant heart monitoring, improved collateral circulation, increased oxygen supply to the heart, and dilating coronary resistance vessels.

■ Discourage the patient over 35 years of age from doing strenuous exercises without having a stress/exercise test or a cardiac evaluation.

■ Inform the patient that he or she can resume activity as indicated.

Exercise Thallium Perfusion Test

■ Explain the procedure for the test (*See Procedure*). Explain that the difference between the routine stress test and the exercise thallium perfusion test is an injection of thallium during the routine stress test followed by scans and/or x-rays.

■ Nursing implications are the same for both tests.

THERMOGRAPHY (BREAST)
Mammothermography

Normal Finding

No hot "white" spots; symmetric appearance of the breasts (photograph)

Description

Mammothermography (breast thermography), an infrared photographic test, measures and records heat energy from the skin surface of the breast. Lesions of the breast, especially cancerous ones, cause increased breast metabolism, resulting in an increased breast surface temperature and vascularity. If hot spots are recorded, then additional tests (such as low-dose mammography, ultrasonography, and/or biopsy) should be performed to confirm breast cancer.

Approximately 80% of positive thermograms are accurate for diagnosing lesions of the breast (35% of positive thermograms show benign breast lesions). The remaining 20% of the tests give false-positive results. Because one-fifth of the results are false positive, mammothermography is not commonly used, except for screening purposes. Usually it cannot detect small or deep breast-cancer lesions. Mammothermography should be used in conjunction with a physical examination of the breast.[2,11]

Clinical Problems

Indications: to detect cancer of the breast, abscesses of the breast, fibrocystic disease of the breast; to analyze the progression of breast lesion(s)

Procedure

- Food and fluids are not restricted. Immediately before the test, hot or very cold drinks should be avoided.
- The patient should remove jewelry and clothes from the neck to the waist. The patient is given a cloth or paper gown, and the gown should be worn with the opening in the front.
- Ointment or powder on the breast should be removed before the test.
- The patient usually sits in a cool room (68°F) for 10 to 15 minutes before the test. This helps to equalize body temperature.
- The patient is seated and will be asked to place her hands over her head or on her hips.
- Usually three photographs of different angles are taken of each breast. The procedure takes about 15 minutes.
- The films are checked for readability before the patient removes the gown.

- Factors Affecting Diagnostic Results

- Ointment, powder, and recent sunburn could change skin temperature and cause false-positive results.
- Fluctuations in room temperature could affect the test results.
- Menstruation (immediately before or during) could increase vascular engorgement of the breasts.

NURSING IMPLICATIONS WITH RATIONALE

- Explain the procedure to the patient. Procedure in hospitals and in private laboratories may differ slightly, so check before discussing the procedure with the patient. Tell the patient the test is not painful.
- Instruct the patient not to use ointment or powder on the breast the day of the test. These could cause false-positive results. Check the skin for recent exposure to sunlight.
- Obtain a menstrual history. Ask the patient when she had her last menstrual period. She should not have the thermogram if she is pregnant or if she is menstruating or close to her period. The vascularity of the breasts increases at these times.
- Inform the patient that the test takes about 15 minutes; however, she will be asked to wait for several minutes after the pictures are taken to be sure

---

they are readable. Tell the patient not to be alarmed if one of the pictures needs to be repeated.
- Encourage the patient to express her concerns. Answer questions, if possible, or refer questions to other appropriate health professionals.
- Inform the patient that the mammothermography is generally a screening test and that if the test is positive, other tests will be conducted to confirm the test results. Inform the patient that approximately one third of the positive results are benign lesions and one fifth of the positive results could be false positives.

Patient Teaching

- Encourage the patient to perform breast examination after each menstrual period and to keep routine medical appointments. If necessary, demonstrate breast examination technique.

ULTRASONOGRAPHY (ABDOMINAL AORTA, BRAIN, DOPPLER—ARTERIES AND VEINS, GALLBLADDER, HEART, KIDNEY, LIVER, PREGNANT UTERUS, PANCREAS, SPLEEN, AND THYROID)
Ultrasound, Echography (Echogram), Sonogram

Normal Finding

A normal pattern image of the organ or normal Doppler analysis

Description

Ultrasonography (ultrasound) is a diagnostic procedure used to visualize body tissue structure or wave-form analysis of Doppler studies. An ultrasound probe called a transducer is held over the skin surface or in a body cavity to produce an ultrasound beam in the tissues. The reflected sound waves or echoes from the tissues can be transformed by a computer into either scans, graphs, or audible sounds (Doppler).

Diagnostic ultrasound examination, a noninvasive test, is relatively inexpensive and fast and does not cause any known harm to the patient. There are limitations, since it cannot be used to determine bone abnormalities or for air-filled organs. The ultrasound beam cannot penetrate air. In obese persons it is difficult for sound waves to pass through fat layers.

Ultrasound can detect tissue abnormalities (ie, masses, cysts, edema, stones). Most ultrasound studies (eg, gallstones) do not need other modalities for confirmation; however, CT, MRI, or radionuclide scanning may be used to confirm certain ultrasound results.

Some of the body structures that this procedure examines are the abdominal aorta, the brain, the arteries and veins (Doppler), the gallbladder, the heart, the kidney, the liver, pregnant uterus (pelvic), the pancreas, the spleen, and the thyroid.

Abdominal Aorta: The area for abdominal scanning includes the xyphoid process to the umbilicus. Ultrasound can detect aortic aneurysms with 98% accuracy.

Brain: Brain echoencephalography is ultrasound of the brain. If the third ventricle, which is normally midline, is shifted to one side, then pathologic findings, such as intracranial lesions or intracranial hemorrhage, may be suspected. It is most useful for evaluating hydrocephalus and intracranial hemorrhage in newborns.

Arteries and Veins (Doppler): Doppler ultrasonography evaluates the blood flow in arteries and veins anywhere in the body. The Doppler transducer can detect decreased blood flow caused by partial arterial occlusion or by deep-vein thrombosis. It can be used in fetal monitoring during labor and delivery. Doppler instrument is available to nurses for monitoring blood flow for those who have altered circulation. Low-frequency waves usually indicate low-velocity blood flow.

Gallbladder and Bile Ducts: Ultrasonography can evaluate the size, structure, and position of the gallbladder and can determine the presence of gallstones.

Heart: Echocardiography is ultrasound of the heart. It can determine the size, shape, and position of the heart and the movement of heart valves and chambers. The methods commonly used are the M-mode and the two dimensional. The M-mode records the motion of the intracardiac structures, such as valves, and the two-dimensional records a cross-sectional view of cardiac structures. The echocardiogram is useful in detecting mitral stenosis, pericardial effusion, congenital heart disease, and enlargement of a heart chamber.

Kidneys: Ultrasound is a reliable test to identify and to differentiate renal cyst and tumor. The cyst is echo free, and the tumor and renal calculi record multiple echoes. This test is highly recommended when the patient is hypersensitive to iodinated contrast dye used in x-ray tests (eg, IVP).

Liver: The liver was one of the first organs examined by ultrasound, since it was large in size and difficult to x-ray. It is useful for distinguishing between a cyst or tumor and for determining the size, structure, and position of the liver. With cysts, the echogram reflects an echo-free response, whereas with a tumor, multiple echoes are recorded. Ultrasound is very helpful in differentiating obstructive from nonobstructive jaundice.

Pregnant Uterus or Pelvic: The pelvic ultrasound may be used to distinguish between a cyst and tumor. In pregnancy the amniotic fluid enhances reflection of sound waves from the placenta and fetus, thus identifying their size, shape, and position. Echoes from the pregnancy may be seen as early as 4 weeks amenorrhea. For better visualization of pelvic structures, a full bladder is indicated. The uterus is sometimes evaluated with a transvaginal transducer with the bladder empty.

Pancreas The pancreas is a difficult organ to examine. Ultrasound does not measure pancreatic function, but it can detect pancreatic abnormalities, such as pancreatic tumors, pseudocysts, and pancreatitis.

Spleen: Ultrasound can be used for determining the size, structure, and position of the spleen. This procedure can identify splenic masses. In some cases it is a useful tool for evaluating a need for a splenectomy.

Thyroid: Ultrasonography of the thyroid is 85% accurate in determining the size and structure of the thyroid gland. This procedure can differentiate between a cyst and a tumor and can determine the depth and dimension of thyroid nodules.[2,4,9,26]

Clinical Problems

ORGAN	ABNORMAL FINDINGS
Abdominal aorta	Aortic aneurysms, aortic stenosis
Brain	Intracranial hemorrhage, lesions (tumors, abscess), hydrocephalus
Arteries and veins (Doppler)	Arterial occlusion (partial or complete), deep-vein thrombosis (DVT), chronic venous insufficiency, arterial trauma
Gallbladder	Acute cholecystitis, cholelithiasis, biliary obstruction
Heart	Cardiomegaly, mitral stenosis, aortic stenosis and insufficiency, pericardial effusion, congenital heart disease
Kidney	Renal cysts and tumors, hydronephrosis, perirenal abscess, acute pyelonephritis, acute glomerulonephritis
Liver	Hepatic cysts, abscesses, tumor; hepatic metastasis; hepatocellular disease
Pelvic and pregnant uterus	Uterine tumor, fibroids; fetal death; placenta previa; abruptio placenta; hydrocephalus; breech fetal presentation
Pancreas	Pancreatic tumors, pseudocysts, acute pancreatitis
Spleen	Splenomegaly; splenic cysts, abscesses, tumor
Thyroid	Thyroid tumors (benign or malignant), thyroid goiters or cysts

Procedure

- Obtain a signed consent form.
- Restrict food and fluids for 8 to 12 hours before test for abdominal aorta, gallbladder, liver, spleen, and pancreas ultrasound studies.
- Mineral oil or conductive gel is applied to the skin surface at the site to be examined. The transducer is hand held and is moved smoothly back and forth across the oiled or gel-skin surface.
- The patient lies still during procedure in a supine position on the examining table. The procedure usually takes 10 to 30 minutes.
- Premedications are seldom given unless the patient is extremely apprehensive or has nausea and vomiting.
- Patient should not smoke before ultrasound to prevent swallowing air.

Doppler
- BP will be taken at certain limb sites.

Obstetrics (first and second trimester), Pelvic and Renal
- The patient should drink four glasses of water and should not urinate until after the test. Third-trimester patients can be tested with an empty bladder.

Brain
- Remove jewelry and hairpins from neck and head.

Heart and Liver
- Ask patient to breathe slowly and to hold breath after deep inspiration.

- Factors Affecting Diagnostic Results

  - Dressings (bandages) and scar tissue inhibit and interfere with the transmission of ultrasound.
  - Residual barium sulfate in the GI tract from previous x-ray studies will interfere with ultrasound results. Ultrasonography should be performed before barium studies.
  - Air and gas (bowel) will not transmit the ultrasound beam.

NURSING IMPLICATIONS WITH RATIONALE

- Explain the purpose and procedure to the patient (*see Description and Procedure above*). Tell the patient that an oil or lubricant is applied to the skin surface at the site of the organ and that a probe will move with light pressure back and forth over the area.
- Inform the patient that this is a painless procedure unless there has been trauma (injury) to the area. Tell the patient that there will be no exposure to radiation, and that the ultrasound test is considered to be safe and fast.
- Instruct the patient to remain still during the procedure. Inform him or her that the test usually takes 30 minutes or less, except for a few ultrasound tests (eg, kidney), which could take 1 hour.
- Encourage the patient to ask questions and to express any concerns. Refer questions you cannot answer to the ultrasonographer or the physician.
- Be supportive of the patient and the family.

VENOGRAPHY (LOWER LIMB)
Phlebography

Normal Finding

Normal, patent deep leg veins

Description

Lower-limb venography is a fluoroscopic and/or x-ray examination of the deep leg veins after injection of a contrast dye. This test is useful for identifying venous obstruction caused by a deep-vein thrombosis (DVT). A thrombus formation usually occurs in the deep calf veins and at the venous junction and its valves. If DVT is not treated, it can lead to femoral and iliac venous occlusion, or the thrombus can become an embolus and cause pulmonary embolism.

This procedure is frequently done after Doppler ultrasonography to confirm a positive or questionable DVT. *Radionuclide venography* using I-125 fibrinogen with scintillation scanning may be done for patients who are too ill for venography or are hypersensitive to contrast dye. The I-125 fibrinogen is given intravenously, and the tagged fibrinogen collects at the site of the thrombus. It may take 6 to 72 hours for the isotope to collect at the thrombus site; thus the scanner will be used to check the leg daily for 3 days. This test should not be performed for screening purpose.[1,2]

Clinical Problems

Indications: to detect DVT; to identify congenital venous abnormalities, a vein for arterial bypass grafting

Procedure

- A consent form should be signed.
- The patient should be NPO for 4 hours before the test; some hospitals permit clear liquids before the test.
- Anticoagulants may be temporarily discontinued.
- A skin test , antihistamine, and/or steroids may be ordered for patients who have a history of allergies to iodine, seafood, or x-ray dye from other tests (eg, IVP).
- The patient lies on a tilted radiographic table at a 40- to 60-degree angle. A tourniquet is applied above the ankle, a vein is located in the dorsum of the patient's foot, a small amount of normal saline is administered intravenously into the vein, and then the contrast dye is injected slowly over a period of 2 to 4 minutes. A cutdown may be necessary if a vein in the foot cannot be located or is not suitable. Fluoroscopy may be used to monitor the flow of the contrast dye, and spot films are taken.
- Normal saline is used after the procedure to flush the contrast dye from the veins.
- A sedative may be indicated prior to the test for patients who are extremely apprehensive and for those who have a low threshold of pain.
- The test takes 30 minutes to 1 hour.

- **Factors Affecting Diagnostic Results**

  - Weight on the leg being tested can cause a decrease in the flow of the contrast dye.
  - Movement of the leg being tested can interfere with the clarity of the film.

NURSING IMPLICATIONS WITH RATIONALE

- Explain the purpose and procedure to the patient.
- Inform the patient that he or she may have a slight burning sensation when the dye is injected. Inform the patient not to move the leg being tested during the injection of the dye or during x-ray filming.
- Obtain a patient history of allergies to iodine, iodine substances (x-ray dye), and seafood. Antihistamines or steroids (eg, cortisone) may be given for 2 to 3 days before the test.
- Record base-line vital signs. Have the patient void before the test.

Post-test

- Monitor vital signs until stable and as ordered.
- Check the pulse in the dorsalis pedis, popliteal, and femoral arteries for volume intensity and rate.
- Observe for signs and symptoms of latent allergic reaction to the contrast dye (ie, dyspnea, skin rash, urticaria [hives], and tachycardia).
- Observe the injection site for bleeding, hematoma, and signs and symptoms of infection (ie, redness, edema, and pain). Report abnormal changes and problems to the physician, and record the observations on the patient's chart.
- Elevate the affected leg as ordered. If the venogram is positive for DVT, the physician most likely will order bed rest, blood laboratory tests, heparin infusion, leg elevation, and warm, moist compresses.
- Be supportive of the patient. Answer the patient's questions, or refer them to the physician.

VENTILATION SCAN
Pulmonary Ventilation Scan

Normal Finding
Normal lung tissue with normal gas distribution in both lungs.

Description
The ventilation scan is a nuclear scan of the lungs. The patient inhales a mixture of air, oxygen, and radioactive gas (xenon [Xe-127 or Xe-133] or krypton-85 [Kr-85]). A single-breath scan is taken first. Then three phases of scanning follow: (1) the wash-in phase, which is the buildup of gas distribution in the lungs; (2) the equilibrium phase, in which radioactive gas reaches a steady state; and (3) the washout phase, in which room air is breathed to remove radioactive gas from the lungs.

The pulmonary ventilation scan is usually performed with the pulmonary perfusion scan to differentiate between a ventilatory problem and vascular abnormalities in the lung. The pulmonary perfusion scan indirectly evaluates problems related to blood flow to the lungs (eg, pulmonary embolism). The radioactive substance used is technetium or iodine, and images are displayed by a scintillator. A ventilation scan can reveal decreased ventilation (uptake of radioactive gas) caused by chronic obstructive lung disease, atelectasis, and pneumonia, although the pulmonary perfusion scan is normal. However, pulmonary embolus can cause an abnormal perfusion scan and a normal ventilation scan.[2,9]

Clinical Problems
Indications: to differentiate between parenchymal lung disease (chronic obstructive lung disease) and vascular abnormalities (pulmonary emboli); to detect

419

tuberculosis, sarcoidosis, lung cancer; to locate hypoventilation resulting from excess smoking and chronic obstructive lung disease

Procedure

- There is no food or fluid restriction.
- Remove all metal objects (jewelry) from around the neck and chest.
- The patient inhales gas (radioactive xenon or krypton). The patient will be asked to take a deep breath and to hold it for a short time (single breath) while the scanner takes an image of the lung. Other images will be recorded during three phases of the test; wash-in, equilibrium, and washout.

■ Factors Affecting Diagnostic Results

- Metal objects could cause inaccurate recorded images.

NURSING IMPLICATIONS WITH RATIONALE

- Explain the procedure to the patient (*see Procedure*). Tell the patient that the amount of radioactive gas is minimal.
- Instruct the patient to remove all jewelry from the chest and neck area.
- Assess respiratory status. Note and report changes in rate and difficulty in breathing. Check breath sounds.
- Assess communications for verbal and nonverbal expressions of anxiety and fear about tests and/or potential or actual problem.
- Report if patient is having chest pain, especially if pulmonary embolism is suspected.
- Be supportive of patient and family members prior to the test. Answer questions, or refer the questions to appropriate health professionals.

X-RAY (CHEST, HEART, FLAT PLATE OF ABDOMEN, KIDNEY, URETER, BLADDER, AND SKULL)
Roentgenography, Radiography

Normal Finding

Chest: normal bony structure and normal lung tissue

Heart (cardiac): normal size and shape of the heart and vessels

Flat Plate of Abdomen: normal abdominal structures

Kidney, Ureter, Bladder (KUB): normal kidney size and structure

Skull: normal structure

Description

In November of 1895, Wilhelm Konrad Roentgen, a German physicist, discovered x-radiation for diagnosing diseases. Adequate control of the rays (roentgen rays) for the patient and the operator did not occur until 1910, and it was then when the machines and techniques were greatly improved. Today x-ray studies cause only small amounts of radiation exposure because of the high quality of x-ray film and procedure.

There are four densities in the human body—air, water, fat, and bone—that will absorb varying degrees of radiation. Air has less density, causing dark images on the film, and bone has high density, causing light images. Bone contains a large amount of calcium and will absorb more radiation, thus allowing less radiation to strike the x-ray film; thus a white structure is produced.

The chest x-ray is one of the diagnostic tests most often ordered by the physician. A skull x-ray is usually ordered following head trauma. The requests for cardiac, flat plate of abdomen, and kidney-ureter-bladder (KUB) x-rays have increased in the last two decades. X-ray studies are requested primarily for screening purposes and then are followed by other extensive diagnostic tests.[1,2,5,11]

Clinical Problems

TEST	ABNORMAL FINDINGS
Chest	Atelectasis, pneumonias, tuberculosis, tumors, lung abscess, pneumothorax, sarcoma, sarcoidosis, scoliosis/kyphosis
Heart	Cardiomegaly, aneurysms, anomalies of the aorta
Abdominal (flat plate)	Abdominal masses, small bowel obstruction, abdominal tissue trauma, ascites
KUB	Abnormal size and structure of KUB, renal calculi, kidney and bladder masses
Skull	Head trauma (intracranial pressure, skull fractures), congenital anomalies, bone defects
Skeletal	Fractures, arthritic conditions, osteomyelitis
Abdominal (flat plate)	Abdominal masses in the liver, stomach, pancreas, intestines
	Small bowel obstruction
	Abdominal tissue trauma
	Ascites (abnormal fluid)
KUB	Abnormal size and structure of KUB
	Renal calculi
	Kidney and bladder masses
Skull	Head trauma: intracranial pressure, skull fractures, etc
	Congenital anomalies
	Bone defects

Procedure

Chest

■ Food and fluids are not restricted.

■ A posteroanterior (PA) chest film is usually ordered with the patient standing. An anteroposterior (AP) chest film may be ordered when PA film cannot be obtained. With an AP chest film, the patient is sitting or lying down. A lateral chest film may also be ordered.

■ Clothing and jewelry should be removed from the neck to the waist, and a paper or cloth gown should be worn.

■ The patient should take a deep breath and hold it as the x-ray is taken.

Heart

■ Food and fluids are not restricted.

■ PA and left-lateral chest films are usually indicated for evaluating the size and shape of the heart. The left anterior oblique (LAO) 60-degree rotation with the PA position may be ordered for cardiac evaluation.

■ Clothing and jewelry should be removed from the neck to the waist, and a paper or cloth gown should be worn.

■ Patient instructions will include body position (usually standing) and when to take a deep breath and hold it.

Abdomen and KUB

■ Food and fluids are usually not restricted.

■ X-rays should be taken before an IVP or GI studies.

■ Clothes are removed, and a paper or cloth gown is worn.

■ The patient lies in the supine position with his or her arms away from the body on a tilted x-ray table.

■ The testes should be shielded as an added precaution.

Skull

■ Food and fluids are not restricted.

■ The patient should remove hairpins, glasses, and dentures before the x-ray tests.

■ The patient will be asked to assume various positions so that different areas of the skull can be x-rayed. X-rays may include the facial bones and sinuses.

Skeletal

■ NPO if a fracture is suspected.

■ Immobilize suspected fracture site.

■ Factors Affecting Diagnostic Results

■ Radiopaque materials for IVP and GI studies administered within 3 days of routine x-rays (ie, chest, flat plate or abdomen, and KUB) could distort the pictures.

■ Incorrect positioning of the patient could produce distorted pictures.

■ Obesity and ascites could affect the clarity of the x-ray film.

NURSING IMPLICATIONS WITH RATIONALE

■ Describe the x-ray procedure to the patient.

■ Inform the patient that the x-ray test usually takes 10 to 15 minutes.

■ Inform the patient that there may be several x-rays taken, one or two chest films, or five skull films. The patient may be asked to remain in the waiting room for 10 to 15 minutes after x-rays are taken to be sure the films are readable.

- Encourage the patient to ask questions or to express his or her concerns to the nurse, physician, and the technician. Also, if the patient does not understand the directions, he or she should ask to have them repeated.
- Ask the female patient if she is pregnant or if pregnancy is suspected. X-rays should be avoided during the first trimester of pregnancy. If x-ray of the chest is necessary, the female patient should wear a lead apron covering the abdomen and pelvic areas. Some dentists have women of childbearing age (12 to 48 years old) wear lead aprons.
- Explain to the patient that the x-ray equipment and film today are of good quality and decrease the exposure to radiation.

Diagnostic Tests

REFERENCES

1. Brunner, L.S., & Suddarth, D.S. *Medical-surgical nursing* (6th ed.). Philadelphia, Penn: Lippincott, 1988.
2. *Diagnostic tests handbook.* Springhouse, Penn: Springhouse Corp, 1987.
3. Whaley, L.F., & Wong, D.L. *Nursing Care of Infants and Children* (3rd ed.). St. Louis, Mo: Mosby, 1987.
4. Phipps, W.J., Long, B.C., & Woods, N.F. *Medical-surgical nursing* (3rd ed.). St. Louis, Mo: Mosby, 1987.
5. Thompson, T.T. *Primer of Clinical Radiology* (2nd ed.). Boston, Mass: Little, Brown, 1980.
6. Farrell, J. Arthroscopy. *Nursing'82 ,* 1982 *12*(5),73–75.
7. Kee, J.L. *Handbook of laboratory and diagnostic tests with nursing implications.* Norwalk, Conn: Appleton & Lange, 1990.
8. Pagana, K.D., & Pagana, T.J. *Diagnostic testing and nursing implications.* St. Louis, Mo: Mosby, 1982.
9. Tilkian, S.M., Conover, M.B., & Tilkian, A.G. *Clinical implications of laboratory tests* (4th ed.). St. Louis, Mo: Mosby, 1987.
10. *Manual of radiology service.* Wilmington, Del: Veterans Administration Center, 1978.
11. Fischbach, F. *A manual of laboratory diagnostic tests* (3rd ed.). Philadelphia, Penn: Lippincott, 1988.
12. Grossman, W. *Cardiac catheterization and angiography* (2nd ed.). Philadelphia, Penn: Lea and Febiger, 1980.
13. Haughey, C.W. CT scans. *Nursing'81 ,* 1981 *11* (12), 72–77.
14. Rodibaugh, D. Choosing an imaging technique. *Emergency Medicine,* 1987, *19* (4), 26–36.
15. Goldberger, A.L., & Goldberger, E. *Clinical electrocardiography* (2nd ed.). St. Louis, Mo: Mosby, 1981.
16. Davis, G.R., Santa Ana, C.A., & Morawski, S.C. Development of a lavage solution associated with minimal water and electrolyte absorption or secretion. *Gastroenterology,* 1980, *78,* 991–995.
17. Hyman, R.A., & Gorey, M.T. Imaging strategies for MRI of the brain. *Radiologic Clinics of North America,* 1988, *26* (3), 471–502.
18. Kramer, D.M. Basic principles of magnetic resonance imaging. *Radiologic Clinics of North America,* 1984, *22* (4),765–778.
19. National Multiple Sclerosis Society. (1987). MRI—no mystique. *Inside,* 1987, *5* (4), 24–27.
20. Reed, J.D., & Soulen, R.L. Cardiovascular MRI: Current role in patient management. *Radiologic Clinics of North America,* 1988, *26* (3), 589–600.
21. Young, S.W. *Nuclear magnetic resonance imaging* (2nd ed.). New York, NY: Raven Press, 1988.

22. Early, P.J., & Sodee, D.B. *Principles and Practice of Nuclear Medicine* St. Louis, Mo: Mosby, 1985.
23. Hoffer, P.B. (Ed.). *The yearbook of nuclear medicine.* Chicago, Ill: Year Book Medical Publisher, 1988.
24. Matin, P. *Clinical nuclear medicine.* New York, NY: Medical Examination Publishing, 1981.
25. Walker, J.M., & Margouleff, A. *Clinical manual of nuclear medicine.* Norwalk, Conn: Appleton & Lange, 1984.
26. Corbett, J.V. *Laboratory tests and diagnostic procedures with nursing diagnoses* (2nd ed.). Norwalk, Conn: Appleton & Lange, 1987.
27. Brooks, D.J., Beaney, R.P., & Thomas, D.G.T. The role of positron emission tomography in the study of cerebral tumors. *Seminars in Oncology,* 1986, *13,* 83–93.
28. Goldstein, R.A., Mullani, N.A., & Wong, W.H. Positron imaging of myocardial infarction with rubidium-82. *Journal of Nuclear Medicine,* 1986, *27,* 1824–1829.
29. Cohen, S. Pulmonary function tests in patient care. *American Journal of Nursing,* 1980, *80* (6), 1135–1161.
30. Intermountain Thoracic Society. *Clinical Pulmonary Function Testing, A Manual of Uniform Laboratory Procedures* (2nd ed.)., 1984.
31. Jones, N.L. *Clinical Exercise Testing* (3rd ed.). Philadelphia, Penn: Saunders, 1988.
32. Miller, W.F., Scacci, R., & Fast L.R. *Laboratory evaluation of pulmonary function.* Philadelphia, Penn: Lippincott, 1987.
33. Ellenstad, M. *Stress testing* (2nd ed.). Philadelphia, Penn: F.A. Davis, 1980.
34. Janz, N., & Lampman, R.M. Treadmill stress test: Coaching your cardiac patient along the path to recovery. *Nursing '81,* 1981, *11* (12), 36–41.

Part III

Laboratory/Diagnostic Assessments of Body Function

Numerous laboratory and diagnostic tests are ordered to assist in the diagnosis of disease entities and to determine organ function. The purpose of Part III is to provide a listing of groups of tests, with explanations, used for diagnosing body dysfunction. Twelve categories related to organ, body structure, and clinical condition are presented. In each categoric section, the laboratory and diagnostic tests frequently performed are explained as they relate to the disorder. Nursing processes follow with nursing diagnoses, nursing implications, and evaluation at the end of each of the 12 categories. Nursing diagnoses are stated according to the Fourth National Conference on Nursing Diagnoses; Carpenito, *Nursing Diagnosis: Application to Clinical Practice*[32] and Gordon, *Manual of Nursing Diagnosis.*[33]

For a more detailed description, procedure, and specific nursing implications of each test, the nurse should refer to Parts I and II of the text.

Cardiac Function
Respiratory Function
Renal Function
Liver, Gallbladder, and Pancreatic
  Function
Gastrointestinal Function
Neurologic and Musculoskeletal
  Function

Endocrine Function
Reproductive Function
Arthritic and Collagen Conditions
Shock
Neoplastic Conditions
Hematologic Conditions

CARDIAC FUNCTION

LABORATORY TESTS	DIAGNOSTIC TESTS
Cardiac Enzymes	ECG/EKG
CK/CPK	Echocardiography
AST/SGOT	Phonocardiography
LD	X-ray
Electrolytes (Serum)	Exercise/Stress Testing
Lipoproteins (Serum Lipids)	Cardiac Catheterization (Cardiac
Clotting Times	Arteriography)
PT	Magnetic Resonance Imaging (MRI)
PTT, APTT	Positron Emission Tomography (PET)
Coagulation Time	
ESR	
Glucose (Blood, Serum)	
Leukocytes (WBC)	
ABGs	
TDM	

Introduction

Numerous laboratory and diagnostic tests are performed to detect cardiac problems and the extent of myocardial injury. Serum enzyme levels are generally ordered immediately upon complaint of cardiac discomfort. Enzyme levels are frequently repeated later to determine if significant changes have occurred. Other tests ordered include: serum electrolytes, blood glucose, blood lipids, sedimentation rate, PT, PTT, ECG, cardiac x-ray, cardiac catheterization, etc.

Laboratory Tests

Cardiac Enzymes: Since serum cardiac enzyme levels might be normal immediately following cardiac trauma, the first set of enzyme levels acts as base-line measurement for comparison of changes. Following heart injury, creatine kinase (CK/CDK) and isoenzyme CK-MB band, lactate dehydrogenase (LD) and LD isoenzymes with a $LD_1:LD_2$ shift, and aspartate aminotransferase (AST/SGOT) increase in the blood in proportion to the extent of the injury. Each enzyme has its own time course of release after injury. Table 1 is a list of cardiac enzymes including significant changes that can occur.

Electrolytes (Serum): Norms: Potassium: 3.5–5.0 mEq/L; sodium: 135–145 mEq/L

Serum electrolyte levels could be normal immediately following myocardial damage. Cellular potassium is lost, and so serum potassium level might be elevated if urinary output is decreased. It could be normal or decreased if urinary output is increased. Serum sodium level could be normal or decreased if sodium shifts into heart cells. Potassium-wasting diuretics (ie, hydrochlorothiazide (HydroDIURIL), furosemide (Lasix) used for treating congestive heart failure could cause a loss of potassium and sodium.

Lipoproteins (Serum Lipids): Norms: Adult: Total: 400–800 mg/dL, 4–8 g/L (SI units). Cholesterol: 150–240 mg/dL. Triglycerides: 30–39 years: 20–150 mg/

TABLE 1. CARDIAC ENZYME TESTS

Enzyme	Reference Values	Changes	Comments
Creatine kinase (CK) or creatine phosphokinase (CPK)	*Norms:* Male: 5–35 μg/mL 30–180 IU/L 55–170 U/L at 37°C Female: 5–25 μg/mL 25–150 IU/L 30–135 U/L at 37°C CPK-MB: 0%–6%	Early detection after heart damage: 4–6 hours. Maximal levels for 24 hours. Maximum level rise is five to eight times normal. CK-MB: 5–15 times normal. Return to normal 3–4 days.	Increased CK is an indicator of muscle damage (cardiac or skeletal). Differentiation between cardiac and skeletal involvement is determined by the CK isoenzymes: CK-MB (heart) CK-MM (skeletal muscle) CK-BB (brain)
Asparatate aminotransferase (AST) or SGOT	*Norms:* Adult: 5–40 U/mL (Frankel) 4–36 IU/L 16–60 Karmen U/mL 30°C 8–33 U/L at 37°C, SI units	AST/SGOT increases within 6–10 hours after heart damage. Peak within 24–48 hours. Returns to normal in 4–6 days. Rise is three to five times normal.	AST/SGOT is not the first enzyme to rise after severe heart damage.
Lactic dehydrogenase (LD/LDH)	*Norms:* Adult, total: 100–190 IU/L, 70–250 U/L 70–200 IU/L	LD elevation occurs 6–12 hours after heart damage. Peak 2–5 days. Returns to normal 6–12 days.	Rise in LD is later than CK/CPK and AST/SGOT. The prolongation of serum level makes it valuable for diagnosing a late MI.
Isoenzymes: LD_1, LD_2	Isoenzymes: LD_1 14%–26% LD_2 27%–37%	Isoenzymes: 12–24 hours after heart damage. Flipped LD ratio LD_1:LD_2.	Normally LD_2 has a higher level than LD_1 with a ratio LD_2:LD_1. After acute myocardial infarction, LD_1 increase is greater than LD_2.

dL; 40–49 years; 30–160 mg/dL; >50 years: 40–190 mg/dL. Phospholipids: 150–325 mg/dL. There could be laboratory differences with these ranges.

Elevated lipid levels (cholesterol, triglycerides, and phospholipids) could be the major factor in the cause of coronary artery disease (CAD). Since most lipids are bound to protein (lipoproteins), electrophoresis is used to separate the lipoproteins. Low-density lipoprotein (LDL) is composed of 45% cholesterol, and very-low-density lipoprotein (VLDL) is composed of 70% triglycerides. Both LDL and VLDL are strongly associated with CAD.

Clotting Times: The tests frequently used to monitor clotting time are prothrombin time (PT), partial thromboplastin time (PTT), activated partial thromboplastin time (APTT), and coagulation time (CT) or Lee-White clotting time (LWCT). Table 2 explains these tests, gives the reference values, and their purposes.

Sedimentation (Sed) Rate, Erythrocyte Sedimentation Rate (ESR): Norms: Adult: Under 50 years (Westergren method): 0–10 mm/hr; female: 0–20 mm/hr. Over 50 years (Westergren method): male: 0–20 mm/hr; female: 0–30 mm/hr.

Elevated sedimentation rate might occur after a myocardial infarction (MI) or bacterial endocarditis.

Blood Glucose: Norms: 60–100 mg/dL

Serum or Plasma Glucose (Fasting): Norms: 70–110 mg/dL

A slight to moderate increase in blood or serum glucose level (blood 150 mg/dL or serum 160 to 180 mg/dL) could be the result of stress caused by release of glucogen and catecholamines. A continuous elevation in blood or serum glucose level is a risk factor for CAD.

Leukocytes, White Blood Cells (WBC): Norms: 5000–10000 mm^3; (μL) 5–10 $\times$ 10^3/μL; 5–10 $\times$ 10^9/L (SI units)

Elevated WBC could occur after MI because of an inflammatory response secondary to the infarction or could occur as the result of bacterial endocarditis.

Arterial Blood Gases (ABGs): Norms: Adult: pH: 7.35–7.45; Pco_2: 35–45 mm Hg; Po_2: 75–100 mm Hg: HCO$_3$: 24–28 mEq/L; BE: +2 to −2

Abnormal ABGs could occur after an acute myocardial infarction; Po_2

TABLE 2. TESTS FOR MONITORING CLOTTING TIMES

Test	Reference Values	Purpose
Prothrombin time (PT)	*Norms:* 11–15 seconds or 70% *Anticoagulant therapy:* 2 to 2.5 times control in seconds or 20%–30%	PT is used to monitor clot formation and oral anticoagulant therapy. The PT is kept 2 to 2.5 times the control for anticoagulant therapy.
Partial thromboplastin time (PTT) or Activated partial thromboplastin time (APTT)	*Norms:* 60–70 seconds Anticoagulant therapy: 1.5 to 2.5 times the control *Norms:* 20–35 seconds	PTT and APTT are primarily used to detect clotting factor defects and to monitor heparin therapy. Following a myocardial infarction, many patients receive heparin therapy, and later some take oral anticoagulants.
Coagulation time (CT) or Lee-White clotting time (LWCT)	*Norms:* 3-tube method: 5–15 minutes	An infrequently used test to determine coagulation problems. It can be used to regulate heparin therapy. It is a time-consuming test.

decreased, Pco_2 decreased because of hyperventilation, normal or increased because of hypoventilation, HCO_3 and base excess (BE) decreased.

Therapeutic Drug Monitoring (TDM): Drugs taken for cardiac conditions should be closely monitored through blood samples to determine therapeutic levels and peak time to avoid drug toxicity. Most drug levels should be checked after serum drug level is at a steady state, approximately in 12 to 72 hours. Lidocaine is usually checked in 12 hours after administration and then daily. Propranolol (Inderal), procainamide (Pronestyl), and quinidine are checked 24 to 72 hours after administration; digoxin after 5 days. A schedule for TDM is suggested to maintain therapeutic levels and to prevent drug toxicity.

NAME OF DRUG	THERAPEUTIC RANGE	PEAK TIME	TOXIC LEVEL
Digitoxin	10–25 ng/mL	12–24 hours	>30 ng/mL
Digoxin	0.5–2 ng/mL	6–8 hours	2.5 ng/mL
Lidocaine	1.5–5.0 μg/mL	10 minutes	>6 μg/mL
Propranolol (Inderal)	50–100 ng/mL	1–2 hours	>150–1000 ng/mL
Procainamide (Pronestyl)	4–10 μg/mL	1 hour	>10 μg/mL
Procainamide + NAPA	5–20 μg/mL		>30 μg/mL
Disopyramide (Norpace)	2–5 μg/mL	2 hours	>7 μg/mL
Quinidine	2–5 μg/mL	1–3 hours	>5–6 μg/mL
Diazepam (Valium)	400–600 ng/mL	1–2 hours	>1000 ng/mL
Verapamil (Isoptin)	100–300 ng/mL	1–2 hours	>300 ng/mL
Nifedipine (Procardia)	50–100 ng/mL	30 minutes	100 ng/mL
Diltiazem (Cardizem)	50–200 ng/mL	2–3 hours	>200 ng/mL

Diagnostic Tests

Electrocardiography (ECG, EKG): ECG records the electrical impulses of the heart by means of electrodes attached at appropriate sites on the chest. Abnormal P waves, QRS complexes, ST segments and/or T waves indicate a possible cardiac problem. A depressed ST segment and an inverted T wave could indicate myocardial ischemia.

Echocardiography, Ultrasound Cardiography: This test is useful in detecting enlargement of a heart chamber, changes in heart dimensions during cardiac cycle, valvular disease (eg, mitral stenosis, pericardial effusion, and congenital heart disease). It is considered a noninvasive test.

Phonocardiography, Phonocardiogram: It is a graphic recording of sounds from the heart. The phonocardiogram is considered superior to examination by stethoscope in that it can record low-frequency sounds (eg, gallop sounds). It is useful to detect cardiac valvular damage and to record the shape of various murmurs heard.

X-ray of Heart and Chest: X-rays of the chest to determine heart size are taken in posteroanterior (PA) and left-lateral positions. The x-ray films from these positions are helpful for identifying cardiomegaly and anomalies of the aorta.

Exercise/Stress Testing: Stress testing is a diagnostic tool that provides information about the cardiac function during exercise (stress). From the results of the test, decisions can be made about the degree of work level considered safe and how soon the individual should return to work after the MI.

Left Cardiac Catheterization, Cardiac Angiography/Arteriography: This is an invasive procedure to determine the patency of the coronary arteries and functions of aortic and mitral valve. Dye is injected to determine left ventricular functioning while video film is recording the activity of the coronary arteries and heart valves.

Magnetic Resonance Imaging (MRI): MRI, a noninvasive test, is useful for evaluating the cardiovascular system. It can detect atrial and ventricular septal defects, myocardial infarction, aortic and ventricular aneurysms, plaque formation, and blood flow through coronary branches and through extremities.

Positron Emission Tomography (PET): This test is useful for myocardial perfusion imaging. It can evaluate myocardial perfusion after 72-hour MI and postmyocardial infarction with angina; it can also be used to determine if the ischemic area in the myocardium is viable or is infarcted after an acute MI.[1–10]

■ Nursing Diagnoses

- Anxiety related to pain and the unknown
- Knowledge deficit related to lack of understanding of the laboratory or diagnostic procedure, disease process, and/or outcome
- Potential for noncompliance to prescribed laboratory test related to lack of adequate explanation
- Decreased tissue perfusion related to coronary artery insufficiency
- Alteration in comfort related to chest pain secondary to cardiac tissue ischemia
- Ineffective coping with disease process and laboratory and diagnostic test procedures
- Potential alteration in mobility related to perceived or actual chest pain
- Disturbance in self-concept related to dependence and/or role change

---

NURSING IMPLICATIONS WITH RATIONALE

- Explain the purpose of the laboratory and diagnostic tests.
- Give a detailed explanation concerning the laboratory and diagnostic procedures and the need for the client's compliance with the procedure(s). Explanation might be brief or in-depth depending upon the individual's unfamiliarity with the test.
- Explanation of the tests and procedures to the family members could be helpful with test compliance.
- Inform the patient of any food, beverage, or drug restrictions (*see Parts I and II*).
- Listen to the patient's expressed anxiety or fear concerning the tests and potential clinical problems. Clarification of test procedure might alleviate fear and anxiety and promote test compliance.
- Assess the patient's chest discomfort by eliciting the intensity, duration, and location of the pain from the patient. Check skin color and vital signs. Report findings immediately to the physician.

- Provide care to the patient as prescribed by the physician (ie, oxygen, drugs).
- Suggest to the patient and family members the community resources available to them (eg, American Heart Association).

Evaluation

- Determine if the test was completed correctly according to the procedure. Notify the laboratory of any changes that occurred during the test.
- Check to see that patient's discomfort was alleviated. If not, notify the physician.
- Evaluate the status of the patient's anxiety and fear in regard to the test(s) and clinical problem.
- Assist the patient and family member in making changes regarding activity, recreation, future tests, and health care.
- Contact dietitian and social service for their participation in patient's health care in hospital and home.

RESPIRATORY FUNCTION

LABORATORY TESTS	DIAGNOSTIC TESTS
ABGs	Chest X-ray
Sputum Culture	Pulmonary Function Studies
α-1-Antitrypsin (Serum)	Tomography
TDM	Thoracic CT
Skin Tests	Bronchoscopy
	Bronchography
	Mediastinoscopy
	Radionuclide Thoracic Scan
	Lung Scan
	Ventilation Scan
	Pulmonary Angiography/Arteriography
	Lung Biopsy
	Thoracentesis
	Magnetic Resonance Imagine (MRI)

Introduction

Chest x-ray, arterial blood gases (ABGs), and pulmonary function studies are usually ordered for respiratory problems. If abnormalities are reported, other diagnostic tests are performed (ie, thoracic computerized tomography [CT], radionuclide thoracic scan, bronchoscopy, and others).

Laboratory Tests

Arterial Blood Gases (ABGs): Norms: Adult: pH: 7.35–7.45; Pco_2: 35–45 mm Hg; Po_2: 75–100 mm Hg; HCO_3: 24–28 mEq/L.

TABLE 3. USES OF SPUTUM CULTURE

Sputum Test	Comments
Culture and sensitivity (C&S)	Sputum specimens are useful for diagnosing microorganisms causing respiratory infection and the appropriate antimicrobial sensitive to the pathogens.
Acid-fast bacilli (AFB)	When tuberculosis (TB) is suspected, sputum specimens are checked (over 3 days) to determine the presence of *Mycobacterium tuberculosis.*
Cytology	Cytologic examination of slough cells from the lung are checked. If malignant cells are *not* present, this means lung cancer is unlikely. However, the malignancy may be in its early stage and not shedding cancer cells.

A decreased P_{CO_2} less than 35 mm Hg, and an elevated pH greater than 7.45 mm Hg indicate respiratory alkalosis. An increased P_{CO_2} greater than 45 mm Hg and a decreased pH less than 7.35 indicate respiratory acidosis. The latter acid-base imbalance is the result of many respiratory problems (ie, chronic obstructive lung disease, pneumonia, drug-induced repiratory depression).

Culture (Sputum): Sputum specimens are useful for diagnosing microorganisms causing respiratory infection and for detecting malignant cells in lung tissue. Table 3 explains three studies conducted on sputum that are associated with respiratory problems.

α-1-Antitrypsin (Serum): Norms: Adult: 78–200 mg/dL; 0.78–2.0 g/L. Child: same as adult.

Antitrypsin inhibits proteolytic enzymes in destroying lung tissue. With a lack of this protein, the alveoli are damaged, resulting in chronic obstructive lung disease (eg, emphysema). A nonsmoker with a decreased antitrypsin level could develop pulmonary emphysema.

Therapeutic Drug Monitoring (TDM); Theophylline: Serum theophylline: Therapeutic Range: Adult: 5–20 μg/mL; 28–112 μmol/L (SI units). *Toxic level:* Adult: >20 μg/mL; >112 μmol/L (SI units). Child: same as adult.

Patients with bronchoconstriction (eg, asthma) are usually given one of the theophylline preparations (ie, aminophylline, Theo-dur, Slo-phyllin). Serum theophylline levels should be closely monitored to maintain therapeutic levels and to avoid toxic levels.

Skin Tests: Skin tests are useful for determining the presence of suspected bacterial or mycotic organisms that can infect lung tissue. This test is one of the methods used to diagnose tuberculosis and histoplasmosis.

Diagnostic Tests

Chest X-ray: Chest x-ray is a frequently ordered diagnostic test. It is useful in diagnosing pneumonia, neoplasms (malignant and benign tumors), lung abscess, tuberculosis, atelectasis, and pneumothorax.

Pulmonary Function Studies: these tests are routinely ordered for patients with respiratory disorders or for those suspected of having a respiratory problem

Pulmonary function studies are helpful for assessing the progression of lung disease and for evaluating the response to drug and rehabilitative therapies.

Tomography, Laminography, Planigraphy: Tomography is used to detect lung tumors and mediastinal lesions. The x-ray machine or tube and film moves around the patient. Since it emits high radiation levels, this test is not used as a routine screening test to diagnose lung disorders.

Thoracic Computerized Tomography (CT): CT scanning is useful for detecting questionable chest masses—lesions and tumors. It identifies metastasis in the lung. Contrast media (dye) may or may not be used.

Bronchoscopy: Either a standard metal or flexible fiberoptic bronchoscope is inserted into the tracheobronchial tree to visualize the larynx, trachea, and bronchi for abnormalities, (ie, strictures, inflammation, tumors). Also bronchial secretions may be aspirated for bacteriologic, cytologic, and histologic examination. To remove a foreign object or to excise a small lesion or growth, a large metal bronchoscope would be necessary. Complications as a result of the test procedure might be bleeding, infection, or pneumothorax.

Bronchography: A bronchography may be done in conjunction with bronchoscopy. Contrast media (radiopaque iodine dye) is injected through a catheter into the tracheobronchial tree, followed by x-rays. This test is not frequently performed because of newer, more effective diagnostic tests (eg, CT scan). However, the purposes for the test are to detect bronchial obstruction, tumors, cysts, and bleeding sites.

Mediastinoscopy: The mediastinoscope is inserted through a small incision at the suprasternal notch for the purposes of examining mediastinal lymph nodes and of obtaining biopsy specimen(s). This test is frequently indicated when other diagnostic tests (ie, chest x-ray, sputum cytology, bronchoscopy) fail to confirm a diagnosis. It is also useful to determine if the lung cancer is inoperable because of metastatic spread to the lymph nodes. Other uses of this test include detecting lymphoma (eg, Hodgkin's disease, and sarcoidosis).

Radionuclide Thoracic Imaging (Scan)

> *Lung Scan:* Radionuclide imaging is useful for evaluating pulmonary blood perfusion and for diagnosing perfusion obstruction (eg, pulmonary embolism). A radionuclide, such as technetium tagged with macroaggregated albumin or technetium tagged with human albumin microspheres, is injected into the patient's peripheral vein.
> *Ventilation Scan:* When the perfusion problem is due to an airway obstruction causing decreased ventilation, a ventilation scanning may be ordered. The patient inhales radioactive gas, such as xenon. A nuclear scanner checks the distribution of the gas in the lungs at intervals.

Pulmonary Angiography/Arteriography: Contrast medium (radiopaque dye) is injected into the pulmonary arteries to detect vascular abnormalities (eg, pulmonary embolus). Usually pulmonary angiography/arteriography is performed when other diagnostic tests fail to confirm a diagnosis.

Lung Biopsy: Biopsy specimens from the tracheobronchial tree and lymph nodes are usually obtained during bronchoscopy (if ordered) and mediastinoscopy. A transbronchial lung biopsy may be obtained through the use of a bronchoscope by wedging a small biopsy forcep into the lung tissue.

Thoracentesis; Pleural Fluid Aspiration: This test is used to remove fluid from the pleural cavity and to examine the fluid for the cause of pleural effusion.

Magnetic Resonance Imaging (MRI): MRI helps to supplement CT examination of the chest in lung cancer. It can evaluate recurrent or residual lung masses.

Pulmonary Function Tests (PFTs): Various pulmonary studies evaluate pulmonary function. These include: slow vital-capacity groups, lung-volume groups, forced vital capacity, diffusion study, bronchodilator response studies, exercise studies, and nutritional studies.[1,5,7,9–14]

- **Nursing Diagnoses**

  - Anxiety related to breathlessness
  - Knowledge deficit related to lack of understanding of laboratory and diagnostic procedures, disease process, and/or outcome
  - Potential for noncompliance to prescribed laboratory and diagnostic tests related to lack of adequate explanation
  - Potential inability to perform diagnostic tests related to breathlessness
  - Activity intolerance related to breathlessness and/or fatigue
  - Impaired gas exchange relate to obstructive lung disease (eg, chronic obstructive lung disease)
  - Impaired verbal communication related to dyspnea
  - Potential for infection related to excessive, tenacious, mucous secretions
  - Potential alterations in sleep and rest related to dyspnea secondary to chronic lung disease
  - Potential for injury related to allergic reactions to contrast medium (dye) secondary to diagnostic test (ie, bronchography, radionuclide scan, pulmonary angiography)
  - Disturbance in self-concept related to dependence and/or role change

---

NURSING IMPLICATIONS WITH RATIONALE

- Explain the purpose of the laboratory and diagnostic tests.
- Give detailed explanation concerning the test procedures and the need for patient's compliance. Explanation may be brief or in-depth, depending upon the patient's familiarity with the test.
- Inform the patient of any food, beverage, or drug restrictions (*see Parts I and II*).
- Elicit from the patient or family member a history of any allergies, especially to contrast medium (dye), iodine, or seafood.
- Assess respiratory status in regard to breathlessness and dyspnea caused by acute and chronic lung diseases.
- Be supportive of the patient with dyspnea during the procedure. Remain with the patient and provide adequate time; this reduces anxiety and increases test compliance.
- Assist the patient with breathing difficulty as needed.

- Check bleeding sites at incisional areas (eg, mediastinoscopy test).
- Monitor vital signs before, during, and following invasive tests (ie, bronchoscopy, pulmonary angiography).
- Listen to patient's expressed anxiety or fear concerning the tests and potential clinical problems. Clarification of the test procedure might alleviate fear and anxiety and promote compliance.

Evaluation

- Determine if the test was correctly performed according to the procedure. Notify laboratory and physician of any changes that occur during the test.
- Check the patient's vital signs for changes.
- Evaluate patient's activity in regard to breathlessness.
- Determine if support measures to patient and family have been effective.
- Clarify or answer any questions the patient and family members might have.
- Encourage the patient to use resources for information and support, such as the American Lung Association.
- Reinforce the importance of seeking health care assistance whenever changes in health status occur.

RENAL FUNCTION

LABORATORY TESTS	DIAGNOSTIC TESTS
Urinalysis	Kidney, Ureter, Bladder (KUB) X-ray
BUN	IVP
Creatinine (Serum)	Retrograde Pyelography
Creatinine Clearance	Cystoscopy
Inulin Clearance	Cystography
Protein (24-Hour Urine)	CT
Electrolytes (Serum & Urine)	Nephrotomography
Osmolality (Serum & Urine)	Renal Ultrasound
Complement C_3 (Serum)	Radionuclide Renal Scan
Complement C_4 (Serum)	Renal Angiography
Aldosterone (Serum)	Renal Biopsy
Renin (Plasma)	
Urine Culture	
Antiglomerular Basement	
Membrane Antibody (Serum)	
Uric Acid (Serum and Urine)	

Introduction

The first set of laboratory tests performed to determine renal function are urinalysis, blood urea nitrogen (BUN), and serum creatinine. These tests are ordered routinely when renal insufficiency is suspected. If any of these are

TABLE 4. URINALYSIS

Components	Results
Color	Color can indicate lack of body fluids (dark yellow), excess of body fluids (pale yellow), or the result of blood, drugs, and food (red, red-brown).
pH	Urine pH is usually 4.5–8. The urine would be acidic if pH is 4.5 and alkalotic if pH is >7.5. Bacteria multiply rapidly in alkalotic urine.
Specific gravity (SG)	A low SG is related to diluted urine, and a high SG is associated with concentrated urine.
Protein	Urine protein >8 mg/dL could indicate renal disorder. However, an athlete's urine protein (single sample) level might be 10–20 mg/dL. This could be normal after strenuous activity.
Glucose	Glycosuria could indicate diabetes mellitus. Normally glucose is not a measureable quantity in urine.
Blood cells (BCs)	Urine should not contain BCs. The presence of BCs in urine could indicate a renal disorder.

abnormal, other Laboratory and diagnostic tests would be necessary (ie, creatinine clearance, inulin clearance, serum and urine osmolality, serum and urine electrolytes, intravenous pyelography [IVP], kidney, ureter, bladder [KUB] x-ray, renal ultrasound, renal computerized tomography [CT] scan, and others).

Laboratory Tests

Urinalysis: A urinalysis is routinely performed in a variety of settings (hospitals, clinics, and physician's office) for checking kidney and endocrine function. The components it measures are color, pH, specific gravity (SG), protein, glucose, and blood cells. Table 4 shows the components that are usually checked during urinalysis and their significant results. For more comprehensive data on urinalysis, *see Part I*

Blood Urea Nitrogen (BUN): Norms: 5–25 mg/dL; Child: 5–20 mg/dL

Urea is a by-product of protein metabolism excreted by the kidneys. If the BUN is slightly elevated, 25 to 35 mg/dL, the cause could be dehydration caused by hemoconcentration. Elevated BUN that remains elevated after hydration is an indicator of renal disorder.

Creatinine (Serum): Norms:

ADULT:	INFANT	2–6 YEARS	OLDER CHILD
0.5–1.5 mg/dL 45–132.5 umol/L (SI units)	0.7–1.7 mg/dL	0.3–0.6 mg/dL	0.4–1.2 mg/dL 36–106 umol/L (SI units)

Creatinine, a by-product of muscle creatinine phosphate, is excreted entirely by the kidneys. Serum creatinine is a more reliable test to determine renal function, since it is less affected, if at all, by dehydration or malnutrition than BUN. After renal damage or insult, the serum creatinine would rise because the kidneys could not excrete this by-product. Monitoring serum creatinine is important for determining kidney function.

Creatinine Clearance: Norms:

PERSON	CREATININE CLEARANCE	URINE CREATININE
Adult:		
Male	85–135 mL/min	20–26 mg/kg/24 h
		0.18–0.23 mmol/kg/24 h
Female	somewhat lower values	14–22 mg/kg/24 h
		0.12–0.19 mmol/kg/24 h
Child:		
Male	98–150 mL/min	
Female	95–123 mL/min	

The creatinine clearance test (12- or 24-hour) is performed to determine glomerular filtration rate (GFR) and renal insufficiency. Usually this test includes serum creatinine level on the morning of or at the beginning of the test. Serum and urine creatinine levels are assessed, and creatinine clearance rate is calculated (*see Part I*). If less than 40 mL/min, the test is suggestive of moderate to severe renal impairment.

Inulin Clearance: Norms: Male: 125 mL/min/1.73 m^2, 124 ± 15 mL/min; Female: 110 mL/min/1.73 m^2, 110 ± 15 mL/min

Inulin, a small, inert sugar that is not bound to protein, is freely filtered by the glomeruli and can be used to determine GFR. This is not a routine clinical test because it involves an initial IV injection of inulin and a continuous controlled infusion rate to achieve a constant plasma level. It is a reliable test for GFR and is often compared with other urine clearance procedures. Decreased levels are indicative of renal impairment.

Protein (24-hour Urine): Norms: 25–150 mg/24 h.; Random: 0–5 mg/dL

If urinalysis report indicated proteinuria, a 24-hour protein-urine test might be ordered. The presence of protein in the urine, more than 150 mg/24 h, could indicate glomeruli damage or disease.

Electrolytes (Serum and Urine): Both serum electrolytes and urine electrolytes are closely monitored in renal disorders. Table 5 explains the effects of serum and urine potassium and sodium as they relate to renal dysfunction.

Osmolality (Serum): Norms: Adult: 280–300 mOsm/kg/H_2O. Child: 270–290 mOsm/kg/H_2O

Serum and urine osmolality are used in assessing distal tubular response to circulating antidiuretic hormone (ADH). An increased serum osmolality could be due to an inadequate ADH release or due to the distal renal tubules inadequate response to circulating ADH.

TABLE 5. SERUM AND URINE ELECTROLYTES

Electrolytes	Reference Values	Cause and Effect
Serum Potassium (K)	*Norms:* Adults: 3.5–5.0 mEq/L Child: 3.5–5.5 mEq/L Infant: 3.6–5.8 mEq/L	Primary cause of hyperkalemia; >5.5 mEq/L is renal insufficiency
Sodium (Na)	*Norms:* Adult, child: 135–145 mEq/L Infant: 134–150 mEq/L	Hypernatremia, >145 mEq/L, might be caused by anuria due to acute renal failure. Hyponatremia, <135 mEq/L, might result from tubular disorders when there is an inability to reabsorb sodium.
Urine Potassium (K)	*Norms:* Adult: 25–120 mEq/24 h 25–120 mmol/24 h (SI units)	Decreased urine potassium level <25 mEq/24 h, with an increased serum potassium level, could be indicative of acute renal failure. Elevated urine potassium level could be due to chronic renal failure. *Note:* Urine potassium range depends on the amount of potassium consumed in the diet.
Sodium (Na)	*Norms:* Adult: 40–220 mEq/24 h 40–220 mmol/24 h (SI units)	A low urine sodium level occurring with oliguria could be due to acute renal failure from decreased perfusion of the kidneys. An increased urine sodium level could result from the inability of the kidney tubules to reabsorb sodium (ie, polycystic disease, chronic pyelonephritis).

Osmolality (Urine): *Norms:* Adult: 50–1200 mOsm/kg/H_2O (average 200–800 mOsm/kg/H_2O. Child: same as adult. Newborn: 100–600 mOsm/kg/H_2O

Urine osmolality is a more accurate indicator of the kidneys' ability to concentrate and dilute urine than specific gravity. In advanced, renal medullary disease, the urine osmolality could be decreased because of the inability of the kidneys to concentrate urine.

Complement C_3(Serum): *Norms:* Male: 80–180 mg/dL; Female: 76–120 mg/dL

Complements contribute about 10% of the total plasma proteins and play an important role in the immunologic system. Serum C_3 (the most abundant complement) is decreased in certain renal conditions (ie, glomerulonephritis and acute renal transplant rejection).

Complement C_4 (Serum): *Norms:* 15–45 mg/dL

Serum C_4, the second most abundant component of the complement system, is significantly decreased in lupus nephritis and acute poststreptococcal glomerulonephritis.

Aldosterone (Serum): Norms: Adult 1–9 ng/dL (supine position)

An increased serum aldosterone level can be associated with renal disease and chronic renal failure.

Renin (Plasma): Norms: Adult: 1.3–4.0 ng/mL (upright position, normal salt intake)

Renin, an enzyme secreted by the kidneys, is a test used for diagnosing renal vascular hypertension. The result of this hypertension could lead to renal failure.

Urine Culture: Urine cultures are commonly performed to determine the type of microorganism present in the genitourinary tract. To avoid urine contamination, the urine should be obtained using the procedure for midstream specimen collection or by catheterization.

Antiglomerular Basement Membrane Antibody (AGBM): This test detects GBM antibodies that can damage the glomerular basement membrane in the glomeruli. Beta-hemolytic streptococcus is the major organism responsible for antibody response.

Uric Acid (Serum): Serum: Male: 3.5–8.0 mg/dL; Female: 2.6–6.8 mg/dL. *Urine:* 250–750 mg/24 h (normal diet)

Serum and urine uric acid level is dependent upon renal function. Elevated serum uric acid can be attributed to renal disease such as glomerulonephritis and renal failure. A decreased urine uric acid is associated with renal disease.

Diagnostic Tests

Kidney, Ureter, Bladder (KUB) X-ray: KUB x-ray is a flat plate of the lower abdomen to identify the size, shape, and position of the kidneys, ureters, and bladder. If abnormalities (ie, tumors, calculi, or malformations) are noted, more extensive diagnostic tests are performed. Usually the x-ray is taken while the patient is in the supine position; however, an upright KUB may be requested for better visualization of the area.

Intravenous Pyelography (IVP): During the IVP, radiopaque contrast medium (dye) is injected intravenously. A series of x-rays is taken at specified times as the dye circulates and is collected by the renal glomeruli and passed throughout the urinary tract. The purpose is to visualize the kidneys, kidney pelvis, ureters, and bladder. This test is useful for determining kidney dysfunction and for locating renal tumors and calculi. A test dose of the dye is given first because some patients may be allergic to the dye.

Retrograde Pyelography: During the retrograde pyelography (pyelogram) test, contrast medium (dye) is injected through a ureteral catheter to visualize the ureters and kidney. X-rays are taken. This test is usually done during cystoscopy to determine the cause of unilateral kidney disease (eg, ureteral obstruction). The retrograde pyelogram gives better visualization of the ureter and problems than the IVP test.

Cystoscopy: A cystoscope, lighted, telescopic tube, is transurethrally inserted into the bladder for numerous purposes, including the following: to visualize the bladder wall; to obtain tissue biopsy of the bladder, urethra, or prostate; to remove calculi from the bladder or urethra; to remove small lesions and/or growths; or to obtain a urine specimen directly from the kidney(s). If ureter examination is necessary, dye is injected through an ureteral catheter into the ureters and x-rays are taken (retrograde pyelogram).

Cystography: The bladder is instilled with contrast medium (dye) to detect a rupture in the bladder, a neurogenic bladder, fistulas, or tumors. X-rays are taken. The patient voids, if able, or the dye is withdrawn through the catheter.

Computerized Tomography (CT) Scan: CT, also known as computerized axial tomography (CAT), provides an image of the kidneys for the purpose of identifying tumors, malformations, cysts, and calculi. Contrast medium (dye) might be used during the CT scan to enhance better visualization of the kidneys. Usually renal CT scan is done after abnormal IVP results have been reported.

Nephrotomography: The nephrotomography test combines IVP and CT. It provides a clearer picture of the kidneys, identifying and differentiating between cysts and solid tumors.

Renal Ultrasound, Ultrasonography: Renal ultrasonography (considered a noninvasive test) passes high-frequency sound waves through a transducer to the kidneys and perirenal area. An image of the kidneys and surrounding structures is displayed on an oscilloscope screen. The purpose of this test is to detect abnormalities (ie, masses [cyst, tumor]) or to clarify findings from other tests.

Radionuclide Renal Scan: A radionuclide, such as technetium compounds (Tc-99m), Tc-99m–pertechnetate, Tc-99m–diethylenetriamine-penta-acetic acid (Tc-99m–DTPA), and I-131 hippuran, is administered intravenously. The purpose of the test is to detect renal lesions or masses and to determine the presence of acute or chronic renal diseases. This test may be used instead of IVP for patients who are allergic to contrast medium (dye).

Renal Angiography: A contrast medium (dye) is injected into the renal artery to visualize renal arterial, capillary, and venous systems. Rapid-sequence x-ray filming detects renal vascular malformations (eg, stenosis, nonfunctioning kidney, renal masses, and obstructive uropathy).

Renal Biopsy: Microscopic examination of kidney tissue provides data concerning renal disease (eg, glomerulonephritis caused by streptococcal infection or lupus). The renal biopsy test is useful for diagnosing primary or metastatic cancer of the kidney. Complications that could result are hematuria, uncontrolled bleeding, and kidney damage.[1,2,7,9,15–18]

- ■ Nursing Diagnoses

  - ■ Knowledge deficit related to lack of understanding of the laboratory and diagnostic procedures, disease process, and/or outcome
  - ■ Potential for noncompliance to prescribed laboratory and diagnostic tests related to lack of or inadequate explanation
  - ■ Alteration in urinary elimination related to decreased urine output secondary to urinary tract obstruction, renal lesions or masses, acute or chronic renal failure

- Potential alteration in renal tissue perfusion related to renal vascular obstruction, drug toxicity, or tumors
- Fluid volume excess related to sodium and fluid retention secondary to renal damage or insufficiency
- Potential fear related to kidney status, the unknown, and/or dependence on others
- Potential impairment of skin integrity related to peripheral edema secondary to renal failure
- Potential for injury related to allergic reactions to contrast medium (dye) secondary to diagnostic test (eg, IVP)
- Potential disturbance in self-concept related to dependence and/or role change

---

NURSING IMPLICATIONS WITH RATIONALE

- Explain the purpose of the laboratory and diagnostic tests.
- Give detailed explanation of the test procedures and the need for the patient's compliance. Explanation might be brief or in-depth, depending upon the patient's familiarity with the test.
- Inform the patient of any food, beverage, or drug restriction (*see Parts I and II*).
- Collect specimen(s) at specific times according to the procedures.
- Elicit from the patient a history of any allergies, especially to contrast medium (dye) or iodine.
- Assess renal function (ie, changes in urinary output, abnormal laboratory results—elevated BUN and serum creatinine, hematuria).
- Monitor the patient's intake and output and vital signs before and after laboratory and diagnostic tests.
- Listen to the patients' expressed anxiety or fear about the tests and potential clinical problems. Clarification of test procedure might alleviate fear and anxiety and promote compliance.

Evaluation

- Determine if the test was correctly performed according to the procedure. Notify the laboratory or physician of any changes that occur during the test.
- Check the patient's urinary output and vital signs for changes: improvement or deterioration.
- Determine if the patient's fear and/or anxiety has been lessened or alleviated.
- Clarify or answer any additional questions patient might have.
- Encourage the patient to use resources available (eg, National Kidney Foundation).
- Encourage the patient and family members to participate in the decision-making process concerning the patient's long-term needs.

LIVER, GALLBLADDER, AND PANCREATIC FUNCTION

LABORATORY TESTS	**DIAGNOSTIC TESTS**

Liver
Bilirubin (Serum)
Bilirubin (Urine)
Urobilinogen (Urine)
Liver Enzyme Tests
   ALP and Isoenzyme (Serum)
   5′ N (Serum)
   ALT SGPT (Serum)
   LDH and Isoenzymes (Serum)
   GGT/GGTP (Serum)
Protein (Serum)
   Protein Electrophoresis
Ammonia (Plasma, Blood)
PT (Plasma)
Cholesterol (Serum)
HB_sAg (Serum)
HB_sAb/anti-HB_s (Serum)
HB_cAb/anti-HB_c (Serum)

Diagnostic Tests (Liver)
X-ray of Abdomen
Ultrasonography of Liver
Liver and Spleen Scan
CT, Liver
Liver Biopsy
Hepatic Angiography

Gallbladder
X-ray of Abdomen
Cholecystography (Oral)
Cholangiography
   Intravenous
   Percutaneous
   T tube
ERCP
Ultrasonography of
Gallbladder and Biliary System
HIDA Scan
CT: Gallbladder and Biliary System

Pancreas
Amylase (Serum)
Amylase (Urine)
Lipase (Serum)
Secretin Test

Diagnostic Tests (Pancreas)
ERCP
Ultrasonography of Pancreas
Hypotonic Duodenography
CT, Pancreas

Introduction

Since the liver, gallbladder, and pancreas are in close proximity, several diagnostic tests (ie, computerized tomography [CT]; ultrasound of the liver, gallbladder, and pancreas; and endoscopic retrograde cholangiopancreatography [ERCP]) are performed on two or three of these organs at the same time. However, assessment of these organs will be represented separately.

Liver Assessment

Laboratory Tests

Bilirubin (Serum): Norms:

PERSON	INDIRECT UNCONJUGATED	DIRECT CONJUGATED	TOTAL
Adult	0.1–1.0 mg/dL 1.7–17.1 µmol/L (SI units)	0.1–0.3 mg/dL 1.7–5.1 µmol/L (SI units)	0.1–1.2 mg/dL 1.7–20.5 µmol/L (SI units)
Child >6 months	Same as adult	Same as adult	0.2–0.8 mg/dL
Newborn			1–12 mg/dL

Bilirubin is derived from hemoglobin and results from the breakdown of red blood cells (RBCs). There are two forms of bilirubin in the body: indirect or unconjugated, and direct, or conjugated.

Indirect, or Unconjugated: Elevated indirect bilirubin is related to increased destruction of RBCs.

Erythroblastosis fetalis in newborns results from massive hemolysis of RBCs, resulting in a possible serum indirect bilirubin level of 20 mg/dL or greater. Other causes include sickle cell anemia, drug toxicity, transfusion reaction caused by blood incompatibility, and autoimmune diseases.

Direct, or Conjugated: Bilirubin is conjugated (transformed) by the liver and made water soluble. There are smaller amounts of conjugated bilirubin than unconjugated bilirubin in the blood. Only water-soluble bilirubin (conjugated) can be excreted in the urine. Causes of an increase in direct bilirubin are cirrhosis, biliary obstruction, infectious hepatitis, carcinoma of the pancreas, and drugs (ie, oral contraceptives, sulfonamides, rifampin, aspirin, morphine, thiazides, and procainamide).

Bilirubin (Urine): Norms: negative to 0.02 mg/dL

Unconjugated bilirubin (fat soluble) cannot be excreted in the urine because it is not water soluble. If urine bilirubin test is positive, then conditions causing conjugated hyperbilirubinemia are likely to be the cause.

Urobilinogen (Urine): Norms: Adult: Random: 0.3–3.5 mg/dL. 24-hour specimen: 0.05–2.5 mg/24 h, 0.09–4.23 µmol/24 h (SI units)

Conjugated bilirubin from bile is changed in the duodenum to urobilinogen. Decreased urobilinogen level might indicate severe liver damage, biliary obstruction, and/or severe inflammatory disease. Elevated levels may be indicative of hemolytic disease, early cirrhosis of the liver, toxic or infectious hepatitis.

Liver Enzyme Tests: As the result of liver damage by insult or disease, most of the liver enzymes are released into the blood stream, resulting in increased enzyme levels. Some of these enzymes are also found in other organs and are considered nonspecific. Examples of the nonspecific enzymes are alkaline phosphatase and lactic dehydrogenase. Usually several liver enzyme tests are performed at the same time to confirm liver disorder. Table 6 compares the enzyme studies that are usually ordered to evaluate suspected liver diseases:

TABLE 6. LIVER ENZYME TESTS

Enzyme (Serum)	Reference Values	Comments
Alkaline phosphatase (ALP) and isoenzyme	*Norms:* Adult: 30–120 IU/L 25–97 U/L at 37°C (SI units), 4–13 U/dL (King-Armstrong) ALP$_1$ 20–120 U/L	ALP is found mainly in bone and liver and also in intestine, kidney, and placenta. Since ALP is produced by several systems and cells in the body, its activity is classified as nonspecific; therefore other liver function tests should be performed to confirm the diagnosis. In severe liver damage (ie, cancer of liver, hepatocellular problems) serum ALP is greatly increased. ALP isoenzymes assist in identifying the origin of the problem. ALP$_1$ is of liver origin, and ALP$_2$ is of bone origin.
5'Nucleotidase (5'NT or 5'N)	*Norms:* <14 U/L	5'NT is specific to liver cells. ALP and 5'NT are measured at the same time, since both enzymes are found in liver cells and are elevated in hepatocellular disease. However, serum ALP will be elevated in bone disease, but 5'NT will *not* be increased.
Leucine aminopeptidase (LAP)	*Norms:* 8–22 mU/mL, 12–33 IU/L, 18–40 U/L (SI units)	LAP enzyme is found mainly in liver tissue. Serum LAP is elevated in liver disease (ie, cancer of the liver, viral hepatitis, acute necrosis of the liver, and extrahepatic biliary obstruction). LAP, 5'NT, and ALP tests are frequently ordered together to confirm liver disease. If only ALP is elevated and the other two enzymes are not, bone disease would be probable.
Alanine aminotransferase (ALT or SGPT)	*Norms:* Adult: 5–35 U/mL (Frankel) 5–25 mU/mL (Wroblewski) 4–35 U/L at 37°C (SI units)	ALT/SGPT is found primarily in liver cells and is effective in diagnosing hepatocellular obstruction. AST/SGOT is found in liver cells; however, it is more specific to cardiac muscle and skeletal muscle. Serum ALT is slightly to moderately increased in cancer of the liver and cirrhosis. It is highly increased during viral hepatitis and drug hepatotoxicity
Lactic Dehydrogenase (LD/LDH) Isoenzymes	*Norms:* Adult: 100–190 IU/L Isoenzyme LDH$_5$ 6%–16% Child: 50–150 IU/L	LDH is elevated in heart, lung, liver, and renal disease. To determine if the increased LDH is due to liver disease, LDH isoenzymes are measured. LDH$_5$ rises before jaundice occurs and falls before bilirubin level does.

TABLE 6. LIVER ENZYME TESTS (*Continued*)

Enzyme (Serum)	Reference Values	Comments
Gamma-glutamyl transferase/ transpeptidase (GGT/GGTP)	*Norms:* Adult: Male: 10–80 IU/L Female: 5–25 IU/L Average: 0–45 IU/L	GGT/GGTP is found mostly in the liver and kidney and small amounts in heart muscle, spleen, and prostate gland. It is a more sensitive indicator for liver disease than other liver enzymes (ie, ALP and AST/SGOT). Elevated GGT/GGTP occurs in cirrhosis of the liver, alcoholism, cancer of the liver, viral hepatitis, and acute pancreatitis.

alkaline phosphatase (ALP), alanine aminotransferase (ALT or SGPT), 5′ nucleotidase (5′ NT), leucine aminopeptidase (LAP), LDH_5, and gamma-glutamyl transferase (GGT).

Protein (Serum), Protein Electrophoresis: Norms: Adult: Total protein: 6–8 g/dL; albumin: 3.5–5.0 g/dL; globulin: 1.5–3.5 g/dL. (*For other values, see protein electrophoresis.*)

Serum protein is an indirect measure of albumin and globulin. Albumin and globulin are indicators of liver function and diseases. Protein electrophoresis gives the breakdown of albumin and globulin. Albumin level is decreased, and gamma globulin level is elevated in cirrhosis of the liver. α_2-Globulin fraction is elevated in inflammatory disease of the liver and cancer of the liver. An elevated β-globulin might occur in biliary obstruction. In chronic liver disease the A/G ratio is reversed.

Ammonia (Plasma, Blood): Norms: Adult (depends on method used): 15–45 μg/dL 3.2–4.5 g/dL or 32–45 g/L, 11–35 μmol/L (SI units); Child: 21–50 μg/dL; Newborn: 64–107 μg/dL.

Ammonia, a by-product of protein metabolism, is converted to urea by the liver. Ammonia levels are elevated in severe liver diseases (ie, cirrhosis, acute hepatic necrosis, or when blood flow to the liver is altered).

Prothrombin Time (PT) (Plasma): Norms: Adult: 11–15 seconds or 70%–100%. PT levels might differ in institutions.

Prothrombin, factor II of the coagulation factors, is produced by the liver and requires vitamin K for its synthesis. Increase in PT time frequently occurs in liver disease.

Cholesterol (Serum): Norms: Adult: 150–240 mg/dL, <200 mg/dL (desired level); 3.90–6.50 mmol/L (SI units). Child 130–185 mg/dL. Infant: 90–130 mg/dL

Cholesterol is a blood lipid that is synthesized in the liver. In chronic liver disease, serum cholesterol could be decreased. In biliary obstruction and pancreatitis, serum levels could be increased.

Hepatitis B Surface Antigen (HB_sAg) (Serum): Norms: Negative.

A positve HB_sAG is an indicator of acute hepatitis B, chronic active hepatitis, or a carrier of hepatitis B.

Hepatitis B Surface Antibody (HB$_s$Ab/anti-HB$_s$): Norms: Negative.

A positive HB$_s$Ab test indicates a *previous* infection of hepatitis B virus. Years after an acute hepatitis B infection, the HB$_s$Ab test might still be positive.

Hepatitis B Core Antibody (HB$_c$Ab/anti-HB$_c$) (Serum): Norms: Negative.

This test is performed following negative serum HB$_s$Ag and HB$_s$Ab results when hepatitis is suspected. A positive Hb$_c$Ab might indicate a recent hepatitis B infection.

Diagnostic Tests

X-ray of Abdomen: A flat plate x-ray of the abdomen is used to detect abdominal masses in the liver, pancreas, stomach, and intestine. It could indicate small-bowel obstruction and ascites.

Ultrasonography, Ultrasound (Liver): This is a noninvasive procedure useful in locating cysts, abscesses, and tumors. Liver ultrasound can differentiate between obstructive and nonobstructive jaundice. It is useful with liver scanning to define the cold spots. This test is usually ordered for patients with jaundice of unknown cause and unexplained hepatomegaly.

Liver and Spleen Scan: In nuclear liver imaging, a radionuclide (eg, technetium [Tc] compound [Tc-99m pertechnetate, Tc-99m sulfide]) is administered intravenously to determine the size and structure of the liver and to detect abnormalities. If the liver has less radionuclide uptake than the spleen, cirrhosis or chronic hepatitis could be suspected. If cold spots (areas that do not take up radionuclide) appear, cysts, abscesses, and tumors might be suspected. Follow-up diagnostic tests (ie, ultrasound, CT scan, and/or biopsy) are needed to confirm diagnosis.

Computerized Tomography (CT) (Liver): CT visualizes the liver and biliary tract with or without contrast medium. It can detect hepatic cysts, abscesses, tumors, and can differentiate between obstructive and nonobstructive jaundice. CT should be performed before or four days after barium studies. Ultrasound is cheaper than CT and can detect liver and biliary disorders equally as well.

Percutaneous Liver Biopsy: Liver cells can be obtained for microscopic examination by needle biopsy. The needle is inserted through the skin to the liver. It is used to confirm diagnosis of hepatocellular diseases (ie, cirrhosis, hepatitis, tumors). Liver biopsy should not be performed on patients with bleeding disorders or having obstructive jaundice caused by possible bile leakage.

Hepatic Angiography, Celiac and Mesenteric Arteriography: Hepatic angiography is used to evaluate cirrhosis and portal hypertension and to evaluate vascular damage after abdominal trauma.

Gallbladder Assessment

Diagnostic Tests

X-ray of Abdomen: Flat plate x-ray of the abdomen can visualize gallbladder stones. The stones that are not calcified and are composed of cholesterol will not be seen. Therefore contrast medium tests should be ordered.

Cholecystography (Oral), Gallbladder Series: Oral cholecystography is an x-ray test to visualize stones and to diagnose inflammatory disease and tumors of the gallbladder. The patient ingests radiopaque iodinated dye tablets the night before. This dye is concentrated in the gallbladder 12 to 14 hours after ingestion. This test should be performed before or 2 to 4 days after upper GI and small-bowel series, since the barium would hamper visualization.

Cholangiography (Intravenous, Percutaneous, and T tube or Postoperative): Cholangiography is an x-ray examination of the bile ducts using contrast medium either intravenously or percutaneously or through the T tube. Table 7 describes the cholangiography tests used for visualizing the biliary ducts.

Endoscopic Retrograde Cholangiopancreatography (ERCP): Through a fiberoptic endoscope, contrast medium (dye) is injected into the duodenal papilla to visualize the biliary tract for cause of obstructive jaundice. The use of ERCP has increased, since the development of the fiberoptic side-view endoscope. This test is used when other diagnostic tests fail to determine cause of jaundice (ie, stones, tumors).

Ultrasonography, Ultrasound of the Gallbladder, and Biliary System: Ultrasound of the gallbladder and biliary tract is useful for diagnosing cholelithiasis and cholecystitis and to differentiate between obstructive and nonobstructive jaundice. It can detect polyps and tumors. Advantages for the use of ultrasound include the fact that it is cheaper than CT scan with equal results, there is no risk of radiation, and no contrast media is used.

HIDA Scan: Technetium 99m dimethyacetanilide iminodiacetic acid (Tc-99m HIDA) is injected intravenously to visualize the hepatobiliary system. It is useful in detecting biliary obstruction and also hepatocellular disease.

Computerized Tomography of the Gallbladder and Biliary System: CT test of the right upper quadrant includes the visualization of the liver, gallbladder, and biliary tract. It can detect stones in the gallbladder and biliary ducts. Although

TABLE 7. CHOLANGIOGRAPHY TESTS

Tests	Comments
IV cholangiography	With IV cholangiography, contrast medium (eg, meglumine iodipamide) is injected intravenously. The dye is filtered by the liver and passes into the gallbladder and biliary ducts for visualization. There are more reported side effects with the use of IV contrast media than with oral tablets. This test is not indicated if hepatocellular disease is highly suspected or serum bilirubin is > 3 mg/dL.
Percutaneous transhepatic cholangiography (PTHC)	A needle is passed through the skin to the liver and into a dilated bile duct. Contrast medium is injected. Purpose is to visualize the biliary tract and to determine the cause of obstructive jaundice.
T-tube or postoperative cholangiography	Dye is injected into the T tube, which was inserted during surgery. Purpose is to check for retained gallstones in the common bile duct.

ultrasound is cheaper, CT is preferred for obese patients and for those who have livers high in the rib cage.

Pancreas Assessment

Laboratory and diagnostic tests for diabetes mellitus will be covered in the section on assessment of endocrine function.

Laboratory Tests

Amylase (Serum): Norms: Adult: 60–160 Somogyi U/dL, 25–125 U/L (SI units). Child: usually not done

Amylase is a pancreatic enzyme that changes starch to sugar. In acute pancreatitis, serum amylase level is elevated in 2 to 12 hours after onset and remains elevated for 2 to 3 days. Levels are also increased in biliary duct obstruction, (eg, gallstones).

Amylase (Urine): Norms: Adult: 4–37 U/L/2h

When serum amylase is slightly to moderately elevated and pancreatitis is suspected, a 24-hour urine amylase level may be ordered. Urine amylase level is useful to confirm the diagnosis of acute pancreatitis.

Lipase (Serum): Norms: Adult: 20–180 IU/L, 14–280 mU/mL, 14–280 U/L (SI units). Child: 20–136 IU/L at 37°C

Lipase is a pancreatic enzyme that aids in the digestion of fats in the duodenum. Serum lipase level is elevated early in acute pancreatitis and remains elevated longer than serum amylase level.

Secretin Test: This test assesses pancreatic exocrine function and is helpful in diagnosing pancreatic tumor, obstruction of the pancreatic duct, and chronic pancreatitis. It is a 3-hour test and requires a double-lumen tube; one lumen is inserted into the duodenum for aspiration of duodenal secretions and the other lumen into the stomach for aspiration of gastric secretions. Three samples are collected for base-line determination. Then secretin is administered intravenously and four more samples are collected.

Diagnostic Tests

Endoscopic Retrograde Cholangiopancreatography (ERCP): At the duodenal papilla, ERCP procedure visualizes the biliary tract and the pancreatic duct. This test can detect pancreatic tumor and stricture of the pancreatic duct caused by chronic pancreatitis. A complication that might result from this procedure is pancreatitis.

Ultrasonography, Ultrasound of the Pancreas: Ultrasound is helpful in the detection of pancreatic abscess, cysts, and tumors. It could support the diagnosis of pancreatitis after serum amylase and lipase levels have returned to normal.

Hypotonic Duodenography: The purpose of this test is to detect pancreatic and duodenal diseases (ie, tumor at the head of pancreas, stricture caused by chronic pancreatitis, and small duodenal lesion). A catheter is passed through the nose to the duodenum, and barium sulfate and air are injected. Spot x-ray films are taken.

Computerized Tomography (CT) of the Pancreas: CT of the pancreas is useful to distinguish between pancreatic tumors and cysts and to detect suspected pancreatitis. The use of oral or IV contrast media during the test provides a more detailed visualization of the pancreas. Recent barium studies could hamper visualization of the pancreas.[1,2,5,9,11,15,17,18]

■ Nursing Diagnoses

- ■ Knowledge deficit related to lack of understanding of laboratory and diagnostic procedures, disease process, and/or outcome
- ■ Potential for noncompliance to prescribed laboratory and diagnostic tests related to lack of or inadequate explanation and/or anxiety about physical condition
- ■ Alteration in nutrition related to anorexia, reduced food intake, and/or impaired metabolism
- ■ Potential for injury related to bleeding tendencies secondary to decreased prothrombin production
- ■ Potential for injury related to allergic reactions to contrast medium (dye) secondary to diagnostic tests (ie, CT with contrast medium, angiography)
- ■ Fluid volume excess (peripheral and peritoneal) related to sodium and fluid retention and fluid volume shift secondary to liver disorders (eg, cirrhosis)
- ■ Potential impairment of skin integrity related to peripheral edema
- ■ Potential activity intolerance related to peripheral edema and ascites
- ■ Ineffective coping with disease process and laboratory and diagnostic test procedures
- ■ Potential disturbance in self-concept related to body changes (eg, ascites)
- ■ Potential alteration in family processes related to social problems from alcoholism

---

NURSING IMPLICATIONS WITH RATIONALE

- ■ Explain that the purpose of the laboratory and diagnostic tests is to aid in diagnosing liver, gallbladder, and pancreatic disorders. Be specific with explanation as indicated.
- ■ Give an explanation, in detail if indicated, about the laboratory and diagnostic procedures. Provide written instruction sheet to reinforce verbal instructions. Emphasize the importance of the patient's compliance to the test procedures. Stress that tests might need to be repeated if the procedure is improperly performed.
- ■ Inform the patient of any food, beverage, or drug restrictions. Each test should be checked for specific restrictions (*see Parts I and II*).
- ■ Inform the physician if the patient has had recent barium studies or if ultrasonography, CT, ERCP are ordered. Barium sulfate can hinder visualization, and a 2- to 4-day waiting period after barium studies is usually required.
- ■ Listen to the patient's expressed anxiety concerning the tests and potential patient problems. Clarification of test procedure might alleviate fear and anxiety and promote test compliance.

- Be prepared to repeat information to the patient and family if anxiety and/or fear level is determined to be high.
- Elicit from the patient awareness or knowledge of any allergies to contrast medium (dye), iodine, or seafood.
- Monitor the patient's vital signs before and following laboratory and diagnostic tests.
- Assess lower extremities and abdomen for signs of or changes in peripheral edema and/or ascites.
- Notify the physician if the patient's serum bilirubin is greater than 3 mg/dL prior to cholecystography or intravenous cholangiography. An elevated serum bilirubin can prevent contrast medium uptake and excretion.
- Check the laboratory results, and notify physician of abnormal test reports.
- Assess for bleeding from the nose, rectum, and skin. Liver disorders can cause prolonged prothrombin time resulting in bleeding tendencies.
- Check gag reflex for endoscopic procedures (eg, ERCP, before giving fluids and food).

Evaluation

- Determine if the test was correctly performed according to the procedure. Notify laboratory and/or physician of any changes that occur during the test.
- Check the patient's vital signs for changes, worsening and deterioration, or improvement.
- Check lower extremities and abdomen for decrease in pitted edema and ascites.
- Provide ongoing assessment (before, during, and after procedure) of critical changes; document them; and report them to the physician.
- Clarify or answer any additional questions the patient might have.
- Encourage the patient to seek health care assistance whenever changes in health status occur.
- Encourage the patient and family members to participate in the decision-making process concerning long-term plans.

GASTROINTESTINAL FUNCTION

LABORATORY TESTS	DIAGNOSTIC TESTS
Upper GI	
Electrolytes (Serum)	Esophageal Studies
Gastrin (Serum)	Acid Perfusion (Bernstein Test)
	Esophageal Acidity
	Esophageal Manometry
	Gastric Analysis Studies
	Basal Gastric Secretion
	Gastric Cytologic Examination
	Gastric Acid Stimulation

LABORATORY TESTS	DIAGNOSTIC TESTS
Upper GI *(cont.)*	
	Esophagogastroduodenoscopy
	Esophagoscopy
	Gastroscopy
	Barium Swallow
	Fluoroscopy
	Cineradiography
	Upper GI Series and Small Bowel
	Celiac and Mesenteric Angiography/
	Arteriography
Lower GI	
CEA	X-ray of Abdomen
Carotene (Serum)	Barium Enema
Electrolytes (Serum)	Proctosigmoidoscopy
D-xylose Absorption	Proctoscopy
Lactose Intolerance	Sigmoidoscopy
Fecal Analysis	Biopsy
Occult Blood	Colonoscopy
Fat Content	Peritoneal Analysis
Ova and Parasites	Paracentesis

Introduction

There are numerous gastrointestinal (GI) tests performed for assessing GI disorders. When the problem is of the esophagus, stomach, or duodenum, a series of upper GI tests (ie, gastric analysis, upper GI series, and/or esophago-gastroduodenoscopy) might be performed. When the problem is of the colon, a series of lower GI tests (ie, fecal analysis, barium enema, proctosigmoidoscopy, and/or colonoscopy) might be performed.

Endoscopy is a method using an endoscope, a metal or fiberoptic tube, for visualizing abnormalities of the GI tract. Many upper and lower GI tests are classified as endoscopic tests or procedures. Tests for GI disorders are classified as upper GI and lower GI.

Upper GI Assessment

Laboratory Tests

Electrolytes: Potassium, Sodium, Magnesium (Serum): Norms: Adult: Potassium: 3.5–5.0 mEq/L; Sodium: 135–145 mEq/L; Magnesium 1.5–2.5 mEq/L. Child: *See individual tests.*

Electrolytes are plentiful in the GI tract. Continuous vomiting or gastric intubation can cause a loss of the cations (ie, potassium [K], sodium [Na], and magnesium [Mg]). Electrolyte replacement through IV fluids is essential to restore electrolyte balance and to prevent life-threatening problems, (eg, cardiac arrhythmias). Serum electrolyte levels should be monitored, and any changes, decreases, or elevations, should be reported immediately.

Gastrin (Serum): *Norms:* Adult: Fasting: <100 pg/mL; Nonfasting: 50–200 pg/mL

Gastrin is a hormone secreted from the distal part of the stomach. This hormone stimulates the secretion of gastric juices, mainly hydrochloric acid (HCl). Serum gastrin levels are slightly to moderately elevated in patients having gastric ulcer or pernicious anemia and are highly elevated in patients with Zollinger Ellison syndrome (pancreatic islet-cell tumor that secretes excess gastrin.)

Diagnostic Tests

Esophageal Studies: One or more esophageal studies are usually performed for determining the cause of heartburn (pyrosis) and swallowing difficulty (dys-

TABLE 8. ESOPHAGEAL STUDIES

Test	Reference Values	Results
Acid perfusion (Bernstein test)		Epigastric or retrosternal pain that radiates to the back or arms is usually associated with myocardial infarction; however, these symptoms could be due to juices from the stomach backflowing into the esophagus. This test is useful to determine if chest pain or epigastric discomfort is caused by a cardiac condition or by esophagitis. Normal saline and hydrochloric acid (HCl) are dripped at different times into the esophagus. If the patient has pain during the HCl drip, the test is a positive for esophagitis.
Esophageal acidity	*Norms:* pH >5.0	This test measures the pH level of fluid in the lower esophagus. When patients complain of frequent heartburn, a pH electrode attached to a catheter is inserted through the mouth into the esophagus. If the intra-esophageal pH is 1.0–3.0, gastroesophageal reflux (backflow of gastric acid into esophagus) caused by an incompetent sphincter is highly probable.
Esophageal manometry	*Norms:* 15–25 mm Hg (lower esophageal sphincter [LES])	Esophageal manometry measures esophageal sphincter and intraluminal pressures and records the sequence and duration of esophageal peristaltic contractions. When LES pressure is 0–5 mm Hg, incompetent or hypotensive sphincter is likely to be the cause; gastroesophageal reflux results. High LES pressure (>50 mm Hg) could indicate hypertensive sphincter caused by achalasia, esophageal diverticula, or tumor.

TABLE 9. GASTRIC ANALYSIS TESTS

Test	Reference Values	Result
Basal gastric secretion	Basal (fasting): 1–5 mEq/h	No fluid or food for 8–12 hours before the test. High gastric acid levels suggest peptic ulcer (gastric or duodenal), and very high levels could be indicative of Zollinger-Ellison syndrome. Low levels might suggest gastric carcinoma.
Gastric acid stimulation	Stimulation: 10–25 mEq/h	Usually this test follows the basal gastric test. A stimulant such as betazole HCl (Histalog) or pentagastrin is administered. After 15 minutes, four to eight 15-minute specimens are taken. High levels suggest duodenal ulcer and very high levels indicate Zollinger-Ellison syndrome. Low levels might suggest gastric carcinoma.

phagia). Most of these tests check for the pH in the esophagus and esophageal sphincter pressure. Table 8 explains the purposes of three esophageal tests with abnormal results.

Gastric Analysis Studies: Norms: Basal (fasting): 1–5 mEq/h. Stimulation: 10–25 mEq/h

Gastric analysis studies determine the quantity of gastric acid secreted between meals or feedings and during gastric acid stimulation. Stimulants used include histamine phosphate, betazole HCl (Histalog), pentagastrin, caffeine. Table 9 describes the two tests performed for gastric analysis.

Gastric Cytologic Examination: Gastric aspiration for cytologic examination is obtained either during gastroscopy or after nasogastric catheter/tube insertion. If secretions aspirated through the tube are insufficient, then 100 mL of saline is instilled to facilitate specimen collection.

Esophagogastroduodenoscopy, Gastroscopy, Esophagoscopy: This endoscopic test examines the esophagus, stomach, and duodenum to determine cause of epigastric or substernal pain and hematemesis. It is one of the most effective methods in diagnosing GI disorders (ie, peptic ulcer [gastric or duodenal], esophageal varices, tumors, inflammatory conditions, hiatal hernia, Mallory-Weiss syndrome, and for obtaining biopsy, foreign body, cells for cytology, or gastric acid secretions). Esophagogastroduodenoscopy should be done before or 2 days after an upper GI series, since the barium sulfate retention would inhibit visualization. This test is useful to confirm a diagnosis, especially when contrast radiography procedures (eg, upper GI series) fail to detect the GI problem.

Gastroscopy: This test, part of the esophagogastroduodenoscopy, can detect gastric disorders. A metal gastroscope could be used instead of the fiberoptic endoscope.

Esophagoscopy: It is used to visualize only the esophagus.

Barium Swallow: This diagnostic procedure is ordered to assess the pharynx and the esophagus for abnormalities. Usually it is part of the upper GI series, although it could be a separate test. The patient swallows a thick mixture of barium sulfate, followed by cineradiographic examination of the pharynx and fluoroscopic examination of the esophagus. Barium swallow is useful for detecting esophageal strictures, tumors, polyps, ulcers, hiatal hernia, diverticula, and motility disorders.

Fluoroscopy: This can be part of the upper GI series. It is x-ray viewing from the time barium sulfate or meglumine diatrizoate (Gastrografin) is ingested and passes from the esophagus to the stomach. Fluoroscopic viewing can also take place during the barium enema test as the contrast agent goes through the large bowel.

Cineradiography: This is a filming method used for detecting esophageal motility problems.

Upper GI Series: The upper GI series uses barium sulfate or meglumine diatrizoate (Gastrografin) as the contrast medium to visualize abnormalities in the esophagus and stomach. Usually barium sulfate is more effective for visualizing the mucosa, and meglumine diatrizoate is preferred when perforation is suspected because it is a water-soluble agent. This test is useful for detecting causes of dysphagia (difficulty in swallowing), epigastric pain and discomfort, hematemesis, and melena. It is primarily used to diagnose gastric or duodenal ulcers, strictures, and tumors. Double-contrast studies (barium and air) give a better view of the mucosa for detecting polyps, early carcinoma, and gastritis.

Angiography, Celiac and Mesenteric Arteriography: This is an invasive procedure in which a catheter is threaded from the femoral artery to the celiac or mesenteric artery to detect the site of GI bleeding or to detect ischemic areas. Contrast medium is injected for visualization. When the GI bleeding site is identified, vasopressin is infused slowly to the site of bleeding. If vasopressin is not effective in stopping bleeding, then arterial embolization might be necessary. This test is performed when endoscopy and barium studies fail to determine the cause of a GI bleeding problem.

Lower GI Assessment

Laboratory Tests

Carcinoembryonic Antigen (CEA) (Plasma): Norms: Nonsmokers: <2.5 ng/mL; Smokers: <3.5 mg/mL

High plasma CEA levels are found in patients with colorectal cancer. The test should not be the sole criterion for diagnosing colon cancer, since this antigen is relatively nonspecific. The usefulness of this test is to monitor plasma CEA levels following surgical intervention or therapeutic treatment for colon cancer. A decreased CEA level indicates effective response to surgery or treatment. A rise in plasma CEA later might indicate a recurrence of the cancer.

Carotene (Serum): Norms: Adult: 60–200 μg/dL, 0.74–3.72 μmol/L (SI units). Child: 40–130 μg/dL

A decreased serum carotene could be a result of intestinal fat malabsorption. This could affect the absorption of fat-soluble vitamins.

Electrolytes: Potassium, Sodium, Magnesium (Serum): Norms: Adult: Potassium: 3.5–5.0 mEq/L; sodium: 135–145 mEq/L; magnesium: 1.5–2.5 mEq/L. child: *See individual tests.*

Potassium, sodium, and magnesium are plentiful in the intestine as well as the stomach. Loss of intestinal secretions because of diarrhea or intestinal intubation could cause serum electrolyte deficits (ie, hypokalemia, hyponatremia, hypomagnesemia).

D-xylose Absorption (Serum and Urine): Norms: Adult: Serum: 25–40 mg/dL/2 h; urine: >3.5 g/5 h and >5 g/24 h. Older adult: Serum: 25–40 mg/dL/2 h urine: >4g/5 h. Child: Serum: 30 mg/dL/1 h

Good urine function is needed for this test. It evaluates absorption of D-xylose, a pentose sugar, in the small intestine. Eighty percent to 95% of the D-xylose dose is excreted in 5 hours. Decreased serum and urine levels could indicate malabsorptive disorder of the small intestine, jejunal enteritis, or jejunal diverticula.

Lactose Tolerance: Norms: Adult: blood glucose increase of 20 mg/dL/2 h

This test is to identify patients who have a deficiency of the intestinal enzyme lactase. With a decreased intestinal lactase activity, lactose ingested (eg, milk products) is inadequately absorbed. As a result of lactose deficiency, diarrhea, abdominal cramps, and flatus occur, especially after ingestion of milk and/or milk products.

Fecal Analysis Various studies can be performed on stool specimens (ie, occult blood, fat content, and ova and parasites). Table 10 shows substances that are analyzed in feces.

Diagnostic Tests

X-ray of Abdomen: Flat x-ray films of the abdomen are ordered to identify abdominal masses of the stomach, liver, and intestine. Suspected abnormal findings are confirmed with other GI tests.

TABLE 10. FECAL ANALYSIS STUDIES

Fecal Substances	Values	Comments
Occult blood	Negative	When bleeding from the GI tract is not evident but is suspected, a stool sample is examined for occult (hidden) blood. Either microscopic examination or chemical tests (ie, guaiac or orthotolidine) are used for identifying fecal occult blood.
Fat content	Norms: <6 g/24 h	This can be a screening test when malabsorption syndrome is suspected. If fecal fat content is >6 g/24 h, then malabsorption syndrome is the probable cause. A very small stool could cause false test results.
Ova and parasites	Negative	Ova and parasites (O&P) may be present in the intestine. Usually three stool specimens are evaluated to identify and to confirm the organism present, so that appropriate treatment can be ordered.

Barium Enema: This is a test that has been used for years in diagnosing lower bowel disorders. Barium sulfate is the contrast agent used and when a more detailed visualization is needed, barium sulfate and air (double contrast) is given. Barium enema is ordered when patients complain of abnormal bowel habits, lower abdominal pain or cramps, blood in the stool, or changes in stool formation. This test is useful for diagnosing polyps and intestinal masses (eg, tumors, diverticula, strictures, and ulcerations). Barium should not be used when perforation of the bowel is strongly suspected.

Proctosigmoidoscopy: This is an endoscopic procedure for visualizing the anus, rectum, and sigmoid colon. Usually a flexible fiberoptic proctosigmoidoscope is used instead of a rigid metal sigmoidoscope. Abnormalities detected by this procedure include polyps, tumors, hemorrhoids, and inflammatory process.

> *Proctoscopy:* Usually this test is performed during a proctosigmoidoscopy; however, the conventional rigid proctoscope, 3 in. in length, could be used to examine the lower rectum and anal canal.
>
> *Sigmoidoscopy:* For years, the sigmoidoscope (a rigid 10- to 12-inch instrument) was used to examine the rectum and sigmoid colon. The proctosigmoidoscope (fiberoptic endoscope) is the instrument of choice today for this test procedure.
>
> *Biopsy and Cytologic Examination:* During a proctosigmoidoscopy, specimens can be obtained by the use of biopsy forceps, cytology brush, or culture swab.

Colonoscopy: This is another endoscopic procedure, and its use has markedly increased in recent years. It is an inspection of the large intestine (colon) using a long, flexible fiberscope (colonoscope). Colonoscopy can detect lesions in the proximal colon that would be missed by sigmoidoscopy. Biopsy forceps and cytologic brush can be used during this test. It should not be done before or 2 days after a barium enema because the barium sulfate would inhibit visualization.

Colonoscopy is effective in detecting early cancerous lesions, which have a good prognosis. It can detect advanced cancerous tumors and determine the extent of inflammatory tissue. Polyps can be removed with the use of an electrocautery snare during the colonoscopy.

Peritoneal Analysis/Paracentesis Draining copious amounts of fluid from the peritoneal cavity is not done unless the large abdominal fluid volume is causing respiratory distress. Loss of large quantities of peritoneal fluid could cause severe fluid and electrolyte imbalance. Fluid samples may be requested for analyzing the fluid content (ie, electrolytes, blood cells, sugar, protein, organisms, and cancer cells).[1,2,7,9,11,15,16,19,20]

- Nursing Diagnoses

  - Knowledge deficit related to lack of understanding of laboratory and diagnostic procedures, disease process, and/or outcome
  - Potential for noncompliance with prescribed laboratory and diagnostic tests related to lack of or inadequate explanation and/or anxiety about physical condition
  - Alteration in nutrition related to anorexia, nausea, vomiting, and/or diarrhea

- Potential impairment of skin integrity related to poor nutritional intake
- Alteration in comfort related to endoscopic examination(s)
- Ineffective coping with laboratory and diagnostic test procedure
- Alteration in bowel elimination related to diarrhea, constipation or barium sulfate
- Fluid volume and electrolyte deficits related to vomiting, diarrhea, or gastric/intestinal intubation
- Potential disturbance in self-concept related to body changes (eg, colostomy)

NURSING IMPLICATIONS WITH RATIONALE

- Explain that the purpose for the laboratory and diagnostic tests is to aid in the diagnosis of esophagus, stomach, or colon disorders. Be more specific in explanation if indicated.
- Give an explanation (in detail if indicated) about the laboratory and diagnostic procedures. Emphasize the importance of the patient's compliance to the test procedures. Stress that tests might need to be repeated if the procedure was improperly performed.
- Inform the patient of any food, beverage, or drug restrictions. Each test should be checked for specific restrictions (*see Parts I and II*).
- Inform the physician if the patient has had recent barium studies (ie, upper GI series, barium enema), especially if esophagogastroduodenoscopy, proctosigmoidoscopy, and colonoscopy are ordered. Barium sulfate can hinder visualization and a 2- to 4-day waiting period after barium studies is usually required.
- Listen to patient's expressed anxiety and fear concerning the tests and potential patient problems. Clarification of test procedure might alleviate fear and anxiety and promote test compliance.
- Monitor the patient's vital signs before and after laboratory and diagnostic tests. Report significant changes.
- Obtain stool specimen for occult blood analysis. Determine frequency of bowel movements.
- Assess for throat discomfort (ie, soreness, swallowing difficulty after oral endoscopic procedure).
- Check gag reflex before giving fluids and food after endoscopic procedures.
- Check laboratory results, and notify physician of abnormal test findings.

Evaluation

- Determine if the test was correctly performed according to the procedure. Notify the laboratory and/or physician of any changes that occur during the test.
- Check the patient's vital signs and frequent bowel movements for changes and improvement.
- Evaluate the status of the patient's anxiety and fear in regard to the test(s) and clinical problem.
- Clarify or answer any additional questions the patient may have.

■ Encourage the patient to seek health assistance when changes in health status occur. Continue with assessing the patient's state of health.

NEUROLOGIC AND MUSCULOSKELETAL FUNCTION

LABORATORY TESTS	DIAGNOSTIC TESTS
Neurologic	
CSF	X-rays
Pressure, Cells, Protein, Glucose,	Skull
Culture, Cytology	Lumbosacral Spine
TDM—Anticonvulsants	EEG
	Echoencephalography
	Brain Scan
	CT, Brain
	Cerebral Angiography
	MRI
	PET
	Electroneurography
	Myelography
	Thermography of Spine
	Oculoplethysmography
Musculoskeletal	
Muscle Enzymes	X-ray, Bone and Joints
ALD (Serum)	Synovial Fluid Aspiration
AST/SGOT (Serum)	Arthrography
CPK/CK (Serum)	Bone Scan
Bone Enzymes—ALP	Arthroscopy
Electrolytes (Ca)	EMG
(Serum)	Muscle Biopsy
	MRI

Introduction

With suspected neurologic disorders, a group of diagnostic tests is performed to confirm a diagnosis. When there are frequent headaches, the tests usually ordered to determine their origin include cerebrospinal fluid (CSF) examination, skull x-rays, and electroencephalography (EEG). If headaches intensify and persist, echoencephalogram, computerized tomographic (CT) scan of the head, brain scan, or cerebral angiogram or MRI or PET might be requested. For seizure disorders, EEG, echoencephalography, and CT scan of the head usually are ordered. After acute head injury, skull x-rays are immediately taken. CT scan and MRI of the head might be requested.

Musculoskeletal disorders are evaluated by using various diagnostic procedures (ie, synovial fluid analysis, electromyography [EMG] arthrography, bone scan, and arthroscopy). Neurologic assessment will be presented first, then musculoskeletal.

Neurologic Assessment

Laboratory Tests

Cerebrospinal Fluid (SCF): Norms: See reference values in Part I.

Analysis of CSF usually includes color, pressure, white blood cell (WBC) count, protein, chloride, glucose, culture, cytologic cells. Table 11 lists the component found in CSF and the result of the analysis.

Therapeutic Drug Monitoring (TDM): Anticonvulsants are ordered for seizure disorders (ie, grand mal, psychomotor, and/or petit mal), and therapeutic drugs levels should be closely monitored. The following drug outline gives the name of anticonvulsant, type of seizure, therapeutic range, and toxic level for adults (child as indicated).

DRUG NAME	SEIZURE DISORDER	THERAPEUTIC RANGE	TOXIC LEVEL
Carbamazepine	Grand mal	4–12 μg/mL	>12–15 μg/mL
Ethosuximide	Petit mal	40–100 μg/mL	>100 μg/mL
Phenytoin	Grand mal	Adult: 10–20 μg/mL Child: 4–8 mg/kg/day	Adult: >20 μg/mL Child: 15–20 μg/mL
Primidone	Grand mal and psychomotor	Adult: 5–12 μg/mL Child: 7–10 μg/mL	Adult: >12–15 μg/mL Child: >12 μg/mL
Valproic acid	Grand mal and petit mal	Adult: 50–100 μg/mL Child: Same as adult	Adult: >100 μg/mL Child: Same as adult

Diagnostic Tests

X-rays

Skull: Skull x-rays are usually ordered after head trauma to detect fracture of the skull. Skull x-rays are also useful to visualize primary and metastatic tumors of the skull, to confirm the existence of increased intracranial pressure, and to diagnose pituitary tumors.

Lumbosacral Spine: Spinal x-rays are frequently ordered to determine cause of pain radiating from back to leg(s). Spinal x-rays could show narrowed intervertebral disk spaces and/or calcified spurs in intervertebral foramina, which could be indicative of degenerated disks.

Electroencephalography, Electroencephalogram (EEG): EEG measures the electrical activity of the brain cells to determine abnormalities (eg, cerebral lesions [tumor, hemorrhage, abscess]). It is useful in locating the cause of seizure disorders. Another use is to confirm cerebral death. It is not the test of choice for evaluating head injuries.

Echoencephalography, Ultrasonography of the Brain, Brain Echogram: Ultrasound of the brain, a noninvasive procedure, is helpful in detecting cerebral

TABLE 11. ANALYSIS OF CSF

Component of CSF	Abnormal Results
Pressure	A pressure >200 mm H$_2$0 is considered abnormal and could be due to increased intracranial pressure caused by meningitis, subarachnoid hemorrhage, and tumors.
Color	Pink or red color could be due to subarachnoid or cerebral hemorrhage or a traumatic spinal tap. Yellow color might indicate old blood (4 to 5 days after cerebral hemorrhage).
WBC	WBC differential count may be ordered. An increased number of neutrophils could be indicative of bacterial meningitis or cerebral abscess. An increased number of lymphocytes could be indicative of viral meningitis or encephalitis.
Protein	In acute bacterial meningitis, protein levels could be >250 mg/dL. Increased protein levels indicate infections or inflammatory processes (ie, meningitis, encephalitis, and tumors).
Glucose	Glucose levels in CSF are 40–80 mg/dL, two thirds of blood/plasma levels. When there is a decrease in CSF glucose, there is usually an increase of other cells (ie, bacterial, tumor cells in the spinal fluid). A decrease in glucose, <40 mg/dL, might be indicative of bacterial meningitis, leukemia, or tumors.
Culture	A culture specimen of spinal fluid is withdrawn to determine the type of organism present.
Cytology	Slough cells from tumor sites in the brain or spinal column could flow into the spinal fluid. Examination of CSF for cancerous cells might be requested.

midline shifts characteristic of an intracranial hemorrhage. It is used in neonatal intensive care units, checking infants suspected of having intracranial hemorrhage. Follow-up studies using CT and radionuclides might be indicated.

Brain Nuclear Scan: Brain scans may be ordered for patients complaining of severe headaches or having frequent seizures. This test can detect intracranial lesions (ie, abscess, tumors [benign or malignant], metastasis to the brain, subdural hematoma, aneurysms, and cerebrovascular accident [CVA]). A technetium compound, Tc-99m-O$_4$ or Tc-99m-DTPA, is given intravenously prior to cranial scanning. The blood-brain barrier is disrupted at the pathologic lesion site, thus increasing the amount of radionuclide agent uptake.

Computerized Tomography (CT) of the Head: CT of the head is useful for diagnosing cerebral lesions (ie, tumors, hematomas caused by intracranial bleeding, abscess, cerebral infarction [obstruction], hydrocephalus, and cerebral edema). For detailed visualization of the lesion, IV contrast medium (iodinated dye) is used. CT scan of the head is replacing more invasive procedures, i.e., pneumoencephalography, cerebral angiography.

Cerebral Angiography, Arteriography: Iodinated contrast medium is injected into the carotid or vertebral artery, usually through the femoral or brachial artery, to visualize the cerebral blood vessels for abnormalities (ie, occlusions, aneurysms, abnormal vascularization resulting from neoplasms [tumors]). This is an invasive procedure, and there are patients who are allergic to the contrast medium.

Magnetic Resonance Imaging (MRI): This is a sensitive test for detecting edema, hemorrhage, blood flow, tumors, and infection sites in the brain tissue. MRI is useful in detecting demyelinating diseases, such as multiple sclerosis.

Positron Emission Tomography (PET): PET is an effective test in determining blood flow to the brain. Radiation from PET is about one fourth of that received by CT. It is useful in studying the epilepsy focal areas, viable brain tissue after a CVA (stroke), brain tumor, migraine headaches, and parkinsonism, and in differentiating between Alzheimer's disease and other types of dementia.

Electroneurography, Nerve Conduction Studies: Norms: normal conduction velocity: 50–60 meters/sec

This test is useful in determining peripheral nerve injury. It measures the time required for a nerve impulse to travel from the proximal site to the distal site. The distance per time the nerve impulse takes to travel from the proximal site of stimulation (shock) to the muscular contraction is known as the *conduction velocity*. The conduction velocity frequently varies with different nerves.

Myelography, Myelogram: Myelography is a fluoroscopic and radiologic examination of the spinal subarachnoid space (spinal column). The purpose of this test is to identify herniated intervertebral disks, cysts, metastatic tumors, neurofibromas, and meningiomas and to detect spinal nerve root injury.

Thermography (Lumbar, Thoracic, and Cervical): Irritated nerve root and musculoligamentous spasm may be detected by the use of thermography. An abnormal thermogram could include asymmetrical heat patterns that would be indicative of nerve root injury. This test might be ordered for patients with severe or chronic back pain. Usually other diagnostic tests are ordered to aid in the diagnosis (ie, electromyography [EMG], myelography).

Oculoplethysmography: This is a noninvasive test to evaluate carotid blood flow to the ophthalmic artery. It may be used in patients with CVA to determine size of carotid occlusion. Oculoplethysmographic techniques could also be used in patients with asymptomatic bruits, symptoms of transient ischemic attacks (TIA) and syncope, for detecting occlusions, and for preventing CVA.[1,6,9,10,15,21–23]

Musculoskeletal Assessment

Laboratory Tests

Muscle and Bone Enzyme Tests: Certain enzymes are present in muscles, such as aldolase, creatine phosphokinase (CPK/CK), and aspartate aminotransferase (AST or SGOT) and in bones, such as alkaline phosphatase (ALP) and isoenzyme ALP_2. Table 12 explains the uses of these enzyme tests.

Electrolyte (Calcium) (Serum): Norms: Adult: 4.5–5.5 mEq/L, 9–11 mg/dL, 2.3–2.8 mmol/L (SI units). Child: 4.5–5.8 mEq/L, 9–11.5 mg/dL. Infant: 5.0–6.0 mEq/L.

Calcium is found abundantly in bones. Frequently in bone disorders, calcium leaves bones and becomes plentiful in circulating body fluid; thus serum

TABLE 12. ENZYME TESTS OF MUSCLES AND BONES

Enzyme (Serum)	Reference Values	Results
Muscle: Aldolase (ALD)	*Norms:* Adults: <6 U/L 3–8 U/dL (Sibley-Lehninger) 22–59 mU/L at 37°C (SI units) Child: 6–16 U/dL	Aldolase is abundant in skeletal and cardiac muscles. Serum aldolase is elevated in muscular dystrophy but not in muscle diseases of neural origin (ie, multiple sclerosis, myasthenia gravis).
Aspartate aminotransferase (AST or SGOT)	*Norms:* Adult: 5–40 U/mL (Frankel) 4–36 IU/L 16–60 (Karmen) U/mL at 30°C 8–33 U/L at 37°C (SI units)	AST/SGOT is less sensitive than CPK/CK for determining muscle disorder. This enzyme is assessed in suspected myopathic diseases.
Creatine phosphokinase (CPK/CK)	*Norms:* Adult: Male: 5–35 μg/mL 30–180 IU/L; Female: 5–25 μg/mL 25–150 IU/L Child: Male: 0–70 IU/L at 30°C Female: 0–50 IU/L at 30°C	CKP/CK is more sensitive than AST/SGOT for determining muscle disorder. Actually CPK/CK is a better indicator of cardiac diseases than muscle diseases; however, this enzyme is assessed in suspected myopathic diseases.
Isoenzyme: (CPK-MM)	94%–100%	
Bone: Alkaline phosphatase (ALP)	Adult: 30–120 IU/L, 25–97 U/L at 37°C (SI units) Child: 60–270 U/L Infant: 40–300 U/L	ALP is an enzyme produced primarily in the bone and liver. In bone disorders, ALP level is increased because of abnormal osteoblastic activity (bone cell production). High ALP levels can be found in children during prepuberty and puberty ages because of bone growth. Elevated ALP levels are found in cancer of the bone, Paget's disease (osteitis deformans), healing fractures, multiple myeloma, osteomalacia.
Isoenzyme ALP$_2$	20–110 U/L	Isoenzyme ALP$_2$ is of bone origin.

calcium level is elevated (hypercalcemia). Elevated calcium levels occur as the result of bone tumors, multiple myeloma, multiple fractures, and prolonged immobilization.

Diagnostic Tests

X-rays of Bone and Joint: X-rays are frequently taken of bones and joints to determine presence of disease (ie, arthritis, spondylitis, bone lesions, and fractures).

Synovial Fluid Aspiration, Arthrocentesis: Samples of synovial fluid are aspired from joint cavity for analysis of cells (WBC, rheumatoid arthritic cells, lupus cells), protein, glucose, uric acid, and for culture.

Arthrography, Arthrogram: Arthrography uses contrast medium and/or air (both: double contrast) to visualize joint structure. This test is able to detect tears, derangements of joints, and synovial cysts. X-rays are taken during the procedure.

Bone Scan: Radionuclide, technetium-labeled phosphate compounds (eg, Tc-99m diphosphonate given intravenously) are absorbed into bone tissue and concentrated in abnormal bone cells. The scanner can pick-up hot spots months before x-rays can note abnormal bone area. This procedure is primarily used to diagnose metastatic bone disease. Bone scans are also useful to monitor bone response to radiation therapy and/or chemotherapy. This test may be used for early detection of osteomyelitis and for detection of degenerative bone disorders.

Arthroscopy: This is an endoscopic procedure usually performed in an operating room. An incision is made into the knee joint cavity, and a fiberoptic endoscope is inserted for visualization and/or removal of loose particles. It is an invasive procedure, but the findings are more inclusive than with other diagnostic tests. Biopsy of the synovium could be taken during this procedure.

Electromyography (EMG): EMG measures the electrical activity of muscles at rest and during voluntary muscle contraction. When the muscle is at rest, normally there is no electrical activity. Abnormal EMG results occur in neuropathic and myopathic disorders (ie, peripheral neuropathy (diabetes mellitus, alcoholism), myasthenia gravis, muscular dystrophy, amyotropic lateral sclerosis [ALS]).

Muscle Biopsy: The purpose for the muscle biopsy is to provide histopathologic information that could be used in the diagnosis of myopathic disorders. EMG is usually performed at the affected muscle site prior to the biopsy.

Magnetic Resonance Imaging (MRI): MRI can be used to identify muscle disease and skeletal abnormalities.[1,9–11]

- Nursing Diagnoses

  - Knowledge deficit related to lack of understanding of laboratory and diagnostic procedures, disease process, and/or outcome
  - Potential for noncompliance with prescribed laboratory and diagnostic tests related to lack of adequate explanation and/or anxiety about physical condition
  - Potential for injury related to allergic reactions to contrast medium (dye)

secondary to diagnostic test (ie, CT of the head with contrast medium, angiography)
- Impaired physical mobility related to neuromuscular impairment
- Diversional activity deficit related to inability to move freely
- Social isolation related to impaired mobility, inability to communicate
- Potential for alteration in bladder and bowel elimination related to lack of bladder and bowel control secondary to neurologic impairment
- Alteration in thought process related to impaired cerebral circulation
- Impaired verbal communication related to aphasia or brain damage
- Potential for powerlessness related to inability to communicate, dependence on others
- Ineffective coping with disease process and laboratory and diagnostic test procedures
- Disturbance in self-concept related to dependence and/or role change

---

NURSING IMPLICATIONS WITH RATIONALE

- Explain that the purpose of the laboratory and diagnostic tests is to aid in the diagnosis of brain, muscle and/or bone disorders. Be specific with explanation as indicated.
- Give an explanation of the test procedures, and emphasize the need for the patient's compliance. Explanation might be brief or in-depth, depending upon the patient's ability to comprehend.
- Inform the patient of any food, beverage, or drug restrictions (*see Parts I and II*).
- Elicit from the patient or family member information about any allergies to dye (contrast medium), iodine, or seafood.
- Listen to the patient's expressed anxiety about the tests and potential patient problems. Clarification of test procedure might alleviate fear and anxiety and promote test compliance.
- Assess muscle strength in all extremities. Weak or lacking muscle strength might indicate a neurologic (eg, CVA) or muscular problem.
- Assess the patient's ability to talk. Inability to communicate could hinder the patient's compliance to the test regime.
- Assist the patient with ambulation as needed.
- Observe for seizures prior to or after test procedure.
- Monitor the patient's vital signs before and following diagnostic procedures (ie, cerebral angiography, myelography, lumbar puncture, pneumoencephalography, arthroscopy).

Evaluation

- Determine if the test was correctly performed according to the procedure. Notify the laboratory and physician of any changes that occur during the test.
- Check the patient's vital signs for changes.
- Monitor changes in muscle strength, ambulation, and speech. Report changes and abnormal findings to the physician.

- Clarify or answer any additional questions the patient or family member might have.
- Encourage patients to use resources available (eg, National Muscular Dystrophy Society).
- Reinforce the importance of seeking health care assistance whenever changes in health status occur.

ENDOCRINE FUNCTION

LABORATORY TESTS	DIAGNOSTIC TESTS

Thyroid

T_4 (Serum)
T_3 (Serum)
T_3 Resin Uptake
Free T_4 Index
Calcitonin (Serum)
TA (Serum)
TSH (Serum)
Provocative Tests
   TSH Stimulation Test
   Thyroid Suppression Test
   TRH Stimulation Test

RAIU Test
Thyroid Scan
Ultrasonography of Thyroid

Parathyroid

Electrolytes (Ca, P) (Serum)
PTH (Serum)
cAMP (Urine)
Prednisone Suppression Test

Ultrasonography of Parathyroid

Adrenal

Electrolytes (K, NA, Ca) (Serum)
Cortisol (Plasma)
Cortisol (Urine)
ACTH (Plasma)
Aldosterone (Serum)
Aldosterone (Urine)
17-OCHS (Urine)
17-KS (Urine)
17-KGS (Urine)
Pregnanetriol (Urine)
VMA (Urine)
Provocative Tests
   ACTH Stimulation Test
   ACTH Suppression Test
   Dexamethasone Suppression Test
   Metyrapone Suppression Test
   Aldosterone Stimulation Test
   Aldosterone Suppression Test

X-ray of Sella Turcica
Adrenal Arteriography
Adrenal Venography
Ultrasonography of Adrenal
CT Scan

(continued)

467

LABORATORY TESTS	DIAGNOSTIC TESTS

Pancreas (Beta Cell)
Electrolytes (K, Na) (Serum)
BUN (Serum)
Creatinine (Serum)
Acetone/Ketone Bodies (Serum, Plasma, Urine)
Chemstrip bG and Destrostix
Glucose: FBS and PPBS (Blood)
Glucose Tolerance Test
Insulin (Serum)
Tolbutamide Tolerance Test

Introduction

Usually there is a battery of laboratory and diagnostic tests ordered for suspected endocrine disorders of the thyroid, parathyroid, adrenal, and pancreas (beta cell) glands. Laboratory tests include serum, plasma, blood, urine, and provocative tests. Provocative tests assess glandular function by stimulating or suppressing secretions. Diagnostic tests are ordered to confirm suspected glandular disorders.

Thyroid Assessment

Laboratory Tests

Thyroxine (T_4) (Serum): Norms: Adult: T_4 (RIA); 5–12 μg/dL; T_4 by column: 4.5–11.5 μg/dL; free T_4: 1.0–2.3 ng/dL. Child: 1–6 Years: T_4: 5.5–13.5 μg/dL; 6–10 years: T_4: 5–12.5 μg/dL.

T_4 a major hormone secreted by the thyroid gland, is an effective indicator of thyroid function. Elevated serum T_4 levels are found in patients with hyperthyroidism, acute thyroiditis, thyrotoxicosis. Decreased levels are found in patients with hypothyroidism. Most thyroxine is bound to thyroxin-binding globulin (TBG).

Triiodothyronine (T_3) (Serum): Norms: Adult: 80–200 ng/dL. Child: 6–12 years: 115–190 ng/dL

T_3, a hormone of the thyroid, is more potent, shorter acting, and of less quantity than T_4. It is helpful in diagnosing thyrotoxicosis, especially when serum T_4 is in normal range. In hypothyroidism, serum T_3 levels may be within normal range; therefore T_4 would be more reliable.

T_3 Resin Uptake: Norms: 25%–35%.

This test indirectly measures free T_4 levels by determining protein-binding sites present for T_4. T_3 resin uptake and serum T_4 (RIA) give free T_4 index. In hyperthyroidism there is a high T_3 resin uptake and the percentage is increased; in hypothyroidism, there is a low T_3 resin uptake and the percentage is decreased.

Free T_4 Index: Norms: Adult: 0.9–2.2 ng/dL

Free T_4 index is unaffected by TBG and correlates more with the true hormonal status. It is difficult to measure T_4 directly, so T_3 resin uptake and serum T_4 give the free thyroxine index.

Calcitonin, Thyrocalcitonin (Plasma): *Norms:* Basal: Adult: Male: <40 pg/mL; Female: <20 pg/mL

Calcitonin is a hormone secreted by the C cells of the thyroid gland. Calcitonin lowers calcium levels. Elevated plasma calcitonin levels could indicate medullary carcinoma of the thyroid.

Thyroid Antibodies, Thyroglobulin Antibodies (TA) (Serum): *Norms:* Adult: negative to 1:20,0–50 ng/mL (RIA). Child: same as adult

A high titer of thyroglobulin antibodies is indicative of thyroid autoimmune disease. In Hashimoto's thyroiditis, the titer is high, 1:5000. Titer can also be elevated in carcinoma of the thyroid and thyrotoxicosis.

Thyroid-Stimulating Hormone (TSH) (Serum): *Norms:* Adult: 2–5.4 μIU/mL, <10 μU/mL (RIA), <3 ng/mL

TSH is secreted from the anterior pituitary gland in response to thyroid-releasing hormone (TRH) from the hypothalamus. Secretion of TSH is dependent on negative feedback system that promotes the release of TRH when the level of T_4 is decreased; this in turn stimulates TSH secretion. An elevated TSH level and a decreased T_4 indicate hypothyroidism.

Thyroid Provocative Tests: These tests are useful for evaluating thyroid function.

TSH Stimulation Test, Thyroid Stimulation Test: This test is useful in distinguishing between *primary,* or thyroidal, hypothyroidism and *secondary,* or hypothalamic-pituitary, hypothyroidism. After an injection of TSH, radioactive iodine uptake (RAIU), serum TSH, and/or serum T_4 are measured. In primary hypothyroidism, the RAIU will remain about the same, TRH and TSH will be increased, and T_4 will show no response. In secondary hypothyroidism, the RAIU will increase about 10%, TRH and TSH will not be increased, and T_4 will rise >1.5 μg/dL.

Thyroid Suppression Test: *Norms:* Adult: 25% decrease in RAIU; T_4 <50% of base line

This test is useful to confirm borderline hyperthyroidism. Base-line RAIU and T_3 or T_4 levels are first obtained. The patient is given T_4 or T_3 for 7 days. Normally TSH production should be depressed, thus decreasing RAIU and T_4. In hyperthyroidism, the RAIU and T_4 will *not* be decreased.

Thyrotropin-Releasing Hormone (TRH) Stimulation Test: The purpose for the TRH stimulation test is to differentiate between hypothalamic and pituitary insufficiency in patients with hypothyroidism with low serum TSH levels. This test can be used to confirm equivocal thyrotoxicosis, since free thyroid hormone suppresses pituitary production of TSH. A base-line value for serum TSH is obtained. TRH is injected intravenously, followed by serum TSH measurements. A serum TSH increase is indicative of hypothalamic disorder, however, no response in serum TSH is indicative of pituitary disorder. Decreased TRH and TSH levels occur when aspirin and steroids are being taken.

Diagnostic Tests

Radioactive Iodine Uptake Test (RAIU): *Norms:* Adult: 2 hours: 1%–13%; 6 hours: 2%–25%; 24 hours: 15%–45%.

The RAIU test is primarily used in detecting hyperthyroidism. I-131 or I-123 is given orally or I-125 is given intravenously. The patient's thyroid gland is scanned at three different times to determine the concentration of radioactive iodine uptake in the thyroid gland. An elevated RAIU indicates hyperthyroidism or Graves' disease. A low RAIU could mean hypothyroidism; however, if T_3 and T_4 are elevated, then it could be caused by thyrotoxicosis or chronic thyroiditis.

Thyroid Scan: The purpose for thyroid scanning is to determine size, structure, and position of thyroid gland, to detect thyroid masses (eg, tumors), and to evaluate thyroid function. Thyroid nodules are easily detected; cold spots could indicate hypofunction and thyroid tumor, and hot spots could indicate hyperfunction (ie, Graves' disease, thyrotoxicosis).

Ultrasonography of Thyroid, Thyroid Echogram, Thyroid Sonography: Ultrasound of the thyroid gland is helpful in distinguishing between solid and cystic nodules. It is a noninvasive procedure and considered safe for pregnant women.

Parathyroid Assessment

Laboratory Tests

Electrolytes: Calcium and Phosphorus (Serum): *Norms:*

PERSON	CALCIUM	PHOSPHORUS
Adult	4.5–5.5 mEq/L	1.7–2.6 mEq/L
	9–11 mg/dL	2.5–4.5 mg/dL
Child	9–12 mg/dL	2.5–6.0 mg/dL
		7.0 mg/dL during bone growth

Parathyroid hormone (PTH) promotes calcium absorption from the GI tract and promotes a release of calcium from bone when there is a deficit. Hypocalcemia could be attributed to hypoparathyroidism and hypercalcemia to hyperparathyroidism. If the patient is in renal failure, the serum calcium level is usually low, and the serum phosphorus (phosphate) is elevated. Secondary hyperparathyroidism can occur because of low calcium levels stimulating the secretion of PTH. Decreased serum phosphorus level (hypophosphatemia) is associated with hyperparathyroidism and hypercalcemia. An elevated phosphorus level (hyperphosphatemia) is associated with hypoparathyroidism, hypocalcemia, and renal failure.

Parathyroid Hormone (PTH) (Serum): *Norms;* Adult: 400–900 pg/mL
PTH is released according to serum calcium levels. Decreased circulating calcium stimulates PTH release, and elevated or normal circulating calcium inhibits PTH release. PTH levels might be elevated as the result of parathyroid hyperplasia or tumor. Decreased PTH level could be due to parathyroid trauma or postparathyroidectomy.

Cyclic Adenosine Monophosphate (Cyclic AMP, cAMP) (Urine): PTH promotes production of cAMP in the kidneys. After an IV infusion of PTH, urine cAMP is measured. In primary hyperparathyroidism, cAMP excretion is increased. Poor renal function can decrease cAMP excretion; thus this test may not be the most accurate one for evaluating parathyroid function.

Prednisone/Cortisone Suppression Test: The purpose of this test is to determine the cause of hypercalcemia. Oral prednisone or cortisone is administered daily for 10 to 14 days. If the serum calcium level is lowered in patients with hypercalcemia, then the cause of elevated calcium level is not hyperparathyroidism but might be bone metastasis, sarcoidosis, or excess vitamin D. In hyperparathyroidism, prednisone or cortisone will not lower calcium levels.

Diagnostic Tests

Ultrasonography of the Parathyroid Gland: In ultrasound of the parathyroid gland the echo pattern is of less amplitude than that of thyroid tissue. Enlargement of the gland(s) might be caused by hyperplasia or tumor growth.

Adrenal Assessment

Laboratory Tests

Electrolytes (Potassium, Sodium, Calcium) (Serum): Norms: Adult: Potassium: 3.5–5.0 mEq/L; Sodium: 135–145 mEq/L; Calcium: 4.5–5.5 mEq/L, 9–11 mg/dL

Steroids (eg, cortisone, secreted from the adrenal gland) promote sodium retention and potassium excretion. Adrenal hyperfunction causes an elevated serum sodium level (hypernatremia), a decreased serum potassium level (hypokalemia), and a decreased serum calcium level (hypocalcemia). Adrenal insufficiency causes hyponatremia and hyperkalemia.

Cortisol (Plasma): Norms: Adult: 8 AM–10 AM: 5–23 μg/dL, 138–635 nmol/L (SI units); 4 PM–6 PM: 3–13 μg/dL, 83–359 nmol/L (SI units)

Cortisol is a potent glucocorticoid released from the adrenal gland. Cortisol levels are higher in the morning than in the afternoon. The diurnal variation ceases in early adrenal hyperfunction. In Addison's disease, the plasma cortisol levels are decreased.

Cortisol (Urine): Norms: Adult: 24–108 μg/24 h

Urine cortisol levels usually reflect the secretion of cortisol. With an elevated plasma cortisol level, excess free cortisol enters the urine, increasing urine cortisol level. Elevated plasma and urine cortisol are significant of adrenal hyperfunction.

Adrenocorticotropic Hormone (ACTH) (Plasma): Norms: Adult: 8 AM: 20–80 pg/mL. 4 PM: 10–40 pg/mL

This test is used to determine the cause of Cushing's syndrome or Addison's disease; however, ACTH stimulation and suppression tests are usually needed to confirm the diagnosis of adrenal disorders. Elevated ACTH could be due to pituitary tumors or nonpituitary ACTH-producing tumor (ie, of the pancreas, lung, ovary), or it could be due to primary adrenal insufficiency in those with Addison's disease. A decreased ACTH level in Addison's disease could indicate hypofunction of the pituitary gland.

Aldosterone (Serum): Norms: Adult with normal salt intake: 1–9 ng/dL (supine), 4–30 ng/dL (sitting)

Aldosterone, a potent mineralocorticoid, promotes sodium reabsorption from the kidneys and potassium excretion. Thus this hormone affects electrolyte balance, especially sodium and potassium. A 24-hour urine aldosterone level is more reliable than the serum aldosterone test. A decreased serum aldosterone level is indicative of adrenal hypofunction and an elevated level is indicative of adrenal hyperfunction. Serum aldosterone may be checked with serum renin; an elevated aldosterone and a decreased serum renin is usually due to primary hyperaldosteronism. If both serum aldosterone and serum renin are elevated, secondary hyperaldosteronism is suspected.

Aldosterone (Urine): Norms: Adult: 6–25 μg/24 h

The 24-hour urine aldosterone test eliminates diurnal variation that occurs with serum aldosterone. Decreased urine aldosterone levels can indicate adrenal hypofunction and elevated levels can indicate primary or secondary hyperaldosteronism, stress, or adrenal hyperfunction.

17-Hydroxycorticosteroids (17-OHCS) (Urine): Norms: Adult: Male: 5–15 mg/24 h; Female: 3–13 mg/24 h. Child: lower than adults

The 17-OHCS are a group of steroids, cortisone and hydrocortisone, excreted in the urine. Urine 17-OHCS and serum cortisol frequently are the tests of choice for assessing adrenal function. Elevated urine 17-OHCS level is indicative of adrenal hyperfunction (eg, Cushing's syndrome), and a decreased urine 17-OHCS is indicative of adrenal hypofunction (eg, Addison's disease).

17-Ketosteroids (17-KS) (Urine): Norms: Adult: Male: 5–25 mg/24 h; Female: 5–15 mg/24 h. Adolescent: 3–14 mg/24 h. *For other reference values, see Part I.*

The 17-KS are metabolites of male hormones secreted from the adrenal cortex and testes. Urine 17-KS levels are higher in male than female. An elevated urine 17-KS could indicate adrenal cortical hyperfunction (eg, hyperplasia, Cushing's syndrome, adrenal tumors), and a decreased urine 17-KS could indicate adrenal cortical hypofunction (eg, Addison's disease).

17-Ketogenic Steroids (17-KGS) (Urine): Norms: Adult: Male: 4–22 mg/24h; Female: 2–15 mg/24 h. Adolescent: 2–9 mg/24

The 17-KGS are a group of steroids that are used to assess adrenal cortical function. An elevated urine 17-KGS level occurs in adrenal hyperfunction and a decreased level occurs in adrenal hypofunction.

Pregnanetriol (Urine): Norms: Adult: Male: 0.4–2.4 mg/24 h; Female: 0.5–2.0 mg/24. Child: 0–1.0 mg/24 h

Pregnanetriol comes from adrenal corticoid synthesis. Elevated level is indicative of adrenal cortical hyperfunction (ie, congenital hyperplasia, adrenal gland tumor).

Vanillylmandelic Acid (VMA) (Urine): Norms: Adult: 1.5–7.5 mg/24 h, 7.6–37.9 μmol/24 (SI units)

VMA is a byproduct of catecholamines (epinephrine and norepinephrine). Elevated urine VMA levels might indicate adrenal medulla tumor. Certain foods and drugs can give false positive test results.

Adrenal Provocative Tests: These tests help evaluate adrenal function.

ACTH Stimulation Test: With the administration of ACTH, the plasma cortisol level should double in 1 hour. If the plasma cortisol level remains the same or is lower, adrenal gland insufficiency or Addison's disease is the cause.

ACTH Suppression Test: When a synthetic, potent cortisol, dexamethasone (Decadron), is given, the ACTH production should be suppressed. If an extremely high dose is needed for ACTH suppression, the cause is of pituitary origin, such as pituitary tumor.

Dexamethasone Suppression Test: Norms: Adult: plasma cortisol: 8 AM, <10 μg/dL; 4 PM, <5 μg/dL

This is an overnight screening test to evaluate the pituitary feedback system and to determine the presence of adrenal hyperfunction (eg, Cushing's syndrome). Dexamethasone (Decadron), a potent adrenal steroid, is given at 12 midnight, and plasma cortisol levels are measured at 8 AM and 4 PM (17-OHCS may be measured also).

With Cushing's syndrome, the adrenals will continue to secrete cortisone despite the ACTH suppression by the pituitary gland.

Metyrapone Suppression Test: Norms: Adult: 17-OHCS should be twofold.

This test evaluates the pituitary feedback system and determines the presence of adrenal hyperfunction. Metyrapone is a potent blocker of cortisol production. After administration of metyrapone, cortisol production should decline, and a decreased plasma cortisol should increase the ACTH secretion. If urine 17-OHCS levels are markedly increased, adrenal hyperplasia is suspected. If there is not an increase in urine 17-OHCS, adrenal tumor might be suspected. Adrenocortical insufficiency (eg, Addison's disease) is a complication of this test.

Aldosterone Stimulation Test: Norms: Adult: Plasma aldosterone increases twofold to fourfold. Urine aldosterone increases twofold to threefold.

This provocative test using furosemide (Lasix) differentiates between adrenal disorder and essential hypertension. As body fluids deplete, aldosterone secretion increases and so does renin secretion. Increased plasma and urine aldosterone levels suggest primary aldosteronism and decreased levels suggest hypoaldosteronism.

Aldosterone Suppression Test: Norms: Adult: approximately 50% decrease in secretion or excretion of aldosterone.

IV saline infusion expands extracellular fluid volume, thus decreasing aldosterone secretion. If aldosterone levels are not suppressed, primary hyperaldosteronism is suspected. Deoxycorticosterone (DOCA) may be substituted for saline. After normal saline diet and DOCA injections for 3 to 5 days, the plasma aldosterone level should decrease by approximately 70%.

Diagnostic Tests

X-ray of Sella Turcica: X-raying this site can detect destruction of the sella turcica, which would be suggestive of an ACTH-producing tumor of the pituitary gland. An overproduction of ACTH caused by the pituitary tumor results in secondary adrenal hyperfunction (eg, Cushing's syndrome).

Adrenal Angiography, Arteriography: Radiopaque dye is injected into the adrenal arteries to visualize the adrenal gland and adrenal arterial system. This is an invasive test and should not be performed if patient is allergic to iodine or dye. This test will detect adrenal tumors and hyperplasia. If pheochromocytoma is suspected, beta- and alpha-adrenergic blockers should be given several days before the test to decrease the chance of hypertensive crisis.

Adrenal Venography: This test detects adrenal vein and adrenal disorders. Plasma cortisol levels from both adrenal glands are obtained to determine the involved gland causing Cushing's syndrome (eg, unilateral tumor). If cortisol levels are bilaterally elevated, then adrenal hyperfunction is caused by bilateral adrenal hyperplasia. If pheochromocytoma is suspected, then adrenal venous blood is tested for catecholamines.

Adrenal Ultrasonography, Sonography: Ultrasound is useful in detecting adrenal gland abnormalities (eg, tumors).

Computerized Tomography (CT) of the Adrenal Gland: CT scan determines the size and shape of the adrenal gland. It is useful in detecting adrenal abnormalities (eg, tumors).

Pancreas (Beta Cell) Assessment

Laboratory Tests

Electrolytes (Potassium and Sodium) (Serum): *Norms:* Adult: Potassium: 3.5–5.0 mEq/L; Sodium: 135–145 mEq/L

In diabetic ketoacidosis, serum potassium could be normal or elevated, depending upon the patient state of body fluid balance. If severe dehydration is present because of polyuria and glycosuria, there would be elevated potassium value resulting from hemoconcentration secondary to dehydration.

Serum sodium level could be normal or low, depending on body fluid balance. Frequently sodium is lost with fluid as a result of osmotic diuresis because of increased blood sugar.

Blood Urea Nitrogen (BUN) (Serum): *Norms:* Adult: 5–25 mg/dL

In diabetic ketoacidosis with dehydration, the BUN is slightly to moderately elevated because of hemoconcentration. After hydration, the BUN should return to normal; if not, then renal disorder should be suspected.

Creatinine (Serum): *Norms:* Adult:0.5–1.5 mg/dL, 53–106 μmol/dL (SI units). Child: 0.4–1.2 mg/dL

A serum creatinine level greater than 2.5 mg/dL could be indicative of renal impairment. In diabetic ketoacidosis, BUN and creatinine levels are usually compared. If BUN is elevated and serum creatinine is in normal range or less than 2.5 mg/dL, dehydration is likely to be the problem.

Acetone, Ketone Bodies (Serum, Plasma, Urine): *Norms:* Adult: Serum acetone: 0.3–2.0 mg/dL; serum ketones: 2–4 mg/dL

Ketone bodies, by-products of fat metabolism and fatty acids, are greatly increased during uncontrolled diabetes mellitus and starvation. Urine should also be checked with reagent strips or tablets for ketone bodies. Positive acetone and ketone tests are indicative of ketoacidosis.

Chemstrip bG, Dextrostix (Blood): Dextrostix has been a useful screening test for blood sugar for 20 years. With this method a drop of blood is placed on the Dextrostix, and after 1 minute the strip is compared to a color chart with many ranges (40 mg to 240 mg). It is not as accurate as the Chemstrip bG. The use of Chemstrip bG for hospital and home blood-sugar monitoring is popular and is considered accurate. Follow directions on set.

Glucose: Fasting Blood Sugar (FBS) and 2-Hour Postprandial Blood Sugar (PPBS), or Feasting: FBS: Serum/plasma: 70–100 mg/dL; blood: 60–100 mg/dL. *PPBS:* Serum/plasma: <140 mg/dL/2 h; blood: <120 mg/dL/2 h

Insulin is needed for transportation of glucose into the cells. A decrease in insulin production increases blood glucose level. A decrease glucose level (hypoglycemia) frequently results from too much circulating insulin. An elevated glucose level greater than 200 mg/dL indicates not enough insulin, the condition known as diabetes mellitus.

Glucose Tolerance Test (GTT) (Serum, Blood): GTT is a test to diagnose diabetes mellitus. This test should not be performed if the fasting blood sugar is greater than 200 mg/dL.

Insulin (Serum): Norms: Adult: 10–250 µIU/mL; 5–25 µU/mL

Serum insulin and blood glucose levels are compared to determine the glucose disorder. If the serum insulin level is elevated or the insulin: glucose ratio is greater than 0.3, tumor or hyperplasia of the islet cells of the pancreas should be suspected.

Tolbutamide (Orinase) Tolerance Test: This test determines the insulin and glucose response to the hypoglycemic agent tolbutamide. After IV injection of tolbutamide, the blood glucose level should decrease and remain low for 30 minutes. Blood samples are drawn for base-line value and then 5, 10, 20, 30, 60, and 120 minutes after IV injection. Serum insulin may also be drawn. With a high serum insulin level and severe hypoglycemia resulting, insulinoma should be suspected. A diminished response could mean possible diabetes mellitus, thus, further studies would be necessary.[1,2,9,11,15,18,24]

- ■ Nursing Diagnoses

  - ■ Knowledge deficit related to lack of understanding of laboratory and diagnostic procedures, disease process, and/or outcome
  - ■ Potential for noncompliance to prescribed laboratory and diagnostic tests related to lack of or inadequate explanation and/or anxiety about physical condition
  - ■ Potential alteration in fluid and electrolyte balance related to fluid volume excess and hypokalemia secondary to increased ADH and aldosterone secretion
  - ■ Potential for injury related to allergic reactions to contrast medium (dye) secondary to diagnostic tests (eg, angiography)
  - ■ Potential ineffective coping with disease process and laboratory and diagnostic test procedure
  - ■ Potential disturbance in self-concept related to body changes secondary to hypofunction and hyperfunction of the thyroid gland and adrenal gland
  - ■ Potential alteration in nutrition related to insufficient insulin production and inadequate glucose metabolism secondary to diabetes mellitus

■ Potential alteration in family processes related to exacerbation of glandular dysfunction and hospitalization

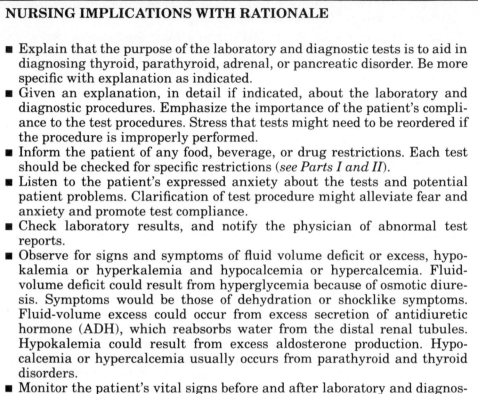

NURSING IMPLICATIONS WITH RATIONALE

■ Explain that the purpose of the laboratory and diagnostic tests is to aid in diagnosing thyroid, parathyroid, adrenal, or pancreatic disorder. Be more specific with explanation as indicated.
■ Given an explanation, in detail if indicated, about the laboratory and diagnostic procedures. Emphasize the importance of the patient's compliance to the test procedures. Stress that tests might need to be reordered if the procedure is improperly performed.
■ Inform the patient of any food, beverage, or drug restrictions. Each test should be checked for specific restrictions (*see Parts I and II*).
■ Listen to the patient's expressed anxiety about the tests and potential patient problems. Clarification of test procedure might alleviate fear and anxiety and promote test compliance.
■ Check laboratory results, and notify the physician of abnormal test reports.
■ Observe for signs and symptoms of fluid volume deficit or excess, hypokalemia or hyperkalemia and hypocalcemia or hypercalcemia. Fluid-volume deficit could result from hyperglycemia because of osmotic diuresis. Symptoms would be those of dehydration or shocklike symptoms. Fluid-volume excess could occur from excess secretion of antidiuretic hormone (ADH), which reabsorbs water from the distal renal tubules. Hypokalemia could result from excess aldosterone production. Hypocalcemia or hypercalcemia usually occurs from parathyroid and thyroid disorders.
■ Monitor the patient's vital signs before and after laboratory and diagnostic tests.
■ Provide support to the patient and family members during and after test procedure.

Evaluation

■ Determine if the test was correctly performed according to procedure. Notify the laboratory and physician of any changes that occur during the test.
■ Check the patient's vital signs and intake and output after the laboratory or diagnostic procedure. Assess for significant changes.
■ Clarify or answer any additional questions the patient and family members might have.
■ Identify resources that would provide information, service, and support to the patient and family at home. Be available to answer questions.
■ Reinforce the importance of health care to maintain wellness. Assist the patient and family with health plans as needed.

REPRODUCTIVE FUNCTION

LABORATORY TESTS	DIAGNOSTIC TESTS

Female Reproductive

Estrogen (Serum and Urine)

Estradiol (E_2) (Serum)

FSH (Serum and Urine)

LH (Serum)

Progesterone (Serum)

Pregnanediol (Urine)

Prolactin (Serum)

DIAGNOSTIC TESTS (Female)

Colposcopy

Laparoscopy

Hysterosalpingography

Cytogenetic Studies
  Sex Chromatin Mass
  Chromosome Analysis

PAP Smear

Cervical Biopsy

Mammography

Thermography

Male Reproductive

Testosterone (Serum)

Semen Examination

17-KS (Urine)

Cytogenetic Studies

Pregnancy

HCG

Home Pregnancy Test Kits

HPL (Serum)

Estriol (E_3) (Serum and Urine)

Progesterone (Serum)

Pregnanediol (Urine)

AFP (Serum and Amniotic Fluid)

Genetic Defect Tests: Down's Syndrome, Sickle Cell Anemia, Neural Tube Defects, Tay-Sachs Disease

Rubella Antibody Detection

Maternal Enzymes (Serum)

Blood Type, Rh Screen

L/S Ratio (Amniotic Fluid)

Nitrazine Paper Test

CK/CPK (Serum)

Renin (Plasma)

Albumin (Serum)

Hormone Changes

Hematologic Changes

RPR (Serum)

HSV 2 (Serum)

Cytogenetic Studies

DIAGNOSTIC TESTS (Pregnancy)

Amniocentesis

Pelvic Ultrasonography

External Fetal Monitoring

Internal Fetal Monitoring

Breast Massage Stress Test

Chorionic Villi Biopsy

Neonate

Glucose (Blood)

Cord Blood: Type and Rh

Bilirubin (Blood)

PKU (Serum and Urine)

TORCH Test

Introduction

The focus on reproductive function in this section is on reproductive processes and products involving male and female. Certain tests in the discussion of the female reproductive function, such as cytogenetic studies, also apply to the male reproductive function and pregnancy. Laboratory tests for reproductive function include serum, plasma, urine, and amniotic fluid. The number of tests in pregnancy has greatly increased in the last 10 to 20 years.

Female Reproductive Assessment

Laboratory Tests

Estrogen (Serum): Norms: Early menstrual cycle: 60–400 pg/mL; Midmenstrual Cycle: 100–600 pg/mL; Late Menstrual Cycle: 150–350 pg/mL; Postmenopausal: <30 pg/mL. Male: 40–115 pg/mL

This test is useful for evaluating gonadal hypofunction in females, timing ovulation, and determining hormonally active tumors. Serum estrogen measures estrone (E_1) and estradiol (E_2), but measures small amounts of estriol (E_3); therefore it is *not* a test used in pregnancy to determine fetal well-being.

Estrogen (Urine): Norms: Female: Preovulation: 5–25 μg/24 h; Follicular: 24–100 μg/24 h, Luteal Phase: 22–80 μg/24 h; Postmenopausal: 0–10 μg/24 h. Male: 4–25 μg/24 h

Urine estrogen test includes estrone (E_1), estradiol (E_2), and estriol (E_3). This 24-hour urine test is useful for diagnosing ovarian disorders, tumors, hypogonadism, hypopituitarism, and adrenal hyperplasia. It is not a test for assessing fetal well-being.

Estradiol (E_2) (Serum): Female Follicular Phase: 20–150 pg/mL; Midcycle: 100–500 pg/mL; Luteal Phase: 60–260 pg/mL. *Male:* 15–20 pg/mL. *Child:* 3–10 pg/mL

E_2 evaluates gonadal dysfunction, such as amenorrhea syndromes and testicular tumors. It is decreased in primary amenorrhea and ovarian failure and is elevated in testicular tumors, ovarian tumors and adrenal tumors.

Follicle-Stimulating Hormone (FSH) (Serum): Norms: Female: Preovulation Postovulation: 4–30 mU/mL; Midcycle: 10–90 mU/mL; Luteal Phase: 4–30 mU/mL; Postmenopausal: 40–250 mU/mL Male: 4–25 mU/mL Child: 5–12 mU/mL.

Serum FSH is useful for diagnosing infertility and menstrual disorders. FSH is responsible for developing ovarian follicles for ovulation. A decreased serum FSH can indicate anovulation, causing infertility or secondary hypogonadotropic state caused by panhypopituitarism or anorexia nervosa. Elevated serum FSH might indicate primary hypogonadism (Turner's syndrome) or precocious puberty. It may be elevated in postmenopausal women.

Follicle-Stimulating Hormone (FSH) (Urine): Norms: Female: Preovulation, Postovulation: 4–25 IU/24 h; Midcycle: 8–60 IU/24 h; Postmenopausal: 50–150 IU/24 h. Male: 4–18 IU/24 h. Child: <10 IU/24 h.

A decreased urine FSH level might indicate neoplasms of the ovary, adrenal gland, or testes or anorexia nervosa. An elevated level could indicate gonadal failure caused by postmenopause, FSH-producing pituitary tumor, or Klinefelter's syndrome.

Luteinizing Hormone (LH) (Serum): Norms: Female, Follicular: 3–30 mIU/mL; Midcycle: 30–100 mIU/mL; Postmenopausal: 40–100 mIU/mL. Male: 5–25 mIU/mL. Child: <10 mIU/mL. LH may determine cause of menstrual disturbances, gonadal failure, and infertility. The FSH test is ordered with LH to check on causes of anovulation and infertility. An elevated LH level might indicate ovarian failure associated with Stein-Leventhal syndrome, which is polycystic ovary syndrome, Turner's syndrome (ovarian dysgenesis), or postmenopause.

Progesterone (Serum): Norms: Preovulation: 20–150 ng/dL, 0.1–1.5 ng/mL; Midcycle: 250–2800 ng/dL, 2–28 ng/mL

Purposes of this test are to determine ovulation, to evaluate infertility problems, and to assess placental function. Serum progesterone levels are elevated at time of ovulation, including 5 days postovulation, in early pregnancy, and in adrenal tumors.

Pregnanediol (Urine): Norms: Female: Preovulation: 0.5–1.5 mg/24 h; Midcycle: 2–7 mg/24 h; postmenopausal 0.1–1.0 mg/24 h. Male: 0.1–1.5 mg/24 h. Child: 0.4–1.0 mg/24 h

Pregnanediol is the major metabolite of progesterone. It is produced by the corpus luteum during the latter half of the menstrual cycle and by the placenta. A decreased level could be due to menstrual disorders, ovarian hypofunction, threatened abortion, tumors of the ovary or breast, lutein cell tumors of the ovary, or preeclampsia. Elevated level could be due to pregnancy, ovarian cyst, choriocarcinoma of the ovary, or adrenal hyperplasia.

Prolactin (Serum): Norms: Nonlactating Female: 0–23 ng/dL; Pregnancy: rise of 10- to 20-fold

This test is useful for detecting a suspected pituitary tumor. High prolactin levels, greater than 100 ng/dL, in a nonpregnant female could indicate pituitary adenoma. Hyperprolactinemia may be due to hypothyroidism, acromegaly, or hypothalamic disorders or may occur in patients with galactorrhea and amenorrhea.

Diagnostic Tests

Colposcopy: A colposcope is used to examine the vagina and cervix for precancerous lesions. Colposcopy is performed after an abnormal PAP test, to monitor treatment for dysplasia and cervical lesions, and to monitor females with vaginal and/or cervical tissue changes caused by their mothers taking diethylstilbestrol (DES) during pregnancy.

Laparoscopy: A laparoscope, a small fiberoptic telescope, is inserted through the abdominal wall for the purpose of detecting cysts, fibroids, adhesions, pelvic masses, and for diagnosing cause of pelvic pain (ie, endometriosis, pelvic inflammatory disease [PID]). This procedure may be used for tubal sterilization, ovarian biopsy, and removal of foreign bodies. Laparoscopy has decreased the number of surgical laparotomies performed.

Hysterosalpingography: Ultrasonography has nearly replaced hysterosalpingography. However, this test is still useful for evaluating patency of the fallopian tubes. It is one of the infertility studies. The procedure uses contrast medium and fluoroscopic x-ray filming.

Cytogenetic Studies: Cytogenetic studies for analysis are performed on tissue, blood, bone marrow, and amniotic fluid. Sex chromatin and chromosome analysis are the two tests usually ordered when chromosomal abnormalities are suspected.

Sex Chromatin Mass: Sex chromatin mass or Barr chromatin body (clump of chromatin adhered to nuclear membrane in cells) is represented as an inactive X chromosome in females and not in males. With disturbances of gonadal development or function and/or with disturbance in reproductive function, sex chromosome defect (absence or an increased number of inactivated X chromosomes or Barr chromatin bodies) may be suspected. The purpose of the test is to screen for sex chromosome anomalies such as the following:

- Turner's syndrome: ie, females with poorly developed sex characteristics (amenorrhea, undeveloped breast, sterility) due to XO (no Barr body) or XX/XO mosaics (some with Barr body and some without)
- Klinefelter's syndrome: ie, males with poorly developed sex characteristics (small penis, testes, sterility) due to presence of chromatin body of the Y chromosome with XXY (mostly), XXXY, or XXYY variants

Buccal mucosa is obtained for sex chromosome study. If results are abnormal, chromosome analysis (karyotype) is indicated.

Chromosome Analysis: Blood, tissue, bone marrow, and amniotic fluid are used to identify chromosomal abnormalities (eg, Down's syndrome, congenital anomaly, genetic disorders, and proliferative diseases such as leukemias).

Papanicolaou Smear (PAP): This is a cytologic test to detect precancerous or cancerous cells of the cervix; it is also used to detect some infectious diseases, such as monilia. A positive PAP smear needs further diagnostic test (ie, colposcopy or cervical biopsy) to confirm the PAP result. PAP smears are generally performed during a pelvic examination and during the first prenatal visit if not done previously.

Cervical Biopsy: A cervical biopsy may be indicated for suspicious cervical lesions.

Mammography, Mammogram: This procedure is an x-ray examination of the breast to detect cysts or tumors. Usually it can detect breast lesion(s) 2 years before the lesion is palpable.

Thermography: An infrared photographic test records heat energy from the skin surface of the breast. Increased breast surface temperature may be caused by increased vascularity resulting from a cancerous lesion.

Male Reproductive Assessment

Laboratory Tests

Testosterone (Serum): Norms: Adult: Male: 0.3–1.0 μg/dL, 300–1000 ng/dL. Child: Male (12–14 years): >0.1 μg/dL, >100 ng/dL, Female: 0.03–0.1 μg/dL, 30–100 ng/dL

Testosterone, a male sex hormone, is mostly responsible for male sex characteristics and masculinity. The highest serum testosterone level occurs in the morning.

Decreased level could indicate a testicular disorder, Klinefelter's syndrome alcoholism, estrogen therapy, or hypopituitarism. An elevated level could indicate adrenal hyperplasia or tumor, benign prostatic hypertrophy (BPH), or adrenogenital syndrome in women.

Semen Examination: Semen content is useful for determining sperm count, volume of fluid, percentage of mature spermatozoa (sperms), and percentage of actively mobile sperm cells. This test is ordered to help identify the cause of infertility or to determine the effectiveness of sterilization after a vasectomy.

17-Ketosteroids (17-KS) (Urine): Norms: Adult: Male: 8–25 mg/24 h; over 65 years old: 4–8 mg/24 h; Female: 5–15 mg/24 h. Adolescent: Male; 3–15 mg/24 h

17-KS are metabolites of male hormones from the adrenal cortex and testes. This test is useful in diagnosing adrenal cortex dysfunction and determining pituitary and gonadal hormone function. A decreased level could be indicative of hypogonadism and hypopituitarism. An elevated level could be indicative of adrenocortical hyperplasia or tumor, testicular tumor, hirsutism, or hyperpituitarism.

Cytogenetic Studies: See female Reproductive function.

Pregnancy Assessment

Laboratory Tests

Human Chorionic Gonadotropin (HCG) (Serum and Urine): HCG, glycoprotein hormone, is produced by the trophoblast cell of placental tissue. Serum and urine HCG are early tests for confirming pregnancy. HCG tests are positive in pregnant women only and *not* in nonpregnant women. HCG is present 10 days after egg implantation or 14 to 26 days after conception. It peaks within 8 to 12 weeks.

Home Pregnancy Test Kits: Pregnancy kits were first introduced in 1976, and today there are several commercially prepared kits available for home use (ie, Gravindex [Ortho Diagnostics], Prognosis [Roche], Early Pregnancy Test [EPT; Warner/Chicott], Daisy 2 [Bio Dynamics Home Healthcare] and First Response [Tambrands]). Some tests can be used to detect pregnancy as soon as the day of the first missed menstrual period. False readings can occur. If tests results are negative and menses has not begun a week later, it is suggested that the home pregnancy test be repeated.

Human Placental Lactogen (HPL) (Serum): Norms:

WEEKS OF GESTATION	µg/mL
8–27	<4.6
28–31	2.4–6.0
32–35	3.7–7.7
36–40	5.0–10.0

HPL is produced by the placenta throughout pregnancy. The test is valuable to determine fetal well-being but should not be used as the only test. If HPL value falls below 4 μg/mL after 30 weeks, fetal distress might be present because of impaired placental function. If HPL value falls 50% during late pregnancy, fetal distress is apparent.

Estriol (E_3) (Serum and Urine): Norms:

SERUM		URINE	
Weeks of Gestation	**ng/dL**	**Weeks of Gestation**	**mg/24 Hours**
		16–24	2–6
25–28	25–165	25–28	6–28
29–32	30–230	29–32	6–32
33–36	45–370	33–36	10–45
37–38	75–420	37–40	15–60
39–40	95–450		

E_3 is a major estrogenic compound produced largely by the placenta. It increases in maternal serum and urine after 2 months of pregnancy and continues at high levels until term. If toxemia, hypertension, or diabetes is present after 30 weeks of gestation, E_3 levels are monitored. A decline in serum or urine E_3 levels suggest fetal distress caused by placental malfunction. The test may be repeated to confirm a suspected situation. A cesarean section may be indicated.

Progesterone (Serum): Norms: Pregnancy: >2400 ng/dL

Progesterone is responsible for maintaining pregnancy after fertilization and for placental development. It has little value in evaluating fetal well-being but is useful in assessing placental function during pregnancy.

Pregnanediol (Urine): Norms: Pregnancy: 10–19 gestation weeks: 5–25 mg/24 h; 20–28 gestation weeks: 15–42 mg/24 h; 29–32 gestation weeks: 25–49 mg/24 h

Pregnanediol measures the urinary metabolite of progesterone. At times urine pregnanediol may be of normal range even when fetal distress or fetal death has occurred.

α-1-Fetoprotein (AFP): Norms:

SERUM		AMNIOTIC FLUID	
Weeks of Gestation	**ng/mL**	**Weeks of Gestation**	**μg/mL**
8–12	0–39	14	11.0–32.0
13	6–31	15	5.5–31.0
14	7–50	16	5.7–31.5
15	7–60	17	3.8–32.5
16	10–72	18	3.6–28.0
17	11–90	19	3.7–24.5
18	14–94	20	2.2–15.0
19	24–112	21	3.6–18.0
20	31–122		
21	19–124		

Usually serum AFP is done between 16 and 20 weeks of gestation to detect probability of twins, risk of premature delivery or an infant of low birth weight, or serious birth defects such as open neural tube defect. It is a screening test, and if abnormal results occur, it should be repeated. If a high serum AFP level occurs, amniotic AFP may be done to diagnose neural tube defect in the fetus. Amniocentesis and ultrasound are required to confirm or to rule out the possible condition.

Genetic Defect Tests: Specific laboratory tests are designed to determine genetic disorders. Table 13 shows the defect, specimen, person from which specimen was obtained, and findings.

Rubella Antibody Detection (Serum): Norms: titer >1:64 protection against rubella or German measles

The rubella antibody detection test is done prior to pregnancy or to check pregnant women during their first trimester of pregnancy at time of rubella exposure and again in 3 to 4 weeks.

Maternal Enzymes (Serum): During pregnancy there is an increase in maternal serum enzymes (ie, heat-stable alkaline phosphatase [HSAP], diamine oxidase (DAO), and oxytocinase). Table 14 describes the maternal enzyme and their uses.

Blood Type and Rh Screening: Adult: Rh+ (positive); Rh− (negative)

The Rh-negative pregnant female who carried a fetus that was Rh positive should receive Rho (D) immune globulin or RhoGAM by 72 hours after delivery or abortion to prevent Rh sensitization or Rh antibodies. This is important for prevention of erythroblastosis in future fetus. If the mother is Rh negative and unsensitized, some suggest that Rh immune globulin should be given at 28 weeks gestation.

Maternal blood type should be checked. If mother's type is O positive and

TABLE 13. TESTS FOR GENETIC DEFECTS

Defect	Specimen	Person	Findings
Down's Syndrome	Amniotic fluid	Pregnant female	Trisomy 21 chromosome
Neural tube defects	Serum Amniotic fluid	Pregnant female	Increased serum AFP Increased amniotic AFP
Tay-Sachs disease	Blood	Mother and father (as carriers)	Low level of enzyme hexosaminidase A
	Amniotic fluid	Pregnant female	
Sickle cell anemia	Blood	Mother and father (as carriers)	Hemoglobin S cells
	Cord blood	Newborn	
Galactosemia	Amniotic fluid	Pregnant female	Presence of galactose
Thalassemia (Cooley's or Mediterranean anemia)	Blood	Mother and father (as carriers)	Hemoglobin F cells
	Cord blood	Newborn	
Phenylketonuria (PKU)	Blood	Mother and father (as carriers)	Increased serum phenylalanine

TABLE 14. MATERNAL ENZYMES

Maternal Enzyme	Comments
Heat-stable alkaline phosphatase (HSAP)	HSAP rises in concentration throughout pregnancy. A sudden rise in later pregnancy could indicate placental dysfunction and fetal distress or death. Usually a rise in HSAP occurs before a decrease in E_3.
Diamine oxidase (DAO)	This enzyme protects the pregnant female against histamine produced by the fetus. It rises during early pregnancy but tends to plateau during the third trimester.
Oxytocinase (cystyl-aminopeptidase)	Oxytocinase is produced by the placenta during pregnancy and inactivates oxytocin. It indicates placental function, not fetal well-being.

the baby's type is A or B, there may be potential for ABO incompatibility after delivery.

Lecithin/Sphingomyelin (L/S) Ratio (Amniotic Fluid): Norms: Before 35 weeks of gestation: 1:1; after 35 weeks of gestation 4:1. (L: 15–21 mg/dL; S: 4–6 mg/dL)

L/S ratio is a predictor of fetal pulmonary maturity before delivery. Lecithin is primarily responsible for the formation of alveolar surfactant that lubricates the alveolar lining and inhibits alveoli collapse. A marked rise in amniotic lecithin after 35 weeks is normal, thus decreasing chances for having hyaline membrane in respiratory distress syndrome. Pulmonary maturity occurs earlier in blacks than in caucasians.

Nitrazine Test: Norms: Intact Membranes: pH 5–6 (yellow to olive green). Ruptured Membranes: pH 6.5–7.5 (blue-green to deep blue)

This is a paper test to determine if the amniotic membrane is intact or has ruptured. The pH of amniotic fluid is 7 to 7.5, whereas the pH of vaginal secretions is 4.5 to 5.5.

Creatine Phosphokinase (CPK/CK) (Serum): Norms: Female 5–25 µg/mL; 10–80 IU/L.

Decreased CPK/CK level might occur during the second trimester of pregnancy.

Renin (Plasma): Norms: Upright: 1.3–4.0 ng/mL/h

An elevated plasma renin level might occur during the first trimester of pregnancy, preeclampsia, and eclampsia. This could be due to a kidney problem.

Albumin (Serum): Norms: 3.5–5 g/dL

Albumin levels may decrease by 0.5 to 1.0 g/dL. This could be due to increased plasma volume or acceleration of albumin degradation.

Hormone Changes: Thyroid, parathyroid, and adrenal hormone alterations usually accompany pregnancy. Table 15 shows the increases and decreases of these hormones during pregnancy.

Hematologic Changes: Hematologic values should be monitored during pregnancy. Changes in laboratory values are expected. Table 16 shows the expected changes of hematologic tests.

TABLE 15. HORMONAL CHANGES DURING PREGNANCY

Hormone	Changes	Comments
TBG	Increased markedly	Rise begins after fertilization and continues until 12 weeks of gestation. Failure of TBG rise might indicate hypothyroidism or estrogen deficiency.
T_4	Increased	T_4 rise is not as great as that of TBG.
Resin T_3 uptake	Decreased	T_3 uptake decreases slightly during pregnancy.
TSH	Normal	TSH remains normal in the euthyroid pregnant female.
ACTH	Decreased	Markedly decreased during first trimester of pregnancy.
Cortisol	Increased	Cortisol production slightly declines during pregnancy; however, the plasma half-life is increased. If cortisol value is in the normal range, adrenal hypofunction might be suspected.
Aldosterone	Increased	Aldosterone is increased throughout pregnancy which increases plasma volume and sodium retention.
PTH	Increased	Reason unknown

Rapid Plasma Reagin (RPR) (Serum): Norms: nonreactive
The RPR test is a rapid screening test for syphilis. A positive RPR should be verified by VDRL and/or FTA-ABS tests.

Herpes Simplex Virus (Type 2) (HSV 2) (Serum): HSV 2 is sexually transmitted and infects the urogenital tract. It also can be transmitted to the newborn during vaginal delivery. Neonatal herpes can result in minor to severe complications (eg, from skin rash or eye infection to central nervous disorder). If the mother has active HSV 2 at the time of birth, a cesarian delivery may be indicated.

Cytogenetic Studies: See Female Reproductive Assessment.

Diagnostic Tests

Amniocentesis, Amniotic Fluid Analysis: The purposes for analysis of amniotic fluid are to detect chromosomal abnormalities such as Down's syndrome (trisomy 21), neural tube defects, sex-linked disorders, and fetal and pulmonary maturity. *See Female Reproductive Assessment above and Amniotic Fluid Analysis (Part II).*

Pelvic Ultrasonography: The numerous uses for pelvic ultrasound are to detect multiple fetuses or fetal anomalies; to determine the location of the placenta (rule out placenta previa) or fetal and placenta locations during an amniocentesis; and to evaluate fetal viability, gestational age, and fetal growth. This test procedure is considered noninvasive because contrast media is *not* used.

TABLE 16. HEMATOLOGIC CHANGES DURING PREGNANCY

Blood Tests	Changes	Comments
Red blood cells (RBCs)	Increased	RBC mass increases slightly during pregnancy even with increased plasma volume.
Hemoglobin and hematocrit	Decreased	Plasma volume increase causes hemodilution.
Platelets	Slightly decreased or normal value	Decreased platelet count could result from increased plasma volume.
Reticulocytes	Increased	There is a slight rise in reticulocytes during the second trimester of pregnancy.
White blood cells (WBCs)	Increased	Slightly elevated WBCs. During the last half of pregnancy, granulocytes increase and lymphocytes remain unchanged.
Fibrinogen	Increased	Fibrinogen level increases throughout pregnancy.
Plasminogen	Increased	Reason unknown
Prothrombin time (PT) and partial thromboplastin time (PTT)	Slightly decreased or normal	Reason unknown
Erythrocyte sedimentation rate (ESR)	Increased	ESR increases markedly because of increase in fibrinogen level.
Folate (folic acid)	Decreased	Mother's tissues absorb more folic acid.
Vitamin B_{12}	Decreased	Mother's tissues absorb more vitamin B_{12}.
Iron	Decreased	Fetal use and increased plasma volume (hemodilution).

External Fetal Monitoring: External fetal monitoring records the fetal heart rate and uterine contractions. It is considered a noninvasive test. It can be used as a nonstress test to determine fetal well-being during stressful and nonstressful conditions. Also it can be used as a stress test using oxytocin to determine fetal well-being.

Internal Fetal Monitoring: This is an invasive procedure in which an electrode is attached to the scalp of the fetus to measure fetal heart rate and a catheter is placed in the uterine cavity to measure uterine contractions. Internal fetal monitoring is performed during labor after the membranes have ruptured. It is indicated when external fetal monitoring provides inadequate information.

Breast Massage Stress Test: Breast massage is a relative new contraction stress test (CST) for assessing fetal well-being in high-risk pregnancies. If a nonstress test is *not* effective in determining fetal well-being, then a CST is indicated. CST can be done using the standard stress test with IV infusion of oxytocin or breast massage.

Neonate Assessment

Laboratory Tests

Glucose (Blood): *Norms:* >40 mg/dL

Neonatal hypoglycemia may occur 4 to 6 hours after birth. Chemstrip bG or Dextrostix are useful for monitoring blood glucose in the newborn. Blood sugar falls rapidly during the first few hours of life but stabilizes in 6 hours in the healthy newborn. Newborns who are at high risk (eg, born of diabetic mothers, erythroblastotic newborns or pregnant women taking terbutaline) should have blood glucose monitored closely. In some institutions Chemstrip bG is used as a routine screening test for all newborns.

Cord Blood: At the time of birth a blood sample from the umbilical cord is tested for blood type and Rh (factor) antibody titer.

Bilirubin: Neonatal (Blood): *Norms:* <12 mg/dL. *Critical Range:* 15 mg/dL

Blood is drawn from the newborn's heel by means of a capillary pipette.

Neonatal jaundice could be due to erythroblastosis fetalis, hemorrhage, or physiologic jaundice (caused by increased RBC breakdown and immature liver cells). Repeated heel stick may be needed to monitor bilirubin levels in the newborn.

Phenylketonuria (PKU) (Urine) or Phenylalanine (Blood): *Norms:* 1–3 mg/dL (blood). *Critical Range:* >4 mg/dL

Blood phenylalanine is checked 48 to 120 hours after birth following milk or protein feedings. A positive test indicates that the newborn lacks the enzyme needed to metabolize phenylalanine, an amino acid found in protein foods.

PKU testing of the urine is checked between 2 to 4 weeks of life. Phenistix (Ames) is a dipstick for testing the infant's urine for PKU. Green color is an indicator of a positive PKU test.

TORCH Test (TORCH Screen, TORCH Battery, TORCH Titer): TORCH stands for toxoplasma, rubella, cytomegalovirus, and herpes virus. It is used to determine the presence or exposure of a TORCH agent that could cause congenital or neonatal infections, which could result in central nervous system (CNS) impairment. The test identifies past infection, immunity, or recent infection. It can be done on pregnant women as well as newborns and infants. The number of TORCH testings has grown, with more than 20 TORCH kits produced for laboratory and physician's use. Accuracy of test results has been questioned, as there is often a variation in TORCH titers.[1,5,11,15,25–30]

- Nursing Diagnoses

  - Anxiety related to health status and the unknown
  - Knowledge deficit related to lack of understanding of laboratory and diagnostic procedure, disease process, and/or outcome of pregnancy
  - Potential for noncompliance to prescribed laboratory and diagnostic tests related to lack of or inadequate explanation and/or anxiety about physical condition
  - Ineffective coping with laboratory and diagnostic test procedures

- Fluid volume excess related to hormonal changes as evidenced by fluid retention
- Potential alteration in comfort related to procedure as evidenced by back hurting when lying flat for various test procedures
- Urinary elimination, alteration in patterns related to bladder compression by enlarged pregnant uterus
- Anxiety related to the consequences of the tests that could result in alterations in parenting, coping, and self-concept
- Potential alteration in parenting related to lack of effective coping mechanisms
- Potential for sexual dysfunction related to altered body structure or function, including pregnancy, disease process, and/or diagnostic procedure

---

NURSING IMPLICATIONS WITH RATIONALE

- Explain that the purpose for the laboratory and diagnostic tests is to aid in establishing base-line data regarding previous male or female disease, existing disease, predisposition to disease, or complications in pregnancy.
- Give an explanation (in detail if indicated) about the laboratory and diagnostic procedures. Emphasize the importance of the patient's compliance with the test procedure (*see procedures for individual tests in Parts I and II*).
- Assess the patient's communication for verbal and/or nonverbal expressions of anxiety or fear concerning tests and/or potential sexual problems.
- Determine if anxiety level needs to be reduced before the patient will be able to absorb information concerning test procedure.
- Encourage expression of feelings through provision of private, calm environment; use quiet, steady speech patterns when interacting; and employ touch if appropriate.
- Be prepared to repeat information to the patient and family briefly and clearly if anxiety or fear level is determined to be high. Attempt not to appear irritated with the patient's behavior; plan time to be with the patient.
- Answer questions, or refer the questions to appropriate health professionals.
- Check laboratory results, and notify physician of abnormal test findings.

Evaluation

- Determine if the test was correctly performed according to the procedure. Notify the laboratory and/or physician of any changes that occur during the test.
- Check the patient's vital signs and fetal heart rate for changes.
- Provide ongoing assessment before, during and after the procedure. Document and communicate any alteration.
- Determine if support measures to the patient and family have been effective.

- Evaluate the status of the patient's anxiety and fear in regard to the tests, problems related to pregnancy or infertility.
- Clarify or answer any additional questions the patient and family members might have.

ARTHRITIC AND COLLAGEN CONDITIONS

LABORATORY TESTS

Rheumatoid Arthritis	Lupus Erythematosus
RA Factor	Lupus Erythematosus (LE) Cells
ESR/Sed Rate	ANA
CRP	Anti-DNA
Complements C_3, C_4	Complements C_3, C_4
ASO	Cryoglobulins
Cryoglobulins	RA Factor
Synovial Fluid Analysis	Synovial Fluid Analysis

Introduction

The majority of laboratory tests for arthritic and collagen disorders are to confirm the diagnosis or progression of rheumatoid arthritis and lupus erythematosus. Several of the same laboratory tests are ordered for both suspected conditions; these tests are complements C_3, C_4, and rheumatoid arthritis (RA) factor; cryoglobulins; and synovial fluid analysis.

Rheumatoid Arthritis

Laboratory Tests

Rheumatoid Factor (RF), Rheumatoid Arthritis (RA) Factor: Norms: Adult: <1:20 titer, >1:80 positive for rheumatoid arthritis

RA factor is a screening test used to detect antiglobulin antibodies in patients with suspected rheumatoid arthritis. It is not uncommon to have positive RA factor test results in patients with collagen diseases (eg, lupus erythematosus). Approximately 75% of those with rheumatoid arthritis have a positive RA factor. Other tests are needed to confirm diagnosis.

Erythrocyte Sedimentation Rate (ESR, Sed Rate) (Serum): Norms: See reference values in Part I

Sed rate, or ESR, is a nonspecific test that usually increases during an acute inflammatory process. Frequently the ESR is elevated in patients with rheumatoid arthritis: however, it is not the most reliable test. C-reactive protein (CRP) test is considered more useful than ESR.

C-Reactive Protein (CRP) (Serum): Norms: not usually present; >1:2 titer considered positive

CRP is a nonspecific test similar to ESR; however, during an inflammatory process, CRP elevates sooner than ESR and returns to normal faster than ESR. This test is useful in monitoring the progression of rheumatoid arthritis.

Complements C_3 and C_4 (Serum): Norms: C_3: Adult: 83–177 mg/dL C_4: Adult: 15–45 mg/dL

Both C_3 and C_4 could be slightly elevated in patients with rheumatoid arthritis.

Antistreptolysin O (ASO) (Serum): Norms: Adult: <100 IU/mL

Serum ASO levels can be mildly elevated in patients with rheumatoid arthritis.

Cryoglobulins (Serum): Norms: negative

Cryoglobulins are proteins that are present in the immunoglobulins IgG and IgM. They may be present in rheumatoid arthritis and also in systemic lupus erythematosus.

Synovial Fluid Analysis: Examination of the synovial fluid for rheumatoid factor, complements, leukocytes (WBC), and glucose gives additional information about the possibility of the presence of rheumatoid arthritis. In rheumatoid arthritis, synovial fluid analysis could include a positive RA factor, decreased complements because of complement binding, slightly elevated leukocytes, and decreased glucose level.

Lupus Erythematosus

Laboratory Tests

Lupus Erythematosus (LE) Cell Test: LE cell test is an in vitro procedure used either to aid in the diagnosis of systemic lupus erythematosus (SLE) or to monitor the treatment for this condition. It is not the most reliable test; however, LE cells can be found in 60% to 80% of patients with SLE. If it is used for the purpose of diagnosing SLE, then other laboratory tests, such as antinuclear antibodies (ANA) and anti-DNA, should be ordered to confirm SLE.

Antinuclear Antibodies (ANA) (Serum): Norms: negative

The ANA for assessing tissue-antigen antibodies is frequently used for diagnosing SLE. A positive titer can indicate SLE; however, other clinical conditions such as rheumatoid arthritis, scleroderma, myasthenia gravis, and infectious mononucleosis may have positive titers.

Anti-Deoxyribonucleic Acid (Anti-DNA): Anti-DNA, an antinuclear antibody, is almost always present in SLE and is in lupus nephritis 95% of the time. Anti-DNA values may fluctuate according to the remission and exacerbation of the disease.

Complements C_3 and C_4 (Serum): Norms: See complements under Rheumatoid Arthritis

C_3 and C_4 of the complement system (group of 11 serum proteins) are measured during acute and/or chronic inflammatory process. In SLE, both serum C_3 and C_4 will be decreased.

Cryoglobulins (Serum): Norms: negative

Positive cryoglobulin findings may be reported in patients with SLE.

Cryoglobulins are also present in other conditions, such as rheumatoid arthritis, multiple myeloma, and leukemia.

Rheumatoid Factor (RF, RA Factor) (Serum): Norms: 1:20–1:80 positive for collagen diseases

Even though RA factor is a serum test used to detect antibodies in patients with rheumatoid arthritis, positive findings are common in patients with collagen disease (eg, SLE, scleroderma).

Synovial Fluid Analysis: Examination of synovial fluid might reveal positive LE cells and decreased complement levels in patients with SLE.[1,2,5,11,15]

- Nursing Diagnoses

  - Knowledge deficit related to lack of understanding of the laboratory test procedure, disease process, and/or outcome
  - Potential for noncompliance with prescribed laboratory and diagnostic tests related to lack of adequate explanation
  - Potential fear related to disability (RA), kidney impairment (LE), and/or dependence on others
  - Impaired physical mobility related to stiff, swollen, painful joints secondary to rheumatoid arthritis
  - Disturbance in self-concept related to dependence and/or role change

---

NURSING IMPLICATIONS WITH RATIONALE

- Explain the purpose of the laboratory tests.
- Give an explanation concerning the test procedures and the need for the patient's compliance. Explanation might be brief or in-depth, depending upon the patient's familarity with the test.
- Inform the patient of any food, beverage, or drug restrictions (*see Part I*).
- Assess urinary output in patients with SLE.
- Assess the patient's ability to ambulate. Elicit from the patient the times of day when mobility is not as much of a problem.
- Listen to the patient's expressed anxiety concerning tests and potential clinical problems. Clarification of test procedures might alleviate fear and anxiety and promote test compliance.
- Be supportive to the patient and family members and answer questions or refer the questions to appropriate professionals.

Evaluation

- Determine if the test was correctly performed according to the procedure. Notify the laboratory and physician of any changes that occur during the test.
- Determine if the patient and family members' fear and/or anxiety have been lessened or alleviated.
- Clarify or answer any additional questions the patient and family members might have.

- Encourage the patient to contact resources for additional information and support. Examples are Arthritis Foundation, Meals on Wheels, and others as related to the patient's needs.
- Develop an activity and care plan with the patient and family members.

SHOCK

LABORATORY TESTS	DIAGNOSTIC TESTS
Electrolytes (Serum)	ECG/EKG
Lactic Acid (Serum)	Central Venous Pressure (CVP)
Anion Gap	Pulmonary Arterial Pressure (PAP)
Glucose (Blood/plasma)	Pulmonary Capillary Wedge Pressure (PCWP)
Osmolality (Serum)	X-rays, Chest or Abdominal
CBC (Hg, Hct, WBC, Platelets)	CT
Type and Cross Match (T&C)	
ABGs	
Enzymes (Cardiac)	
BUN	
Creatinine (Serum)	
Protein (Total) (Serum)	
Fibrin Degradation Products (Serum)	
PT and PTT	
Urinalysis (Specific Gravity)	
Urine Electrolytes	

Introduction

Laboratory and diagnostic assessment of shock is extremely important for evaluation and management of shock syndrome. Laboratory studies, ordered immediately, usually include electrolytes, lactic acid/lactate, glucose, osmolality, complete blood count (CBC), type and cross match, and arterial blood gases. Other laboratory tests used to determine the state and progression of shock include serum enzymes, especially if cardiogenic shock is likely, blood urea nitrogen (BUN), creatinine, total protein, prothrombin time, and urine electrolytes. Diagnostic tests performed to determine cardiac and circulatory status are electrocardiogram (ECG), central venous pressure (CVP) or pulmonary arterial pressure (PAP), and x-ray. Later computerized tomography (CT) might be ordered.

Laboratory Tests

Electrolytes (Serum): Serum electrolytes—potassium, sodium, and calcium— are closely monitored during shock. Changes in electrolytes can occur quickly, such as in the levels of potassium and sodium. Table 17 shows the electrolytes associated in shock, with reasons for their decreases and increases.

TABLE 17. ELECTROLYTE CHANGES

Electrolyte (Serum)	Reference Values	Comments
Potassium (K)	3.5–5.0 mEq/L	During shock, potassium leaves the cells because of tissue injury and hypoxia. If urinary output is adequate, potassium is excreted by the kidneys, thus causing a serum potassium loss, or hypokalemia. If kidney shutdown occurs during shock, potassium builds up in the vascular fluid, causing serum potassium excess, or hyperkalemia.
Sodium (Na)	135–145 mEq/L	Serum sodium level can be normal, decreased, or elevated. During cellular damage, potassium shifts out of the cells and sodium shifts in, contributing to the serum sodium loss, or hyponatremia. Also in massive tissue injury, sodium goes to the injured site. If the patient is receiving liters of saline solutions and kidney shutdown occurs, serum sodium level is increased and hypernatremia occurs.
Calcium (Ca)	4.5–5.5 mEq/L	With massive tissue damage, calcium leaves the extracellular fluid and accumulates at the injured site, causing serum calcium deficit, or hypocalcemia. A calcium loss will increase cellular permeability, thus permitting electrolyte and fluid loss from cells.
Ionizing Calcium (iCa)	4.4–5.0 mg/dL, 2.2–2.5 mEq/L	Only ionized calcium can be used by the body. A decrease in iCa leads to tetany symptoms or neuromuscular irritability.
Chloride (Cl)	95–105 mEq/L	Chloride combines with sodium and potassium, and as these cations are lost, so is chloride. Result is hypochloremia.

Lactic Acid, Lactate (Blood): Norms: Adult: 0.5–2.0 mEq/L, 5–20 mg/dL

Elevated blood lactic acid is related to cellular hypoxia. In shock, lactic acid/lactate levels increase greatly and quickly, greater than 5 mEq/L, before blood pressure (BP) falls and urine output decreases. Lactic acidosis occurs when blood lactic acid level is greater than 2.5 mEq/L or greater than 25 mg/dL. As lactic acid level increases, cells need more oxygen.

Anion Gap: 11–17 mEq/L

Anion gap is an interrelationship between serum electrolytes in determining metabolic acid-base imbalances. An elevated anion gap >17 mEq/L is indicative of metabolic acidosis, a complication of shock. Formula for calculating anion gap is:

(sodium + potassium) − (chloride + Co_2) =

Glucose (Blood, Plasma): Norms: Adult: blood: 60–100 mg/dL; plasma: 70–110 mg/dL. Child: 60–100 mg/dL. Newborn: 30–80 mg/dL

During acute trauma and shock, blood/plasma glucose levels could rise to

200 mg/dL. After correction of shock, hypoglycemia could result. An elevated glucose level occurs as the result of an increase in epinephrine and steroid response because of tissue damage.

Osmolality (Serum): Norms: Adult: 280–300 mOsm/kg H_2O. Child: 270–290 mOsm/kg H_2O

Serum osmolality is an indicator of body fluid concentration, mainly the vascular fluid. If shock is due to massive fluid loss, serum osmolality is increased, and fluid replacement is necessary. Care should be taken not to administer massive fluids for mild shock, since overhydration could result. In overhydration, a low serum osmolality occurs.

Complete Blood Count (CBC) (Blood): Abnormal hematology values in hemoglobin (Hgb/Hb), hematocrit (Hct), WBCs, and platelet count can occur in shock. Therefore a CBC is taken in early shock and is monitored for changes during treatment and recovery. Table 18 shows the changes that can occur with these four blood values in shock.

Type and Cross Match (T&C): Although method for type and cross match is more expedient today, blood sample for (T&C) should be obtained immediately when blood loss and shock are determined.

Arterial Blood Gases (ABGs): Norms: Adult: pH: 7.35–7.45; Pco_2: 35–45 mm Hg; Po_2: 75–100 mm Hg; Hco_3: 24–28 mEq/L; BE: +2 or −2

In shock ABGs are helpful in evaluating respiratory and metabolic status. Normally metabolic acidosis occurs in shock as the result of tissue breakdown (release of acid metabolites from cells). Indicators of acidosis are pH less than 7.35, Hco_3 less than 24 mEq/L, Pco_2 of greater than 45 mm Hg. If the pH is less

TABLE 18. COMPLETE BLOOD COUNT

Hematology	Reference Values	Comments
Hgb	Male: 13.5–18.0 g/dL Female: 12–16 g/dL Child: 11–16 g/dL	Hemoglobin levels decrease after hemorrhage, but change may not occur until hours later.
Hct	Male: 40%–54% Female: 36–46%	Hematocrit is an effective indicator of body fluid volume. If shock is due to a large fluid loss, increased hematocrit level occurs because of hemoconcentration. It usually takes 4–8 hours for the hematocrit to increase after fluid loss.
WBC	Adult: 5000–10,000 μL Child, 2 years old: 6000–17,000μL	If WBC levels are slightly increased, the change could be due to tissue damage. If levels are markedly increased, the change could be due to infection.
Platelet count	Adult: 150,000–400,000 μL	Platelet count is monitored during and after blood loss and acute trauma. A low platelet count, thrombocytopenia, will cause bleeding. If platelet count is markedly decreased, hemorrhage might occur. Shock is intensified.

than 7.35 and the HCO_3 is less than 24 mEq/L, *metabolic* acidosis is present. If the pH is less than 7.35 and the Pco_2 is greater than 45 mm Hg, *respiratory* acidosis is present.

Enzymes: CPK/CK, LDH/LD, AST/SGOT (Serum): Norms: See individual reference values in Part I.

Cardiac enzyme levels are obtained when cardiac damage is suspected and in cardiogenic shock. After a myocardial infarction, serum CPK/CK rises first, then serum AST/SGOT, and last LDH/LD.

Blood Urea Nitrogen (BUN): Norms: Adult: 5–25 mg/dL

BUN should be assessed during shock. A BUN of 30 to 40 mg/dL could be indicative of fluid loss and dehydration. If the BUN is greater than 50 mg/dL and does not decrease substantially with the administration of IV fluids, kidney damage is highly suspected. Renal insufficiency or failure can result from prolonged shock.

Creatinine (Serum): Norms: Adult: 0.5–1.5 mg/dL. Older child: 0.4–1.2 mg/dL. Infant to 6 Years: 0.3–0.6 mg/dL

The laboratory test most effective in evaluating kidney function is serum creatinine. As kidney function diminishes, serum creatinine level rises. Creatinine level greater than 3 mg/dL is indicative of kidney disorder.

Protein (Total) (Serum): Total protein count is composed mostly of albumin and globulins. With severe body fluid loss, elevated serum protein (total) level could be present because of hemoconcentration.

Fibrin Degradation Products (FDP) (Serum): Norms: Adult: 2–10 ug/mL

FDP test indicates the activity of the fibrinolytic system. This test is performed when the patient is hemorrhaging following a severe injury. An elevated FDP, >10 ug/mL, is usually indicative of DIC.

Prothrombin Time (PT) and Partial Thromboplastin Time (PTT) (Plasma): Norms: Adult: PT: 11–15 seconds; PTT: 60–70 seconds

PT and PTT are ordered to evaluate clotting time. With prolonged PT and PTT times, bleeding can occur. These levels usually are monitored during shock.

Urinalysis/Specific Gravity (SG): In shock, patients frequently have a Foley catheter inserted, and so urine specific gravity can easily be checked. A specific gravity greater than 1.026 is indicative of fluid volume deficit (dehydration). In certain renal diseases (eg, glomerulonephritis, polynephritis), the specific gravity is less than 1.005.

Urine Electrolytes (Potassium and Sodium): Norms: Adult: Potassium: 40–80 mEq/24 h (average); sodium: 40–220 mEq/L/24 h

In renal failure the urine potassium and sodium levels could be increased (chronic failure) or decreased (acute failure). Urine electrolytes are frequently monitored.

Diagnostic Tests

Electrocardiography (ECG/EKG): ECG can detect cardiac changes occurring prior to or following shock. It is performed immediately in suspected cardiogenic shock.

Central Venous Pressure (CVP): *Norms:* Adult: 4–10 cm of H_2O

CVP is monitored during shock to determine fluid imbalance. A decreased CVP is indicative of hypovolemia (fluid volume deficit), and an increased CVP is indicative of hypervolemia (fluid volume excess). As an indicator of left ventricular pressure, CVP is not as accurate as pulmonary arterial (PA) pressure but is considered safer and accompanied by fewer complications.

Pulmonary Arterial Pressure (PAP) and Pulmonary Capillary Wedge Pressure (PCWP): *Norms:* Adult: PAP: 10–20 mm Hg mean, 20–30 mm Hg systolic, 10–15 mm Hg diastolic; PCWP: 4–12 mm Hg mean

PAP indicates the pulmonary blood volume and the pulmonary vascular resistance. A low PAP is indicative of fluid volume deficit (hypovolemia) or vasodilation, and an elevated PAP is indicative of fluid volume overload or increased pulmonary vascular resistance, possibly due to pulmonary embolism. A decreased PCWP is indicative of fluid volume deficit (hypovolemia). An elevated PCWP can occur in fluid volume overload (hypervolemia) because of excess IV fluids or because of increased preload from fluid retention in cardiac failure. Increased afterload, vascular resistance to left ventricular ejection, will also increase PCWP.

X-rays: Chest or abdominal x-rays at a suspected trauma site might be helpful in detecting cause of shock.

Computerized Tomography (CT): Emergency CT might be ordered to determine cause of shock.[1,2,5,7,9,11,15,31]

- Nursing Diagnoses

  - Potential for noncompliance to prescribed laboratory and diagnostic tests related to lack of understanding and adherence to the procedures
  - Anxiety related to fear of death and the unknown
  - Ineffective coping with disease process and laboratory and diagnostic test procedures
  - Fluid-volume deficit related to loss of body fluid and blood, inadequate circulation, or body-fluid volume shift
  - Decreased tissue perfusion related to ineffective blood circulation, loss of blood, or hypotension
  - Alteration in elimination (renal) related to inadequate circulation and hypotension
  - Ineffective breathing patterns related to dyspnea, anxiety, pain, or impaired gas exchange secondary to trauma

---

NURSING IMPLICATIONS WITH RATIONALE

- Explain the purpose for the laboratory and diagnostic tests briefly to the patient and family members. A detailed explanation during a crisis might not be appropriate.
- Obtain blood sample collection and send to the laboratory immediately. Check that results are returned and notify the physician of the laboratory results.

- Monitor the patient's intake and output and vital signs before and after laboratory and diagnostic tests and at specified times. Report changes immediately to the physician.
- Listen to the patient and family members' expressed anxiety and/or fear concerning the tests and the patient's outcome from trauma.
- Assess for excess bleeding and apply pressure if appropriate. Report changes to the physician.
- Be supportive of the patient and family members during and after the crisis.

Evaluation

- Determine if the test was correctly performed according to the procedure. Notify the laboratory of any changes that occur during the test.
- Check the patient's urinary output and vital signs for changes and improvement.
- Determine if the patient and family members' anxiety and fear have been lessened or alleviated. Continue being supportive of the patient and family members.
- Clarify or answer any additional questions the patient and family members might have.

NEOPLASTIC CONDITIONS

LABORATORY TESTS

ACTH (Plasma)
ADH (Serum)
Bence-Jones Protein (Urine)
Bilirubin (Serum)
Calcitonin (Serum)
Calcium (Serum)
Carcinoembryonia Antigen (Plasma)
Ceruloplasmin (Serum)
Cold agglutinins (Serum)
Complements C_3, C_4 (Serum)
Copper (Serum)
Cortisol (Plasma)
C-Reactive Protein (Serum)
Cryoglobulins (Serum)
Cytology: sputum, gastric washing, colon, pleural fluid, bronchial secretions, urine, Pap smear, CSF
Enzymes: ACP, ALP, ALT/SGPT, AST/SGOT, GGTP, LDH, LAP
ESR (Blood)
Estradiol (E_2) (Serum)

DIAGNOSTIC TESTS

X-rays: Chest, Bone, GI Series, Barium Enema, IVP, Bronchography
Mammography
Thermography
Lymphangiography
Endoscopy: Bronchoscopy, Esophagogastroscopy, Proctosigmoidoscopy, Colonoscopy, Colposcopy, Cystoscopy, ERCP
Ultrasonography/Ultrasound
Nuclear Scans
CT
Angiography/Arteriography
Biopsy
Bone Marrow Aspiration
MRI

(continued)

LABORATORY TESTS	DIAGNOSTIC TESTS

Estrogen/Total (Serum and Urine)
FSH (Serum and Urine)
Gastrin (Serum)
Haptoglobin (Serum)
HCG (Serum, Urine)
5-HIAA (Urine)
Immunoglobins (Serum)
17-KS (Urine)
LH (Serum)
Occult Blood (Feces)
PTH (Serum)
PTT (Plasma)
Platelet Count (Blood)
Pregnanediol (Urine)
Pregnanetriol (Urine)
Prolactin (Serum)
Protein Electrophoresis (Serum)
Renin (Plasma)
Testosterone (Serum)
Thyroid antibodies (Serum)
Uric Acid (Serum)
WBC/Leukocytes (Blood)

Introduction

Numerous laboratory and diagnostic tests are performed to identify and to confirm the presence of cancer (ie, carcinomas, sarcomas, leukemias, lymphomas). One test only is not sufficient to diagnose cancer. Although most laboratory tests are ordered to determine function of body organs and glands, there are many elevated and decreased test values associated with cancer. Usually diagnostic tests are necessary to confirm cancer site and diagnosis. In this section abnormal laboratory values, elevated or decreased, as they relate to cancer are given instead of the norms for the test. Laboratory tests are arranged in alphabetic order. Refer to Part I for the reference values of these laboratory tests.

A summarized chart of laboratory and diagnostic tests used for diagnosing specific cancers follows the brief description of the tests.

Laboratory Tests

Antidiuretic Hormone (ADH) (Serum): ADH may be elevated, greater than 5 pg/mL in syndrome or secretion of inappropriate antidiuretic hormone (SIADH) as a result of ectopic secretion by bronchogenic carcinoma.

Adrenocorticotropic Hormone (ACTH) (Plasma): Decreased plasma ACTH could occur in patients with cancer of the adrenal gland, and elevated plasma ACTH could occur in patients with pituitary tumor. ACTH could be elevated with any tumor that secretes ACTH ectopically (eg, bronchogenic carcinoma).

Bence-Jones Protein (Urine): Increased Bence-Jones protein greater than 1.0 mg/dL is commonly found in the urine of patients with multiple myeloma, and increased levels are also associated with metastatic carcinoma, bone cancer, and leukemia.

Bilirubin: Total (Serum): Elevated serum total bilirubin greater than 1.2 mg/dL could occur in patients with tumors of the liver or liver metastasis. Elevated bilirubin level could occur in pancreatic carcinoma secondary to common duct obstruction.

Calcitonin (hCT) (Serum): A high serum calcitonin level, > 2000 pg/mL, indicates thyroid medullary carcinoma.

Calcium (Serum): Hypercalcemia, elevated serum calcium level greater than 5.5 mEq/: or greater than 11 mg/dL, occurs in 10% to 20% of all cancer patients. Metastatic tumors can cause bone destruction, which elevates serum calcium level. Common causes of hypercalcemia are metastatic breast cancer, multiple myeloma, ectopic secretion of parathyroid hormone (PTH), and bony metastasis.

Carcinoembryonic Antigen (CEA) (Blood, Plasma): CEA has been extracted from tumors in the GI tract. CEA has been frequently found in patients with cancer of the large intestine and pancreas. Plasma CEA might be elevated in other cancers (eg, esophagus, stomach, lung, breast, bladder, kidney, cervix, testes, and leukemia). CEA is used to evaluate the effectiveness of cancer therapies and to monitor patients in remission for early signs of recurrence. CEA will be increased before clinical symptoms are evident.

Ceruloplasmin (Cp) (Serum): Cp is produced in the liver and binds with copper. An elevated serum ceruloplasmin level greater than 50 mg/dL could occur in patients with cancer of the bone, stomach, or lung and in patients with Hodgkin's disease.

Cold Agglutinins (CA) (Serum): Elevated serum CA, greater than 1:16 to 1:32, might be present in lymphatic leukemia and multiple myeloma.

Complements C_3, C_4 (Serum): Elevated serum C_3 and C_4 could be found in patients with malignant neoplasms of the esophagus, stomach, colon, rectum, pancreas, lungs, breast, cervix, ovary, prostate, and bladder.

Copper (Cu) (Serum): Elevated serum copper levels greater than 140 μg/dL (male) might be present in cancer of the bone, stomach, large intestine, liver, lung, and in Hodgkin's disease and leukemias.

Cortisol (Plasma): Plasma cortisol level could be elevated in patients with cancer of the adrenal gland.

C-Reactive Protein (CRP) (Serum): Positive CRP titer might occur in patients with cancer of the breast with metastasis. Patients with Hodgkin's disease might also have positive CRP titer.

Cryoglobulins (Serum): Positive cryoglobulin findings might be present in patients having Hodgkin's disease, lymphocytic leukemia, or multiple myeloma.

Cytology: Cells that have been sloughed from neoplasms/tumors can be found in body secretions. These secretions are obtained from sputum, gastric washing, colon, pleural fluid, bronchial tract, urine, Pap smear, and cerebrospinal (CSF) for cytologic examination.

Enzymes: When cancer affects organs that produce enzymes, enzyme values are checked. The enzyme *acid phosphatase (ACP)* is plentiful in the prostate gland, and an elevated serum ACP level usually indicates carcinoma of the prostate gland. If ACP is markedly elevated, metastasis to the bone is suspected. Also elevated serum ACP can be associated with multiple myeloma and Paget's disease. The enzyme *alkaline phosphatase* (*ALP*), produced by the bone and liver, is usually elevated in patients with cancer of the bone and liver. An elevated ALP might occur in patients with multiple myeloma. *Alanine aminotransferase* (*ALT/SGPT*) and *aspartate aminotransferase* (*AST/SGOT*) might be noted in patients with cancer of the liver. *Gamma-glutamyl* (*transpeptidase*) *transferase* (*GGTP*) could be elevated in cancer of the liver, kidney, pancreas, prostate, breast, lung, and brain. Elevated *lactic dehydrogenase* (*LD/LDH*) might occur in patients with cancer of the lung, bone, intestines, liver, breast, cervix, testes, kidney, stomach, and melanoma of the skin. Serum LDH could be elevated in acute leukemia. *Leucine aminopeptidase* (*LAP*) is an enzyme produced by the liver. Elevated serum LAP could indicate cancer of the liver.

Erythrocyte Sedimentation Rate (ESR, Sed Rate) (Blood): Patients with Hodgkin's disease, multiple myeloma, and lymphosarcoma might have increased ESR.

Estradiol (E₂) (Serum): E_2 is useful in evaluating gonadal dysfunction. Elevated E_2 level in female, >500 pg/mL, may be present in ovarian tumor, and elevated E_2 level in male, >50 pg/mL, can indicate a testicular tumor.

Estrogen/Total (Serum and Urine-24-Hour): An elevated serum or urine estrogen test might indicate adrenocortical tumor, ovarian tumor, or some testicular tumor.

Follicle-Stimulating Hormone (FSH) (Serum and Urine): Decreased serum and urine FSH, less than 4 mU/mL (serum), or 4 IU/24h. (urine), could indicate tumor of the adrenal gland, testes, or ovary. Increased level could indicate FSH-producing pituitary tumor.

Gastrin (Serum): Elevated serum gastrin level, greater than 200 pg/mL, might be present in patients with malignant neoplasm of the stomach.

Haptoglobin (Serum): Elevated haptoglobin level, greater than 270 mg/dL, might be found in patients with cancer of the lung, large intestine, stomach, breast, and liver and in patients with Hodgkin's disease.

Hormones: Any hormone may be elevated with cancer, since many cancers secrete inappropriate hormones (ectopic hormone secretion) because of bizarre differentiation of cancer cells.

Human Chorionic Gonadotropin (HCG) (Serum, Urine): Usually positive HCG levels indicate pregnancy, but they might indicate hydatidiform mole or choriocarcinoma.

5-Hydroxyindolacetic Acid (5-HIAA) (Urine): Elevated urine 5-HIAA, 10 to 100 mg/24 h, could indicate carcinoid tumors of the appendix and intestine. Usually these carcinoid tumor cells, which secrete excess serotonin, are of low-grade malignancy. When metastasis occurs, 5-HIAA could be greater than 100 mg/24 h. Food and certain drugs could give false-positive results. Several random or spot urine specimens should be tested.

Immunoglobulins (Ig) (Serum): Patients with lymphocytic leukemia could have decreased serum IgG, IgA, IgM levels. Patients with lymphosarcoma might have an increased IgM level.

17-Ketosteroids (17-KS) (Urine): Elevated urine 17-KS, greater than 25 mg/24 h (male), greater than 15 mg/24 h (female), could be associated with neoplasms of the adrenal gland, testes, and ovary.

Luteinizing Hormone (LH) (Serum): In pituitary and testicular tumors, LH is elevated.

Occult Blood (Feces): Hidden blood in the stools could indicate cancer in the upper or lower GI tract. Orthotoluidine (Occultest) is considered more sensitive than the guaiac test.

Parathyroid Hormone (PTH): PTH is secreted ectopically by many carcinomas (ie, squamous cell lung cancer [most common cause], renal carcinoma, pancreatic carcinoma, and ovarian carcinoma). Also PTH might be elevated in parathyroid carcinoma.

Partial Thromboplastin Time (PTT) (Plasma): Increased PTT could be present in patients with myelocytic and monocytic leukemias.

Platelet Count (Blood): decreased platelet count, less than 100,000 mm^3 may occur in patients with cancer of the bone, gastrointestinal tract, and brain, and in multiple myeloma, lymphatic, myelocytic, and monocytic leukemias. An elevated platelet count, greater than 400,000 mm^3 might occur in metastatic carcinoma. Many types of chemotherapy cause temporary thrombocytopenia.

Pregnanediol (Urine): elevated urine pregnanediol, higher than 7 mg/24 h may be present in choriocarcinoma of the ovary.

Pregnanetriol (Urine): malignant neoplasm of the adrenal gland may have an elevated urine pregnanetriol, greater than 2.4 mg/24 hours.

Prolactin (PRL) (Serum): In nonpregnant women and in men, an elevated prolactin level could indicate pituitary adenoma.

Protein Electrophoresis (Serum): The following cancerous conditions could be reflected in protein fractions.

PROTEIN	DECREASED LEVEL	ELEVATED LEVEL
Albumin	Leukemia Liver cancer (primary or metastatic)	
Globulin		
β		Malignant hypertensive
γ	Lymphocytic leukemia Lymphosarcoma	Hodgkin's disease Chronic lymphocytic leukemia Multiple myeloma

Renin (Plasma): Patients with cancer of the kidney may have an elevated plasma renin level.

Testosterone (Serum): Increased testosterone in women after menopause can be caused by malignant neoplasm of the breast.

Thyroid Antibodies (TA) (Serum): elevated serum TA titer could indicate carcinoma of the thyroid gland.

Uric Acid (Serum): Elevated serum-uric acid, greater than 7.8 mg/dL, could occur in patients having lymphocytic, myelocytic, and monocytic leukemias, multiple myeloma, and in metastatic cancer (due to tumor lysis syndrome).

White Blood Cells (WBC)/Leukocytes (Blood): Elevated total WBC count frequently is present in lymphocytic, myelocytic, and monocytic leukemias. Differential WBC count is ordered to determine the cause of disease. With elevated lymphocyte count, the disease entities could be chronic lymphocytic leukemia, Hodgkin's disease, or multiple myeloma. In monocytic leukemia, the monocyte count could be elevated. It is not uncommon to see the neutrophil count increased in myelocytic leukemia and Hodgkin's disease. Leukocytes may be decreased in many forms of cancer (immunosuppression occurs by unknown mechanism). Chemotherapy and radiation frequently cause severe, temporary, decreased WBCs.

Diagnostic Tests

X-rays: X-rays are taken of various organs when malignant neoplasms and metastasis are suspected. Chest and bone x-rays are used to detect neoplasm in the lung and bone metastasis. Procedural x-rays taken of body organs include GI series, barium enema, intravenous pyelography (IVP), and bronchography.

Mammography: This is an x-ray examination of the breast to detect cysts and tumors. Malignant tumors are irregular and poorly defined. They tend to be unilateral.

Thermography (Breast): Breast tumors cause increased metabolism, resulting in vascularity and increased breast-surface temperature. This test is used as a screening test; other diagnostic procedures are necessary to confirm breast cancer.

Lymphangiography, Lymphangiogram: This test is an x-ray examination of the lymphatic system (ie, lymphatic vessels and lymph nodes). It is used to identify lymphoma (eg, Hodgkin's disease) and metastasis to the lymph nodes. Lymphangiogram should not be performed on patients who are highly allergic to iodinated dye.

Endoscopy: Endoscopes, rigid (metal) or flexible fiberoptic, are used for direct visualization of body organs and body cavities to detect any abnormalities. The endoscopes are named for the organ that they are designed to view (eg, colonoscope [colon], gastroscope [stomach], bronchoscope [lungs], cystoscope [bladder], colposcope [vagina and cervix]). The following endoscopic examinations are performed to detect neoplasms of the lung: bronchoscopy and mediastinoscopy; the esophagus and stomach: esophagogastroscopy; the colon: colonoscopy; the duodenum and pancreas: endoscopic retrograde cholangiopancreatography (ERCP); the rectum and sigmoid: proctosigmoidoscopy; the vagina and cervix: colposcopy; and the bladder: cystoscopy. Peritoneoscopy is helpful in observing the peritoneum for effectiveness of treatment and recurrence of metastasis.

Ultrasonography, Ultrasound, Echography: This noninvasive test records echoes of sound from tissues of different densities. It is useful in detecting neoplasms of the brain, kidney, liver, pancreas, spleen, and thyroid. However, positive findings need to be confirmed by other diagnostic tests.

Nuclear Scans, Radioisotope Scan, Radionuclide Imaging. Nuclear scanning using radioactive isotopes or radionuclides is used to detect primary or metastatic cancer. If the radionuclide concentrates in the tumor, the involved urea will show up as dark spot or hot spot on the scintigram. But if the tumor does not concentrate the radionuclide, then light-colored area or cold spot is recorded. Radioisotope scans are useful for detecting metastatic tumor of the bone, tumors of the brain, lung, kidney, liver, spleen, and thyroid gland.

Computerized Tomography (CT): CT is effective for detecting tumors of the brain, lung, liver, kidney, pancreas, and adrenals.

Angiography, Arteriography: Angiography is an examination of arteries leading to organs. This test is useful for detecting abnormal vascularization resulting from tumors. Cerebral angiography identifies brain tumors by the increased vascularization; pulmonary angiography can detect tumors of the lung; and renal angiography can identify kidney tumors.

Biopsy: Biopsy, excision of tissue, is a direct method for diagnosing cancer. Tissue specimens for microscopic examination can be obtained from the lung, liver, kidney, bone, thyroid, lymph nodes, skin, and bone marrow.

Bone Marrow Aspiration: Examination of the bone marrow detects abnormal cells. It is a useful test for diagnosing leukemias, lymphomas, and multiple myelomas.

Magnetic Resonance Imaging (MRI): MRI can detect small, primary or metastatic tumors. It can distinguish solid masses from vascular structures better than CT. It is helpful in evaluating recurrent or residual masses. MRI is useful in supplementing CT.[1,5,7,9–11,15,24]

A summary of laboratory and diagnostic tests used in diagnosing cancer is outlined in Table 19.

■ Nursing Diagnoses

- Anxiety related to the unknown and pain
- Knowledge deficit related to lack of understanding of laboratory and diagnostic procedures, disease process, and/or outcome
- Potential for noncompliance to prescribed laboratory and diagnostic tests related to lack of or inadequate explanation and/or anxiety about physical condition
- Alteration in nutrition related to anorexia, vomiting, reduced food intake secondary to treatment regimen for cancer
- Potential for injury related to bleeding tendencies secondary to decreased platelet count
- Potential for injury related to allergic reactions to contrast medium (dye) secondary to diagnostic tests (ie, IVP, CT, with contrast medium, angiography)
- Potential activity intolerance related to diagnostic testing (eg, angiography), pain (eg, bone metastasis).
- Potential alteration in fluid, electrolyte, and acid-base balance related to cellular catabolism, numerous laboratory and diagnostic tests, and/or treatment regimen
- Ineffective coping with disease process and laboratory and diagnostic procedures

TABLE 19. TESTS USED TO DIAGNOSE SPECIFIC CANCERS

Cancer	Laboratory Tests	Diagnostic Tests
Leukemias	Bence-Jones protein CEA Cold agglutinins Cryoglobulins PTT Platelet count Protein fraction Uric acid WBC	Bone marrow aspiration/biopsy
Hodgkin's disease	Ceruloplasmin Copper CRP Cryoglobulins ESR Haptoglobin Protein fraction WBC	Lymphangiography Lymph node biopsy Mediastinoscopy
Multiple myelomas	Bence-Jones protein Calcium Cold agglutinins Enzymes: ACP, ALP Cryoglobulins ESR Platelet count Protein fraction Uric acid WBC	Bone marrow aspiration/biopsy
Stomach	CEA Ceruloplasmin C_3, C_4 Enzyme: LDH Copper Gastrin Haptoglobin	GI series Esophagogastroscopy
Colon	CEA C_3, C_4 Copper Enzyme: LDH Haptoglobin 5-HIAA Occult stool	Barium enema Colonoscopy Proctosigmoidoscopy ERCP Biopsy
Kidney, Bladder	C_3, C_4 Enzymes: GGTP, LDH Renin	IVP Cystoscopy Ultrasound Nuclear scan CT Angiography Biopsy

continues

TABLE 19. TESTS USED TO DIAGNOSE SPECIFIC CANCERS (*Continued*)

Cancer	Laboratory Tests	Diagnostic Tests
Lung	ADH ACTH Calcium CEA Ceruloplasmin Copper Cytology Enzymes: GGTP, LDH Haptoglobin	Bronchography Bronchoscopy Nuclear scan CT Angiography Mediastinoscopy Chest x-ray MRI
Liver	Bilirubin Ceruloplasmin Copper Enzymes: ALP, LAP, ALT/ SGPT, AST/SGOT, GGTP Haptoglobin	Ultrasound Nuclear scan CT Biopsy
Reproductive	Calcium CEA C_3, C_4 CRP Enzymes: ACP, GGTP Estradiol Estrogen FSH HCG 17-KS LH Pap smear Pregnanediol Testosterone	Mammography Thermography Colposcopy Biopsy Peritoneoscopy
Bone	Bence-Jones protein Calcium Ceruloplasmin Copper Enzymes: ALP, LDH	X-ray Biopsy
Brain	Enzyme: GGTP	Ultrasound Nuclear scan CT MRI Angiography
Endocrine	ACTH Calcitonin Cortisol FSH 17-KS LH Pregnanetriol Prolactin Thyroid antibodies	Ultrasound Nuclear scan CT Biopsy

- Potential alteration in comfort related to test procedure and pain secondary to neoplasm
- Potential disturbance in self-concept related to body changes, dependence, and/or role change
- Potential alteration in family process related to numerous laboratory and diagnostic tests, hospitalization, and/or treatment

---

NURSING IMPLICATIONS WITH RATIONALE

- Explain the purpose for the laboratory and diagnostic tests.
- Give detailed explanation concerning the test procedures and the need for patient's compliance. Explanation might be brief or in-depth, depending upon the person's familiarity with the test.
- Inform the patient of any food, beverage, or drug restrictions. Each test should be checked for specific restrictions (*see Parts I and II*).
- Obtain specimen collection at specific times according to the procedures.
- Elicit from the patient, patient history, or family members information about any allergies, especially to contrast medium (dye), iodine, seafood.
- Monitor intake and output and vital signs before and after laboratory and diagnostic tests.
- Listen to the patient's expressed anxiety or fear concerning the tests and potential clinical problems. Clarification of the test procedure might alleviate fear and anxiety and promote compliance. Assess communications for verbal or nonverbal expressions of anxiety and fear.
- Assess the patient's discomfort by eliciting from him or her the intensity, duration, and location of pain. Provide pain relief by positional changes and medication.
- Observe for bleeding caused by decreased platelet count and treatment regimen.
- Check laboratory results, and notify the physician of abnormal test results.
- Provide support to the patient and family members during test procedure, treatment regimen, and in response to expressed fear and anxiety about physical condition and outcome.
- Repeat information to the patient and family briefly and clearly if anxiety and/or fear level is determined to be high.

Evaluation

- Determine if the test was correctly performed according to the procedure. Notify laboratory and/or physician of any changes that occur during the test.
- Provide ongoing assessment before, during, and after procedure. Check the patient's vital signs, intake and output, and for ecchymosis or bleeding site following laboratory or diagnostic procedure. Assess for changes and improvement.
- Determine if the patient and family members' fear and/or anxiety has been lessened or alleviated. Continue providing support measures.

- Clarify or answer any additional questions the patient and family members might have.
- Encourage the patient to seek health care assistance whenever any change in health status occurs (eg, infection, bleeding, skin breakdown, elevated temperature, and others).
- Identify resources that would provide information, service, and support (eg, American Cancer Association) to the patient and family.
- Encourage the patient and family members to participate in the decision-making process concerning plan of care and daily activities.
- Assist the family with the development of a care plan for health management and activities.

HEMATOLOGIC CONDITIONS

LABORATORY TESTS

CBC	PT (Plasma)
RBC Count	PTT and APTT (Plasma)
Hb (Hgb)	Factors Assay (Coagulation Factors)
Hct	Blood Typing
RBC Indices: MCV, MCH, MCHC, RDW	Bone Marrow Aspiration
WBC Count	G-6-PD (Blood)
Differential WBC Count	Haptoglobin (Serum)
Platelet Count	Coomb's—Indirect (Serum)
Platelet aggregation	Ferritin (Serum)
Reticulocyte Count	Iron (Serum)
Hb Electrophoresis	IBC/TIBC (Serum)
Erythrocyte Osmotic Fragility	Transferrin (Serum)
Bleeding Time (Blood)	Bilirubin—Indirect (Serum)
Coagulation Time (Blood)	Sickle Cell Screening Test
Clot Retraction (Blood)	Folic Acid (Serum)
Fibrinogen (Plasma)	Vitamin B_{12} (Serum)
Fibrin Degradation Products (Serum)	ESR (Sed Rate) (Blood)
Euglobulin Lysis Time	Urobilinogen (Urine)
DIC Screening Tests	
Plasminogen (Plasma)	

Introduction

Laboratory tests for hematologic conditions described in this section are done to diagnose anemias such as microcytic (iron deficiency), macrocytic (aplastic, hemolytic, pernicious), bleeding disorders, and blood cell changes.

For leukemias and multiple myeloma, see Neoplastic Conditions.

Laboratory Tests

Complete Blood Count (CBC): The six components of CBC include RBC count; hemoglobin (Hb/Hgb); hematocrit (Hct); RBC (erythrocyte) indices: mean corpuscular volume (MCV), mean corpuscular hemoglobin (MCH), mean corpuscular hemoglobin concentration (MCHC), RBC distribution width (RDW); WBC; and differential WBC count. Usually CBC is ordered to aid in the detection of anemias; to determine blood loss, hydration status, and as part of the routine hospital admission test; to evaluate blood cell status prior to surgery; and as part of a physical examination. RBC count, Hb, Hct, and RBC index values are useful to determine the type of anemia (*see Part I on RBC indices*).

Differential WBC is necessary for determining the type of infection. During an acute bacterial infection, the body's first line of defense is neutrophils. An increased number of lymphocytes occurs in chronic bacterial and acute viral infections. Monocytes increase in number late in acute bacterial infections but continue to function during the chronic phase.

Table 20 shows the norms for CBC tests and clinical problems associated with decreased and elevated levels.

Platelet Count: Norms: Adult: 150,000–400,000 μL

Thrombocytopenia (decreased platelet count) is associated with aplastic, iron deficiency, pernicious, folic acid deficiency, and sickle cell anemias. Thrombocytosis (elevated platelet count) occurs in polycythemia vera.

Platelet Aggregation and Platelet Adhesion (Blood): Norms: 3–5 minutes

Platelet aggregation measures the ability of platelets adhering to one another. A decrease in platelet aggregation time will cause increased bleeding tendencies. Both platelet aggregation and platelet adhesion aid in diagnosing hereditary and acquired platelet diseases, such as von Willebrand's disease.

Reticulocyte Count: Norms: Adult: 25,000–75,000 μL, 0.5%–1.5% of all RBCs. Elderly: 0.4%–3.6%. Child: 0.5%–2.0% of all RBCs

Reticulocytes are immature, nonnucleated RBCs that are formed in the bone marrow. Decreased reticulocyte count might be present in pernicious, folic acid, and aplastic anemias. A persistently low count could be suggestive of bone marrow hypofunction or aplastic anemia. An elevated reticulocyte count could be present in hemolytic and sickle cell anemias and could be due to hemorrhage, hemolysis, or treatment of iron deficiency.

Hb/Hgb Electrophoresis: Norms: See values in Part I.

This test detects abnormal types of Hb (ie, Hb S [sickle cell anemia], Hb C [hemolytic anemia], and Hb F [thalassemia]).

Erythrocyte Osmotic Fragility: Norms: Adult: 0.30%–0.46%

This test determines the ability of RBCs to resist hemolysis (RBC destruction) in hypo-osmolar solutions. Osmotic fragility might be decreased in the anemias—iron deficiency, folic acid deficiency, sickle cell, thalassemia major and minor (Mediterranean anemia or Cooley's anemia)—and also in polycythemia vera. Elevated osmotic fragility might be present in acquired hemolytic anemia.

Bleeding Time: Norms: Adult: 1–6 minutes (Ivy's method), 1–3 minutes (Duke's method)

The bleeding time test is useful in determining abnormal function of platelets. A prolonged bleeding time could be due to decreased platelet count, increased platelet destruction, platelet abnormality, vascular abnormalities, disseminated intravascular coagulation (DIC) disease, aplastic anemia, and factor V, VII, and XI deficiencies.

TABLE 20. HEMATOLOGIC CAUSES FOR ABNORMAL CBC RESULTS

Type	Reference Value	Decreased Level	Elevated Level
RBC count	Adult: 　Male: 4.5–6.0 μL 　Female: 4.0–5.0 μL Elderly: 　Male: 3.7–6.0 μL 　Female: 4.0–5.0 μL Child: 3.8–5.5 μL	Hemorrhage Anemias Hemodilution 　(overhydration)	Hemoconcentration 　(dehydration) Polycythemia vera
Hb	Adult: 　Male: 13.5–18.0 g/dL 　Female: 12.0–16.0 g/dL Elderly: 　Male: 11.0–17.0 g/dL 　Female: 11.5–16.0 g/dL Infant: 10.0–15.0 g/dL Child: 11.0–16.0 g/dL	Anemias: 　Iron deficiency 　Aplastic 　Hemocytic Acute blood loss Hemodilution	Hemoconcentration 　(dehydration) Polycythemia vera
Hct	Adult: 　Male: 40%–54% 　Female: 36–46% Elderly: 　Male: 38–42% 　Female: 38–41% Child, 1–3 years: 　29%–40% Child, 4–10 years: 　36%–38%	Anemias: 　Aplastic 　Hemolytic 　Folic acid 　　deficiency 　Pernicious 　Sickle cell	Hemoconcentration 　(dehydration) Polycythemia vera
RBC indices MCV	Adult: 80–98 μm^3 Elderly: 　Male: 74–110 μm^3 　Female: 78–100 μm^3	Microcytic anemia: 　Iron deficiency	Macrocytic anemias: 　Aplastic 　Hemolytic 　Pernicious
MCH	Adult: 27–31 pg Elderly: 　Male: 24–33 pg 　Female: 23–34 pg	Microcytic, 　hypochromic 　anemia	Macrocytic anemias
MCHC	Adult: 32%–36% 　0.32–0.36 g/dL Elderly: 　Male: 28%–36% 　Female: 30%–36%	Microcytic, 　hypochromic 　anemia Thalassemia	
RDW	11.5–14.5 　Coulter S		Anemias: 　Iron deficiency 　Folic acid deficiency 　Pernicious 　Sickle cell

(continued)

TABLE 20. HEMATOLOGIC CAUSES FOR ABNORMAL CBC RESULTS (*Continued*)

Type	Reference Value	Decreased Level	Elevated Level
WBC count	Adult: 5000–10,000 μL Child, 2 years: 6000–17,000 μL Elderly: Male: 4200–16,000 μL Female: 3100–10,000 μL	Anemias: Aplastic Pernicious	Anemias: Hemolytic Sickle cell
Differential WBC count Neutrophils	Adult: 50%–70% Elderly: 45%–75% Child: 35%	Anemias: Aplastic Folic acid deficiency Iron deficiency	Anemia: Acquired hemolytic
Basophils	Adult: 0.5%–1.0% Elderly, Average: 1%		Anemia: Acquired hemolytic
Lymphocytes	Adult: 25%–35% Elderly, Average: 30% Child: 38%–50%	Anemia: Aplastic	
Monocytes	Adult: 4%–6% Elderly, Average: 10%	Anemia: Aplastic	Anemias: Sickle cell Hemolytic

Coagulation Time (CT), Lee-White Clotting Time (Blood): Norms: Adult: 5–15 minutes.

CT, frequently known as Lee-White clotting time, is one of the oldest tests of coagulation. A prolonged CT might be indicative of afibrinogenemia, hyperheparinemia, or severe coagulation factor deficiencies.

Clot Retraction (Blood): Norms: Adult: 1 h: half its size; 4 h: near completion; 24 h: completely shrunken. Child: same as adult

Clot retraction (shrunken clot) test is useful for detecting platelet disorder (platelet deficit or platelet abnormality). A decreased clot retraction (longer than 4 to 24 hours) could be indicative of thrombocytopenia (decreased platelets); thrombasthenia (platelet abnormality); or pernicious, folic-acid deficiency, or aplastic anemia.

Fibrinogen (Plasma): Norms: 200–400 mg/dL

Fibrinogen produces fibrin strands necessary for clot formation. A deficiency of fibrinogen results in bleeding. A low fibrinogen level may be due to DIC.

Fibrin Degradation Products (FDP) (Serum): Norms: Adult: 2–10 μg/mL

FDP test, also known as fibrin split products (FSP), indicates the activity of the fibrinolytic system. This test is frequently done in an emergency when the patient is hemorrhaging. An increased FDP, greater than 10 μg/mL, is usually indicative of DIC caused by severe injury or trauma.

TABLE 21. DISSEMINATED INTRAVASCULAR COAGULATION SCREENING TESTS

Test	Positive Results
Platelet count	>400,000 μL
Bleeding time	>6 minutes
PT	>15 seconds
PTT	>60 seconds
APTT	>40 seconds
Factor I: fibrinogen	<100 mg/dL
Fibrin degradation products	>10 μg/dL
Euglobulin lysis time	1½–6 hours, or >6 hours
Plasminogen	<2.5 U/mL, <20 mg/dL

Euglobulin Lysis Time (Fibrinolysis Time) Test: Norms: Adult: 1½–6 hours
This test evaluates the activity of the fibrinolytic system by determining the time from clot formation to clot lysis. It is useful in differentiating between primary fibrinolysis (eg, cancer of prostate) and DIC. The lysis time is short in primary fibrinolysis and normal or prolonged in DIC.

Disseminated Intravascular Coagulation (DIC) Screening Tests: This is a group of tests ordered for detecting the presence of DIC. Table 21 shows the screening tests used for suspected DIC.

Plasminogen (Plasma): Norms: 2.5–5.2 U/mL; 20 mg/dL
Plasminogen test is useful in evaluating the fibrinolytic process, a breakdown of fibrin clots in prevention of coagulation. The level is decreased in disseminated intravascular coagulation (DIC), advanced liver disease, and thrombolytic therapy.

Prothrombin Time (PT) (Plasma): Norms: Adult: 11–15 seconds; 70%–100%. Child: same as adult
Prothrombin, factor II, is converted to thrombin by the action of thromboplastin, which is needed to form a clot. A prolonged PT time could be associated with afibrinogenemia, deficiencies of factors II, VII and X. This test is useful for monitoring anticoagulant therapy.

Partial Thromboplastin Time (PTT), Activated Partial Thromboplastin Time (ATT) (Plasma): Norms: Adult: PTT: 60–70 seconds; APTT: 20–35 seconds
PTT is useful for detecting clotting factors and platelet disorders. APTT is more sensitive than PTT. PTT and APTT are commonly used to monitor heparin therapy.

Factor Assay (Coagulation Factors): Factor assay determines the concentration of specific coagulating factors in the blood. Prolonged clotting time occurs when values of factors I, II, V, VII, VIII, IX, X, and XI are decreased.

Blood Typing (Type and Cross Match): Blood typing and cross matching is necessary to provide compatible blood to recipients. Major and minor antigens can be detected through blood typing.

Bone Marrow Aspiration (Biopsy): Bone marrow specimen is useful for evaluating hematopoiesis. The size, shape, and number of RBCs, WBCs, and megakaryocytes (platelet precursors) are examined to diagnose hematologic disorders (ie, aplastic anemia, leukemia, Hodgkin's disease, polycythemia vera, and multiple myeloma).

Glucose-6-Phosphate Dehydrogenase/G-6-PD (Blood): *Norms:* Adult: (varies with method used) 8–18 IU/g Hb, 125–281 U/dL packed RBCs

G-6-PD, an enzyme in RBCs, assists in glucose use in RBCs. A decreased amount of this enzyme causes hemolysis and hemolytic anemia.

Haptoglobin (Hp) (Serum): *Norms:* Adult: 60–270 mg/dL. Infant: 0–30 mg/dL, and then gradually increases

Hp, a group of α_2-globulins, combines with free Hb during intravascular hemolysis. A decreased Hp level occurs in hemolytic anemia because of too much free Hb to bind. Also a decreased level could occur in pernicious, folic-acid deficiency, and sickle cell anemias.

Coombs Indirect (Serum): *Norms:* negative

This test detects free antibodies in the patient's serum and identifies certain red cell antigens. It is done in cross matching blood for transfusion. Positive results mean incompatible cross-matched blood, anti-Rh antibodies, or acquired hemolytic anemia.

Ferritin (Serum): *Norms:* Male: 35–300 ng/mL; Female: 10–125 ng/mL

Serum ferritin level is useful in evaluating the total storage of iron in the body. It can detect early iron deficiency anemia and anemias due to chronic disease.

Iron (Serum): *Norms:* Adult: 50–150 μg/dL. Infant: 40–100 μg/dL

A decreased serum iron level frequently occurs in iron deficiency anemia. An elevated level might be present in hemolytic, pernicious, and folic acid deficiency anemias.

Iron-Binding Capacity (IBC) or Total Iron-Binding Capacity (TIBC) (Serum): *Norms:* Adult: 250–450 μg/dL. Infant: 100–350 μg/dL

IBC is two to three times greater than the serum iron level. When serum iron is decreased, IBC is increased, and when serum iron is increased, IBC is decreased. A decreased IBC level is present in hemolytic, pernicious, and sickle cell anemias. An elevated IBC level is present in iron deficiency anemia.

Transferrin (Serum): *Norms:* 250–430 mg/dL

Transferrin is responsible for transporting iron to the bone marrow for the purpose of hemoglobin synthesis. A decrease in transferrin occurs in anemias of chronic diseases, and an elevated level occurs in iron deficiency anemia.

Bilirubin Indirect (Serum): *Norms:* Adult: 0.1–1.0 mg/dL

An elevated indirect bilirubin is associated with transfusion reaction and with sickle cell, pernicious, and hemolytic anemias.

Sickle Cell Screening Test: *Norms:* negative

Hb S, a crescent- or sickle-shaped cell, is present in sickle cell disease when the RBC is deprived of oxygen. Hb electrophoresis is needed to confirm sickle cell anemia.

Folic Acid Folate (Serum): *Norms:* Adult: 5–20 ng/mL, >2.5 ng/mL (RIA)

A decreased folic acid level is indicative of folic acid deficiency anemia. In pernicious anemia, the serum folic acid level might be elevated.

Vitamin B₁₂ (Serum): *Adult Norms:* 200–900 pg/mL, 132–703 pmol/L (SI Units)

Vitamin B_{12} is essential for RBC maturation. A decreased vitamin B_{12} level is indicative of pernicious anemia.

Erythrocyte Sedimentation Rate (ESR/Sed Rate) (Blood): *Norms: See values in Part I.*

ESR, a nonspecific test, measures the rate at which RBCs settle in unclotted blood. A decreased ESR could be present in sickle cell anemia and polycythemia vera.

Urobilinogen (Urine): *Norms:* Adult: Random: 0.3–3.5 mg/dL; 24 hours: 0.05–2.5 mg/24 h

Increased urine urobilinogen level could be present in hemolytic, pernicious, and sickle cell anemias.[1,2,5,7,9,11,15]

- Nursing Diagnoses

  - Knowledge deficit related to lack of understanding of laboratory procedures, disease process, and/or outcome
  - Potential for noncompliance with prescribed laboratory tests related to lack of adequate explanation
  - Potential for injury related to bleeding tendencies secondary to hematologic disorders
  - Potential alteration in tissue perfusion related to decreased hemoglobin-carrying oxygen
  - Potential ineffective coping with disease process and laboratory test procedure
  - Potential disturbance in self-concept related to dependence and/or role change
  - Potential alteration in family processes related to patient's chronic hematologic disorder

---

NURSING IMPLICATIONS WITH RATIONALE

- Explain that the purpose for the laboratory tests is to identify the cause for the hematologic disorder.
- Give detailed explanation concerning the test procedures and the need for the patient's compliance. Explanation might be brief or in-depth, depending upon the patient's familiarity with the test.
- Inform the patient of any food, beverage, or drug restrictions. Each test should be checked for specific restrictions (*see Part I*).
- Monitor the patient's vital signs before, during, and after laboratory test procedures. Check respiratory status and skin color, since oxygen deficit frequently results from a decreased hemoglobin.
- Listen to the patient's expressed anxiety or fear concerning the tests and potential clinical problems. Clarification of the test procedure might alleviate fear and anxiety and promote compliance.
- Check laboratory results and notify the physician of abnormal test reports.
- Be supportive of the patient and family members during tests and treatment of hematologic disorders.

Evaluation

- Determine if the test was correctly performed according to the procedure. Notify the laboratory or physician of any changes that occur during the test.
- Check the patient's vital signs and skin color for changes: improvement or deterioration.
- Determine if the patient and family members' fear or anxiety has been lessened or alleviated.
- Clarify or answer any additional questions the patient and family members might have.
- Reinforce the importance of seeking health assistance when changes in health status occur.

LABORATORY/DIAGNOSTIC ASSESSMENTS

REFERENCES

1. *Diagnostic tests handbook*. Springhouse, Penn: Springhouse Corp, 1980.
2. Fischbach, F. *A manual of laboratory diagnostic tests* (3rd ed.). Philadelphia, Lippincott, 1988.
3. Goldstein, R.A., Mullani, N.A., & Wong, W.H. Positron imaging myocardial infarction with rubidium-82. *Journal of Nuclear Medicine*, 1986, *27*, 1824–1829.
4. Govoni, L.E., & Hayes, J.E. *Drugs and nursing implications* (6th ed.). Norwalk, Conn: Appleton & Lange, 1988.
5. Jacobs, D.S. *Laboratory test handbook* (2nd ed.). St. Louis, Mo: Mosby, 1988.
6. Kramer, D.M. Basic principles of magnetic resonance imaging. *Radiologic Clinics of North America*, 1984, *22* (4), 765–778.
7. Phipps, W.J., Long, B.C., & Woods, N.F. *Medical-surgical nursing* (3rd ed.). St. Louis, Mo: Mosby, 1987.
8. Reed, J.D., & Soulen, R.L. Cardiovascular MRI: Current role in patient management. *Radiologic Clinics of North America*, 1988, *26*, (3), 589–600.
9. Tilkian, S.M., Conover, M.C., & Tilkian, A.G. *Clinical implications of laboratory tests* (4th ed.). St. Louis, Mo: Mosby, 1987.
10. Young, S.W. *Nuclear magnetic resonance imaging* (2nd ed.). New York, N.Y.: Raven Press, 1988.
11. Byrne, B.J., Saxton, D.F., & Pelikan, P.K. *Laboratory tests* (2nd ed.). Reading, Mass: Addison-Wesley, 1986.
12. Gefter, W. B. Chest applications of magnetic resonance imaging: An update. *Radiologic Clinics of North America*, 1988, *26* (3), 573–586.
13. Intermountain Thoracic Society. *Clinical pulmonary function testing, a manual of uniform laboratory procedures* (2nd ed.).
14. Miller, W.F., Scacci, R., & Fast, L.R. *Laboratory evaluation of pulmonary function*. Philadelphia, Penn: Lippincott, 1987.
15. Corbett, J.V. *Laboratory tests and diagnostic procedures with nursing diagnoses* (2nd ed.). Norwalk, Conn: Appleton & Lange, 1987.
16. Kee, J.L. *Fluids and electrolytes with clinical applications* (4th ed.). New York, NY: Wiley, 1986.
17. Ravel, R. *Clinical laboratory medicine* (5th ed.). Chicago, ILL: Year Book Medical, 1989.
18. Widmann, F. *Clinical interpretation of laboratory tests* (9th ed.). Philadelphia, Penn: Davis, 1983.
19. Davis, G.R., Santa Ana, C.A., & Morawski, S.C. Development of a lavage solution associated with minimal water and electrolyte absorption or secretion. *Gastroenterology*, 1980, 78, 991–995.

20. Henzel, B.S., Smith, C.E., and Sordelett, S.S. Implementing the diagnostic workup. *Gastrointestinal disorders* (pp. 37–51). Springhouse, Penn: Springhouse Corp, 1984.

21. Brooks, B.J., Beaney, R.P., & Thomas, D.G.T. The role of positron emission tomography in the study of cerebral tumors. *Seminars in Oncology,* 1986, *13,* 83–93.

22. Hyman, R.A., & Gorey, M.T. Imaging strategies for MR of the brain. *Radiologic Clinics of North America,* 1988, *26* (3), 471–502.

23. Rodibaugh, D. Choosing an imaging technique. *Emergency Medicine,* 1987, *19* (4), 26–36.

24. Kee, J.L. Implementing the diagnostic workup. *Endocrine* (pp 31–45). Springhouse, PA: Springhouse Corp, 1984.

25. *Amniotic fluid analysis. Nursing '82,* 1982, *12* (2), 76–79.

26. Brucker, M.C., & MacMullen, N.J. What's new in pregnancy tests. *Journal of Obstetric Gynecologic Nursing* 1985, *14* (5), 353–362.

27. Fantazia, D. Neonatal hypoglycemia. *Journal of Obstetric Gynecologic Nursing,* 1984, *13* (5), 297–300.

28. Gantes, M., Kirchhoff, K.T., and Work, B.A. Breast massage to obtain contraction stress test. *Nursing Research,* 1985, *34* (6), 338–341.

29. Harmon, J.S. *High risk pregnancy and delivery.* St. Louis, Mo: Mosby, 1986.

30. Whaley, L.F., & Wong, D.L. *Nursing care of infants and children* (3rd ed.). St. Louis, Mo: Mosby, 1987.

31. Tietz, N. *Clinical guide to laboratory tests.* Philadelphia, Penn: Saunders, 1983.

32. Carpenits, L.J. *Nursing diagnosis* (2nd ed.). Philadelphia, Penn: Lippincott, 1987.

33. Gordon, M. *Manual of nursing diagnosis* 1984–1985. NY: McGraw-Hill, 1985.

Part IV

Therapeutic Drug Monitoring (TDM)

Selective drugs are monitored by serum and urine for the purposes of achieving and maintaining therapeutic drug effect and for preventing drug toxicity. Drugs with a wide therapeutic range, the difference between effective dose and toxic dose, are not usually monitored. Drug monitoring is important in maintaining a drug concentration-response relationship, especially when the serum drug range is narrow, such as with digoxin and lithium. Therapeutic drug monitoring (TDM) is the process of following drug levels and adjusting them to maintain a therapeutic level.

Drug levels are obtained at peak time and trough time after a steady state of the drug has occurred in the patient. Steady state is reached after four to five half-lives of a drug and can be reached sooner if the drug has a short half-life. Once steady state is achieved, serum drug level is checked at the peak level (maximum drug concentration) and/or at trough/residual level (minimum drug concentration). If the trough or residual level is at the high therapeutic point, toxicity might occur. Careful assessment is needed by both physical and laboratory means.

TDM is required for drugs with a narrow therapeutic index or range; when other methods for monitoring drugs are noneffective, such as blood pressure (BP) monitoring; for determining when adequate blood concentrations are reached; for evaluating patient's compliance to drug therapy; for determining whether other drugs have altered serum drug levels (increasing or decreasing) that could result in drug toxicity or lack of therapeutic effect; and for establishing new serum-drug level when dosage is changed.

Drug groups for TDM include analgesics, antibiotics, anticonvulsants, antineoplastics, bronchodilators, cardiac drugs, hypoglycemics, sedatives, and tranquilizers. To effectively conduct TDM, the laboratory must be provided with the following information: the drug name and daily dosage, time and amount of last dose, time blood was drawn, route of administration, and patient's age. Without complete information, serum drug reporting might be incorrect.[1-7]

DRUG	THERAPEUTIC RANGE	PEAK TIME	TOXIC LEVEL
Acetaminophen (Tylenol)	5–20 μg/mL	1–2½ hours	> 50 μg/mL > 200 μg/mL (Hepatoxicity)
Alcohol	Negative		Mild toxic: 150 mg/dL Marked toxic: >250 mg/dL
Amikacin (Amikin)	Peak: 15–30 μg/mL Trough: 5–10 μg/mL	Intravenously: ½ hour Intramuscular: ½–1½ hours	Peak: > 35 μg/mL Trough: > 10 μg/mL
Aminophylline (see Theophylline)			
Amitriptyline (Elavil)	125–200 ng/mL	2–12 hours	> 500 ng/mL
Amobarbital (Amytal)	5–15 μg/mL	2 hours	> 15 μg/mL Severe toxicity: > 30 μg/mL
Amoxapine (Asendin)	200–400 ng/mL	1½ hours	> 500 ng/mL
Amphetamine		Detectable in urine after 3 hours; positive for 24–48 hours	>30 μg/mL Urine
Aspirin (See Salicylates.)			
Bromide	20–80 mg/dL		> 100 mg/dL
Carbamazepine (Tegretol)	4–12 μg/mL	2–6 hours	> 15 μg/mL
Chloramphenicol (Chloromycetin)	10–20 mg/L		>25 mg/L
Chlordiazepoxide (Librium)	1–5 μg/mL	2–3 hours	> 5 μg/mL
Chlorpromazine (Thorazine)	50–300 ng/mL	2–4 hours	> 750 ng/mL
Clonazepam (Klonopin)	10–50 ng/mL	2 hours	> 100 ng/mL
Desipramine (Norpramin)	125–300 ng/mL	4–6 hours	> 500 ng/mL
Diazepam (Valium)	0.5–2 mg/L 400–600 ng/mL	1–2 hours	> 3 mg/L > 3000 ng/mL
Digitoxin	10–25 ng/mL	Noticeable: 2–4 hours Peak: 12–24 hours	> 30 ng/mL
Digoxin	0.5–2 ng/mL	PO: 6–8 hours IV: 1½–2 hours	> 2.5 ng/mL
Dilantin (See Phenytoin.)			

DRUG	THERAPEUTIC RANGE	PEAK TIME	TOXIC LEVEL
Diltiazem (Cardizem)	50–200 ng/mL	2–3 hours	> 200 ng/mL
Disopyramide (Norpace)	2–5 μg/mL	2 hours	> 7 μg/mL
Doxepin (Sinequan)	150–300 ng/mL	2–4 hours	> 500 ng/mL
Ethosuximide (Zarontin)	40–100 μg/mL	2–4 hours	> 100 μg/mL
Flurazepam (Dalmane)	20–110 ng/mL		> 1500 ng/mL
Gentamicin (Garamycin)	Peak: 5–10 μg/mL Trough: 0.5–2 μg/mL	IV: 15–30 minutes	Peak: > 12 μg/mL Trough: > 2 μg/mL
Glutethimide (Doriden)	2–6 μg/mL		> 20 μg/mL
Haloperidol (Haldol)	3–20 ng/mL	2–6 hours	> 50 ng/mL
Imipramine (Tofranil)	150–300 ng/mL	PO: 1–2 hours IM: 30 minutes	> 500 ng/mL
Kanamycin (Kantrex)	Peak: 15–30 μg/mL Trough: 1–4 μg/mL	PO: 1–2 hours IM: 30 minutes–1 hour	Peak: > 35 μg/mL Trough: > 10 μg/mL
Lead	< 20 μg/dL Urine: < 80 μg/24 hours		> 80 μg/dL Urine: > 125 μg/24 hours
Lidocaine (Xylocaine)	1.5–5 μg/mL	IV: 10 minutes	> 6 μg/mL
Lithium	0.5–1.5 mEq/L	½–4 hours	> 2 mEq/L
Maprotiline (Ludiomil)	200–300 ng/mL	12 hours	> 500 ng/mL
Mephenytoin (Mesantoin)	15–30 μg/mL	2–4 hours	> 50 μg/mL
Meprobamate (Equanil, Miltown)	15–25 μg/mL	2 hours	> 50 μg/mL
Netilmicin (Netromycin)	Peak: 0.5–10 μg/mL Trough: < 4 μg/mL	IV: 30 minutes	Peak: > 16 μg/mL Trough: >4 μg/mL
Nifedipine (Procardia)	50–100 ng/mL	30 minutes	> 100 ng/mL
Nortriptyline (Aventyl)	50–150 ng/mL	8 hours	> 200 ng/mL

(continued)

519

DRUG	THERAPEUTIC RANGE	PEAK TIME	TOXIC LEVEL
Pentobarbital (Nembutal)	2–10 μg/mL	½–1 hour	>10 μg/mL Severe toxicity: > 30 μg/mL
Phenmetrazine (Preludin)	5–30 μg/mL (Urine)	2 hours	> 50 μg/mL (Urine)
Phenobarbital (Luminal)	15–40 μg/mL	6–18 hours	> 40 μg/mL Severe toxicity: > 80 μg/mL
Phenytoin (Dilantin)	10–20 μg/mL	4–8 hours	>20–30 μg/mL Severe toxicity: > 40 μg/mL
Primidone (Mysoline)	5–12 μg/mL	2–4 hours	> 12–15 μg/mL
Procainamide (Pronestyl)	4–10 μg/mL	1 hour	> 10 μg/mL
Prochlorperazine (Compazine)	50–300 ng/mL	2–4 hours	> 1000 ng/mL
Propranolol (Inderal)	50–100 ng/mL	1–2 hours	> 150 ng/mL
Protriptyline (Vivactil)	70–170 ng/mL	8–12 hours	> 200 ng/mL
Quinidine	2–5 μg/mL	1–3 hours	> 6 μg/mL
Salicylates (Aspirin)	15–30 mg/dL	1–2 hours	> 30 mg/dL Severe toxicity: > 50 mg/dL
Secobarbital (Seconal)	5–15 μg/mL	1 hour	> 15 μg/mL Severe toxicity: > 30 μg/mL
Theophylline (Thodur, Aminodur)	5–20 μg/mL	PO: 2–3 hours IV: 15 minutes	> 20 μg/mL
Thioridazine (Mellaril)	100–600 ng/mL	2–4 hours	> 2000 ng/mL > 10 mg/L
Tobramycin (Nebcin)	Peak: 5–10 μg/mL Trough: 1–1.5 μg/mL	IV: 15–30 minutes IM: ½–1½ hours	Peak: > 12 μg/mL Trough: > 2 μg/mL
Trifluoperazine (Stelazine)	50–300 ng/mL	2–4 hours	> 1000 ng/mL
Valproic Acid (Depakene)	50–100 μg/mL	½–1½ hours	> 100 μg/mL Severe toxicity: > 150 μg/mL
Verapamil (Calan)	100–300 ng/mL	PO: 1–2 hours IV: 5 minutes	> 300 ng/mL[1-8]

Therapeutic Drug Monitoring

REFERENCES

1. Byrne, B.J., Saxton, D.F., & Pelikan, P.K. *Laboratory tests* (2nd ed.). Reading, Mass: Addison-Wesley, 1986.
2. Corbett, L.J. *Laboratory tests and diagnostic procedures with nursing diagnoses* (2nd ed.). Norwalk, Conn: Appleton & Lange, 1987.
3. *Diagnostic tests handbook*. Springhouse, Penn: Springhouse Corp, 1987.
4. Fischbach, F.A. *A manual of laboratory diagnostic tests* (3rd ed.). Philadelphia, Penn:, 1988.
5. Jacobs, D.S. *Laboratory test handbook* (2nd ed.). St. Louis, Mo: Mosby, 1988.
6. Nierenberg, D.W. Measuring drug levels in the office: rationale, possible advantages, and potential problems. *Medical Clinics of North America*, 1987, *71* (4), 653–663.
7. Ravel, R. *Clinical Laboratory Medicine* (5th ed.). Chicago, ILL: Year Book Medical publishers, 1989.
8. Govoni, L.E., Hayes, J.E. *Drugs and nursing implications* (6th ed.). Norwalk, Conn: Appleton & Lange, 1988.

Appendix A

Abbreviations of Measurements Used for Normal Values

↑	increased
↓	decreased
>	greater than
<	less than
cm³	cubic centimeter
mm³	cubic millimeter
cu μ	cubic microns
dL	deciliter (100 mL)
fL	femtoliter
g	gram
IU	International Unit
kg	kilogram
L	liter
mol (M)	mole
m²	square meter
mCi	millicurie
mEq	milliequivalent
mg	milligram
mg/dL	milligram per deciliter
mIU	milli-International Unit
mL	milliliter
mm	millimeter
mm³	cubic millimeter
mm Hg	millimeter of mercury
mmol (mM)	millimole
mOsm	milliosmole
mU	milliunit
mUU	mouse uterine units
mμ	millimicron
ng	nanogram
nmol	nanomole
pg	picogram

s	second
SI units	International System of Units
U	unit
μm	micron (micrometer)
μ^3	cubic micron
μg	microgram
μIU	micro-International Unit
μL	microliter
μm^3	cubic micrometer
μmol	micromole
μU	microunit

Appendix B

Abbreviations for Laboratory and Diagnostic Tests

ABG	Arterial blood gas
ACP	Acid phosphatase
ACTH	Adrenocorticotropic hormone
ADH	Antidiuretic hormone
AFB	Acid-fast bacillus
AFP	Alpha-fetoprotein
AGBM	Antiglomerular basement membrane antibody
A/G Ratio	Albumin/Globulin Ratio
AHF	Antihemophilic factor
AIDS	Acquired immune deficiency syndrome
ALD	Aldolase
ALP	Alkaline phosphatase
ALT	Alanine aminotransferase (same as SGPT)
α-1-AT	Alpha-1-antitrypsin
ANA	Antinuclear antibodies
Anti-DNA	Anti-deoxyribonucleic acid
APTT	Activated partial thromboplastin time
ARC	AIDS-related complex
ASO	Antistreptolysin O
AST	Aspartate aminotransferase (same as SGOT)
BE	Base excess
BP	Blood pressure
BUN	Blood urea nitrogen
C	Complement (eg, complement C_3)
Ca	Calcium
CA	Cold agglutinins
cAMP	Cyclic adenosine monophosphate
CAT	Computerized axial tomography
CBC	Complete blood count
CEA	Carcinoembryonic antigen
CHF	Congestive heart failure
CHS	Cholinesterase

CHO	Carbohydrate
Cl	Chloride
CO	Carbon monoxide
CO_2	Carbon dioxide
Cp	Ceruloplasmin
CPK or CK	Creatine phosphokinase
CPK-BB	Creatine phosphokinase, brain
CPK-MB	Creatine phosphokinase, heart
CPK-MM	Creatine phosphokinase, skeletal muscle
Cr	Creatinine
CRF	Corticotropin-releasing factor
CRP	C-reactive protein
CSF	Cerebrospinal fluid
CT	Coagulation time
CT	Computerized tomography
CTT	Computerized transaxial tomography
Cu	Copper
DIC	Disseminated intravascular coagulation
E_2	Estradiol
E_3	Estriol
EBV	Ebstein-Barr virus
ECG (EKG)	Electrocardiogram
ECF	Extracellular fluid
EDTA	Ethylenediaminetetraacetate
EEG	Electroencephalogram
ELISA	Enzyme-linked immunosorbent assay
EMG	Electromyography
ERCP	Endoscopic retrograde cholangiopancreatography
ESR	Erythrocyte sedimentation rate
FBS	Fasting blood sugar
FDP	Fibrin degradation products
FSH	Follicle-stimulating hormone
FSP	Fibrin or fibrinogen-split product
FTA-ABS	Fluorescent treponemal antibody absorption
G-6-PD	Glucose-6-phosphate dehydrogenase
GGTP or GTP	Gamma-glutamyl (transferase) transpeptidase
GI series	Gastrointestinal series (upper)
GH	Growth hormone
HAA	Hepatitis-associated antigen
HAI or HI	Hemagglutination inhibition
Hb or Hgb	Hemoglobin
HB_cAb	Hepatitis B core antibody
HB_sAb	Hepatitis B surface antibody
HB_sAg	Hepatitis B surface antigen
HCG	Human chorionic gonadotropin
HCO_3	Bicarbonate
Hct	Hematocrit
hCT	Calcitonin
HDL	High-density lipoprotein

5-HIAA	5-Hydroxyindolacetic acid
HIV	Human immuno-suppressive virus
Hp	Haptoglobin
HLA	Human leukocyte antigen
HPL	Human placental lactogen
HTLV-III	Human T-Lymphotropic Virus-III
IBC	Iron-binding capacity (see TIBC)
Ig	Immunoglobulin
IM	Intramuscular
IV	Intravenous
IVP	Intravenous pyelography
K	Potassium
17-KS	17-Ketosteroid
KUB	Kidney, ureter, bladder
LAP	Leucine aminopeptidase
LAV	Lymphadenopathy-associated virus
LDH (LD)	Lactic dehydrogenase
LDL	Low-density lipoprotein
LE	Lupus erythematosus preparation
LH	Luteinizing hormone
L/S	Lecithin/sphingomyelin
MCH	Mean corpuscular hemoglobin
MCHC	Mean corpuscular-hemoglobin concentration
MCV	Mean corpuscular volume
Mg	Magnesium
MI	Myocardial infarction
5'NT	5'Nucleotidase
Na	Sodium
NPO	Nothing by mouth
17-OHCS	17-Hydroxycorticosteroid
P	Phosphorus
PAP	Pulmonary arterial pressure
P_{CO_2}	Partial pressure of carbon dioxide
PCWP	Pulmonary capillary wedge pressure
pH	Negative logarithm of hydrogen ion concentration
PKU	Phenylketonuria
P_{O_2}	Partial pressure of oxygen
PPBS	Postprandial blood sugar (feasting blood sugar)
PRL	Prolactin
PT	Prothrombin time
PTH	Parathyroid hormone
PTT	Partial thromboplastin time
RA	Rheumatoid arthritis
RAIU	Radioactive iodine uptake
RBC	Red blood cell
RDW	Red blood cell distribution width
RF	Rheumatoid factor
RIA	Radioimmunoassay
RPR	Rapid plasma reagin

SGOT	Serum glutamic oxaloacetic transaminase (same as AST)
SGPT	Serum glutamic pyruvic transaminase (same as ALT)
SIADH	Syndrome of inappropriate antidiuretic hormone
SLE	Systemic lupus erythematosus
So_2	Oxygen saturation
T_3	Triiodothyronine
T_4	Thyroxine
TA	Thyroid antibodies
TB	Tuberculosis
TBG	Thyroxine-binding globulin
TCA	Tricyclic antidepressants
TDM	Therapeutic drug monitoring
TIBC	Total iron-binding capacity (see IBC)
TRH	Thyrotropin-releasing hormone
$T_3 RU$	T_3 resin uptake
TSH	Thyroid-stimulating hormone
UA	Urinalysis
URI	Upper respiratory infections
VCT	Venous clotting time
VDRL	Venereal disease research laboratory
VLDL	Very low-density lipoprotein
VMA	Vanillylmandelic acid
VS	Vital signs
WBC	White blood cell (leukocyte)

Appendix C

Laboratory Test Groups

Groups of laboratory tests, identified as panels, profiles, evaluations, and sequential multiple analyzers (SMAs), are useful for diagnosing and assessing clinical problems. Tests are usually grouped as general tests for determining health status and organ and disease panels/profiles/evaluations. Laboratories, private or in health care institutions, develop test groups according to their equipment for analyzing laboratory values. The majority of these tests require either one 10-mL red-top tube, one 15-mL red-top tube, or two 10-mL red-top tubes of blood.

GENERAL LABORATORY TEST GROUPS

General Health Panel[1]

Albumin
Alkaline phosphatase
AST/SGOT
Bilirubin (total)
BUN
Calcium
Cholesterol
Creatinine
Glucose
LD/LDH
Potassium
Protein (total)
Sodium
Triglyceride
Uric acid

Chemzyme Evaluation,[2] or Profile 22

A/G ratio
Albumin
Alkaline phosphatase
ALT/SGPT
AST/SGOT
Bilirubin (total)
BUN
BUN/creatinine ratio
Calcium
Chloride
Cholesterol
CO_2 (content)
Creatinine
Globulin
Glucose
LD/LDH
Phosphorus
Potassium

Protein (total)   Triglyceride
Sodium   Uric acid

Chemistry Profile[3]

Albumin   Creatinine
Alkaline phosphatase   Glucose
AST/SGOT   LD/LDH
Bilirubin (total)   Phosphorus
BUN   Protein (total)
Calcium   Uric acid

Profile 11[4]

Albumin   CPK/CK
Alkaline phosphatase   LD/LDH
AST/SGOT   Phosphorus
Bilirubin (total)   Protein (total)
Calcium   Uric acid
Cholesterol

Electrolytes (LYTES)

(Might be ordered with SMA_{12}, chemistry profile, or profile 11)

Chloride   Potassium
CO_2 content   Sodium

SMA 12–60

(Laboratory may select any 12 tests to program on their analyzer.)

Albumin   Cholesterol
Alkaline phosphatase   Glucose
AST/SGOT   LD/LDH
Bilirubin (total)   Phosphorus
BUN   Protein (total)
Calcium   Uric acid

SMA 6–60

(Might be ordered with SMA 12 or chemistry profile)
BUN   Creatinine
Chloride   Potassium
CO_2 content   Sodium

Profile 7[4]

(Might be ordered with profile 11)

BUN	Glucose
Chloride	Potassium
CO_2 content	Sodium
Creatinine	

ROUTINE HEMATOLOGY AND URINE TESTS

Complete Blood Count (CBC)

WBC count and differential:	Hematocrit
Neutrophil	Hemoglobin
band	RBC count
segment	RBC indices
Basophils	MCV
Eosinophils	MCH
Lymphocytes	MCHC
Monocytes	RDW

Urinalysis

Appearance	pH
Bacteria	Protein
Casts	RBC
Color	Specific gravity (SG)
Glucose	WBC
Ketones	

ORGAN AND DISEASE PANEL/PROFILE/EVALUATION

Anemia Panel/Profile/Evaluation[1,5]

CBC with RBC indices	Reticulocyte count
Folate/folic acid	TIBC
Hemoglobin electrophoresis	Vitamin B_{12}
Iron	

Arthritis Panel/Profile/Evaluation[1,2,6]

ANA	ESR
ASO	Phosphorus
Calcium	Rheumatoid factor
CRP	Uric acid

Bone/Joint Panel/Profile/Evaluation[1,2]

Albumin
Alkaline phosphatase
Calcium
Phosphorus

Protein (total)
Synovial fluid analysis
Uric acid

Cardiac Panel/Profile/Evaluation[1,5]

AST/SGOT
CPK/CK
CPK isoenzymes

LDH/LD
LDH isoenzymes
Potassium

Coagulation Panel/Profile/Evaluation[1,4–6]

APTT
Bleeding time
Clot retraction
Coagulation time/clotting time

Factor assay
FDP
Platelet count
PT

Coma Panel/Profile/Evaluation[1,5]

Alcohol
Ammonia
Blood gases (pH, Pco_2, HCO_3)
BUN
Creatinine
Drug-abuse toxicology screen

Electrolytes
Glucose
Lactic acid
Osmolality (serum and urine)
Salicylate

Coronary Risk Panel/Profile/Evaluation[1,2,5]

Cholesterol (total)
  HDL
  LDL
  VLDL
Glucose

Lipoprotein phenotyping
Phospholipids
Total lipids
Triglycerides

Diabetes Mellitus Panel/Profile/Evaluation[1,5]

BUN
Cholesterol
Creatinine
Electrolytes (K, Na, Cl, CO_2)
Glucose (fasting/2-hour feasting)

Glucose tolerance (*not* for high blood
  sugar)
Ketones (serum and urine)
Triglycerides

Drug Toxicology/Drug Abuse Panel/Profile/Evaluation[2]

Acetaminophen
Amphetamines

Barbiturates
Benzodiazepines

Cocaine
Codeine
Meperidine (Demerol)
Meprobamate (Equanil)
Methadone
Morphine

Phenothiazines
Phenytoin (Dilantin)
Propoxyphene (Darvon)
Salicylates
Tricylic antidepressants

Hepatic/Liver Panel/Profile/Evaluation[1-5]

A/G ratio
Albumin
Alkaline phosphatase
ALT/SGPT
AST/SGOT
Bilirubin (total and direct)

Cholesterol
GGT/GGTP
LDH/LD
LDH isoenzymes
Protein (total)
PT

Hepatitis Panel/Profile/Evaluation[1,2,3,5,6]

HB$_c$Ab or Anti-HB$_c$ (antibody to hepa-
titis B core antigen)
HB$_e$Ab (hepatitis B e antibody) or
Anti-HB$_e$ (antibody to HB$_e$Ag)
HB$_e$Ag (hepatitis B e antigen)

HB$_s$Ab (hepatitis B surface antibody)
or Anti-HB$_s$ (antibody to Hb$_s$Ag)
HB$_s$Ag (hepatitis B surface antigen)
Anti-HAV (antibody to hepatitis A
virus [IgM])

Hypertension Panel/Profile/Evaluation[1,5,6]

BUN
Creatinine
Cholesterol
Electrolytes (K, Na, Cl, CO_2)
Glucose

LDH/LD
Renin
T$_4$
Triglycerides
VMA

Lipid Panel/Profile/Evaluation[2]

Cholesterol (total)
   HDL
   LDL

Lipids (total)
Phospholipids
Triglycerides

Neonatal Panel/Profile/Evaluation[5]

Albumin
Bilirubin (total)
Blood type (ABO)
BUN

Calcium
Electrolytes (K, Na, Cl, CO_2)
Glucose
Rh typing

Pancreatic Panel/Profile/Evaluation[1,5]

Amylase
Calcium

Glucose
Lipase

Parathyroid Panel/Profile/Evaluation[1,5]

Alkaline phosphatase
Calcium (serum and urine)
Magnesium

Phosphorus
Protein (total)

Prenatal Panel/Profile/Evaluation[2,5,6]

Atypical antibody screen
Blood type (ABO)
CBC with differential
Rh typing

RPR or VDRL
Rubella screen
Urinalysis

Pulmonary/Lung Panel/Profile/Evaluation[1,2]

Blood gases (pH, Pco_2, Po_2, HCO_3)
CO_2 content
So_2

Renal Panel/Profile/Evaluation[1,5]

Albumin
BUN
Creatinine (serum and 24-hour urine)
Creatinine clearance

Electrolytes (K, Na, Cl, CO_2)
Glucose
Protein (total and 24-hour urine)
Uric acid

Thyroid Panel/Profile/Evaluation[1,3,5,6]

Calcitonin
Free thyroxine index (FTI or Free T_4)
T_4 RIA

T_3RIA
T_3 resin uptake
TSH
TA

REFERENCES

1. Henry, J. B. *Todd-Sanford-Davidsohn: Clinical diagnosis and laboratory methods* (17th ed.). Philadelphia, Penn: Saunders, 1984.
2. *Bio-Science directory of services.* Van Nuys, Calif: Bio-Science Laboratories, 1980.
3. Jacobs, D. S., *Laboratory test handbook with DRG index.* (2nd ed.). St. Louis, Mo: Mosby, 1988.
4. *VA Medical Center's laboratory values.* Elsmere, Del: Veteran's Administration, 1985.
5. Byrne, C. J., Saxton, D. F., Pelikan, P. K. *Laboratory tests* (2nd ed.). Reading, Mass: Addison-Wesley, 1986.
6. Upjohn Company. *Laboratory procedures, service manual.* Eastern Region: King of Prussia, Penn: Upjohn, 1981.

Appendix D

Laboratory Test Values for Adults and Children

The laboratory tests and their reference values for adults and children are listed according to the laboratory sections that analyze the specimens. The personnel from the laboratory department and nuclear medicine frequently work together in obtaining blood specimens to be tested by the radioimmunoassay (RIA) method. So that the patient does not receive several venous punctures, the laboratory personnel will collect enough blood for all laboratory tests, including RIA.

Arterial blood gases are analyzed in either the pulmonary function laboratory, critical care units, or chemistry section of the laboratory. The cerebrospinal fluid tubes are distributed to the appropriate laboratory sections (ie, hematology, chemistry, or microbiology).

Reference values differ from laboratory to laboratory, so nurses should refer to the published laboratory values used in their hospitals or private laboratories to check for any differences.

Reference Values

Hematology	Color-top tube	Adult	Child
Bleeding time		Ivy's method: 3–7 minutes Duke's method: 1–3 minutes	Same as adult
Carboxyhemoglobin (CO)—See Chemistry.			
Clot retraction	Red	1–24 hours	Same as adult
Coagulation time (CT)		5–15 minutes	Same as adult
		Average: 8 minutes	
Erythrocyte sedimentation rate (ESR)	Lavender	<50 years old (Westergren) Male: 0–10 mm/h Female: 0–20 mm/h >50 years old (Westergren) Male: 0–20 mm/h Female: 0–30 mm/h Wintrobe method: Male: 0–7 mm/h Female: 0–15 mm/h	Newborn: 0–2 mm/hour 4–14 years old: 0–20 mm/hour
Factor assay	Blue		
I Fibrinogen		200–400 mg/dL	Same as adult
II Prothrombin		Minimum for clotting: 75–100 mg/dL Minimum hemostatic level: 10%–15% concentration	
III Thromboplastin		Variety of substances	
IV Calcium		4.5–5.5 mEq/L or 9–11 mg/dL	
V Proaccelerin labile factor		Minimum hemostatic level: 50%–150% activity; 5%–10% concentration	Same as adult
VI		Not used	
VII Proconvertin stable factor		Minimum hemostatic level: 65%–135% activity; 5%–15% concentration	
VIII Antihemophilic factor (AHF)		Minimum hemostatic level: 55%–145% activity; 30%–35% concentration	
IX Plasma thromboplastin component (PTC, Christmas factor)		Minimum hemostatic level: 60%–140% activity; 30% concentration	
X Stuart factor, Prower factor		Minimum hemostatic level: 45%–150% activity; 7%–10% concentration	
XI Plasma thromboplastin antecedent (PTA)		Minimum hemostatic level: 65%–135% activity; 20%–30% concentration	

Test	Tube color	Normal values	Pediatric values
XII Hageman factor		0% concentration	
XIII Fibrinase, fibrin stabilizing factor (FSF)		Minimum hemostatic level: 1% concentration	Not usually done
Fibrin degradation products (FDP)	Red	2 to 10 µg/mL	
Fibrinogen	Blue	200–400 mg/dL	Newborn: 150–300 mg/dL Child: same as adult
Hematocrit (Hct)	Lavender	Male: 40%–54%; 0.40–0.54 SI units Female: 36%–46%; 0.36–0.46 SI units	Newborn: 44%–65% 1–3 years old: 29%–40% 4–10 years old: 31%–43%
Hemoglobin (Hb or Hgb)	Lavender	Male: 13.5–18 g/dL Female: 12–16 g/dL	Newborn: 14–24 g/dL Infant: 10–15 g/dL Child: 11–16 g/dL
Hemoglobin electrophoresis	Lavender		
A_1		95%–98% total Hb	
A_2		1.5%–4.0%	
F		<2%	Newborn: 50%–80% total Hb Infant: 2%–8% total Hb Child: 1%–2% total Hb
C		0%	
D		0%	
S		0%	
Lymphocytes (T & B) assay	Lavender (2 tubes)	T cells: 60%–80%, 600–2400 cells/µL B cells: 4%–16% 50–250 cells/µL	
Osmotic fragility: erythrocyte			Same as adult

	% Hemolysis	
% Saline (NaCl)	Fresh blood (3 hours)	Incubated at 37°C (24-hour blood)
0.30	97–100	85–100
0.35	90–98	75–100
0.40	50–95	65–100
0.45	5–45	55–95
0.50	0–5	40–85
0.55	0	15–65
0.60	0	0–40

(continued)

Hematology	Color-top tube	Adult	Child (Reference Values)
Partial thromboplastin time (PTT)	Blue	PPT: 60–70 seconds APTT: 25–40 seconds	
Plasminogen	Blue	2.5–5.2 U/mL 3.8–8.4 CTA	
Platelet aggregation and adhesion	Blue	Aggregation in 3–5 minutes	
Platelet count (thrombocytes)	Lavender	150,000–400,000 μL (mean, 250,000 μL) SI units: 0.15–0.4 $\times$ 10^{12}/L	Premature: 100,000–300,000 μL Newborn: 150,000–300,000 μL Infant: 200,000–475,000 μL Same as adult
Prothrombin time (PT)	Blue or black	11–15 seconds or 70%–100% Anticoagulant therapy: 2–2.5 times the control in seconds or 20%–30%	
RBC indices (mil/μL)	Lavender	Male: 4.6–6.0 Female: 4.0–5.0	Newborn: 4.8–7.2 Child: 3.8–5.5
MCV (cuμ)		80–98	Newborn: 96–108 Child: 82–92
MCH (pg)		27–31	Newborn: 32–34 Child: 27–31
MCHC (%)		32–36	Newborn: 32–33 Child: 32–36
RDW (Coulter S)		11.5–14.5	
Reticulocyte count	Lavender	0.5%–1.5% of all RBCs 25,000–75,000 μL (absolute count)	Newborn: 2.5%–6.5% of all RBCs Infant: 0.5%–3.5% of all RBCs Child: 0.5%–2.0% of all RBCs
Sickle cell screening	Lavender	0	0
White blood cells (WBC)	Lavender	4,500–10,000 μL	Newborn: 9000–30,000 μL 2 years old: 6000–17,000 μL
White blood cell differential	Lavender		
Neutrophils		50%–70% of total WBCs	29%–47%
Segments		50%–65%	
Bands		0%–5%	
Eosinophils		0%–3%	0%–3%
Basophils		1%–3%	1%–3%

	Color-top tube	Adult	Child
Lymphocytes		25%–35%	38%–63%
Monocytes		2%–6%	4%–9%
Immunohematology (Blood Bank)			
Coombs direct	Lavender	Negative	Negative
Coombs indirect	Red	Negative	Negative
Cross matching	Red	Absence of agglutination (clumping)	Same as adult
Rh typing	Red	Rh+ and Rh−	Same as adult

		Reference Values	
Chemistry	**Color-top tube**	*Adult*	*Child*
Acetaminophen	Red	Therapeutic: 5–20 μg/mL; 31–124 μmol/L (SI units) Toxic: >50 μg/mL; >305 μmol/L (SI units) >200 μg/mL, possible hepatotoxicity	Therapeutic: same as adult
Acetone (ketone bodies)	Red	Acetone: 0.3–2.0 mg/dL; 51.6–344 μmol/L (SI units) Ketones: 2–4 mg/dL	Newborn: slightly higher than adult Infant and child: same as adult
Acid phosphatase (ACP)	Red	0.0–0.8 U/L at 37°C (SI units)	6.4–15.2 U/L
Adrenocorticotropic hormone (ACTH)	Green	7 AM–10 AM up to 80 pg/mL	
Alanine aminotransferase (ALT, SGPT)	Red	5–35 U/mL (Frankel)	Same as adult
		5–25 mU/mL (Wroblewski) 8–50 U/mL at 30°C (Karmen) 4–36 U/L at 37°C (SI units)	Infant: could be twice as high
Albumin	Red	3.5–5 g/dL	
Alcohol	Red	0%	
Aldolase (ALD)	Red	3–8 U/dL (Sibley-Lehinger) 22–59 mU/L at 37°C (SI units)	Infant: 12–24 U/dL Child: 6–16 U/dL
Aldosterone	Red or green	Normal salt intake: 1–9 ng/dL (supine position); 4–30 ng/dL (sitting position)	
Alkaline phosphatase (ALP)	Red	30–120 IU/L 25–97 U/L at 37°C (SI units) 2–4 U/dL (Bodansky) 4–13 U/dL (King-Armstrong) 0.8–2.3 U/dL (Bessey-Lowry)	Infant: 40–300 U/L Child: 60–270 U/L; 15–30 U/dL (King-Armstrong); 5–14 U/dL (Bodansky)

(continued)

Reference Values

Chemistry	Color-top tube	Adult	Child
ALP[1] ALP[2]	Red	20–120 U/L 20–110 U/L	
Alpha-1-antitrypsin	Red	78–200 mg/dL	Newborn: 145–270 mg/dL Infant and child: same as adult
Alpha-fetoprotein (AFP)	Red	0.78–2.0 g/L	

Weeks of gestation	Serum (ng/mL)	Amniotic fluid (µg/mL)
14	7–50	11.0–32.0
15	7–60	5.5–31.0
16	10–72	5.7–31.5
17	11–90	3.8–32.5
18	14–94	3.6–28.0
19	24–112	3.7–24.5
20	31–122	2.2–15.0

Chemistry	Color-top tube	Adult	Child
Amikacin	Red	Therapeutic: Peak: 15–30 µg/mL Trough: <10 µg/mL Toxic: >35 µg/mL	
Amitriptyline (Elavil)		Therapeutic range: 125–200 ng/mL Toxic level: > 500 ng/mL	
Ammonia	Green	15–45 µg/dL 11–35 umol/L (SI units)	Newborn: 64–107 µg/dL Child: 21–50 µg/dL
Amylase	Red	60–160 Somogyi U/dL 25–125 U/L (SI units)	Not usually done
Anion gap		11–17 mEq/L	
Antidiuretic hormone (ADH)	Lavender	<5 pg/mL	
Arterial blood gases (see Others)			
Ascorbic acid (vitamin C)	Gray or red	0.6–2.0 mg/dL (plasma) 34–114 µmol/L (SI units, plasma) 0.2–2.0 mg/dL (blood) 12–114 µmol/L (SI units, serum)	0.6–1.6 mg/dL (plasma)

Test	Tube	Normal Values	Pediatric/Other
Aspartate aminotransferase (AST, SGOT)	Red	5–40 U/mL (Frankel) 4–36 IU/L 16–60 U/ml at 30°C 8–33 U/L at 37°C (SI units)	Newborn: four times normal level Child: Same as adult
Barbiturate Phenobarbital		0 Therapeutic: 10–30 μg/mL Toxic: >60 μg/mL	0 15–30 μg/mL
Bilirubin (indirect)	Red	0.1–1.0 mg/dL 1.7–17.1 μmol/L (SI units)	
Bilirubin (total and direct)	Red	Total: 0.1–1.2 mg/dL; 1.7–20.5 μmol/L (SI units) Direct (conjugated): 0.1–0.3 mg/dL; 1.7–5.1 μmol/L (SI units)	Newborn, total: 1–12 mg/dL; 17.1–205 μmol/L (SI units) Child, total: 0.2–0.8 mg/dL
Blood urea nitrogen (BUN)	Red	5–25 mg/dL	Infant: 5–15 mg/dL Child: 5–20 mg/dL
Bromide	Green	0	0
Calcitonin	Green or lavender	Therapeutic: <80 mg/dL Toxic: >100 mg/dL Male: <40 pg/mL Female: <20 pg/mL	Newborn: usually higher
Calcium (Ca)	Red	4.5–5.5 mEq/L 9–11 mg/dL 2.3–2.8 mmol/L (SI units)	Newborn: 3.7–7.0 mEq/L; 7.4–14 mg/dL Infant: 5.0–6.0 mEq/L; 10–12 mg/dL Child: 4.5–5.8 mEq/L; 9–11.5 mg/dL
Ionized Calcium (iCa)		4.4–5.9 mg/dL 2.2–2.5 mEq/L 1.1–1.24 mmol/L	
Carbamazepine	Red	Therapeutic: 4–12 μg/mL; 16.9–50.8 μmol/L (SI units) Toxic: >12–15 μg/mL; >50.8–69 μmol/L (SI units)	
Carbon dioxide combining power (CO₂)	Green	22–30 mEq/L 22–30 mmol/L (SI units)	20–28 mEq/L
Carbon monoxide (CO)	Lavender	2.5% saturation of Hb	Same as adult

(continued)

Chemistry	Color-top tube	Adult	Child
Carboxyhemoglobin (may be done in hematology)		2%–9% saturation of Hb (smokers)	
Carotene	Red	60–200 mg/dL	40–130 μg/dL
Ceruloplasmin (Cp)	Red	18–45 mg/dL 0.74–3.72 μmol/L (SI units)	Infant: <23 mg/dL or normal Child: same as adult
Chlordiazepoxide (Librium)	Red	180–450 mg/L (SI units) Therapeutic Level: 1.0–5.0 ug/mL Toxic: > 6 ug/mL	
Chloride (Cl)	Red	95–105 mEq/L 95–105 mmol/L (SI units)	Newborn: 94–112 mEq/L Infant: 95–110 mEq/L Child: 98–105 mEq/L
Cholesterol	Red	Desirable level: < 200 mg/dL Moderate risk: 200–240 mg/dL High risk: > 240 mg/dL	Infant: 90–130 mg/dL 2–19 years: Desirable level: 130–170 mg/dL; Moderate risk: 171–184 mg/dL; High risk: > 185 mg/dL
Cholinesterase	Green	0.5–1.0 U (RBC) 3–8 U/mL (plasma) 6–8 IU/L (RBC) 8–18 IU/L at 37°C (plasma)	Same as adult
Copper (Cu)	Red or green	Male: 70–140 μg/dL: 11–22 μmol/L (SI units) Female: 80–155 μg/dL; 12.6–24.3 μmol/L (SI units) Pregnancy: 140–300 μg/dL	Newborn: 20–70 μg/dL Child: 30–190 μg/dL Adolescent: 90–240 μg/dL
Cortisol	Green	8 AM–10 AM: 5–23 μg/dL; 138–635 nmol/L (SI units) 4 PM–6 PM: 3–13 μg/dL; 83–359 nmol/L (SI units)	8 AM–10 AM: 15–25 μg/dL 4 PM–6 PM: 5–10 μg/dL
Creatine phosphokinase (CPK)	Red	Male: 5–35 μg/mL; 30–180 IU/L, 55–170 U/L at 37°C (SI units) Female: 5–25 μg/mL; 25–150 IU/L; 30–135 U/L at 37°C (SI units)	Newborn: 65–580 IU/L at 30°C Child: Male: 0–70 IU/L at 30°C Female: 0–50 IU/L at 30°C

Test	Tube	Reference Values	
Creatinine	Red	0.5–1.5 mg/dL 45–132.3 umol/L (SI units)	Newborn: 0.8–1.4 mg/dL Infant: 0.7–1.7 mg/dL 2–6 years: 0.3–0.6 mg/dL, 24–54 umol/L (SI units) 7–18 years: 0.4–1.2 mg/dL, 36–106 umol/L (SI units)
Cryoglobulins	Red	Negative	
Diltiazem (Cardizem)	Red	Therapeutic: 50–200 ng/mL Toxic: >200 ng/mL	
Disseminated intravascular coagulation (DIC) screening test		See Part III, Hematologic Conditions.	
Dexamethasone suppression test	Green	Cortisol: 8 AM: <10 µg/dL	
Diazepam (Valium)	Red	Therapeutic: 400–600 ng/mL; 0.5–2.0 mg/L; Toxic: >1000 ng/mL; >3 mg/L	
Digoxin	Red	Therapeutic: 0.5–2 ng/mL; 0.5–2 nmol/L (SI units) Toxic: >2 ng/mL; >2.6 nmol/L (SI units)	Therapeutic: Infant: 1–3 ng/mL; 1–3 nmol/L (SI units) Toxic: >3.5 ng/mL
Doxepin (Sinequan)		Therapeutic range: 150–250 ng/mL Toxic level: > 500 ng/mL	
D-xylose absorption	Red	25–40 mg/dL/2 h Elderly: same as adult	30 mg/dL/1 h
Estradiol (E$_2$)	Red	Female: Follicular: 20–150 pg/mL Midcycle: 100–500 pg/mL Luteal: 60–260 pg/mL Postmenopausal: < 30 pg/mL Male: 15–50 pg/mL	3–10 pg/mL
Estriol/E$_3$	Red	Pregnancy: Serum	

Weeks of Gestation	ng/dL
25–28	25–165
29–32	30–230
33–36	45–370
37–38	75–420
39–40	95–450

(continued)

		Reference Values	
Chemistry	Color-top tube	Adult	Child
Estrogen	Red	Female: Early Menstrual Cycle: 60–400 pg/mL Midmenstrual Cycle: 120–440 pg/mL Male: 40–155 pg/mL	1–6 years: 3–10 pg/mL 8–12 years: <30 pg/mL
Ethosuximide	Red	Therapeutic: 40–100 μg/mL; 283–708 μmol/L Toxic: >100 μg/mL; >708 μmol/L (SI units)	Therapeutic: 2–4 per/mg/kg/day Toxic: same as adult or higher
Fasting blood sugar (FBS)	Gray or red	70–110 mg/dL (serum)	Newborn: 30–80 mg/dL
Feasting blood sugar (see postprandial blood sugar)		60–100 mg/dL (blood)	Child: 60–100 mg/dL
Ferritin	Red	Female: 10–125 ng/mL 10–300 ug/L Male: 35–300 ng/mL 35–300 ug/L	Newborn: 20–200 ng/mL Infant: 30–200 ng/mL 1–16 years: 8–140 ng/mL
Folate (folic acid) (may be done by nuclear medicine)	Red	3–16 ng/mL (bioassay) >2.5 ng/mL (RIA; serum) 200–700 ng/mL (RBC)	Same as adult
Follicle-stimulating hormone (FSH)	Red	Pre-postovulation: 4–30 mU/mL Midcycle: 10–90 mU/mL Postmenopausal: 40–250 mU/mL Male: 4–25 mU/mL	5–12 mU/mL
Gamma-glutamyl transpeptidase (GGTP)	Red	Male: 10–80 IU/L Female: 5–25 IU/L; 5–40 U/L at 37°C (SI units)	
Gastrin	Red or lavender	Fasting; <100 pg/mL	Not usually done

(continued)

Test	Tube Color	Adult Values	Child (6 years or older)
Gentamicin	Red	Therapeutic: Peak: 5–10 μg/mL Trough: <2 μg/mL Toxic: >12 μg/mL	Same as adult
Glucose-6-phosphate dehydrogenase (G-6-PD) (may be done in hematology)	Lavender or green	8–18 IU/gHb 125–281 U/dL (packed RBC) 251–511 U/dL (cells) 1211–2111 mIU/mL (packed RBC)	
Glucose—fasting blood sugar (See *Fasting blood sugar.*)			
Glucagon	Lavender	50–200 pg/mL	
Glucose tolerance test (GTT)	Gray or red	(see table below)	Same as adult
Growth hormone	Red	Average: < 10 ng/mL Male: < 10 ng/mL Female: < 15 ng/mL	< 10 ng/mL
Haloperidol (Haldol)	Red	Therapeutic range: 3–20 ng/mL Toxic: > 50 ng/mL	
Hexosaminidase	Red	Total: 5–20 U/L A: 55%–80%	
Human chorionic gonadotropin (HCG)	Red	Nonpregnant female: <0.01 IU/mL (see table below)	

Glucose tolerance test (GTT):

Time	Serum (mg/dL)	Blood (mg/dL)
Fasting	70–110	60–100
0.5 hour	<160	<150
1 hour	<170	<160
2 hour	<125	<115
3 hour	Fasting level	Fasting level

Human chorionic gonadotropin (HCG):

Pregnant (Weeks)	Values
1	0.01–0.04 IU/mL
2	0.03–0.10 IU/mL
4	0.10–1.0 IU/mL
5–12	10–100 IU/mL
13–25	10–30 IU/mL
26–40	5–15 IU/mL

Chemistry	Color-top tube	Reference Values	
		Adult	Child
Human immunosuppressive virus (HIV)	Red	Negative	
Human leukocyte antigen (HLA)	Green	Histocompatibility match	
Human placental lactogen (HPL)	Red or green	Weeks of gestation ng/mL	
		8–27 4.6 μg/mL	
		28–31 2.4–6.0 μg/mL	
		32–35 3.7–7.7 μg/mL	
		36–40 5.0–10.0 μg/mL	
Imipramine (Tofranil)	Red	Therapeutic range: 150–300 ng/mL Toxic level: > 500 ng/mL	
Immunoglobulins (see serology)	Red		
Insulin	Red	5–25 μU/mL	
Iron	Red	50–150 μg/dL; 10–27 μmol/L (SI units)	6 months–2 years: 40–100 μg/dL Newborn: 100–270 μg/dL
Iron-binding capacity (IBC, TIBC)	Red	250–450 μg/dL	Infant (6 months–2 years): 100–350 μg/dL Child: same as adult
Lactic acid	Green	Arterial blood: 0.5–2.0 mEq/L; 11.3 mg/dL Venous blood: 0.5–1.5 mEq/L; 8.1–15.3 mg/dL	
Lactic dehydrogenase (LDH/LD)	Red	Critical: >5 mEq/L; >45 mg/dL 100–190 IU/L; 70–250 U/L	Newborn: 300–1500 IU/L Child: 50–150 IU/L
LDH isoenzymes	Red		
LDH_1		14%–26%	
LDH_2		27–37%	
LDH_3		20%–26%	
LDH_4		8%–16%	
LDH_5		6%–16%	

(continued)

Lactose tolerance test	Gray	20–50 mg/dL rise from fasting blood glucose	
Lead	Lavender or green	10–20 μg/dL	10–20 μg/dL
		20–40 μg/dL (acceptable)	20–30 μg/dL (acceptable)
LE cells (Lupus) also in hematology	Red or green	Negative	
Lecithin/sphingomyelin ratio (L/ S; amniotic fluid)		1:1 before 35 weeks of gestation	
		L: 6–9 mg/dL	
		S: 4–6 mg/dL	
		4:1 after 35 weeks of gestation	
		L: 15–21 mg/dL	
		S: 4–6 mg/dL	
Leucine aminopeptidase (LAP)	Red	8–22 mU/mL, 12–33 IU/L	
Lidocaine	Red	Therapeutic: 1.5–5.0 μg/mL; 6.0–22.5 μmol/L (SI units)	
		Toxic: >6 μg/mL	
Lipase	Red	20–180 IU/L	Infant: 9–105 IU/L at 37°C
		14–280 mU/mL	Child: 20–136 IU/L at 37°C
		14–280 U/L (SI units)	
Lipoproteins (See cholesterol, phospholipids, and triglycerides.)			
Lithium	Red	0	0
		Therapeutic: 0.5–1.5 mEq/L	
		Toxic: >2 mEq/L	
Luteinizing hormone (LH)	Red or lavender	Pre-postovulation: 3–30 mIU/mL	<10 mIU/mL
		Midcycle: 30–100 mIU/mL	
		Postmenopause: >35 mIU/mL	
		Male: 5–25 mIU/mL	
Magnesium (Mg)	Red	1.5–2.5 mEq/L	Newborn: 1.4–2.9 mEq/L
			Child: 1.6–2.6 mEq/L
Nifedipine	Red	Therapeutic: 50–100 ng/mL	
		Toxic: >100 ng/mL	
Nortriptyline (Aventyl)	Red	Therapeutic range: 50–150 ng/mL	
		Toxic level: > 200 ng/mL	

Chemistry	Color-top tube	Reference Values	
		Adult	**Child**
5'Nucleotidase (5'N)	Red	<14 U/L	
Osmolality	Red	280–300 mOsm/kg/H_2O	270–290 mOsm/kg/H_2O
Parathyroid hormone (PTH)	Red	C Terminal PTH: 400–900 pg/mL; N-Terminal PTH: 200–600 pg/mL	
Phenothiazines (See Part I.)			
Phenytoin (Dilantin)	Red	Therapeutic: 10–20 µg/mL; 39.6–79.3 µmol/L (SI units) Toxic: >20 µg/mL; >79.3 µmol/L (SI units)	Toxic: >15–20 µg/mL; 56–79 µmol/L (SI units)
Phospholipids	Red	150–380 mg/dL	
Phosphorus (P) (inorganic)	Red	1.7–2.6 mEq/L 2.5–4.5 mg/dl	Newborn: 3.5–8.6 mg/dL Infant: 4.5–6.7 mg/dL Child: 4.5–5.5 mg/dL Same as adult
Postprandial blood sugar (feasting: PPBS)	Gray or red	<140 mg/dL 2 hours (plasma) <120 mg/dL 2 hours (blood) Older adult: <160 mg/dL 2 hours (plasma); <140 mg/dL 2 hours (blood)	
Potassium (K)	Red	3.5–5.0 mEq/L	Infant: 3.6–5.8 mEq/L Child: 3.5–5.5 mEq/L
Primidone	Red	Therapeutic: 5–12 µg/mL; 23–55 µmol/L (SI units) Toxic: >12–15 µg/ml; >55–69 µmol/L (SI units)	Therapeutic: Child < 5 years: 7–10 µg/mL; 30–45 µmol/L (SI units) Toxic: >12 µg/mL; >55 µmol/L (SI units)
Procainamide	Red	Therapeutic: 4–8 µg/mL; 17–34 µmol/L (SI units) Toxic: >10 µg/ml; >102 µmol/L (SI units)	
Progesterone	Red	Female: Follicular: 0.1–1.5 ng/mL Luteal: 2–28 ng/mL Pregnancy: First trimester: 9–50 ng/mL Second trimester: 18–150 ng/mL Third trimester: 60–260 ng/mL Male: < 1.0 ng/mL	

Test	Tube color	Reference values
Prolactin	Red	Female: Follicular: 0–23 ng/mL Luteal: 0–40 ng/mL Pregnancy: First trimester: < 80 ng/mL Second trimester: < 160 ng/mL Third trimester: < 400 ng/mL Male: 0–20 ng/mL	
Propranolol (Inderal)	Red	Therapeutic: 50–100 ng/mL; 193–386 nmol/L (SI units) Toxic: >150 ng/mL	
Protein	Red	6.0–8.0 g/dL	Premature: 4.2–7.6 g/dL Newborn: 4.6–7.4 g/dL Infant: 6.0–6.7 g/dL Child: 6.2–8.0 g/dL
Protein electrophoresis	Red	Albumin: 3.5–5.0 g/dL; 52%–68% of total protein Globulin: 1.5–3.5 g/dL; 32%–48% of total protein	Premature: 3.0–4.2 g/dL Newborn: 3.5–5.4 g/dL Infant: 4.4–5.4 g/dL Child: 4.0–5.8 g/dL
Quinidine	Red	Therapeutic: 2–5 μg/mL; 0.2–15.4 μmol/L (SI units) Toxic: >6 μg/mL; >18.5 μmol/L (SI units)	
Renin	Lavender	30 minutes supine: 0.2–2.3 ng/mL upright: 1.3–4.0 ng/mL	
Salicylate	Red	0 Therapeutic: 15–30 mg/dL Toxic: Mild: >30 mg/dL Severe: >50 mg/dL	0 Toxic: >25 mg/dL
Sodium (Na)	Red	135–145 mEq/L 135–142 nmol/L (SI units)	Infant: 134–150 mEq/L Child: 135–145 mEq/L
T₃	Red	80–200 ng/dL	Newborn: 90–170 ng/dL Child, 6–12 years: 115–190 ng/dL
Testosterone	Red or green	Male: 0.3–1.0 μg/dL; 300–1000 ng/dL Female: 0.03–0.1 μg/dL; 30–100 ng/dL	Male adolescent: >0.1 μg/dL Male, 12–14 years old; >100 ng/dL

(continued)

	Color-top tube	Reference Values	
Chemistry		**Adult**	**Child**
Theophyline	Red	Therapeutic: Adult: 5–20 µg/mL; 28–112 µmol/L (SI units) Elderly: 5–18 µg/mL Toxic: Adult: >20 µg/mL; >112 µmol/L (SI Units) Elderly: same as adult	Therapeutic: Premature: 7–14 µg/mL Neonate: 3–12 µg/mL Child: same as adult Toxic: Premature: >14 µg/mL Neonate: >13 µg/mL Child: same as adult
Thyroid-binding globulin (TBG)	Red or green	10–26 µg/dL	
Tobramycin	Red	Therapeutic: Peak: 5–10 µg/mL Trough: <2 µg/mL Toxic: >12 µg/mL	
Thyroxine (T_4)	Red	4.5–11.5 µg/dL (T_4 by column) 5–12 µg/dL T_4 RIA) 1.0–2.3 ng/dL (Thyroxine iodine)	Newborn: 11–23 µg/dL 1–4 months: 7.5–16.5 µg/dL 4–12 months: 5.5–14.5 µg/dL 1–6 years old: 5.5–13.5 µg/dL 6–10 years old: 5–12.5 µg/dL
Transferrin	Red	250–430 mg/dL	
Transferrin percent saturation	Red	Male: 30%–50% Female: 20%–35%	
T_3 resin uptake (may be done by nuclear medicine)	Red	25–35 relative % uptake	Not usually done
Tricyclic antidepressants (See *Part I.*)			
Triglycerides	Red	10–150 mg/dL 0.11–2.09 mmol/L (SI units)	Infant: 5–40 mg/dL Child: 10–135 mg/dL
Uric acid	Red	Male: 3.5–8.0 mg/dL Female: 2.8–6.8 mg/dL	2.5–5.5 mg/dL
Valproic acid	Red	Therapeutic: 50–100 µg/mL; 347–693 µmol/L Toxic: >100 µg/mL; >693 µmol/L (SI units)	Therapeutic: same Toxic: same
Verapamil	Red	Therapeutic: 100–300 ng/mL; 0.08–0.3 µg/mL Toxic: >300 ng/mL; >0.3 µg/mL	
Vitamin B^{12}	Red	200–900 pg/mL	

Serology	Color-top tube	Reference Values	
		Adult	Child
Anti-DNA	Red	<1:85	<1:60 <1:70
Antiglomerular basement membrane antibody (AGBM)	Red	Negative	
Antinuclear antibodies (ANA)	Red	Negative	Negative
Antistreptolysin O (ASO)	Red	100 IU/mL	Negative Newborn: similar to mother's Infant: <60 U/dL Preschool: <100 IU/mL 12–19 years: <200 IU/mL
Carcinoembryonic antigen (CEA) (may be done by nuclear medicine)	Red or lavender	<2.5 ng/mL (nonsmokers) <3.5 ng/mL (smokers)	Not usually done
Cold agglutinins (CA)	Red	1:8 antibody titer	Same as adult
Complement C$_3$	Red	Male: 80–180 mg/dL Female: 76–120 mg/dL	Not usually done
Complement C$_4$	Red	15–45 mg/dL	Not usually done
C-reactive protein (CRP)	Red	0	0
Cryoglobulins	Red	up to 6 mg/dL	Negative
Febrile agglutinins	Red	Febrile group: titers *Brucella:* <1:20 Tularemia: <1:40 *Salmonella:* <1:40 *Proteus:* <1:40	Same as adult
FTA-ABS (fluorescent treponemal antibody absorption)	Red	Negative	Negative
Haptoglobin	Red	60–270 mg/dL 0.6–2.7 g/L (SI units)	Newborn: 0–10 mg/dL Infant: 1–6 months: 0–30 mg/dL, then gradual increase
HB$_s$Ab	Red	Negative	Negative
HB$_c$Ab	Red	Negative	Negative
Hepatitis B surface antigen (HB$_s$Ag)	Red	Negative	Negative

(continued)

Serology

	Color-top tube	Reference Values		
		Adult	Child	
				1–3 years old	7–11 years old

Serology	Color-top tube	Adult	Child	
Heterophile antibody	Red	<1:28 titer	Same as adult	
Immunoglobulins (Ig)	Red			1–3 years old / 7–11 years old
Total Ig		900–2200 mg/dL	400–1500 mg/dL	700–1700 mg/dL
IgG		800–1800 mg/dL	300–1400 mg/dL	600–1450 mg/dL
IgA		100–400 mg/dL	20–150 mg/dL	50–200 mg/dL
IgM		50–150 mg/dL	20–100 mg/dL	30–120 mg/dL
IgD		0.5–3 mg/dL		
Legionnaire antibody test	Red	Negative	Same as adult	
Lyme antibody test	Red	Titer < 1:256	Same as adult	
Rapid plasma reagin (RPR)	Red	Negative	Negative	
Rhematoid factor (RF)	Red	<1:20 titer	Not usually done	
Rubella antibody detection (HAI or HI)	Red	<1:8 titer susceptible; 1:10–1:32 titer, past rubella exposure; 1:32–1:64 titer, immunity; >1:64 titer, definite immunity	Same as adult	
Thyroid antibodies (TA)	Red	Negative or <1:20 titer	Not usually done	
TORCH test	Red	Negative	Negative	
Venereal disease research laboratory (VDRL)	Red	Negative	Negative	

Microbiology

Microbiology		Reference Values	
		Adult	Child
Antibiotic susceptibility (sensitivity)		Sensitive to antibiotic; Intermediate to antibiotic; Resistant to antibiotic	Same as adult
Cultures (blood, sputum, stool, throat, wound, and urine)		No pathogen	Same as adult
Fungal organisms (mycotic infections)		No pathogen or under 8	Same as adult
Malarial smear		Negative	Negative
Occult blood (feces)		Negative	Negative
Parasites and ova (feces)		Negative	Negative

Reference Values

Urine Chemistry	Adult	Child
Aldosterone	6–25 µg/24 h	Not usually done
Amylase	4–37 U/L/2h	Not usually done
Ascorbic acid tolerance (4-, 5-, or 6-hour sample)	Oral: 10% of administered amount IV: 30%–40% of administered amount	Not usually done
Bence-Jones protein	Negative to trace	Same as adult
Bilirubin and bile	Negative to 0.02 mg/dL	Same as adult
Calcium (Ca)	100–250 mg/24 h (average calcium diet) 2.50–6.25 mmol/24 h	Same as adult
Catecholamines	<100 µg/24 h <0.59 µmol/24 h (SI units) 0–14 µg/dL (random)	Lower level than adult—weight difference
Epinephrine	<10 ng/24 h	
Norepinephrine	<100 ng/24 h	
Cortisol	24–105 µg/24 h	
Creatinine clearance	85–135 mL/min	Similar to adult
Creatinine	Male: 20–26 mg/kg/24 h; 0.18–0.23 mmol/kg/24 h (SI units) Female: 14–22 mg/kg/24 h; 0.12–0.19 mmol/kg/24 h (SI units)	
Estriol (E_3)	Pregnant: Weeks of Gestation mg/24 hrs 25–28 6–28 29–32 6–32 33–36 10–45 37–40 15–60	
Estrogens (total)	Preovulation: 5–25 µg/24 h Follicular phase: 24–100 µg/24 h Luteal phase (menstruation): 22–80 µg/24 Postmenopause: 0–10 µg/24 h Male: 4–25 µg/24 h	<12 years: 1 µg/24h >12 years: same as adult
Follicle-stimulating hormone (FSH)	6–50 mUU/24 h > 50 mUU/24 h (postmenopausal)	<10 mUU/24 h (prepubertal)

(continued)

Reference Values

Urine Chemistry	Adult	Child
Human chorionic gonadotropin (HCG)	Positive for pregnancy: no agglutination Negative for pregnancy: agglutination	Usually not done
17-Hydroxycorticosteroids (17-OHCS)	Male: 5–15 mg/24 h Female: 3–13 mg/24 h	Infant: <1 mg/24 h 2–4 years: 1–2 mg/24 h 5–12 years: 6–8 mg/24 h
5-Hydroxyindolacetic acid (5-HIAA)	Random: negative 24 hours: 2–10 mg/24 h	Usually not done
Ketone bodies (acetone)	Negative	Negative

17-Ketosteroids (17-KS)	Male: 5–25 mg/24 h
	Female: 5–15 mg/24 h
	>65 years: 4–8 mg/24 h
		Infant: 1 mg/24 h
		1–3 years: <2 mg/24 h
		3–6 years: <3 mg/24 h
		7–10 years: <4 mg/24 h
		10–12 years:
		  Male: <6 mg/24 h
		  Female: <5 mg/24 h
		Adolescent:
		  Male: <3–15 mg/24 h
		  Female: <3–12 mg/24 h

Osmolality	50–1200 mOsm/kg/H_2O Average: 200–800 mOsm/kg/H_2O	Newborn: 100–600 mOsm/kg/H_2O Child: same as adult
Phenylketonuria (PKU)	Not usually done	PKU: negative (positive when serum phenylalanine is 12–15 mg/dL) Guthrie: negative (positive when serum phenylalanine is 4 mg/dL)
Porphobilinogen	Random: negative 24 hour: 0–2 mg/24 h	Same as adult
Porphyrins Coproporphyrins	Random: 3–20 µg/dL 24 hours: 50–160 µg	0–80 µg/24 h
Uroporphyrins	Random: negative, 24 hours: <30 µg	10–30 µg/24 h
Potassium (K)	25–120 mEq/24 h 25–120 mmol/24 h (SI units)	Same as adult

	Adult	Child
Pregnanediol	Male: 0.1–1.5 mg/24 h Female: 0.5–1.5 mg/24 h (proliferative phase); 2–7 mg/24 h (luteal phase); 0.1–1.0 mg/24 h (postmenopausal) Pregnancy: Gestation weeks	0.4–1.0 mg/24 h mg/24 h
	10–19 20–28 29–32	5–25 15–42 25–49
Pregnanetriol	Male: 0.4–2.4 mg/24 h Female: 0.5–2.0 mg/24 h	Infant: 0–0.2 mg/24 h Child: 0–1.0 mg/24 h
Protein	0–5 mg/dL/24 h	
Sodium (Na)	40–220 mEq/24 h	Same as adult
Uric acid	250–750 mg/24 h (low-purine diet)	Same as adult
Urinalysis		
pH	4.5–8.0	Newborn: 5–7 Child: 4.5–8
Specific gravity (SG)	1.005–1.030	Newborn: 1.001–1.020 Child: Same as adult
Protein	Negative	Negative
Glucose	Negative	Negative
Ketones	Negative	Negative
RBC	1–2/low-power field	Rare
WBC	3–4	0–4
Casts	Occasional hyaline	Rare

	Reference Values	
Others	*Adult*	*Child*
Urobilinogen	Random: 0.3–3.5 mg/dL 0.05–2.5 mg/24 h 0.5–4.0 Ehrlich units/24 h 0.09–4.23 μmol/24 h (SI units)	Same as adult
Vanillylmandelic acid (VMA)	1.5–7.5 mg/24 h 7.6–37.9 μmol/24 h (SI units)	Same as adult

(continued)

| Others | Reference Values | |
	Adult	Child
Bleeding time	Ivy's method: 3–7 minutes	Same as adult
Arterial blood gases (ABGs)		
pH:	7.35–7.45	7.36–7.44
Pco_2	35–45 mm Hg	Same as adult
Po_2	75–100 mm Hg	Same as adult
HCO_3	24–28 mEq/L	Same as adult
BE	+2 to −2 (± 2 mEq/L0	Same as adult
Cerebrospinal fluid (CSF)		
Pressure	75–175 mm H_2O	50–100 mm H_2O
Cell count	0–8 mm^3	0–8 mm^3
Protein	15–45 mg/dL	15–45 mg/dL
Chloride	118–132 mEq/L	120–128 mEq/L
Glucose	40–80 mg/dL	35–75 mg/dL
Culture	No organism	No organism
Chloride (sweat)	<60 mEq/L	<50 mEq/L
Semen examination	60–150 millim/mL	Not usually done
	Volume: 1.5–5.0 mL	
	Morphology: >75% mature spermatozoa	
	Motility: > 60% actively mobile spermatozoa	

Index